Claude R. Rufenacht   Fundamentals of Esthetics

Fundamentals of Esthetics

Dr Claude R. Rufenacht
Medecin Dentiste
Geneva, Switzerland

With the contribution of
Robert P. Berger, CDT
Chatsworth, California
Robert L. Lee, DDS, MS
Private practice, Grand Terrace, California
Robert L. Nixon, DMD
Private practice, Los Angeles, California
Giano Ricci, MD, DDS, MScD
Private practice, Florence, Italy
Harold M. Shavell, DDS
Private practice, Chicago, Illinois

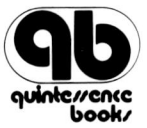

Quintessence Publishing Co, Inc
Chicago, Berlin, London, São Paulo, Tokyo, and Hong Kong

Library of Congress Cataloging-in-Publication Data
Rufenacht, Claude.
  Fundamentals of esthetics / Claude Rufenacht.
    p. cm.
  Includes bibliographical references.
  Includes index.
  ISBN 0-86715-230-3
  1. Dentistry–Aesthetics. I. Title.
  [DNLM: 1. Esthetics, Dental. WU 100 R922f]
  RK54.R84 1990
  617.6–dc20
  DNLM/DLC   90-8621
  for Library of Congress   CIP

qb
quintessence
books

© 1990 by Quintessence Publishing Co, Inc, Chicago, Illinois.
All rights reserved.
1st reprinting, 1992

This book or any part thereof must not be reproduced by any means or in any form without the written permission of the publisher.

Lithography: Scantrans, Singapore
Printing and binding: Toppan Printing Co. Pte., Ltd., Jurong Town, Singapore
Printed in Singapore

Contents

Part I	**Fundamentals of Esthetics**	**9**

Chapter 1   **Introduction to Esthetics**   **11**
Claude Rufenacht

The philosophy of beauty	11
The origins of esthetics and its perception	12
Esthetic principles	15
Personality	31

Chapter 2   **Morphopsychology**   **33**
Claude Rufenacht

Introduction	33
Typologic classifications	34
Biodynamic conception of the personality	37
Laws of adaptation to the environment	38
Facial morphopsychology	39
Morphopsychologic interpretation	45
Affective and sentimental zone	47
Cerebral zone	48
Instinctive and physical zone	52
Mouth and lips	55

Chapter 3   **Morphopsychology and Esthetics**   **59**
Claude Rufenacht

The evaluation of human beauty	59
Youth factor	63
Integration and sublimation	64

Chapter 4   **Structural Esthetic Rules**   **67**
Claude Rufenacht

Facial components	67
Dental components	85
Gingival components	121
Physical components	127

Part II	**Intraoral and Extraoral Means to Rejuvenation**	**135**

Chapter 5   **Esthetics and Its Relationship to Function**   **137**
Robert Lee

Natural permanent crown morphology	137
Physiology of occlusion	145
Mastication	167
Occlusal loading	181
Clinical aspects in bioesthetic function	183

Chapter 6   **Facial Sculpture**   **211**
Claude Rufenacht

Striated muscles: Physical and physiologic characteristics	211
Muscular activity	211
Facial muscle characteristics	212
Perioral anatomy	213
Muscle retraining exercises	214

Contents

Part III — **Esthetic Restoration of the Smile** — 223

Chapter 7 — **Esthetic Management of the Dentogingival Unit** — 225
Claude Rufenacht

- The dentogingival unit — 225
- Passive eruption — 226
- Delayed passive eruption — 226
- Tooth lengthening — 229

Chapter 8 — **Gingival Recessions** — 237
Giano Ricci

- Historical rationale and treatment techniques — 239
- Therapeutic possibilities — 241

Chapter 9 — **Ridge Pontic Relationship** — 263
Claude Rufenacht

- Prevention of ridge collapse — 264
- Morphology of the ridge — 264
- Correction of an increased available space — 266
- Graft material and donor site — 269
- Implant material — 269
- Improved techniques for localized ridge augmentation — 270
- Pontic — 282

Chapter 10 — **Mastering the Art of Tissue Management** — 289
Harold Shavell

- Periodontal esthetics — 291
- Gingival displacement methods — 293
- Biologic final impression — 311
- Globalism and the perioprosthetic gestalt — 317
- Coda: The search for excellence — 318

Chapter 11 — **Metal Ceramic Framework Design** — 319
Robert Berger

- Marginal fit — 319
- Planning for esthetics, physiologic form, and strength — 322
- Interproximal connectors: Design for strength — 323
- Interproximal design: Esthetics — 324
- Pontic-tissue relationship — 325
- Lingual metal band design — 326

Chapter 12 — **Porcelain Veneers: An Esthetic Therapeutic Alternative** — 329
Robert Nixon

- Case evaluation — 330
- Indications for porcelain veneers — 330
- Contraindications for porcelain veneers — 332
- Stratification method — 332
- Tooth preparation and impression taking — 336
- Tooth preparation sequence: Maxillary teeth — 338
- Tooth preparation sequence: Mandibular teeth — 344
- Laboratory communication — 350
- Veneer try-in for individual and collective fit — 352
- Chairside try-in sequence for individual and collective fit — 352
- Veneer try-in for color/color modification — 354
- Cementation and finishing — 360
- Maintenance of porcelain veneers — 366

Index — 369

Preface

Woven into the tradition of Western civilization, from the Ancient Greeks to Aquinas and Kant, beauty has been central to all philosophical thought, deeply rooted in human nature. The appreciation of beauty, far from being related to the subjectivity of individual taste, requires esthetic training for the promotion of individual feelings, in accordance with the objective criteria.

The purpose of this book is to set forth objective criteria for the appreciation of beauty, so that critical discrimination between the beautiful and the ugly may be made. A variety of elements bearing on the structural beauty of the dental, dentofacial, and facial composition will be presented, as well as therapeutic measures including restorative, surgical, or functional procedures designed to reproduce nature.

The reality of human esthetics implies the necessity for a harmonious integration of dental elements with the environment and requires a capability of understanding and interpreting the morphopsychological features manifested by the individual that we are called upon to treat. Modern dentistry, influenced by technology for technology's sake, has all too often neglected to take this reality into consideration.

The principles outlined in this work will provide practitioners with the means to ensure or improve the patient's dentofacial esthetic well-being, within the framework of the aging process.

Dedication and Acknowledgment

This book is dedicated to my wife and daughter for having made this work possible through their love, encouragement, and complaisance, and to my patients and friends for their tolerance.

I also acknowledge the invaluable assistance provided by Mr Rafael Contreras, Head of my Technical Department.

I am deeply indebted to those colleagues, contributors, and friends who joined with me in this project and contributed to its consistency, a fundamental requirement for the scientific credibility of the subjects dealt with.

Finally, I express my gratitude to Mr Eugene Abrams for his help, as well as to all those who participated in this endeavor.

Part I
Fundamentals of Esthetics

Chapter 1

Introduction to Esthetics

Claude R. Rufenacht

The philosophy of beauty

"Beauty is measure and symmetry and virtue all the world over" (Plato, *Dialogues, Philebus*), and if the perfect mixture can rarely be found in man, they feel free to strive towards it, point it out, praise it, because *"ugliness and discord and inharmonious motion are nearly allied to ill words and ill nature, as grace and harmony are the twin sisters of goodness and virtue and bear their likeness"* (Plato, *Republic III*).

The profound respect for beauty as a fundamental measure of perfection and a measure of the divine is not to be taken lightly or to be associated with human vanity when a degree of perfection is sought in humans themselves.

For the Ancient Greeks and throughout the tradition of Western thought, from Plato to Kant, beauty has not only been at the center of all philosophical preoccupation, but it has blended easily with goodness and truth.

This triad of terms — beauty, goodness, and truth — has been called "the three fundamental values" (with the implication that the worth of everything can be judged in reference to these three standards) or "transcendental" (because everything is in some manner subject to denomination as true or false, good or evil, beautiful or ugly).

Greek culture, whose point of perfection lasted only 60 years, from the Median wars (492 BC) to the Peloponnesian War (431 BC), has been considered the highest expression of human spirit. Its impact on human history, gathered in such an incredibly short time, tends to prove that it contained all the elements deeply imbedded in human nature.

"The predominant elements of Athenian existence were the independence of the social units and a culture animated by the spirit of beauty" (Hegel, *Philosophy of History*).

Today the influence of Greek culture on modern society is still predominant, but the individual's legitimate aspiration to beauty has been clouded by the "usefulness spirit" or the necessity to be efficient, which seems to occupy the stage as the only justification of human behavior. Under such conditions the gratuitousness of the human spirit is less considered and, as a result, individuals do not feel free to identify with esthetics if they cannot persuade themselves that it is useful to do so.

This fear, however, is just a screen. Utility or pleasure proposed either as an additional value or as a significant variant of the so-called three fundamentals has been held by Benedict Spinoza (1632–1677) and John Stuart Mill (1806–1873) to be the ultimate criterion of beauty and goodness. With true efficiency always comes a certain degree of beauty that will then bring to the individual some amount of deeply needed moral satisfaction.

We should always remember that, contrary to our masters, we have forsaken the notion that esthetic curiosity as much as intellectual curiosity originally moved us on our path and that the first fields of experimentation we acted upon were our own bodies and minds.

Our primary concern throughout this book will constantly refer to natural and artificial beauty, but we should always keep in mind beauty's numerous manifestations, such as sensitivity and intelligence, both material and spiritual.

Introduction to Esthetics

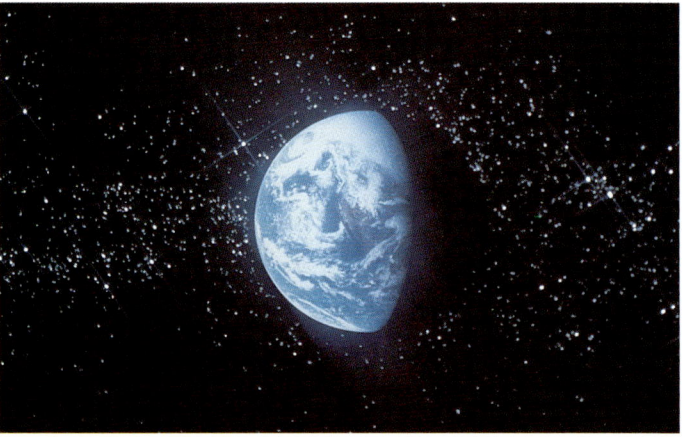

Fig 1-1 Beauty cannot be an exact science (Hegel). Beauty is virtual (Plato).

The origins of esthetics and its perception

Esthetics

What is esthetics and what is the significance of esthetics and dental esthetics? Are the roots of esthetics hidden in a world that we are constantly attempting to apprehend, hoping secretly to discover its nature, dissect its rules, reinforce our understanding, and finally, to master its most innermost elements?

Although a dictionary definition of esthetics — *"the science of beauty in nature and arts"* — appeals to our scientifically oriented education, it does not stand up to Hegel's statement: *"Beauty as the substance of the imagination and feeling, cannot be an exact science"* (Fig 1-1).

The essence of beauty may be the invisible background of the physically perceptive, concrete beauty that rules and decorates the appearance of vegetable and animal species and the constant equilibrium of shapes and colors that can be observed at any time in any geographic location. *"Beauty in nature is the mirror of essential beauty."*

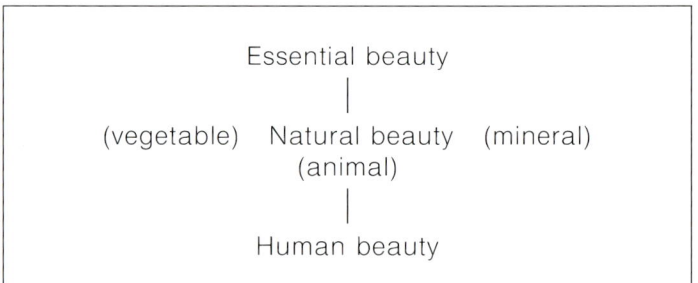

If we accept this fundamental principle, then we must find in nature elements that can be reproduced or integrated in humans to mimic the essential beauty because the esthetic of human forms appears as a microcosm in the universal macrocosm.

This approach will permit us to aim at the development of objective criteria of beauty as well as at the ability to discriminate critically between the beautiful and the ugly. This is not to say that beauty is purely objective. If it were so, no training would seem to be necessary for sharpening our perception of it. There seems to be a middle ground between objectivity and subjectivity of beauty intrinsic to an object without denying the influence of individual sensitivity.

The fact that esthetic judgment requires universal as-

The origins of esthetics and its perception

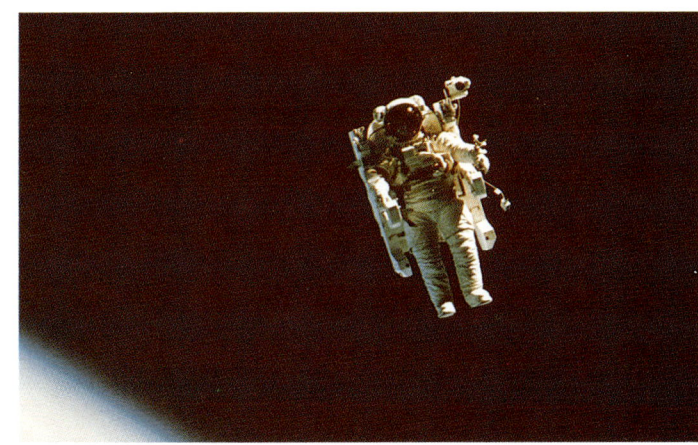

Fig 1-2 Human beings represent the sensitive vector that gives life to virtual or essential beauty (L. da Vinci).

sent does not preclude the necessity to win assent from all individuals. Not all people have good taste, or, having it, have it to the same degree, but the universal character of esthetic judgment in respect of individual feelings tends to refute the notion that in matters of beauty one can seek refuge in the adage: *"Everyone has his own taste"* (Darwin).

Perception

"Human beings represent the sensitive vector that gives life to essential beauty" (Leonardo da Vinci; Fig 1-2).

In a broader sense, esthetics is a phenomenon of the intellect. When the term esthetic or unesthetic is used, it engenders an emotion that connotes that which is pleasant or unpleasant. The process of perception is an organization of sensory data (sight, touch, hearing, taste, and smell stimuli), which are brought to the intellect where an answer is developed in combination with the results of previous experiences or beliefs that are unconsciously interpreted. This is what is known as a *precept*. In visual perception the physiologic functions of rods and cones bring stimuli to the center of vision of the brain where they engender a psychologic response that may be conditioned by a variety of factors.

Visual perception is a prerequisite for esthetic appreciation in the same fashion that visual examination is also a routine in normal clinical investigation.

If the interpretation of clinical results is possible by reason of scientific knowledge, the comprehension of esthetic principles should permit a logical evaluation of the fundamentals of beauty. This necessitates esthetic training to refine our perception and permit the development of individual feelings in accordance with objective criteria. As a result, the objective diagnosis of elements that have been subjectively appreciated or rejected will become progressively possible to the extent that the capacity to please will be restricted to objects or elements that should elicit that reaction.

"This faculty for the appreciation of beauty is related to high tastes acquired though culture and depends upon complex associations" (Darwin).

Scientific investigations into the physiology and psychology of perception have resulted in the formulation of certain principles or parameters of visual perception that provide a basis for an introduction to the elements of esthetics that are part of essential and natural beauty.

Introduction to Esthetics

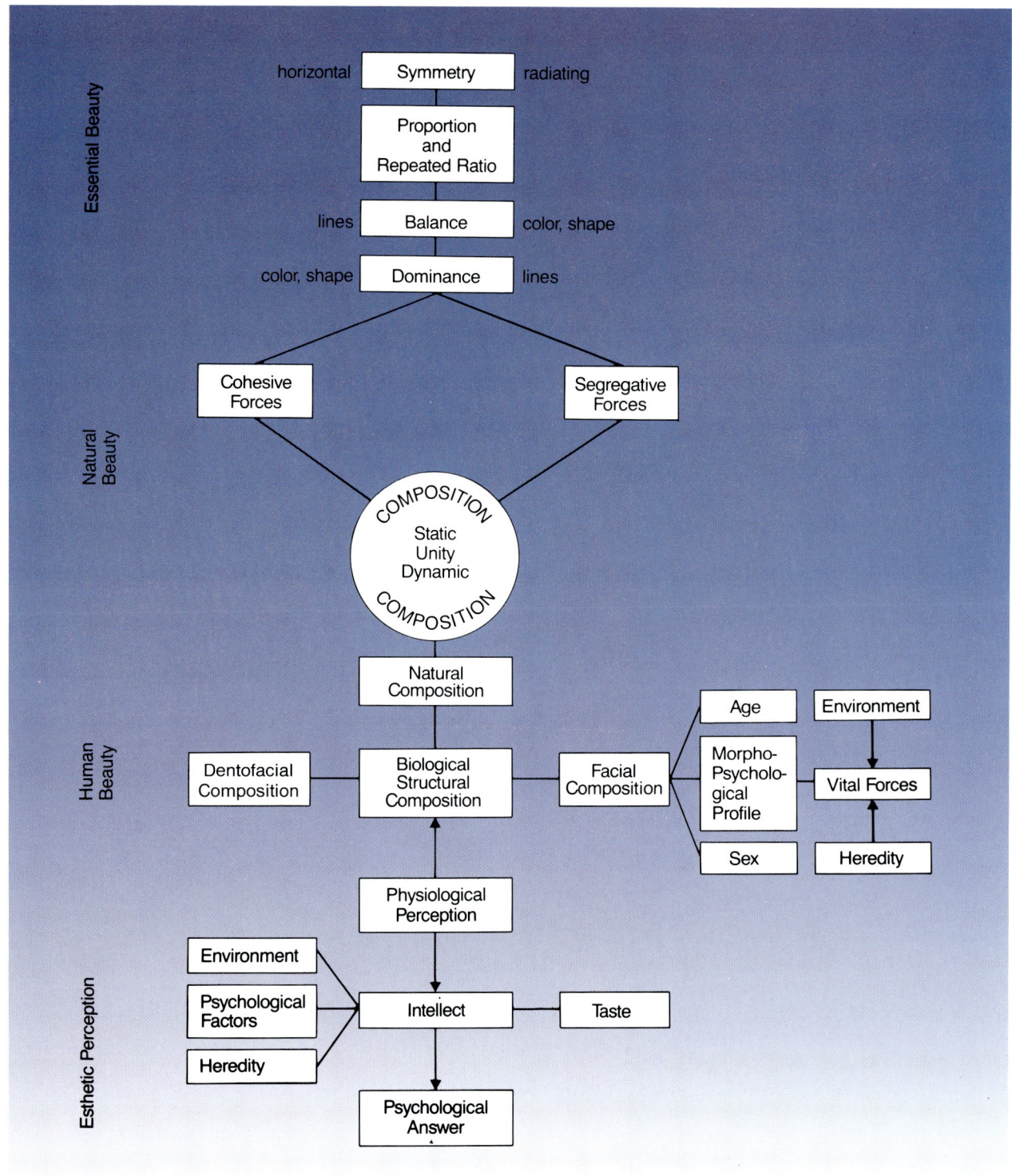

Fig 1-3 Schematic framework of esthetics.

Esthetic principles

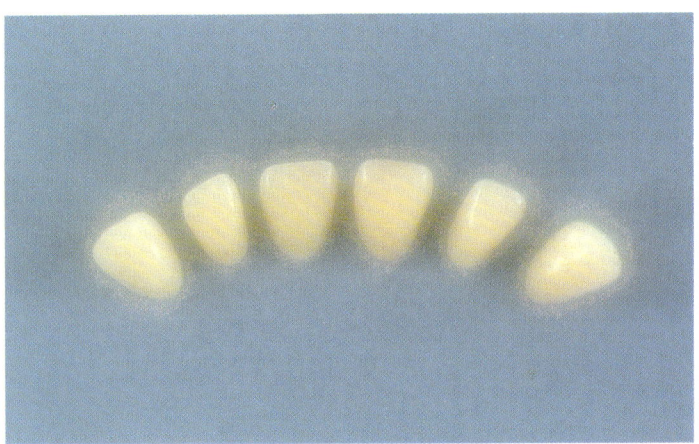

Fig 1-4a

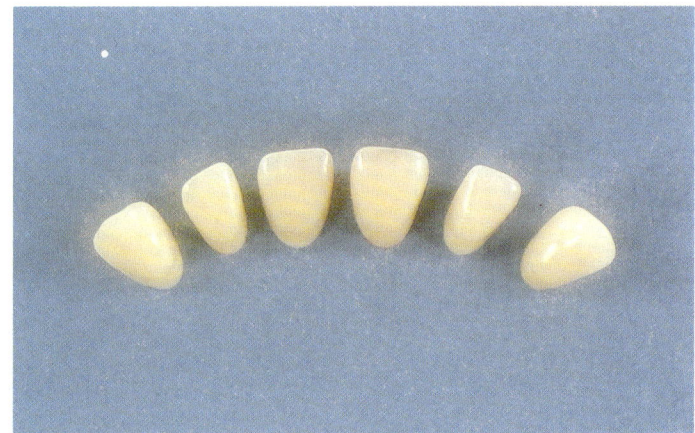

Fig 1-4b

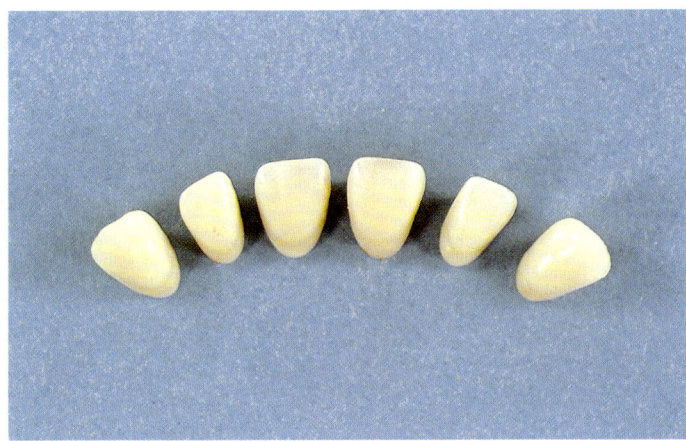

Fig 1-4c

Figs 1-4a to c Objects are made visible by contrast. The increase of visibility is proportional to the increase of contrast.

The schematic framework of esthetic parameters should be used as a reference guide into which everybody should be free to introduce elements that may reveal that which is of importance as well as to ignore others not adapted to the situation.

The evaluation of parameters dealing with human personality, key elements bringing life to human esthetic, should never be ignored because their integration will allow us to fulfill the individual's demand for esthetic self-satisfaction (Fig 1-3).

Esthetic principles

Composition

The physiologic property of the eye is vision. Vision is possible if the eye can differentiate. This is possible only if there is contrast. The increase of visibility is proportionate to the increase in contrast. We are able to see because of the contrasts of colors, lines, and texture (Figs 1-4a to c).

The relationship between objects made visible by contrasts is called *composition*. In our field of interest the following terminology will be used: dental composition, dentofacial composition, and facial composition (Figs 1-5 to 1-7).

Introduction to Esthetics

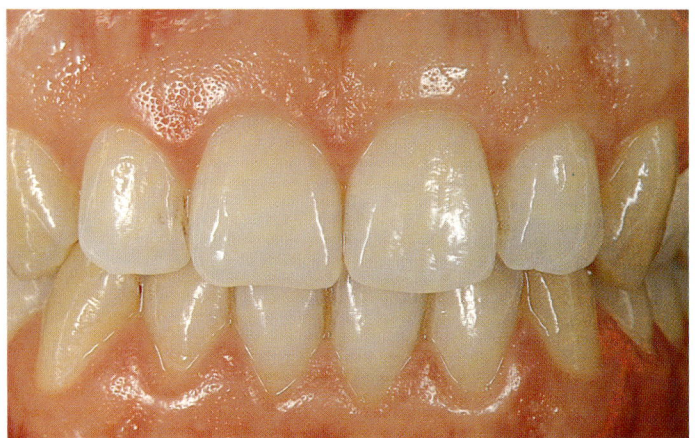

Fig 1-5 Dental composition.

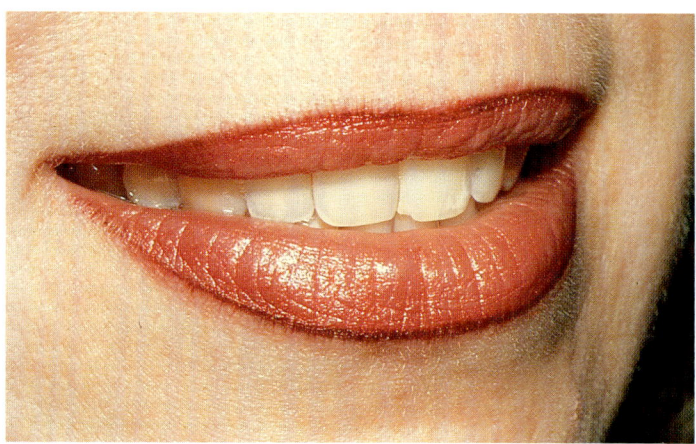

Fig 1-6 Dentofacial composition.

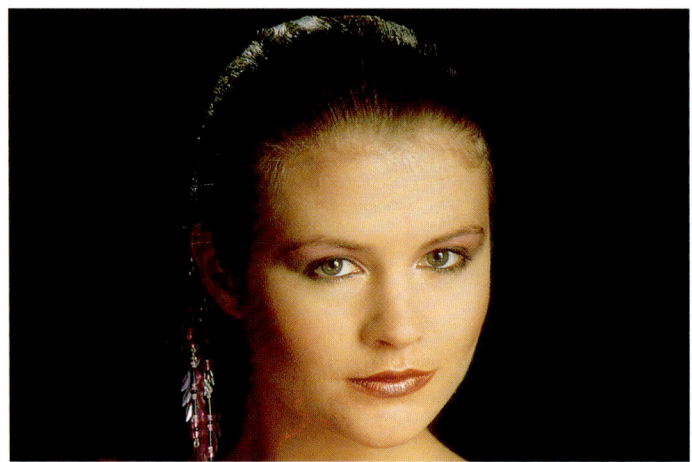

Fig 1-7 Facial composition.

Unity

The prime requisite for a composition is unity that will give the different parts of the composition the effects of a whole.

Two types of unity exist: static and dynamic. Static unity is composed of geometric and regular shapes, such as inorganic shapes and forms, eg, drops of water, snowflakes, and crystals (Fig 1-8). Passive and inert (without motion) static design is based on a regular, repetitive pattern. Plants and animals are dynamic units: active, living, and growing (Fig 1-9).

Cohesive and segregative forces

Cohesive forces

Elements that tend to unify a composition are cohesive forces. A border is a cohesive force as well as arrangements of elements in a definite form or according to a principle (Figs 1-10 and 1-11).

Esthetic principles

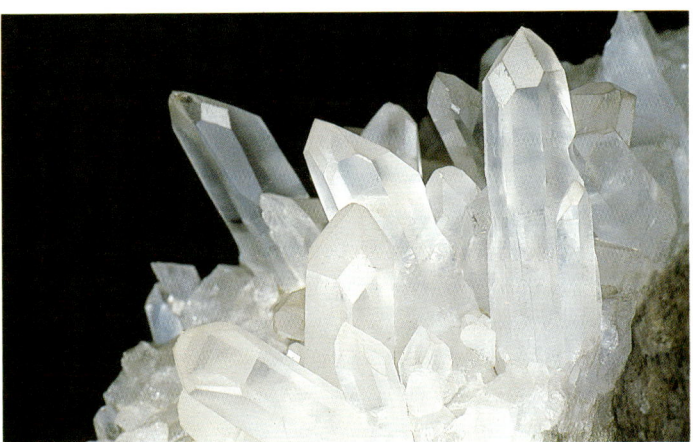

Fig 1-8   Bound together as a "whole," a *static* unity is inert, based on geometric and repetitive patterns.

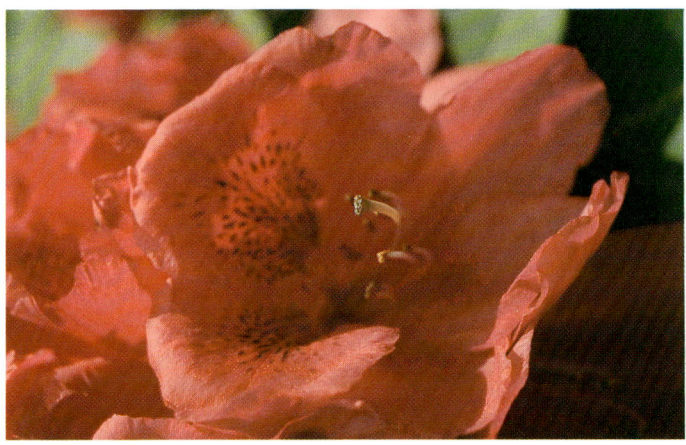

Fig 1-9   Bound together as a "whole," a *dynamic* unity is a living, growing entity, based on dynamic units.

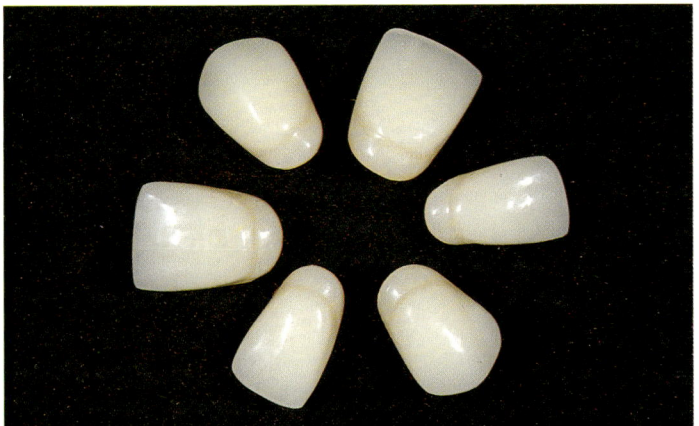

Fig 1-10   Cohesive forces tend to unify a composition. They are represented by elements arranged according to a principle.

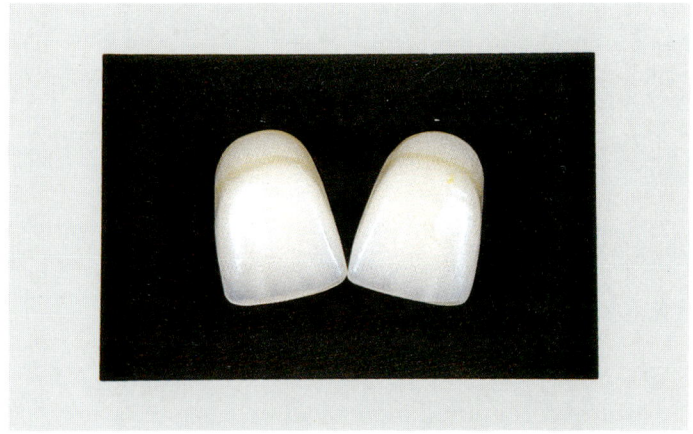

Fig 1-11   A frame or elements arranged in a definite form, giving strength to a composition represent typical cohesive forces.

Introduction to Esthetics

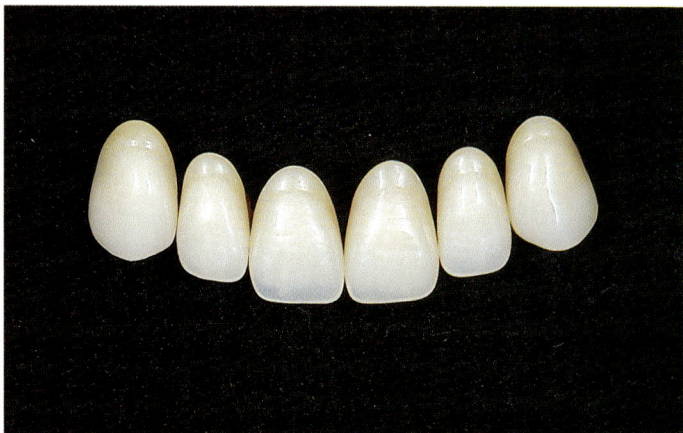

Fig 1-12 Segregative forces are represented by elements arranged in an appealing manner, reminders of an interesting thing or event, such as a Class I tooth arrangement.

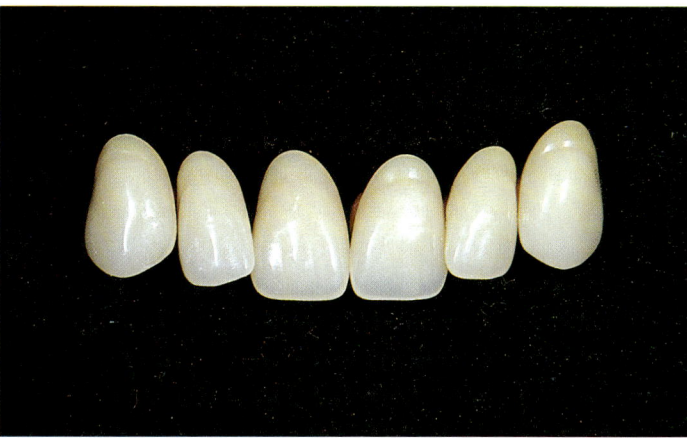

Fig 1-13 Segregative forces are the necessary elements that enhance the esthetic value of a composition. A slight malposition, a reminder of a Class II arrangement, conforms to this definition.

Segregative forces

Segregative forces are the opposite of cohesive forces. They provide variety in the unity, which is required to make a design effective because even if the elements must be bound together in a whole, they must be arranged in an interesting manner (Figs 1-12 and 1-13).

Principle: In a dentofacial composition, harmony depends on the equilibrium created by cohesive and segregative forces (Figs 1-14 and 1-15).

Symmetry

One of the primary concerns in esthetics is symmetry. Symmetry refers to the regularity in the arrangement of forms or objects (Furtwangler, 1964). It is and can be totally differentiated from balance in the sense that in balance things that are farther from the center grow in importance and weight. This is not the case for symmetry where all elements are alike with reference to their position in relation to a central point.

We can differentiate between two kinds of symmetry: *(1)* horizontal, or running symmetry, and *(2)* radiating symmetry. Horizontal symmetry occurs when a design contains similar elements from left to right in a regular sequence. Radiating symmetry is a result of the design of objects extending from a central point and the right and left sides are mirror images. Examples of horizontal or radiating symmetry and asymmetry can be best found in the variety of dental arrangements (Figs 1-16 and 1-17). Horizontal symmetry that is psychologically predictable and comfortable tends to be monotonous (cohesive forces), whereas radiating symmetry generally represents a segregative force that brings life and dynamism to a composition. However, this statement, approved by a majority of dental professionals, does not always conform to patients' preferences, who seem to favor forms and designs that are repetitive and regular. This infers that they may prefer teeth or tooth arrangements that look less natural but conform to their concept of ideal esthetic appearance.

The ideal esthetic appearance is influenced by many factors, and this influence has to be introduced in dental compositions to respect the patient's desire to feel comfortable in reference to the standards they have adopted.

Principle: Symmetry must be introduced in dentofacial composition to create a positive psychologic response.

Esthetic principles

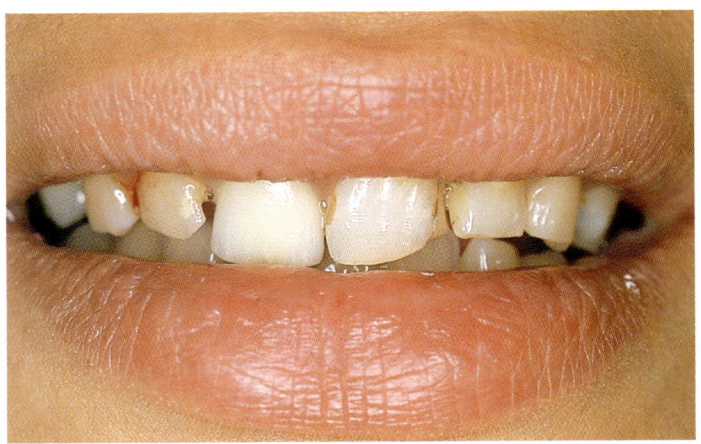

Fig 1-14 When segregative forces that cannot be identified with reality or thinking (eg, tooth design and structure) are introduced in a composition, disharmony can result if cohesive forces (eg, lip frame structure) are not able to restore the necessary equilibrium.

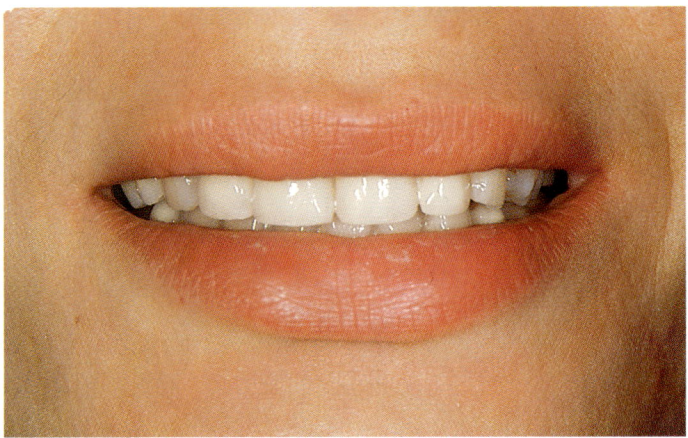

Fig 1-15 The restoration of harmony requires the presence of cohesive and segregative forces. This is a condition necessary to ensure the esthetic equilibrium of a composition.

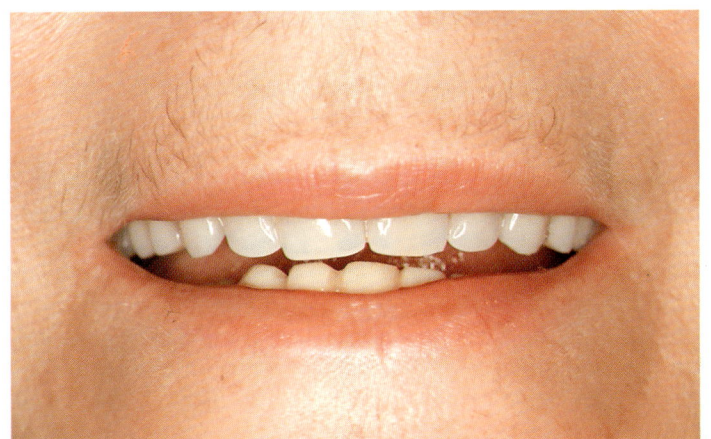

Fig 1-16 Horizontal symmetry can be described as an arrangement in which all elements are alike.

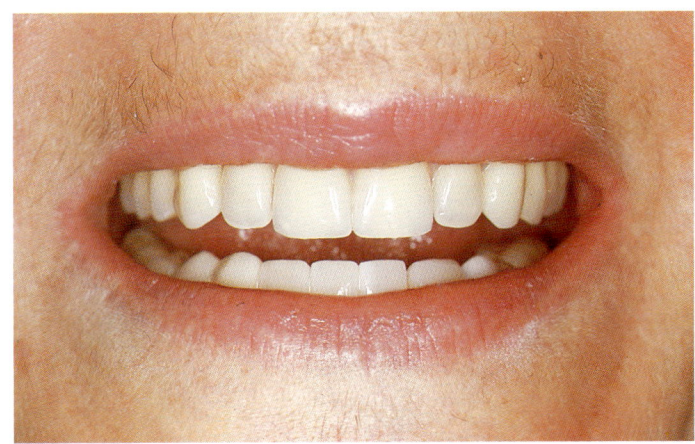

Fig 1-17 When one part of the composition is the mirror image of the other, a radiating type of symmetry is apparent.

Introduction to Esthetics

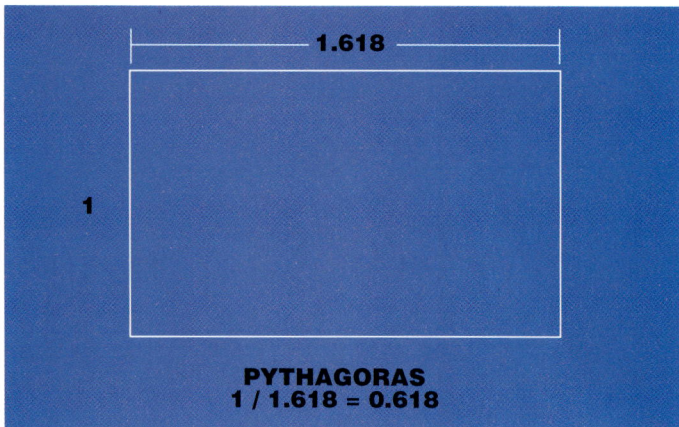

Fig 1-18 Golden proportion (Pythagoras). This proportion of ancient origin has generated esthetic appraisal for many centuries. A rectangular frame, with sides of the ratio of this golden proportion, is said to have a particular beauty.

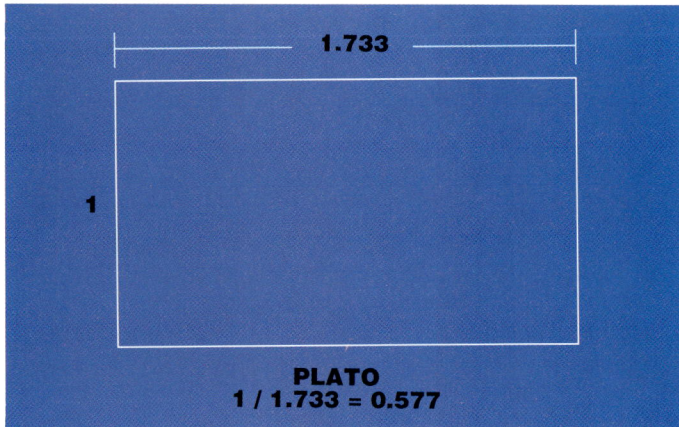

Fig 1-19 Beautiful proportion (Plato). This proportion, linked to another ratio, has been claimed by Plato as reflecting also a particular beauty. Such a proportion can be found in a rectangle formed by two halves of an equilateral triangle.

Proportion and repeated ratio

Proportion

The concept of beauty has most often corresponded to a harmony in proportion. To speak of proportion stems from a notion of relationship, percentage, or measure in its numerical determination and implies the quantification of norms that can be applied to every physical reality. The language of mathematics has always been considered the only reference related to the understanding of nature. The idea of application of this language to arts as an objective criterion of evaluation has focused the attention of generations of philosophers desiring to prove the hypothesis that beauty could also be expressed mathematically.

The elaboration of a formula assessing a ratio in the harmonious relationship between two parts, attributed to Pythagoras and called golden number, gave credit to this hypothesis.

The statement that the division of a surface by the golden number (Fig 1-18) engenders a special appeal explains the constant reference to the basic axiom of the Pythagorean concept:

"Penta en arithmo."

"Everything is in the number."

The dispute originating with Plato, claiming that other ratios not only could but really did exhibit a particular beauty, somehow disqualified the pretentions of the Pythagorean concept without questioning the "universality" of the golden number (Fig 1-19).

It initiated the development of esthetic studies dominated by a psychologic approach: concepts of sympathy (Einfühlung), shape (Gestalt), and behavior (behaviorism) that eclipsed the presuppositions of the mathematical esthetic and made conspicuous the belief that nature and beauty should only depend upon numerical rules originated by a real will of simplification. Although by reason of facts proportion is mathematical, it seems more pertinent today to combine the numerical quantification of beauty with its psychophysical quantification.

Repeated ratio

The satisfactory division of a surface into parts that contrast in shape and size yet are related to each other is called repeated ratio. There are many manifestations of proportion in nature and art, but the division of a surface

Esthetic principles

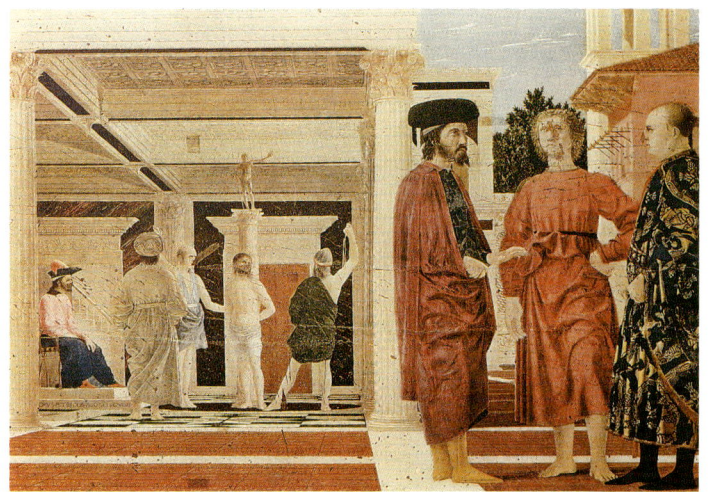

Fig 1-20 *The Flagellation* (Piero della Francesca). The static beauty characterizing this picture has its origin both in the absence of light and shadow and in the use of a geometric concept. The realism of the picture reflects a compromise between the perceptive impulses of the sensibility and the practical application of a pure mental construction. Courtesy of Archivi Alinari, Firenze.

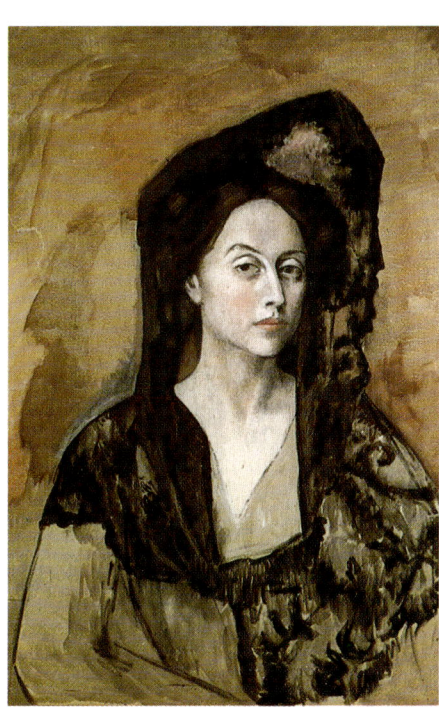

Fig 1-22 *Señora Canals* (Picasso). The respect for morphologic likeness and proportion may be a pretext for the artist to apply a system of lines and volumes that blends with his esthetic requirements. The realism is linked to an intellectual concept. (Courtesy of Museo Picasso, Barcelona.)

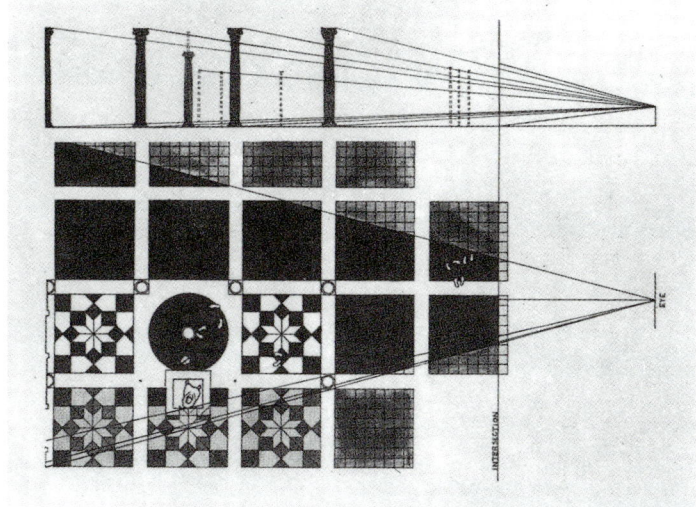

Fig 1-21 Plan and elevation of the scene represented in Piero della Francesca's *The Flagellation*, demonstrating its rational construction by the systematic use of proportional relationships. (Courtesy of B.A.R. Carter.)

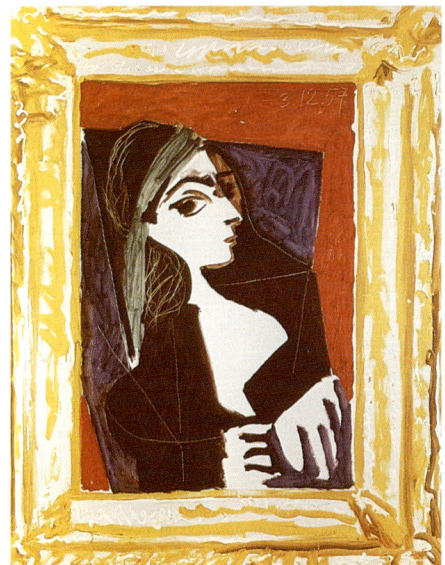

Fig 1-23 *Retrato de Jacqueline* (Picasso). The realism is idealized and represents a compromise between the reflection of feeling and the illustration of an intellectual concept. Proportions are naturally integrated into this composition that rather induce intellectual versus visual tension. (Courtesy of Museo Picasso, Barcelona.)

Introduction to Esthetics

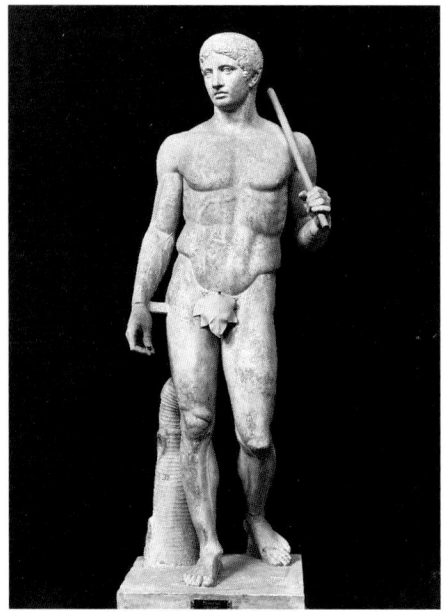

Fig 1-24 *The Doryphorus*. In this statue not only can one see the body of a beautifully restituted athlete, but one is also forced to see the materialization of the first theoretical essay on arts, "The Canon" produced by Polyclitus. Beauty, finality in arts, depends on "the symmetry of all parts of the body, and of the relationships existing between these parts and between each of them related to the whole." (Courtesy of Museo Nazionale, Napoli.)

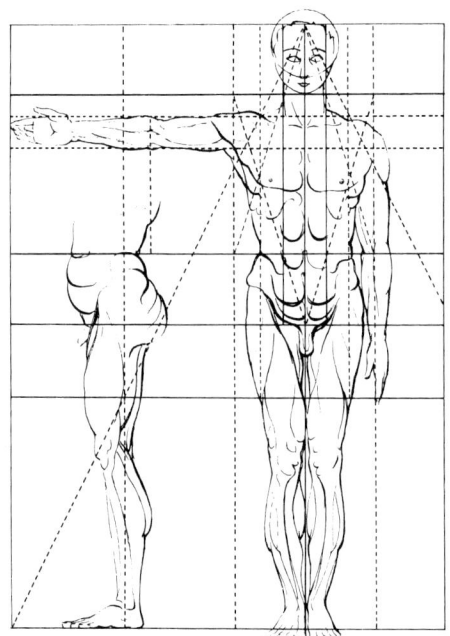

Fig 1-25 The realism of Greek art dissimulates mathematical formulas that are used as a basis for artistic creation, fortifying the intellect in its search for a more precise notion of beauty.

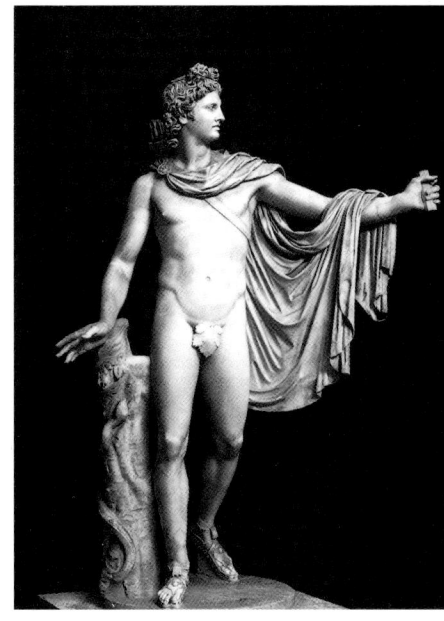

Fig 1-26 *Apollo Belvedere*. Greek art has brought esthetic principles to the level of consciousness. It has made those principles the goals of art and has given strict expression of them, applying proportionate relationships, ie, the foundation of harmony. In the *Apollo Belvedere* the body is proportionate to eight times the height of the head. (Courtesy of Museo Vaticano, Roma.)

through the golden number creates an equilibrium that is not accomplished when divided by any other number and engenders a psychologic effect of esthetic appraisal. It has been observed that this golden number has been intuitively used in the construction of antique monuments from the pyramids to Gothic cathedrals. At a time when the prevalence of the Pythagorean concept was unanimously recognized, Phidias and others, who contributed to the construction of the Parthenon, deliberately used this number. This relationship, which is a constant in the works of the Italian Renaissance, can also be found in the composition of the great classical painters, and a meticulous analysis of some masterpieces has evidenced its masterful application (Figs 1-20 and 1-21). Many modern painters, who give the feeling of distorting proportions, know full well the laws of harmony that are stylized to a sublime degree (Figs 1-22 and 1-23).

Esthetic morphology is based on the notion of beauty and the mathematical theory of the proportionate body naturally linked to the Pythagorean concept. Polyclitus, who produced a mathematical study of beauty, stated that: "Beauty depends upon infinite differences and re-

Fig 1-27 Pictorial realism of Greek art, based on abstraction, was gradually overwhelmed by the naturalism, generator of lassitude and decadence. The esthetic value of the golden section was stressed again by Luca Pacioli in his book "Divina Proportione" (1504) illustrated by Leonardo da Vinci. (Courtesy of Archivi Alinari, Firenze.)

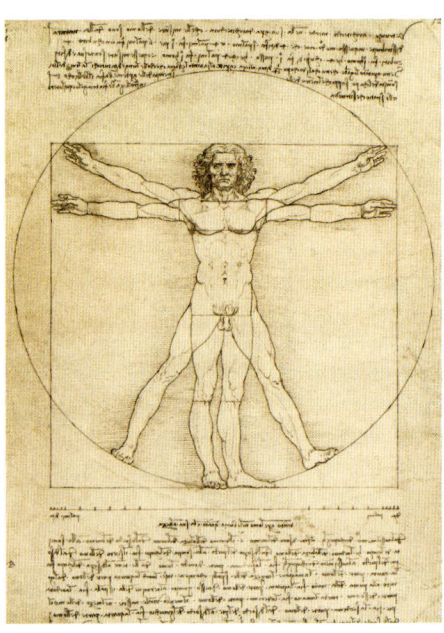

sults of the harmonization of a multitude of numbers." His statue, *The Doryphorus*, based on the calculation of seven and a half times the height of the head for the whole body, was judged by Pliny as the consolidation of the ultimate laws of beauty (Fig 1-24).

The definition of an absolute esthetic physical norm was philosophically envisaged to an extreme (Fig 1-25). Although it blended with the idea of the microcosm of the human body in the macrocosmic harmony, the reasoning did not resist the lack of recognition of the importance of variety existing in geographic and physiologic conditions. The perception of beauty as a corporal expression can vary from one individual to another, from one civilization to another, and from one ethnic group to another. Proportions that are judged beautiful vary with the epoch, but at any given moment there are some that become doctrine or standards of beauty. Magically, under the influence of the Pythagorean concept, Greek sculptors of the Fourth Century used the golden number in the body proportions of their statues. In *Apollo Belvedere*, which made Lysippus a celebrity, the entire body was proportionate to eight times the height of the head (Fig 1-26).

Later Roman standards were imposed by its most famous artist, Vitruvius, whose proportions have been reproduced by Leonardo da Vinci in a classic, *Square of the Ancients* (Fig 1-27).

More recently, modern rules, established scientifically and based on the anatomy and average proportions of the human body, were first set forth in Charles Blanc's *Rules of the Studio*, but many others have also been described.

The most important idea that stems from these works is that good-looking is the norm or average. This was confirmed by the Italian typologist Viola, who, after having established the characteristics of an Italian who would be average in all respects, ascertained that the proportions of this standard type are found in the statues of antiquity.

The evaluation of human proportion can best be assessed by reference to the Greek standards that through their perfection, exactness, and pureness (whatever the epoch) received unanimous esthetic approval. However, the introduction of "updated" parameters will serve as the necessary ingredients to achieve the characterization of human proportion. Do dental elements or dental compositions invariably conform to the golden proportion to be judged as esthetically pleasing? Teeth having their own shape and relation to each other in the vertical and frontal plane may precisely exhibit other proportions and still be favorably perceived. The psychologic effect of shapes, the tension resulting from the integration of various forms, and the phenomenology of perception may easily engender reactions of esthetic appraisal. However, sooner or later, at any given distance, attention will be focused on proportions. The beauty of the dentofacial composition greatly depends on the presence of a number of "golden" relationships and upon elements that are linked to the biologic or structural beauty. This

Introduction to Esthetics

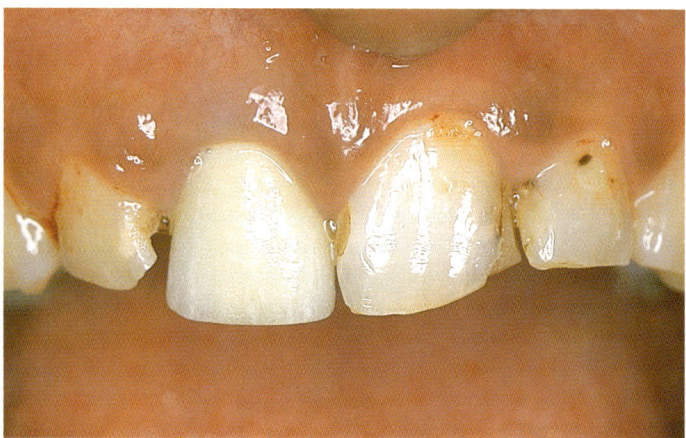

Fig 1-28 The fragility of the composition reflects more from the absence of proportionate relationships than from an apparent pathologic structure.

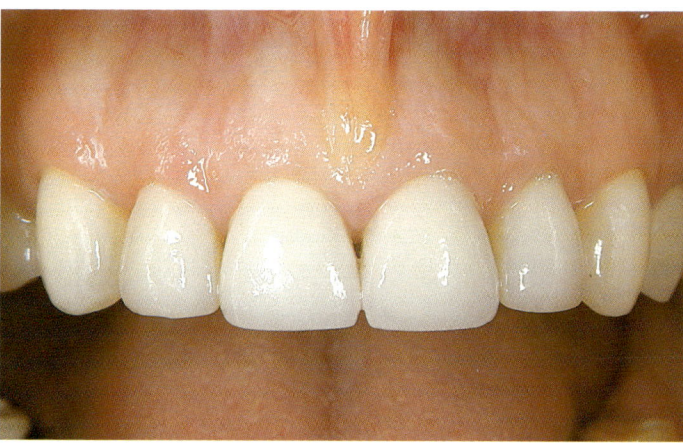

Fig 1-29 The restoration of proportionate relationships gives strength to a composition and produces peaceful appearance and harmony.

may explain why there is a definite and intuitive acknowledgment or mechanical tendency to build up restorations or reestablish proportions of the dentofacial composition in conformity with the golden proportion to achieve a reliable, esthetic result (Figs 1-28 and 1-29).

Principle: The golden proportion appears to be an example of harmony in which cohesive and segregative forces are equally integrated.

Balance

Balance can be defined as the stabilization resulting from the exact adjustment of opposing forces. When all the parts are judiciously adjusted to each other and when none of the constituent elements is out of proportion, it suggests a steady, balanced result. Equilibrium refers not only to forces or weight but also to esthetics. Our perceptive visual sense is used to maintain or induce equilibrium. When the position of an object in its background is perceived with uncomfortable tension, the equilibrium of the composition is not achieved (Fig 1-30). To relieve the tension or reestablish balance two possibilities are left to the viewer or operator:

1. Move the causative element toward the line of forces until the magnitude of the visual tension is totally released (Fig 1-31).
2. Introduce an opposite element along the same line of forces to promote equilibrium (Fig 1-32).

This tension, as opposed to our perception of repeated ratio, is not influenced by the contribution of our fancy or intellect. This tension has a magnitude and direction influenced by the structural features of the surface upon which the causative element is perceived, so that unbalanced compositions look unfinished, accidental, temporary, or transitory. Conversely, a balanced composition looks peaceful, stable, or permanent because visual tension is eliminated. Generally, left and right balance must be considered in terms of visual weights over a centrally located fulcrum. Things farther out from the center have more impact than those closer to it.

For the first time, we feel more comfortable with the manipulation of this basic esthetic element because we have long experienced its effect in dental compositions and provided it whenever possible with appropriate modifications (Figs 1-33 and 1-34). In the simplest examples, a structural map of the field forces present in the com-

Esthetic principles

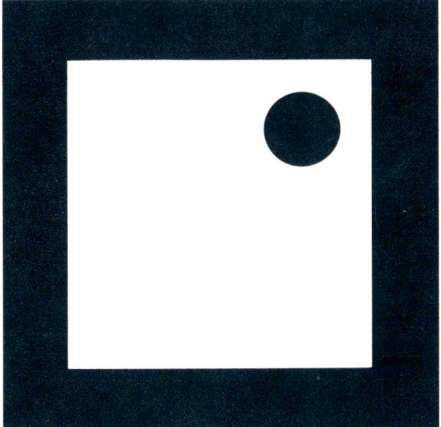 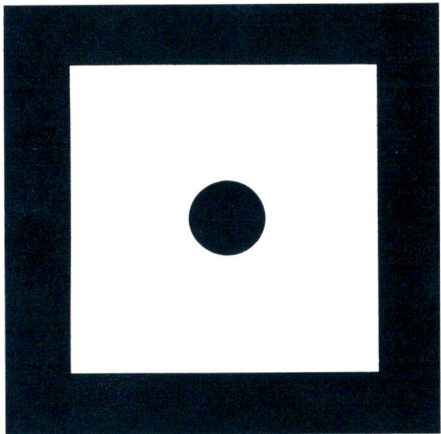 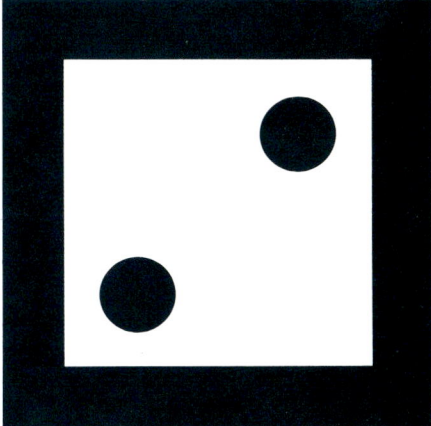

Fig 1-30 The placement of a round form in its background produces visual tension.

Fig 1-31 In moving this form toward the center, visual tension is relieved.

Fig 1-32 The same phenomenon occurs in placing another form in a position of equilibrium.

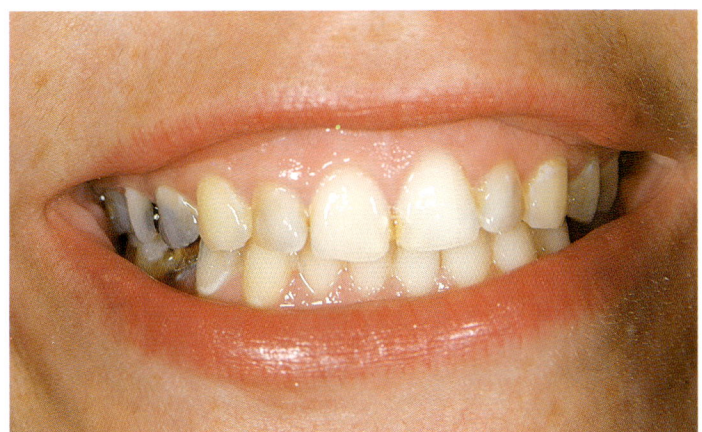 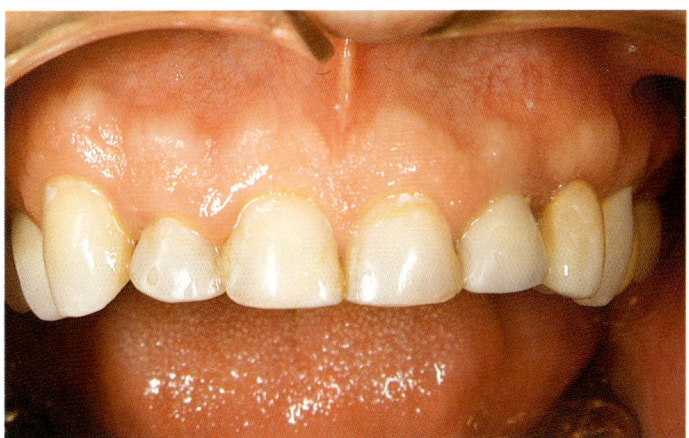

Fig 1-33 Imbalance of color. Equilibrium is not achieved when elements of different colors are placed at various distances from the fulcrum or central point.

Fig 1-34 Imbalance of shape. The farther the elements are located away from the central fulcrum, the more differences of shape grow in importance.

Introduction to Esthetics

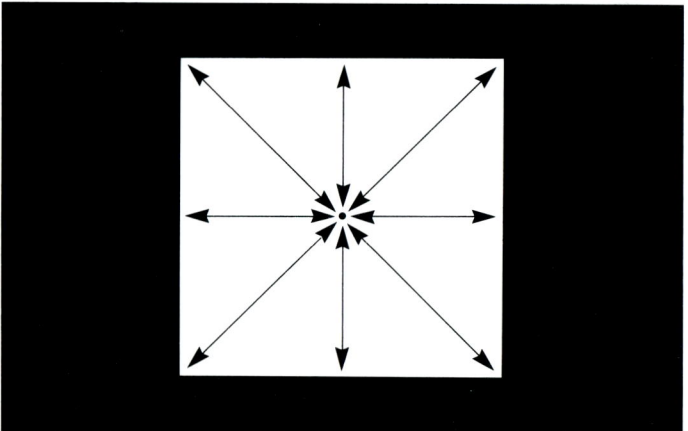

Fig 1-35 A field of forces can always be drawn in a composition, permitting the placement of elements without visual tension.

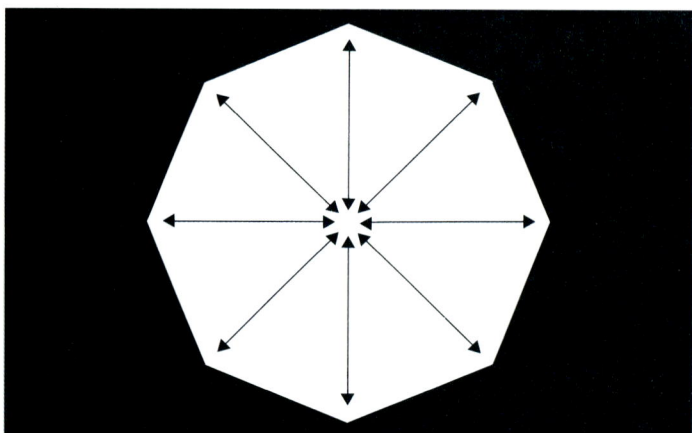

Fig 1-36 A basic field of forces can easily be drawn for this octagonal composition. Its completion becomes more difficult.

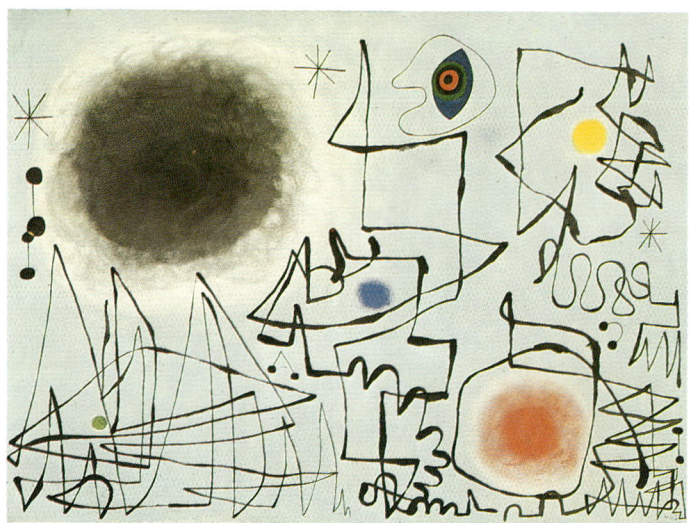

Fig 1-37 *The Diamond Smiles at Dawn* (Miro). The contrasts originating from the nature of the subject, expressed by the extravagant multiplicity of lines and volumes, reflect a magnificent state of harmony by the desire and ability of the artist to generate equilibrium. This implies that final harmony may usually be achieved by means of a variety of factors form the simple to the most complicated. (Courtesy of the Miro Foundation, Barcelona.)

position can be drawn (Figs 1-35 and 1-36). In complicated compositions, only an acute, sensitive sense of visual perception can perceive or achieve balance (Fig 1-37). Perception or achievement of balance may be realized depending on the importance of the offending elements and as a function of the surface upon which they are perceived.

The mouth, face, or head may exhibit complicated and difficult fields of forces that directly depend on the distance from which the viewer focuses to analyze and elaborate esthetic judgment.

Dentofacial compositions exhibiting evading or flaring teeth look, for some obscure reason, both on the frontal and horizontal planes, unbalanced, offending the natural field of forces exerted in the oral cavity (Figs 1-38 and 1-39).

Lines

The importance of lines in dental and dentofacial compositions is far from being negligible and deserves attention because it has been stated that many factors that are part of biologic or structural beauty depend on the visualization of lines. In reality a line does not need to be expressed to be perceived. It can be suggested by two or three points in a directional movement (Fig 1-40).

Esthetic principles

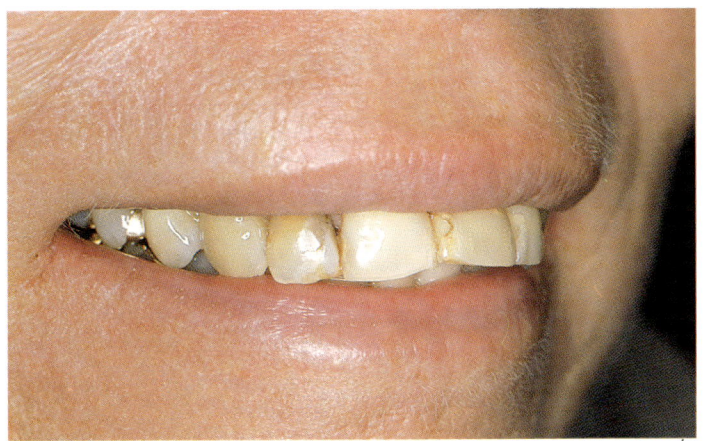

Fig 1-38 The field of forces that develops in the structure of the mouth has yet to be discovered. It should explain why divergent teeth produce visual tension.

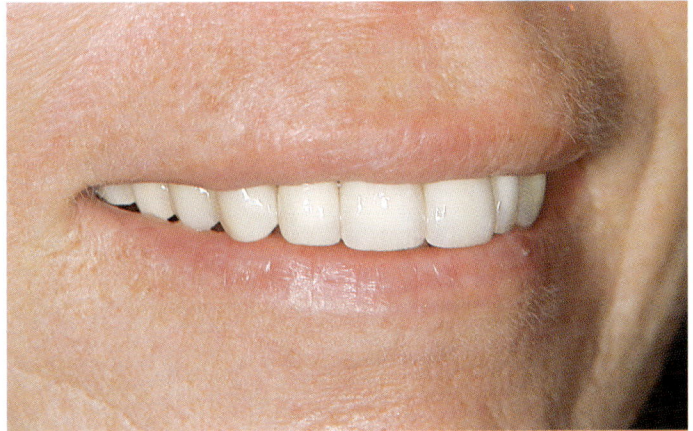

Fig 1-39 The restoration of a more normal tooth direction gives a partial answer to the nature of the field of forces existing in the oral cavity.

The parallel relationship between two lines is the most harmonious because it does not exhibit conflict. The strongest psychologic relationship that lines can engender is a perpendicular relationship. Whereas parallel lines are used as the equals sign, the perpendicular connotes the strong relationship of the plus sign or the cross (Fig 1-41).

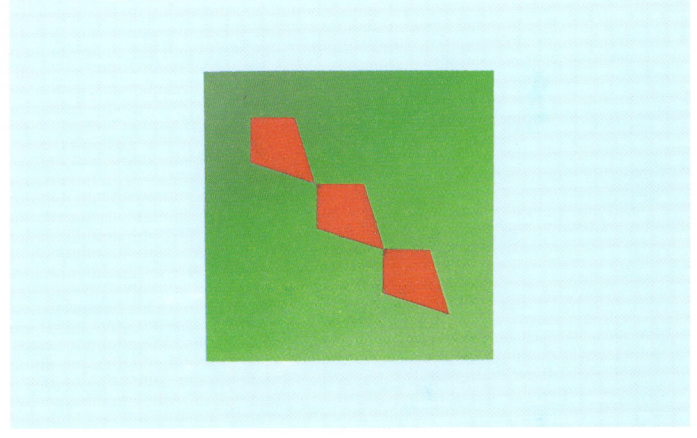

Fig 1-40 Lines do not need to be drawn to be perceived. They reach the level of consciousness by simple suggestion.

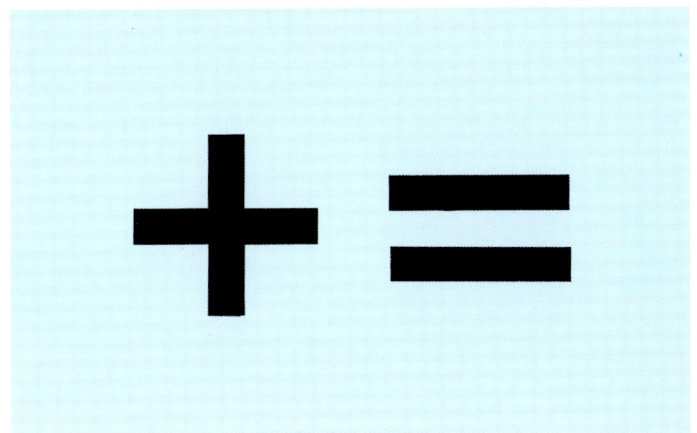

Fig 1-41 Equal lines represent important cohesive forces, whereas crossed lines have the stronger connotation of the segregative forces.

27

Introduction to Esthetics

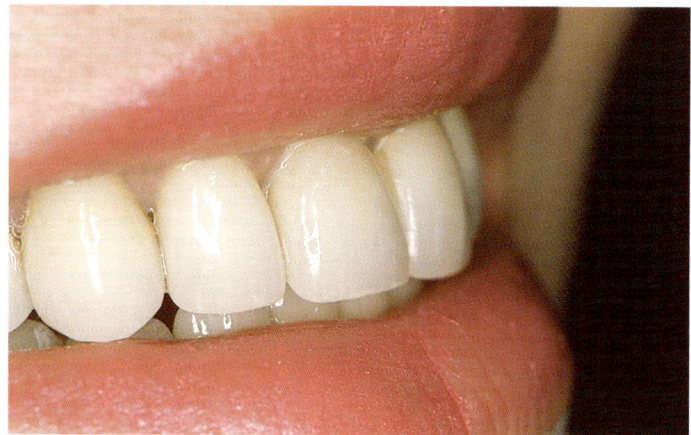

Fig 1-42 The coincidence of incisal and labial lines (cohesive forces) is enhanced by the perception of tooth axial direction (segregative forces).

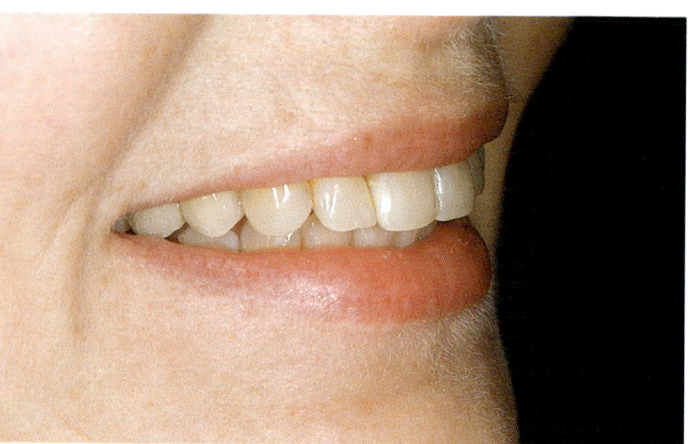

Fig 1-43 The coincidence of a hypothetical line, drawn along the tip of the canines and premolars, with that of the lip margin, is enhanced by the opening of the incisal embrasures.

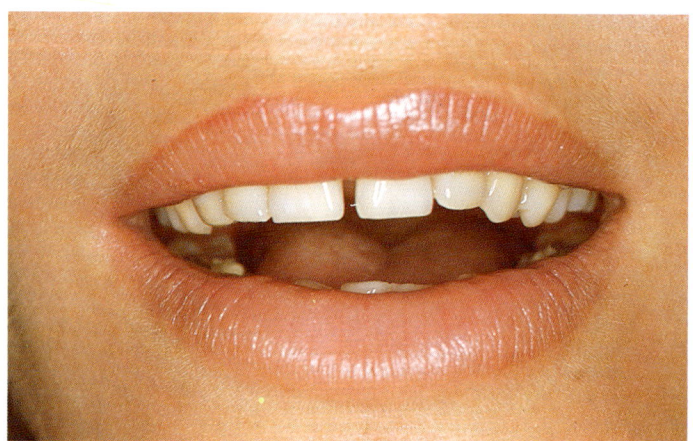

Fig 1-44 Although dominance of axial lines of posterior teeth draws attention, an imbalance of tooth shape (left canine and premolar) indicates functional disturbances.

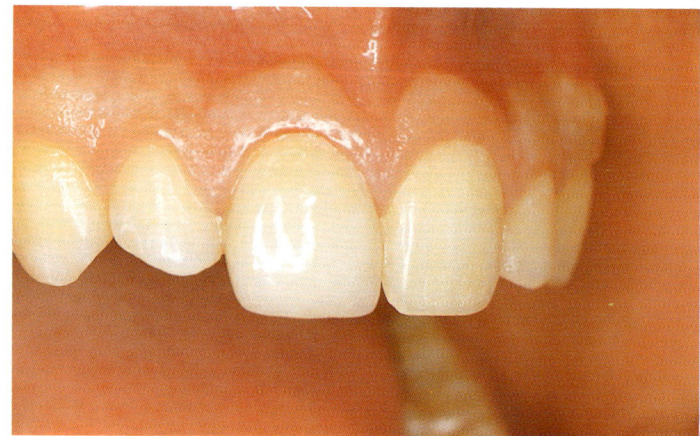

Fig 1-45 The dominance of size of the anterior teeth that can be described as individual can only be evaluated by reference to the size of the subsequent teeth.

Esthetic principles

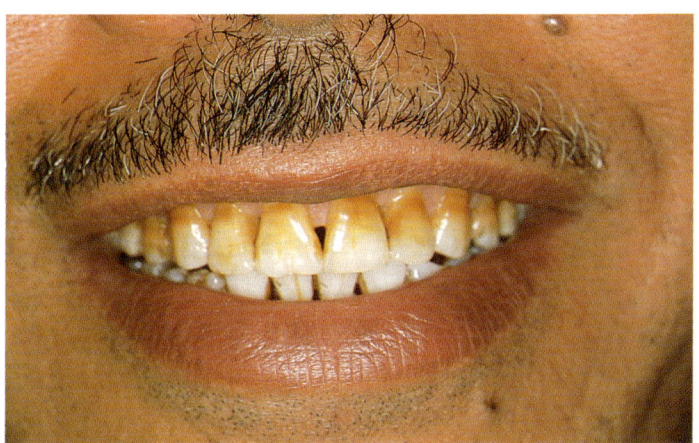

Fig 1-46 A weak dominance takes place when subsequent elements do not provide sufficient factors of contrast.

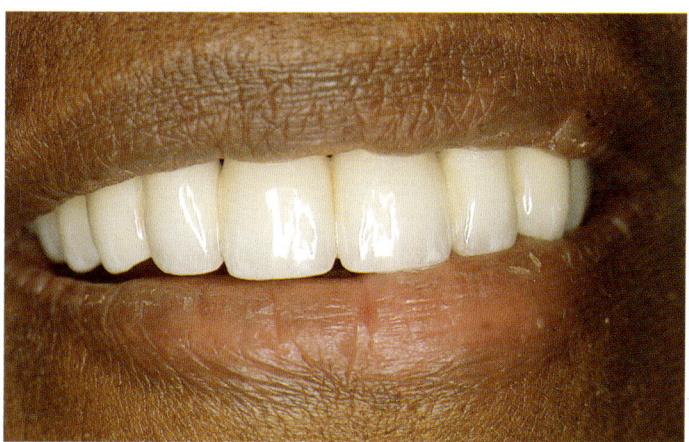

Fig 1-47 A strong dominance requires the presence of subsequent elements providing strong factors of contrast.

Dental compositions contain a multitude of lines that are more or less expressed as the occlusal plane, incisive plane, midline, or tooth direction. Equal and crossed lines are important to the harmony of the composition because of the cohesive or segregative forces that they can produce (Figs 1-42 and 1-43).

Dominance

Dominance is the prime requisite for providing unity because unity is the prime requisite for providing a composition. Dominance provides static (monotonous) or dynamic (vigorous) unity. Color, shape, and lines are factors that can create dominance. They can always be detected in any natural composition, but their importance varies (Figs 1-44 and 1-45).

Dominance implies the presence of subsequent similar elements. The stronger the subsequent element, the stronger the dominating element and the more vigorous the composition will be (Fig 1-46). A weak dominance is a cohesive force that brings static and monotonous unity (Fig 1-47).

Introduction to Esthetics

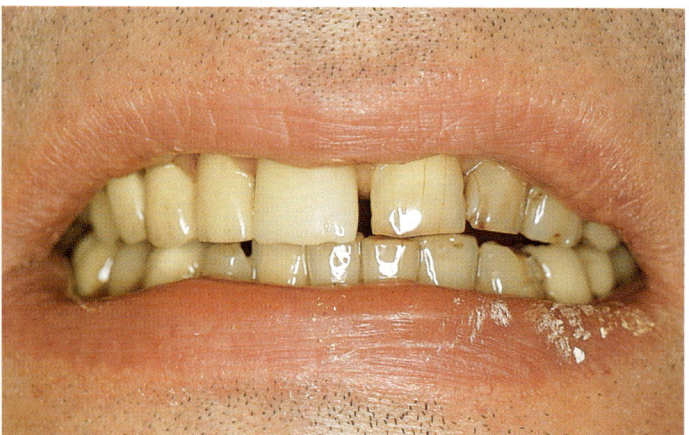
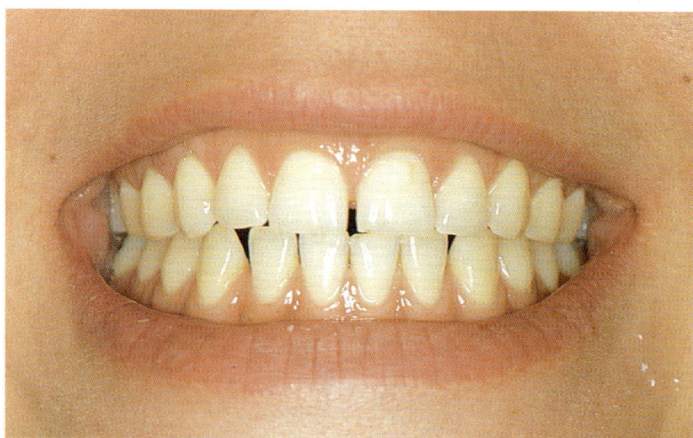

Figs 1-48 and 1-49   These similar square types of tooth shape and arrangements emphasized by the diastema between the central incisors, replicate the psychologic connotation of the cross. They obviously reflect character strength. More will and ambition can be observed in Fig 1-48, which exhibits important anterior tooth wear, a characteristic of the manager type. The dentofacial composition of Fig 1-49, enhanced by the design of upper lip curvature, reflects more accommodating and easygoing character traits.

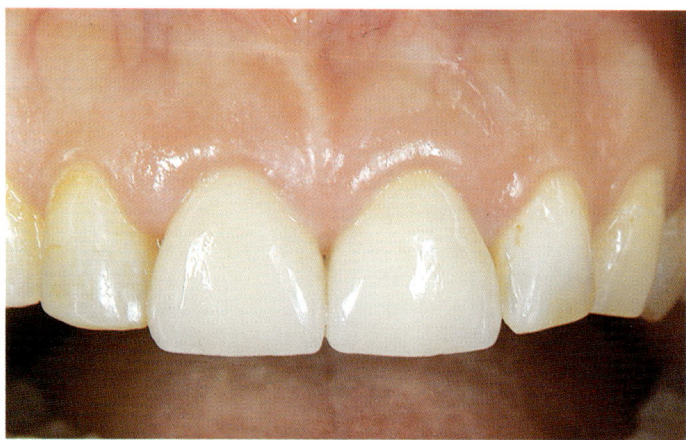
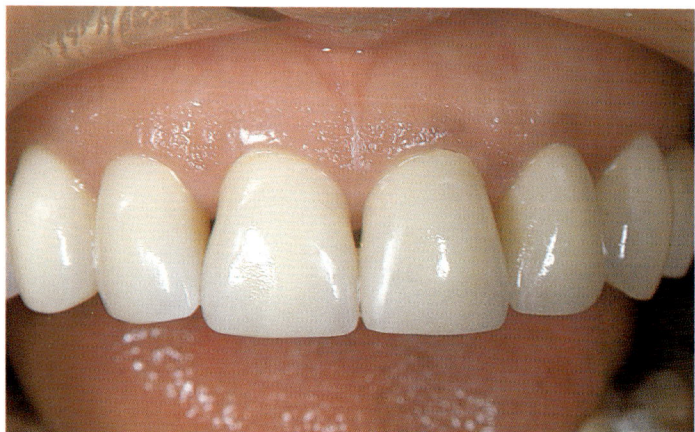

Fig 1-50   In the variety of dental arrangements that characterize a dental composition, one must make a distinction between an individual dominance, which implies the projection of two or multiple dental elements, and a segmental dominance.

Fig 1-51   The segmental dominance that involves the dominance of the whole anterior segment is usually preferred by the public ignoring the particularities and variety of dental compositions. Careful observation shows that in nature, teeth meet with functional requirements and pure segmental dominance does not exist. This type of dominance should imply the arrangement of the dental elements in the vertical plane to meet with functional requirements.

30

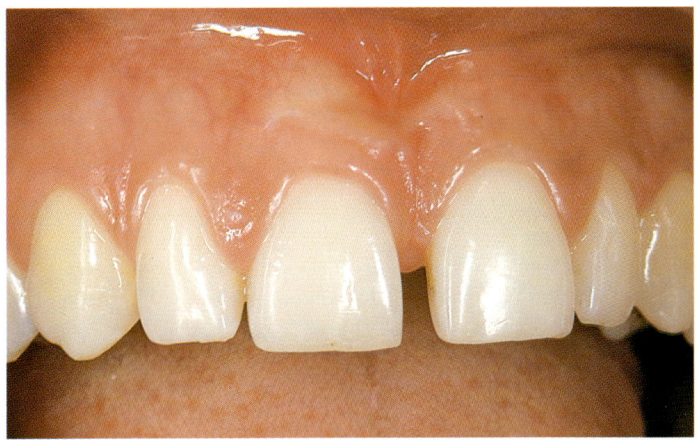

Fig 1-52 Individual dominance of multiple dental elements, a specific ethnic factor, and diastemata that characterize this type of dominance usually do not generate esthetic approval.

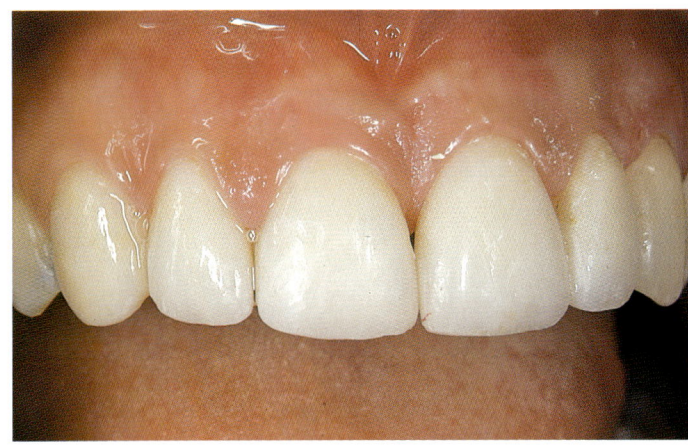

Fig 1-53 It is common practice to modify an individual dominance into a segmental dominance. One must realize that the integration of this new dental composition will be best achieved by respecting specific environmental relationships and by maintaining the morphopsychologic force reflected in this composition.

In decoration harmony is often realized by the presence of a peaceful basic dominant color (cohesive force), to which segregative forces generated by different or opposite colors must be introduced to enhance the beauty of the composition. However, a strong centralized structure, surrounded by appropriately characterized elements, creates an immediate, harmonious composition.

The dominance principle is paradoxical by virtue of the fact that the same ingredients arranged differently will not generate the same psychologic response (Figs 1-48 and 1-49). It also focuses our attention on the fact that in dentistry the evaluation of beauty should not be restricted to the dental composition. Dominance is the key factor required to provide a broadened appraisal of dentofacial composition and the necessity for a harmonious integration of dental composition into facial structure (Figs 1-50 to 1-53). This is only possible by incorporating into the dentofacial composition elements of the patient's personality because the mouth, by its dimension, mobility, and physiologic and psychologic significance, is the dominant element of the face.

Principle: Dominance must be evaluated in the light of its physical and psychologic connotation.

Personality

The structures of personality can be defined according to the following parameters.

1. *Individuality:* identical situations or stimuli produce a variety of emotions that assess the unique distinctiveness of the individual.
2. *Stability:* behavior may change under the influence of the environment without observing structural changes of personality.
3. *Motivations:* look like stimuli, the results of which can only be observed.
4. *Autonomy:* events are never compelling and only exist through the significance they are granted.

Personality only exists through a network of relationships connected by attitudes and behavior that require the body's participation. The maintenance or the deterioration that could effect its most expressive part, the dentofacial composition, greatly depends on the objective perception and integration of these parameters in rehabilitations, assuming that the technical quality assured by the prosthodontist is a reliable constant.

This physical and psychologic link that establishes facial esthetic harmony not only revives an old concept but also focuses attention on the need for a reliable concept of perception in our eyes, best realized through the morphopsychologic concept because it requires the same elements of perception and evaluation as esthetic principles.

References

Academy of Denture Prosthetics. Glossary of Prosthodontic Terms. *J Prosthet Dent.* 1968;20:447, 486.

Albino JE, Tedesco LA, Conny JD. Patient perception of dental-facial esthetics. Shared concerns in orthodontics and prosthodontics. *J Prosthet Dent.* 1984;52:9.

Aquinas, St. Thomas. *Summa Theologica.* (c. 1250).

Arnheim R. *Art and Visual Perception.* Berkeley and Los Angeles, Calif: University of California Press; 1965.

Becker EO. Esthetics — An enigma. *J Prosthet Dent.* June, 1971;588–591.

Bercleid E, Walter E. Beauty and the best. *Psychol Today.* 1972;5:10.

Brigante RF. Patient assisted esthetics. *J Prosthet Dent.* 1981;46:14.

Brisman AS. Esthetics: A comparison of dentists and patients concepts. *J Am Dent Assoc.* 1980;100:345.

Burckett PJ, Christensen LC. Estimating age and sex by using color, form and alignment of anterior teeth. *J Prosthet Dent.* 1988;59:175–179.

Cattel RB. *The Scientific Analysis of Personality.* Chicago, Ill: Aldine Publ; 1965.

Cirici A. *Miro et son temps.* Barcelona, Spain: Ediciones Poligrafia; 1985.

Darwin ChR. *Descent of Man and Selection in Relation to Sex.* 1871.

Fechner GT. *Vorschule der Ästhetik.* Leipzig; 1876.

Fisher RD. Esthetics in denture construction. *Dent Clin North Am.* March, 1957.

Fisher S, Cleveland SE. *Body Image and Personality.* New York, NY: Dover Publications Inc; 1968.

Frush JP, Fisher RD. Introduction to dentogenic restorations. *J Prosthet Dent.* 1955;5:586–595.

Frush JP, Fisher RD. How dentinogenic restorations interpret the sex factor. *J Prosthet Dent.* 1956;6:160–172.

Frush JP, Fisher RD. How dentinogenics interpret the personality factor. *J Prosthet Dent.* 1956;6:441–449.

Frush JP, Fisher RD. The age factor in dentogenics. *J Prosthet Dent.* 1957;7:5–13.

Frush JP, Fisher RD. The dynesthetic interpretation of the dentinogenic concept. *J Prosthet Dent.* 1958;8:560–681.

Furtwangler A. *Masterpieces of Greek Sculpture.* Chicago, Ill: Argonaut; 1964.

Garret HE. *Psychology.* New York, NY: American Book Co; 1950.

Gerber A. Creative and artistic tasks in complete prosthodontics. *Quintessence Int.* 1975;6(2):45.

Goldstein RE. *Esthetics in Dentistry.* Philadelphia, Pa: JB Lippincott; 1976.

Goldstein RE, Fritz M. Esthetics in dental curriculum. *J Dent Educ.* 1981;45:355.

Graber LW, Lucker, GW. Dental esthetics self evaluation and satisfaction. *Am J Orthod.* 1980;77:163.

Hambidge J. *The Elements of Dynamic Symmetry.* New York, NY: Dover Press; 1970.

Hegel GWF. In Montaigne, ed. *Vorlesungen über die Ästhetik.* Paris: 1944.

Hegel GWF. *Philosophy of History.* New York, NY: Collier; 1905.

Hershon LE, Giddon DB. Determinants of facial profile self perception. *Am J Orthod.* 1980;77:279–293.

Honour H, Fleming J. *Histoire Mondiale de l'Art.* Paris: Bordas; 1984.

Huyghe R. *Dialogue avec le Visible.* Paris: Flammarion; 1955.

Kant E. *Critique of Judgment,* 1790.

Lee, JH. *Dental Aesthetics.* Bristol, Conn: John Wright and Sons; 1962.

Lombardi R. Visual perception and denture esthetics. *J Prosthet Dent.* 1973;29:352–382.

Lombardi R. A method for the classification of errors in dental esthetics. *J Prosthet Dent.* 1974;11:501–513.

Lombardi R. Factors mediating against excellence in dental esthetics. *J Prosthet Dent.* 1977;9:243–248.

Meyers B. L'interprétation de l'Art. *Le Lion d'Art.* Grolier; 10:1971.

Miller WH, Ratcliff F, Hartline HK. *Perception: Mechanism and Models.* San Francisco, Calif: WH Freeman and Co; 1961.

Molnar ME. *Forever Young: The Practical Handbook of Youth Extension.* West Hartford, Conn: The Withower Press Inc; 1985.

Palau J, Favre J. *Picasso en Catalogne.* Société Française du Lion, trad. française; 1979.

Peck H, Peck S. A concept of facial esthetics. *Angle Orthod* 1970;40:284.

Plato. *Philebus.* c. 400 BC.

Plato. *Republic.* c. 400 BC.

Pound E, Muriel G. An introduction do denture simplification. *J Prosthet Dent.* 1971;26:571–580.

Preston JD. A systematic approach to the control of esthetic form. *J Prosthet Dent.* 1976;35:393–402.

Reidel RA. Esthetics and its relation to orthodontic therapy. *Angle Orthod.* 1950;20:168–178.

Renner RP. *An Introduction to Dental Anatomy and Esthetics.* Chicago, Ill: Quintessence Publ Co; 1985.

Schärer P, Rinn LA, Kopp FR. *Aesthetische Richtlinien für die Reconstructive Zahnheilkunde.* Berlin: Quintessenz Verlag; 1980.

Shelby DS. Anterior Restoration, Fixed Bridgework and Esthetics. Springfield, Ill: Charles C Thomas Publisher; 1976.

Sobnow I. The emotional significance of loss of teeth. *Dent Clin North Am.* 1962; Nov:641.

Tea E. *La proporzione nelle arti figurative.* Milan; 1945.

Tedesco LA, Albino JE, et al. Variables discriminating individuals who seek orthodontic treatment. A dento-facial attractiveness scale. Part I: Reliability and validity. *Am J Orthod.* 1983;83:36. Part II: Consistency and perception. *Am J Orthod.* 1983;83:38.

Tripodakis AP. Dental esthetics: Oral personality and visual perception. *Quintessence Int.* 1987;7(6):405–418.

Vincent JA. *History of Art.* New York, NY: Barnes and Noble; 1955.

Zeising A. *Neue Lehre von den Proportionen des menschlichen Körpers.* Leipzig; 1854.

Chapter 2

Morphopsychology

Claude R. Rufenacht

Introduction

The objective of morphopsychology is to establish the links between physical or morphologic appearance and characterological or psychologic particulars. "Facial shapes are a reflection of the life forces that are at work within each individual" (Corman). The study of the various facial forms as a concrete and harmonious reflection of the development of thought and spirit should be helpful in understanding the secret nature of these elements. This postulate is the basis for the development of the "science" of morphopsychology, an understanding of which represents one of the means of assessing the personality of our patients.

The human body is characterized by four basic anatomic elements, represented by the digestive, respiratory, nervous, and osteomuscular systems, which respond to four dominant instincts, which can be defined as an internal obligatory impulsion toward a concrete, specific objective.

1. The intuitive, material, and reproductive instincts, represented by the digestive and genital mechanisms.
2. The vital or thoracic instinct, which is the basis for breathing, developed and implemented by the respiratory system.
3. Psychic or cerebral instinct, on which reflection, thought, reason, and understanding are based, represented by the nervous system.
4. The motor or unifying instinct, which is the basis for actions and decisions according to the individual's physiologic and intellectual capabilities and taste, represented by the osteomuscular system.

Segments

The human being appears in a trinity of forces combined within an individual unit because this entity has in itself a directional spirit, an animating life, and a body to execute (Fig 2-1).

The trinity of forces is clearly inscribed within the human organism, which is composed of three segments:

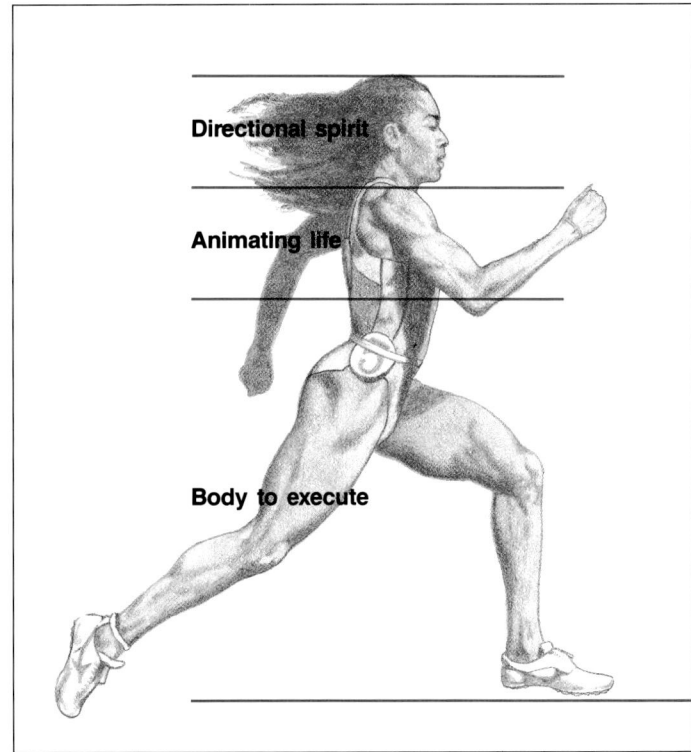

Fig 2-1 The individuality of the human unit appears in a trinity of segmental forces.

Morphopsychology

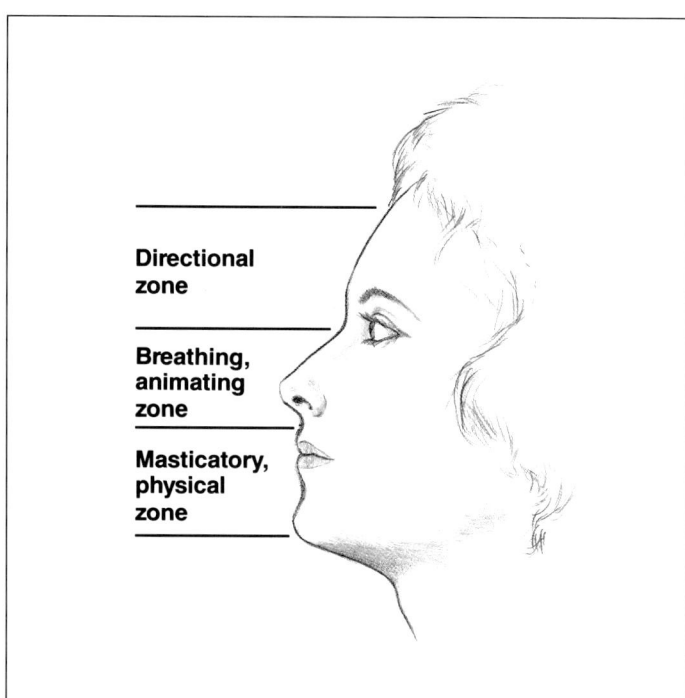

Fig 2-2 The head itself presents the same elements of segmental differentiation.

the head, which directs, the thorax, which vivifies, and the abdomen, which carries out the acts of nutrition.

The head itself is divided into three levels:

1. The upper level (intellectual or cerebral zone) from the upper part of the forehead to the root of the nose, which directs:
2. the middle level (emotional or sentimental zone) from the root to the base of the nose, which breathes and animates:
3. the lower level (instinctive or physical zone) from the base of the nose to the chin, which obeys and masticates (Fig 2-2).

Factors of morphology and morphopsychologic appraisal

There are four means of appraising morphology:

1. Clinical, based on anatomic knowledge, linked to folds and volumes, the indispensable knowledge of which is acquired through our medical training.
2. Esthetics, which allows for an appreciation of harmony and beauty, or disfavor through the knowledge or perception of the esthetic parameters that have been described earlier.
3. Anthropometric, or body measurement techniques.
4. Biometric, or the methods for using and exploiting numerical factors, particularly with respect to the definition of biologic normality, which is the basis of modern orthodontics.

The study of forms is essentially based on observation and is aimed at distinguishing normal from abnormal forms or proportions of the body and face. In the field that is of interest to us, the main focus will be on the face with emphasis on the most obvious elements that mark an individual. One subject will be bony, the other muscular, and a third will be obese. Similarly, the manner in which the person moves, heavily, with alacrity, or decisiveness, can provide an indication of whether the person is an introvert or an extrovert. The distinctive particulars of the same anatomic elements determine the factors of morphologic appraisal designed to identify the fundamental types.

Typologic classifications

Hippocratic classification

According to Hippocrates, the father of typology, the Greek physician Gallien (131–201), and Dr Carton, four fundamental types of persons can be identified: the lymphatic, the sanguine, the nervous, and the bilious (Figs 2-3 to 2-6), each of which presents specific morphologic particulars.

The nervous person scowls, the sanguine is agitated, the bilious acts, and the lymphatic does not move. Although this statement results from an evident will of simplification, it has been attributed to each fundamental type general traits of character behavior (Fig 2-7). How-

Typologic classifications

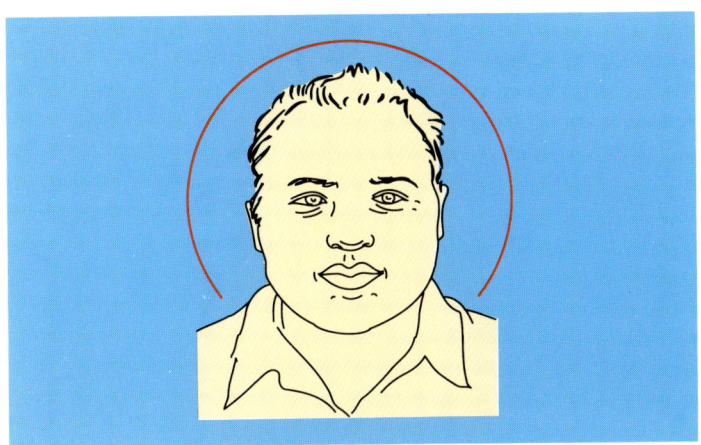

Fig 2-3 The lymphatic, heavy person, with a voluminous abdomen, thick members, and a full face. This individual is slow-moving, with a calm and placid character.

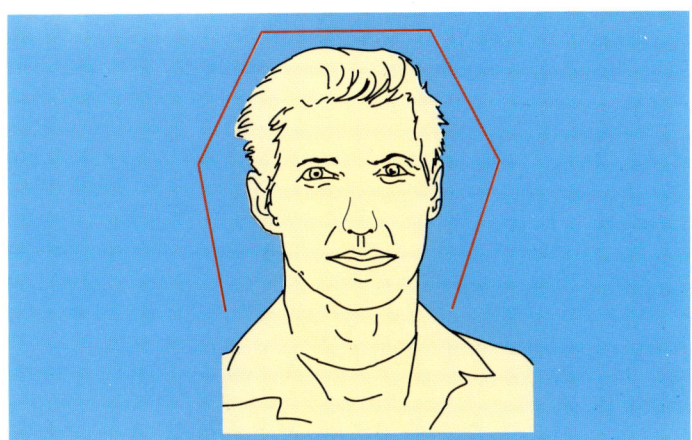

Fig 2-4 The sanguine, strong, and thick-set person has a well-developed thorax, a wide, ruddy complexion, spontaneous gestures, and an ebullient spirit.

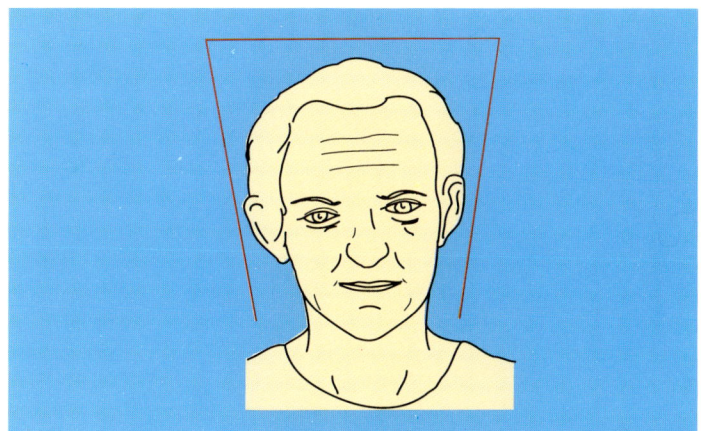

Fig 2-5 The nervous individual presents an elongated, pear-like head, with a wide superior extremity and an ample cerebral volume that contrasts with the others. The body is thin, with tegument of a grayish pallor and a thoughtful, anxious look.

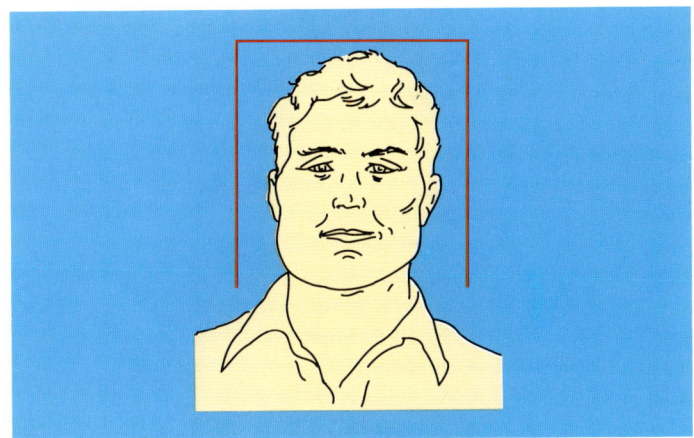

Fig 2-6 The bilious person has a rectangular face, straight eyebrows, an ardent and dominating look, and a firm, prominent musculature.

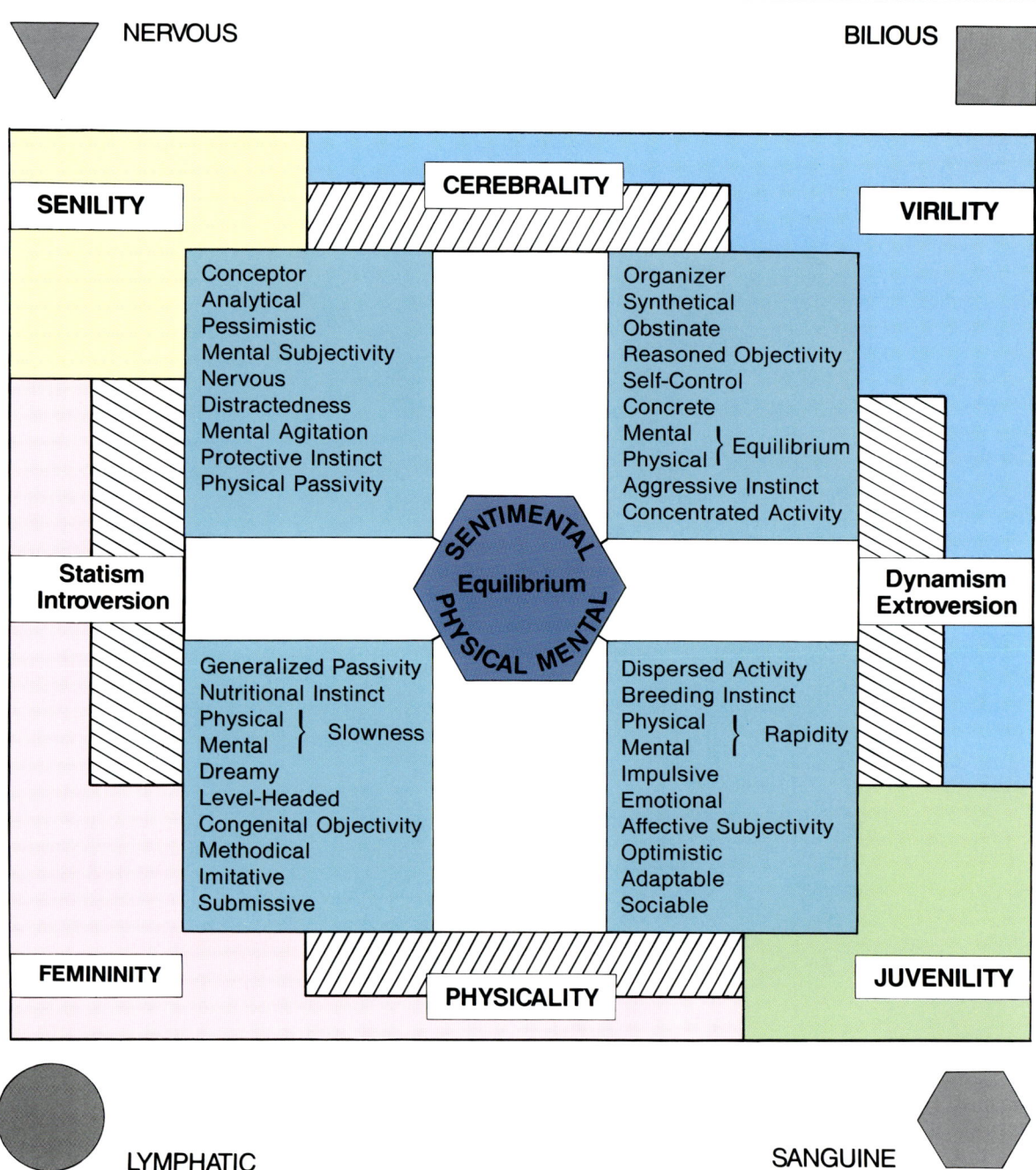

Fig 2-7 The characteral square enumerates general traits of behavior specific to the four fundamental types and underlines the connections and similarities that can exist among them. One must consider that each individual presents a tendency to blend with one of the fundamental types. However, it presents a mixture of secondary characteristics requiring proper evaluation and prudent judgment. (Suggested by "La Rose Caractérielle," Morphopsychologie, Cours de Base, Institut Français de Culture Humaine, Paris, 1982.)

ever, the observation that an individual is far from presenting the specific morphologic particularities of a fundamental type fixes the limits of a strict application of these general traits. Judgment must be modulated, and interpretation should result from a correct evaluation of the mix and variety of accessory types existing within each human being.

In considering the hierarchical origin of the fundamental types according to the chronology of their creation, it can be observed that a child starts living a lymphatic life through the placental roots, and at the moment of birth the respiratory life of the sanguine. The nervous system and thoughts slowly become animated, and the child ends up mastering its locomotion system by creeping and finally walking.

The same chronology can be stated in the different stages of development beginning with the lymphatic and abdominal in the first 15 months of life. One becomes predominantly sanguine through the growth of the thorax until the age of 7 years. The development of the cerebral zone occupies the stage until adolescence, characterized by the final sculpture of the osseous structure and muscular mass.

The Hippocratic classification offers the advantage of simplicity and appears as a necessary step for the introduction to morphopsychology. Even if more specific and precise classifications have been proposed and adopted since then (eg, animal or planetary typologies), it still remains an original basis and standard for all schools.

It must be recognized that although biologic evolution is fundamental to the laws of life, it depends on a number of factors that can deeply modify the basic formula, best ascertained by considerations drawn from the work of different authors that are part of modern morphopsychologic concepts.

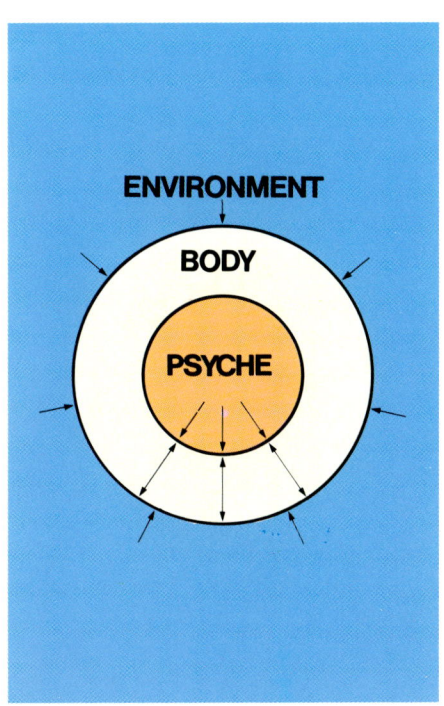

Fig 2-8 Morphologic analysis must be carried out, taking into account environmental influences pertaining to family, profession, climate, and subconscious psychosomatic pulsions. Morphologic appearances are the result of these two evolutive dynamic factors.

Biodynamic conception of the personality

It is difficult to conceive of limiting the morphology of the body and the face, both in the study of humans and in the human's "global beauty." When one's point of view remains static one is limited to the boundaries that are set, and the comparison among the various types of character is reduced to superficial parallels. To create a true synthesis of characterologies, a penetration in depth is required so that the physiologic forces may be understood in their nascent state.

Although there are certain inbred constitutive properties inscribed within each individual, the personality is in constant evolution and in permanent interaction with its environment (Fig 2-8). From this viewpoint, character traits should not be emphasized, but rather the profound tendencies that are the cause of such traits should be stressed. These psychologic forces are within the body, and all duality of body–spirit must be abandoned so that, while keeping in mind their close interdependence, a biodynamic conception of the personality as a whole may be substituted. This dynamist conception allows for the opportunities presented to each person to modify by the choice of environment, as well as through personal, intimate, daily effort, that which is inscribed in one's morphology and psychism. "I was as you said I was, but I dominated my instincts and transformed myself" (Socrates).

Morphopsychology

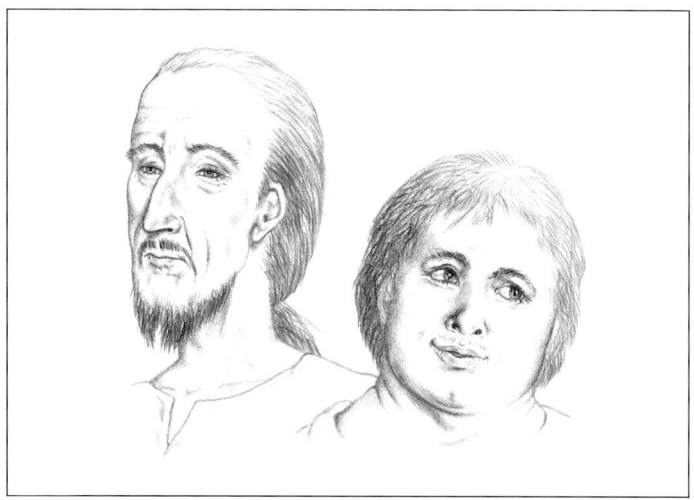

Fig 2-9 Don Quixote and Sancho Panza. According to Corman, the laws of adaptation to the environment have generated two types of person: the retracted and the dilated, best illustrated by these two individuals, made popular by literature. Pure retraction or dilatation rarely exists in the same person. Whereas Sancho Panza seems to behave at ease in any environmental condition and be receptive to life's pleasures with some kind of passive attitude, the movement of retraction, which characterizes his withdrawn companion, seems to escape the influence of visual inputs. Long and sharp sensitive receptors indicate selected social activities.

The components of the character according to this biodynamic conception are best summarized as follows:

1. Character is the whole person in all aspects, a synthesis of life and body.
2. Character is a synthesis of emotional life, will, and intelligence.
3. Character is not immutable. Aside from the acquired and the rejected, there is the environment. The difficulty lies in determining the constants and the variables.
4. A human being cannot be studied outside the environment in which he lives and by which he is influenced.
5. There is only a difference of degree and not of nature between normal and abnormal characters. The former contains the same fundamental elements but distributed evenly.

Laws of adaptation to the environment

The variety marking the development of human morphology has been interpreted by Corman as a sensitive and individual reaction to the environment. This reaction depends on the antagonism existing between two basic instincts that characterize the movements of life: the instinct of expansion and the instinct of preservation, the activities of which are placed under the influence of heredity and environment.

From the moment of birth, hereditary factors will generate in individuals subject to identical environmental conditions, reactions of dilatation or retraction. As a result, two distinct types can be observed: the dilated and the retracted (Fig 2-9).

Open-minded, optimistic, sensual, concrete, adaptable, and uninhibited individuals turn toward social contacts; the dilated type develops and radiates in the environment in a movement of dilatation that characterizes the instinct of expansion.

Conversely, the retracted, hypersensitive person, ready to detect dangers in cutting the roots that connect him with his environment, retires within himself in a movement of retraction. One has to consider that retraction should not be opposed to dilatation, as if one were dealing with two symmetric states. Retraction is not a static but an active process, turned toward interiorization and preservation. This type of personality is far more complex to understand because it contains the duality that enables behavior in a selected environment in a movement of expansion. Thus, according to circumstances, the re-

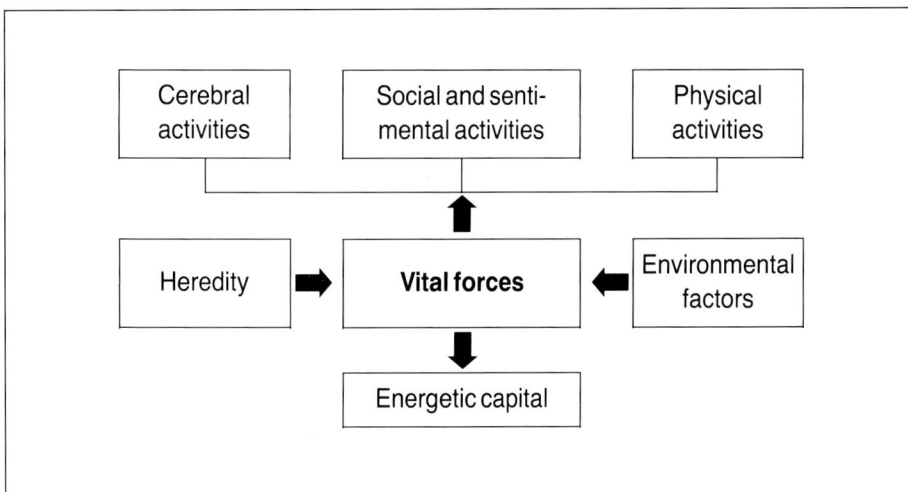

Fig 2-10 Schematic partition of vital forces.

tracted may be an extrovert or an introvert, efficient or indecisive, reasonable or impulsive.

Facial morphopsychology

The evaluation of the different elements of the morphopsychologic profile is directly proportional to the importance of the time dedicated to the patient, the sense of observation, and the degree of receptivity. Our level of knowledge and training may become totally worthless if our attention is focused on mastering technical problems.

Although a detailed analysis of the body cannot be considered here because the diversity of fashions, both of season and culture, often hides volume and proportion, the evaluation will be done on its most significant and important part — the face.

This introduction to morphopsychology, limited to general principles, selected concepts, and laws, states as a basic postulate that our facial frame, originating from our heredity, contains the potentialities necessary to its evolution.

Modeled from generation to generation, the facial framework, analyzed through the variety of typologic classifications, may reveal a number of general traits of character behavior and attest to the energetic possibilities of the individual. However, the variability exerted by vital forces not only determines the overall volume of the facial osseous framework but also the development in length of the different facial zones corresponding to life activities (Fig 2-10).

Facial zones

The distinct significance of the three facial zones (Figs 2-11 and 2-12) has long been recognized by the public and used extensively by caricaturists. However, one must beware of simplistic conclusions because it is common sense that the level of intelligence, for example, cannot be measured by the development of the cerebral zone.

The definition of a facial zone through its quantitative value is not justified unless it has been dictated by the qualitative appreciation of its dilatation or retraction and the tonicity and vitality of the sensitive receptors. The eyes, nose, and mouth occupy the stage of these different zones and determine their importance.

Morphopsychology

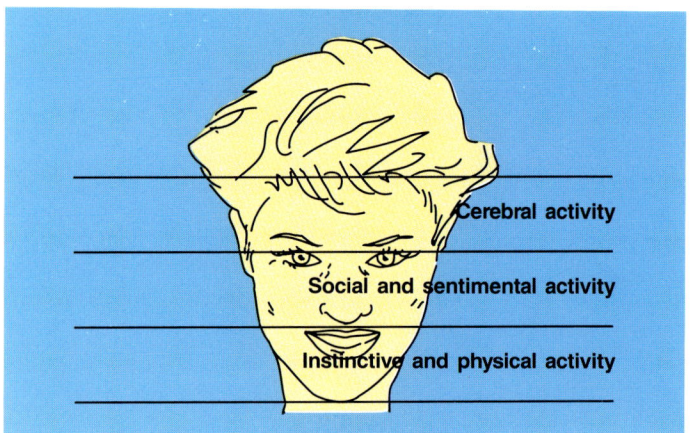

Fig 2-11 Segmental division of the face in three zones called facial zones. The dominance of one facial zone over the others indicates the preferential type of activity.

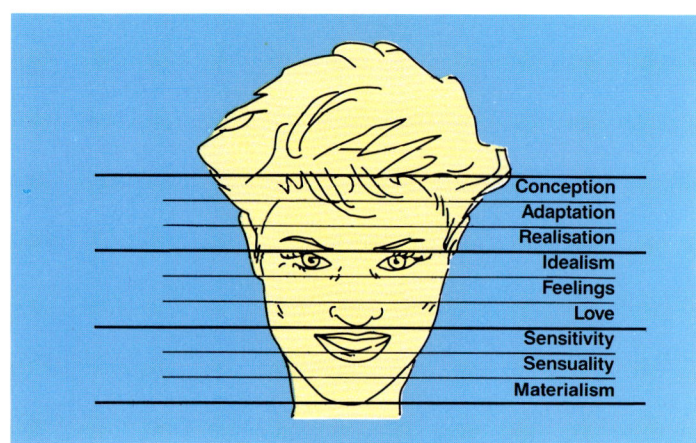

Fig 2-12 A facial zone may be divided into three parts: upper, middle, and lower (segmental division), each of which is related to the corresponding facial zone. The upper part of the lower facial zone, eg, represents the sensitive and reasoning element of the instinctive life.

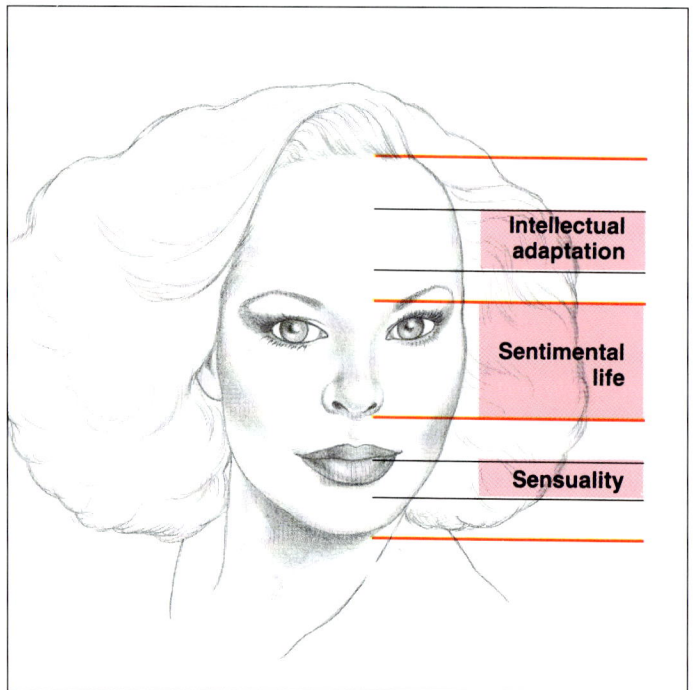

Fig 2-13 *Morphopsychologic equilibrium.* In this type of expansion of the median zone, reflecting the predominant influence of sentimentality, equilibrium can be obtained when feelings, helped by the intellect through the development of the adaptative factor, manifest themselves in the concrete sensuality of physical life.

Equilibrium

The equilibrium existing between the facial zones must be determined and ascertained according to both their qualitative and quantitative value. This implies the elective use of the same elements of dominance, proportion, symmetry, and balance, which are required for esthetic perception and evaluation. Equilibrium still exists when a hierarchical dominance takes place in a zone of expansion that involves the active and nonconflicting participation of the two others. The subdivision of each facial zone into three parts and the presentation of the same elements of differentiation contribute to the understanding of this hierarchy and to a selective type of equilibrium.

Identical developments of the three facial zones engender morphopsychologic equilibrium and esthetic harmony. When a hierarchical dominance of selected facial levels takes place, esthetic harmony and morphopsychologic equilibrium still exist, most often enhanced by the nature of the dominance reflecting from the facial composition (Fig 2-13).

This equilibrium can also be disturbed when the prevalence of one dominating zone overburdens the others quantitatively and qualitatively. As a result, the field of activities induced by vital forces is restricted to life activities reflecting from these zones (Fig 2-14). The dominance factor, the prime requisite for esthetic unity, requires the presence of subsequent elements. The particularities of these elements determine the character and the importance of the dominance factor. The predominance of a facial zone can be determined through the amplitude of its development, the opening and tonicity of its receptors, its reactivity to environmental influences, and the abundance of exchanges in the field of its preferential activities.

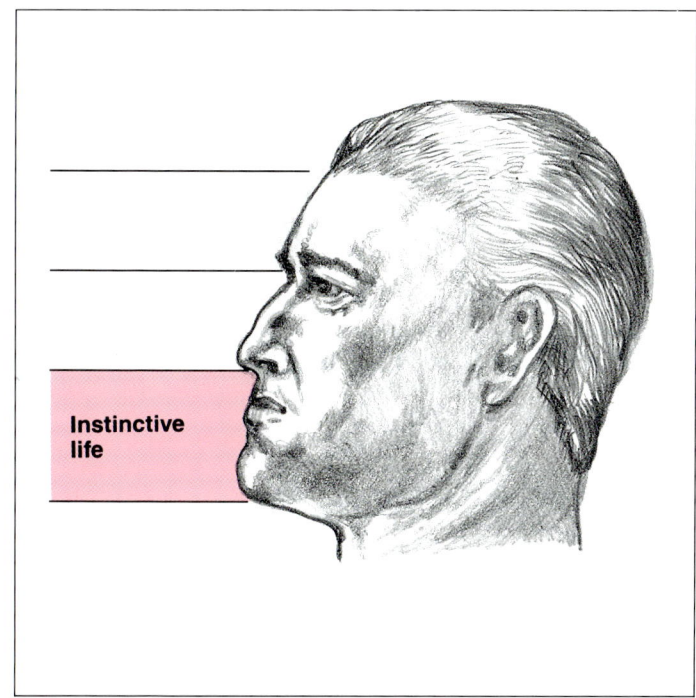

Fig 2-14 *Morphopsychologic disequilibrium.* In this overdevelopment of the mandibular zone, irrational instinctive impulses will generate excessive physical activities and intemperate ambitions, most probably far from being justified by the individual's capabilities.

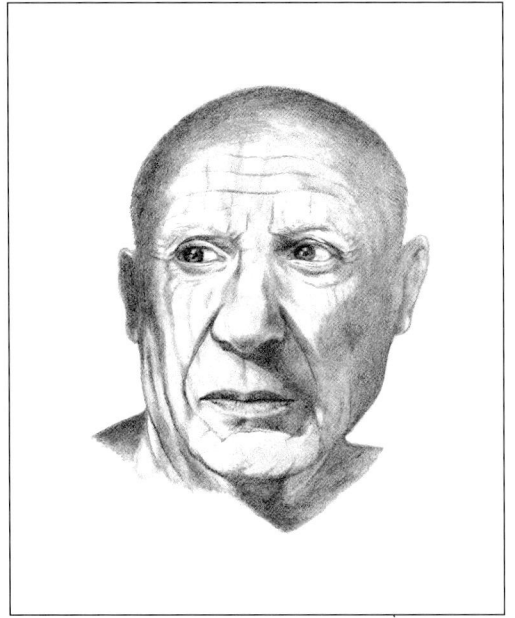 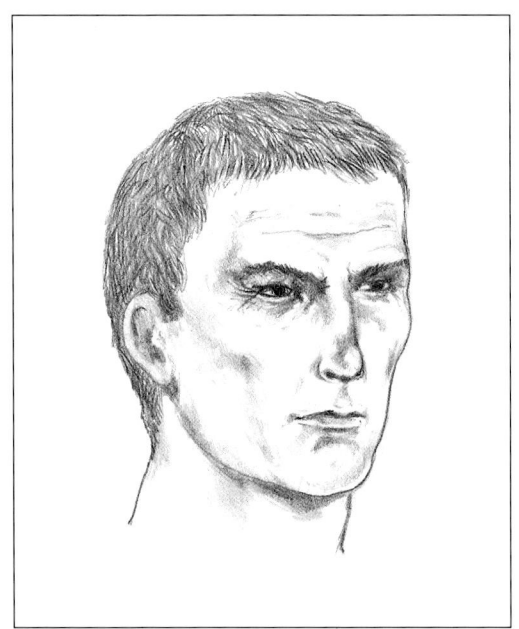

Fig 2-15 *Opened receptors.* Although wide open receptors characterize this individual, a gradation in the quality and quantity of exchanges seems to take place in each receptor. Exchanges are predominantly emotional and, to a lesser degree, instinctive. The ocular receptor appears to ensure a quality of information more cosmic than realistic.

Fig 2-16 *Closed receptors.* Closed receptors are energy-saving, sunken, and protected, filtering information and production. Provided with the necessary elements to ensure integrity, this individual may move in unfavorable environmental conditions with independence and self-control.

The receptors

The receptors are the sensitive elements — eyes, nose, mouth, and ears — that occupy the different facial zones, assuming the functions of exchange. As opposed to the general frame, which fixes the energetic potentials of the individual, the location and importance of the receptors on the facial map determine what has been called the *vestibular frame*.

Receptors have been described as opened or closed. Opened receptors are characterized by prominent and separated eyes, dilated nostrils, and a wide and fleshy mouth. The individual presents the characteristics of the extrovert (Fig 2-15). With closed receptors the eyes are small, sunken, retracted, and close to each other, the mouth is small, and the filtering and saving of energy take place, indicating a tendency of self-protection and selectivity (Fig 2-16).

Sexual type

Every human being is a mixture of male and female types in varied and unequal proportions. There always exists an active, subconscious, and hidden sexual type opposed to that which is morphologically manifested. As a result, this opposed side appears either as a physical image or as a character quality. The statement that females possess one third of heterosexual hormones and men possess only one sixth opens the hypothesis that females may exhibit many more masculine characteristics than males exhibit feminine ones.

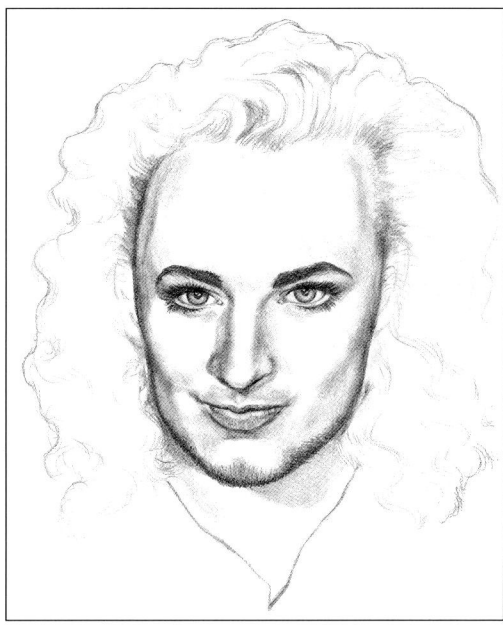 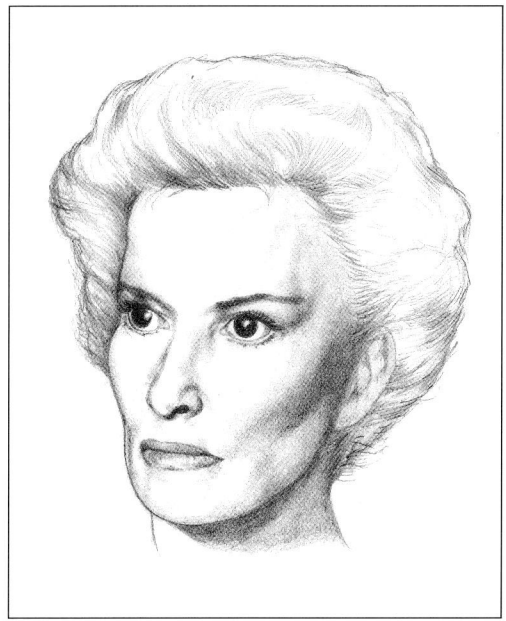

Fig 2-17 *Feminine type*. The effects of make-up, aimed at underlining the sexual duality of morphologic image, have resulted in stressing the "feminine" qualities reflecting from this face. Mainly intellectual and artistic with a high and evading cerebral zone, it is served by the sentimentality of a marked middle facial zone.

Fig 2-18 *Masculine type*. With straight facial angles and a large instinctive zone underlined by the strong protrusion of eyebrows, the realistic part of the intellectual activity, the whole facial image reflects energy, determination, and domination, ie, "masculine" qualities.

Feminine components are characterized by round, oval, and gracile shapes, delicacy in the osseous structures, opened facial angle, vertical overhead, oval jaws, and round chin with soft facial features, sensitivity, and sentimentality. Qualities related to feminine components were traditionally considered as being oriented toward introspection, arts, and esthetics.

Masculine components, on the contrary, show angular and rectangular shapes, strong osseous structures, closed facial angle, oblique forehead, and strong and angular jaws. A square chin with marked facial features exhibits energy, will of action, and aggressivity power (Fig 2-18). Masculine qualities are usually turned toward exterior life.

The words animus or anima refer to individuals, male or female, reflecting in varying degrees masculine or feminine components, and one can state that the sexual type is determined both by morphologic and "temperamental" (psychologic) components, which not only depend on the nature of morphologic features but also on the nature of predilective activity, corporal or intellectual energy, and vitality.

Tegumental relief

The tegumental cover of this osseous framework, a sensitive barrier between inner impulses and outer aggressions, cannot escape our attention during the accomplishment of our activity and should be evaluated according to the particulars of its tonicity, texture, color, and relief.

Morphopsychology

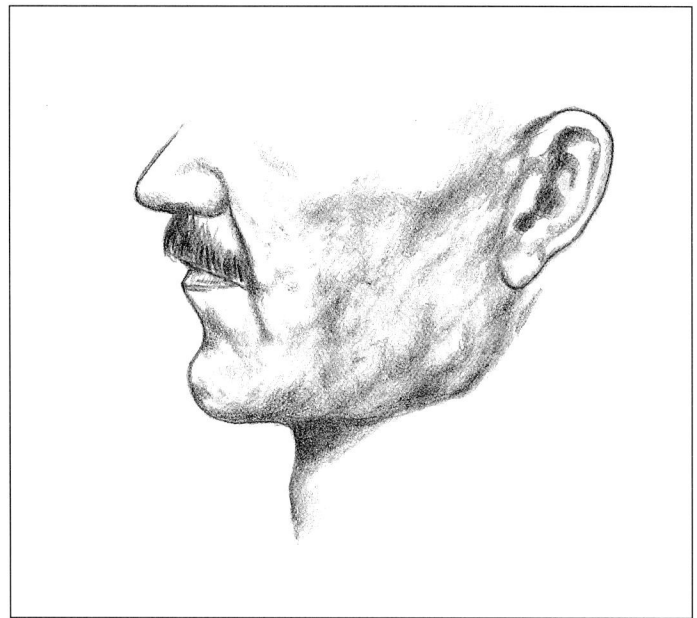

Fig 2-19 Rough skin relief and rough skin structure are easily associated with difficult and irregular character traits.

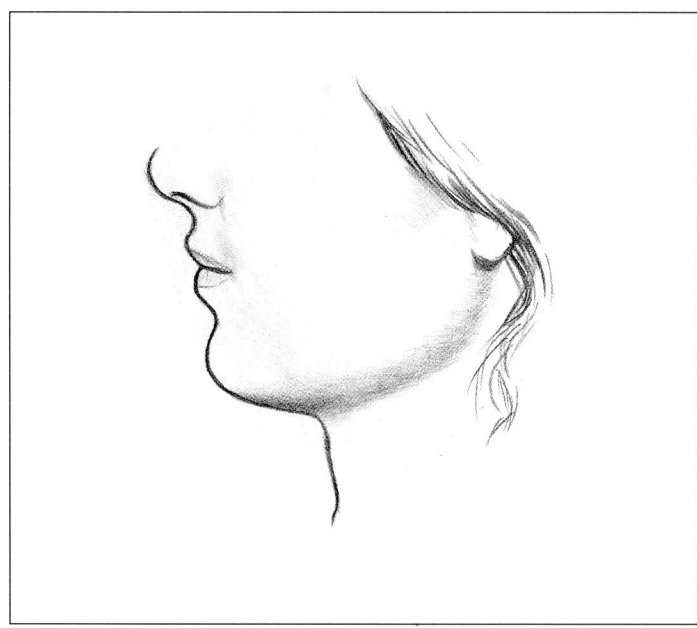

Fig 2-20 Round and undulating skin relief is linked to sweet, charming, and easygoing persons.

While the tonicity may reveal the degree of reactivity, rhythm of action, or state of health of the individual, it constitutes, with the characteristic significance of skin texture and, above all, skin relief, an important and specific means of evaluation (Figs 2-19 and 2-20).

Although one must observe that both tonicity and skin relief may differ from one facial zone to the other, the changes affecting these parameters with the progression of age have long been stated and today constitute an important field of activity of plastic surgeons. The increase of the skin's relief or flaccidity reflecting character hardness or softness is most often evaluated according to its esthetic value by the individual and the individual's milieu. It confirms the links existing between morphopsychologic and esthetic factors, which both must be considered for harmonious integration of any type of reconstruction.

According to the principle of harmony, and even if the literature does not give any credit to the correlation that may exist between skin and tooth texture and relief, one can hardly advocate as a judicious choice the incorporation in a roughly moulded tegumental relief of highly glazed and flat teeth reflecting luminosity. Similarly, teeth showing rippling and stippling, when placed in an environment characterized by the delicacy of skin texture and facial traits, will not be harmoniously integrated.

Hemifaces

The degree of development of the right and left hemifaces should be appreciated not only by reason of the fact that their partition line has an esthetically key function in the perception of the elements of balance and symmetry but also because it will provide information about the differences existing in the brain's dominating action.

The right hemisphere, location of the subconscious heritage and buried past, controlling the development of the left part of the face and body, is confronted with the action of the left hemisphere presiding over the development of the right anatomic part as the result of the constructive impact of the conscious reality (Fig 2-21).

Morphopsychologic interpretation

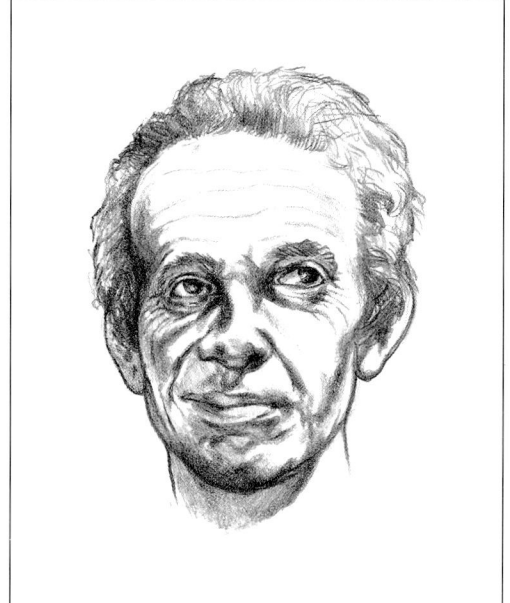

Fig 2-21 Hemifaces. Disparities of the hemifaces not resulting from accidents must be analyzed with respect to their location on the right and left facial hemisphere. The predominant retraction of the middle facial zone affecting this individual underlines the dreadful blow that his sentimental and social activities have suffered despite hereditary factors that would have permitted full realization of his potential.

At this point, one must realize how our therapeutic possibilities, introducing elements of conscious or subconscious needs or compensations, by means of accurately integrated prosthetic devices, reconstructive surgery, or orthodontic corrections that, changing body's image perception, may enhance the reality of the patient's personality.

Morphopsychologic interpretation

The interpretation of the morphopsychologic concept is based on the postulate that there exists a close link and a relationship between the physical morphology and the psychic character, and this infers the following:

1. The more a specific part of the body is developed, the more the tendencies represented by that part of the body become important.
2. There always exists a relationship among the general form of the body, the consistency of the teguments, and the gestures and reactions of an individual. Angular forms and firm teguments are linked to energetic gestures and quick reactions. Rounded forms with softer teguments are associated with sluggish, mild reactions and slow, weak gestures.
3. Two opposite signs do not cancel each other out; they combine and supplement each other or are occasionally effaced and permit nuances in judgment.
4. One single sign has only a relative value. It must be interpreted within the context of the whole.
5. An innate quality always has more influence than an acquired or developed quality.

Guided by the observation of these morphopsychologic laws, it can be stated that the morphopsychologic profile is best interpreted when modulated by the accumulation of available elements of diagnostics.

Whereas a large and solid osseous structure may be associated with strength and slowness of reaction, ra-

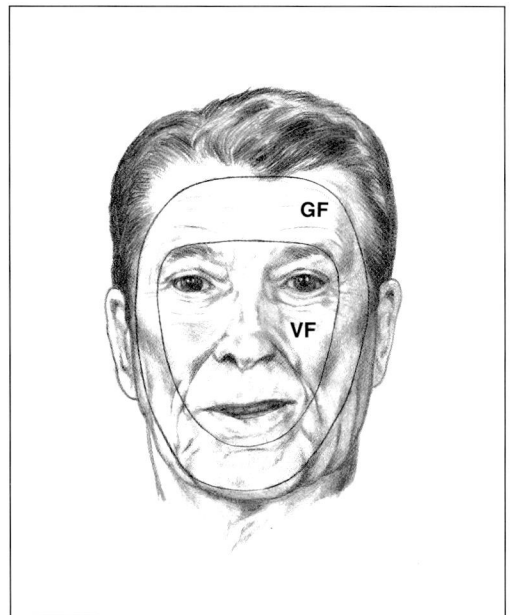 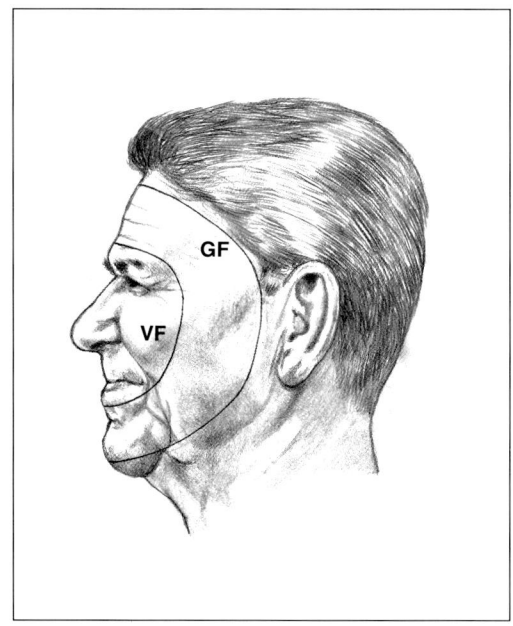

Figs 2-22 and 2-23 *Energetic potential.* The vestibular frame (VF) containing the facial receptors has to be evaluated in relation to the general frame (GF). In this particular case, exhibiting a large osseous framework, receptors seem to increase in importance from eyes to nose and from nose to mouth. This attests to a selective tendency to conserve energy and consequently a selective management of the energetic potential.

pidity and fragility reflect from a narrow and gracile structure. However, this solidity or fragility must be evaluated, considering the relationship that exists between the degree of expansion or retraction of the osseous framework and that of the vestibular frame containing the sensitive receptors, eyes, nose, and mouth, attesting to the real energetic potentials of the individual (Figs 2-22 and 2-23).

These considerations suggest the need for adopting a protocol of morphopsychologic interpretation that, receiving successive refinements by means of appropriate information, will permit the determination of the patient's character and personality, the degree of maturity, and the affective orientation toward oneself or others: *(1)* typologic classification, *(2)* evaluation of facial zones, *(3)* evaluation of their degree and type of expansion, *(4)* analysis of the sensitive receptors, *(5)* analysis of skin texture and relief, and *(6)* determination of the sexual type.

Although this rule of order may greatly help the beginner, one should keep in mind that the basic goal of this determination is the harmonious integration of oral rehabilitation in its morphopsychologic facial frame.

One must also realize that perceptive capabilities, progressively developed by training, can be focused on selective points, using preferential techniques best suited to the professional's individuality.

Affective and sentimental zone

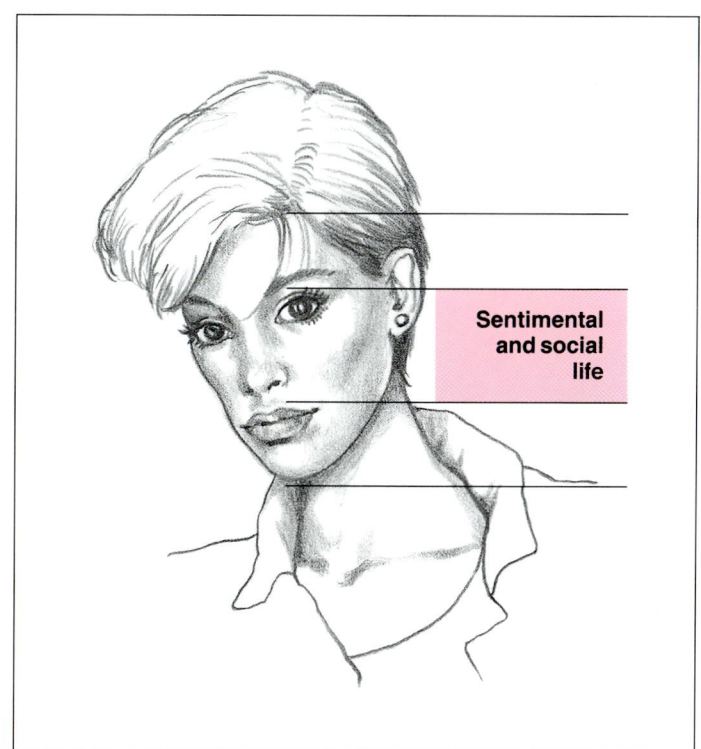

Fig 2-24 The quantitative development of the middle facial zone underlines the predilection type of life activity. It can only be ascertained by proper evaluation of its qualitative value.

Affective and sentimental zone

The median facial zone corresponds to the elective zone, reflecting social and affective activities (Fig 2-24). The quantitative development of this median zone is best evaluated according to the particulars of its receptor. The nose, rather rigid in comparison with the mobility of the other receptors, assures in its verticality the transition between the cerebral and instinctive zone, between eyes and mouth, between thinking and realization. A straight nose line assures an easy connection, whereas a broken, sinuous, or narrow nose line attests the difficulties for actively realizing the movements of ideas and thoughts.

The ridge of the nose that seems to form the extension of the forehead ends up with its tip overhanging the mouth. The distance from nose to mouth suggests the direct relationship existing between social activities and material interest. The further the turned up nose is from the mouth, the less friendship and social contacts are linked to any type of concrete profit. The nose through its dimension assures the individual's involvement in the environment. This penetration illustrates the individual's potential to behave as an actor or an object. This dimensional value, far from affecting social capabilities, attests to an attitude that will induce or favor social contacts, and implies that, in general, persons with big extrovert noses will behave more freely in public and go to others more easily than will those with small noses. One should also consider, according to Corman, the relief of the receptors, characterized by different types of expansion: passive, active, and controlled. In the passive expansion, a plump and soft nose with heavy nostrils is associated with those who are dominated by the passivity of their affective life and the need to receive and be loved. Active expansion, reflecting from individuals ready to respond immediately to events affecting their emotional sensitivities, is characterized by a nose with

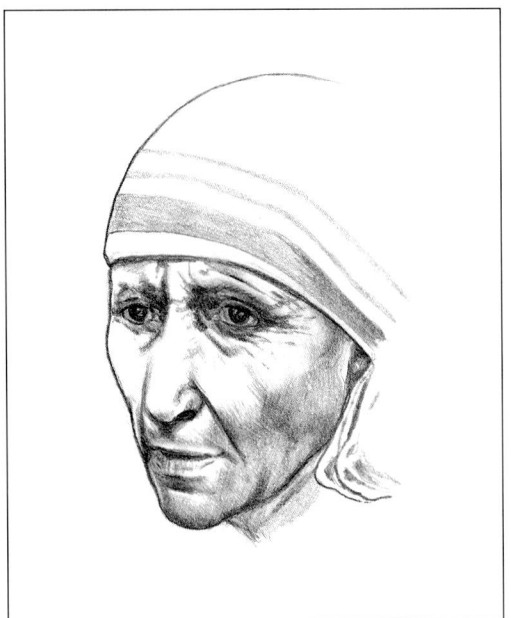

Fig 2-25 Active expansion. The evaluation of the particulars of the nose, a necessary link between thinking and action, brings a qualitative value to the predominant expansion of the middle facial level. Straight, it indicates an absence of barrier between thinking and action. The nostrils are vibrant, slightly closed; social actions are carried out with enthusiasm and obstinacy.

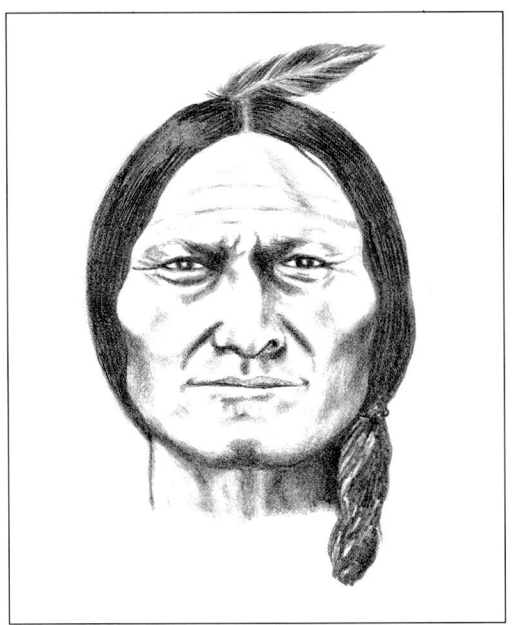

Fig 2-26 Controlled expansion. The development of the middle facial zone takes place both in the vertical and horizontal plane with the lateral projection of the cheekbone. The morphology of the nose suggests a tortuous route from thinking to action. Nostrils that are vibrant and dilated indicate that enthusiastic and demonstrative social actions only take place in specific situations.

rounded relief and thin and vibrating nostrils (Fig 2-25). When the expansion is controlled, the same dynamism in emotional life can be observed but expresses itself only in selective situations and is mastered in others by a cool appearance. The nose's relief is then characterized by more or less rough, undulating movements, nostrils opened or closed, with a lateral projection of the cheekbone (Fig 2-26). In a general sense, a rounded and fleshy ridge of the nose with a soft or delicate tip predisposes to easy and accommodating relationships, which become more difficult with an angulate one.

Cerebral zone

The expansion of the cerebral zone is a characteristic of the human species that can be observed in the young child, constituting the key element of differentiation between humans and animals (Fig 2-27).

In humans the anatomic variations in the development of this zone have contributed to the study of their morphopsychologic significance linked to the following factors: *(1)* expansion type, *(2)* segmental subdivision in three parts, which, like facial divisions, reconstitute a whole by themselves, *(3)* frontal shape, *(4)* frontal inclination, and *(5)* characteristics of its receptors.

In considering the type of expansion marking the pre-

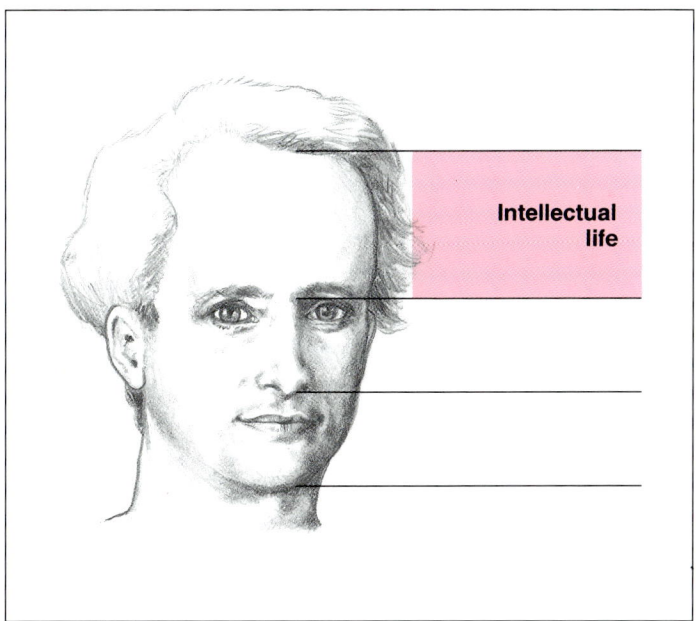

Fig 2-27 Preferential intellectual activities are usually illustrated by the expansion of the upper facial zone. This zone, different from other facial zones, receives information from the ocular receptor situated at a lower facial level.

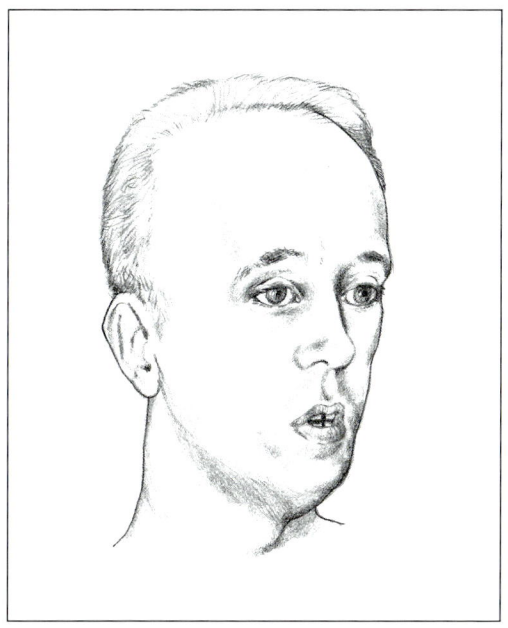

Fig 2-28 This active type is characterized by wide open receptors denoting the important receptive capabilities of a large and round forehead. Provided with a flat transitional zone and a prominent lower level (eyebrows), this type of expansion indicates that what has been received or conceived can be easily adapted to concrete reality.

dominance of the superior zone, cranium, forehead, and ocular receptors, one can observe the passive type, in which the forehead is round with globular and unexpressive eyes. This condition is predominant in the child able to apprehend reality intuitively. When still present in adulthood it distinguishes those who easily assimilate all perceptions without any criticism or analysis.

The active type, which also exhibits a round forehead shape but with a flat transitional zone, gives more strength in this relief. The large eyes show a more intense expression (Fig 2-28). In the active type the important receptive capabilities are linked to a solid adaptation to concrete reality. What has been assimilated can be used or transmitted. When the expansion is controlled, the intelligence level reaches a new step. The individual thinks, calculates, organizes, imagines, and foresees (Fig 2-29).

The forehead is differentiated, and the delimitation of the three zones reflects the scale of intellectual possibilities. Its global shape marks the storage capacities of perceptions and the field of possible application (Figs 2-12 and 2-30 to 2-33). The inferior part of the forehead with its supraorbital prominences is associated with practical and concrete intelligence and indicates a faculty for finding applications for what can be realized with little pure speculation or intellectual abstraction.

The median part of the forehead is a typical zone of exchange between conception and realization and cor-

Morphopsychology

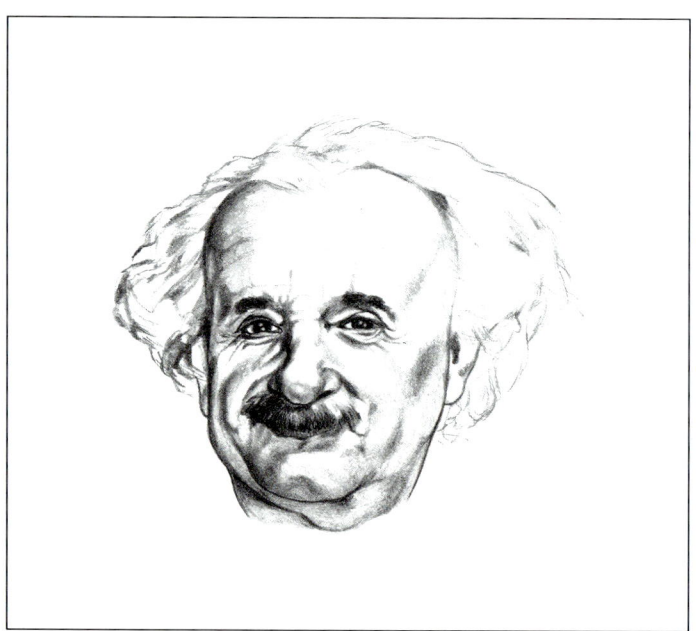

Fig 2-29   In this controlled type, in which the straight forehead exhibits both rounded and flat zones, the intellectual capabilities receiving filtered information from slightly retracted ocular receptors can alternatively evaluate, imagine, conceive, or transmit. Note the retraction of both the middle and lower right hemispheres, indicating a significant reduction of the practical life activities characterizing these zones.

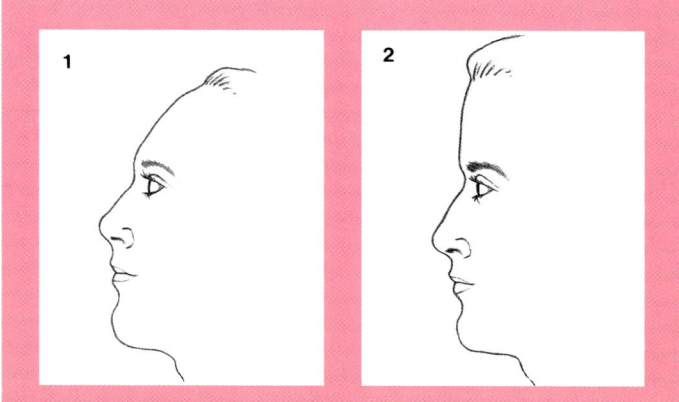

Fig 2-30   A straight or vertical forehead (2) indicates reasoning and carefulness. Action is dictated by thinking rather than by instinct. The rapidity of action and the tendency to take risks are characterized by a proportionate inclination of the forehead (1). In an extreme situation, impulsiveness dictates action and precedes thinking.

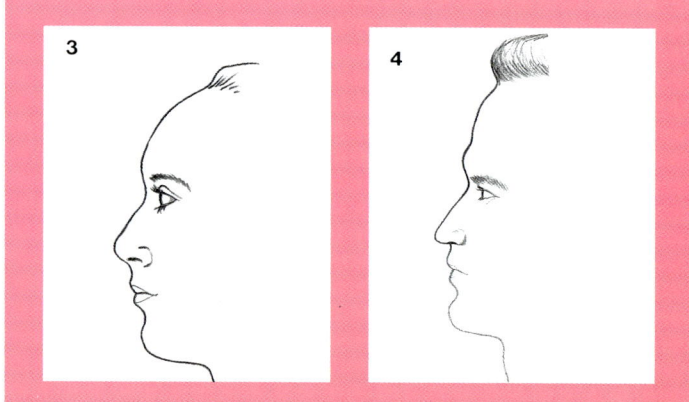

Fig 2-31   A round and convex forehead (3), which is usually observed in young children, reflects juvenescence and ingenuousness. Its persistence in adulthood tends to indicate a suspended maturity. The observation of this type of forehead on a number of painters (see Fig 2-15) or philosophers may indicate a "cosmic" type of intellectual receptivity common to those who create and work in abstractions. Maturity and reflection characterize a flat forehead. The horizontal brow may indicate difficulties in concretizing thoughts (4).

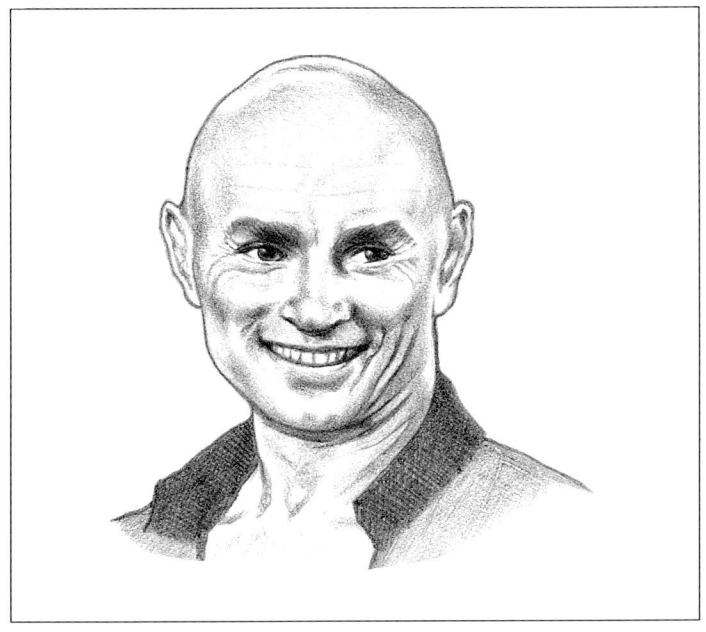 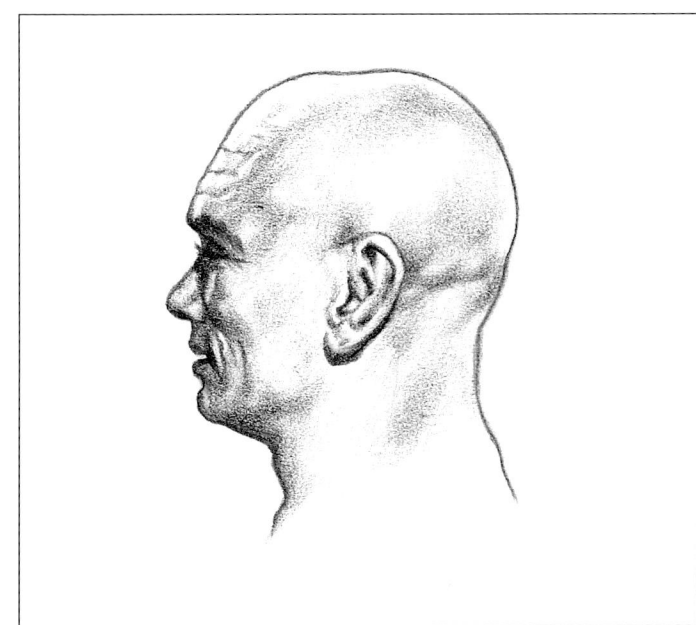

Figs 2-32 and 2-33 The upper level of the forehead corresponds to the intellectual capabilities of imagination, conception, synthesis, and abstraction. The widening of this zone, where two lateral round protuberances may be felt, evidences intellectual qualities of imagination and abstraction. The lower level, close to the eyes and to the vision of concrete realities, is linked to practical, technical, and manual intelligence. Its development, illustrated by the projection of the supraorbital relief, underlines faculties of concentration and realization. The middle level is characterized by a slight depression separating conception from realization. Its profile tends to facilitate or obstruct exchanges between these zones.

responds to the possibilities of adaptation through thinking. Often flat or depressed, its relief indicates whether these exchanges are inhibited or favored.

The upper part, always more extended than the two others, corresponds to the intellectual functions of abstraction, imagination, and conception and represents the part of the child's forehead still persisting in the adult. Thus, the elementary pictorial way of thinking, the cosmic communication by way of the subconscious, when still present in the adult, has been suggested by many to be at the origin of artistic creative power, thus illustrating the link that may exist between essential beauty and the individual's interpretation.

Considering the three cerebral zones, the importance of the notion of harmony present in the controlled expansion type readily becomes apparent. When equilibrium is realized, intelligence, both logical and intuitive, is capable of concrete and abstract thinking. This equilibrium, however, should be ascertained by the degree of inclination of the forehead. This would indicate whether reason or impulsiveness dictates action. Finally, the proportionate relationship existing between the forehead and ocular receptors will assure the conditions necessary to this equilibrium.

The eyes, in providing abundant information necessary for the development of cerebral functions, are by

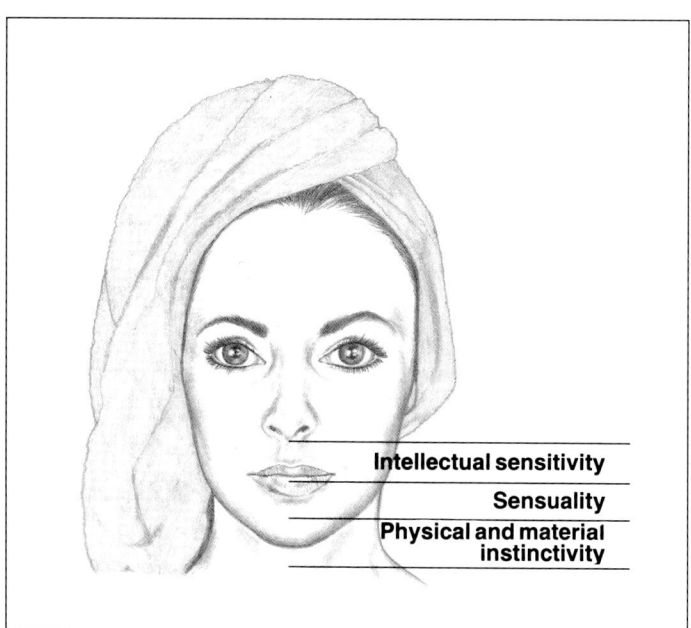

Fig 2-34 Knowledge of the morphopsychologic significance of the different levels of the lower facial zone is extremely important, considering the direct influence exerted on this zone, both by pathologies and by therapeutic measures.

reason of facts closely associated with the cerebral zone, serving as a joint line to the facial affective zone, with which they are automatically integrated. Vision is, above all, a cerebral sense, and the eyes must be appraised depending on their size, measure of the quantity of exchanges, their tonicity, their reflection of intellectual reactivity, and their degree of retraction, an indication of depth of thinking and protective needs regarding exterior ideas and judgments. The importance of the cerebral zone in comparison with the others that are subordinate to it is best comprehended when a state of equilibrium is realized among thinking, feeling, and instinct. Conversely, the relative retraction of the lower facial zones or the overdevelopment of the upper area creates a situation in which intellectual activity, deprived of the weight of the affective and instinctive life, is restricted to abstractions, ideologies, or fantasies, for want of concrete possibilities of achievement. Cut off from its roots, it loses the advantages of its position and no longer deserves the nobleness attributed to it.

Instinctive and physical zone

The morphopsychologic study of the median and upper zones in combination with that of the instinctive or physical zone will provide a number of factors for assessing a patient's personality and permit the evaluation of motivations and the profound reasons of his or her demands. At the same time, it will serve as a training aid for esthetic perception, a necessary condition for esthetic appraisal, which quickly becomes more acute when dealing with the lower facial zone. It has been observed to be electively affected by the impacts of life and materializes the effects of oral pathologies and prosthetic devices that may disturb its equilibrium.

The subdivision in three parts of this instinctive zone (Fig 2-34), which occupies the space from the subnasal point to the tip of the chin, is naturally a part of the elements of morphopsychologic evaluation that should not be obscured by pathologies. Therefore, the coordinated restoration of the importance of this zone, the morphopsychologic significance that reflects from it, and its harmonious integration in the overall facial structure are requirements for the success of rehabilitation.

Instinctive and physical zone

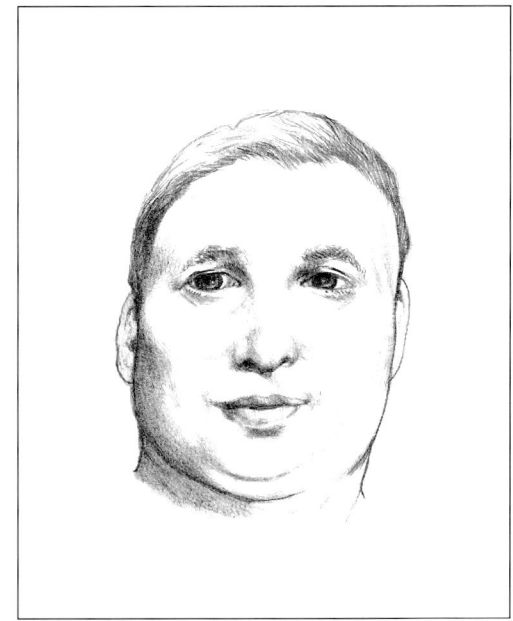

Fig 2-35 The elective expansion of this lower facial zone reflects the acquisition instinct that one expects from this type of expansion, but at the same time a total absence of will of concretization. The expansion, stressed by the tegumental relief, is said to be passive, and the instinctive capabilities are restricted to nutritional and sensual pleasures.

The instinctive zone will be successively evaluated according to the importance of its subdivisions, its kind and degree of expansion, and, finally, the particulars of its receptor, the mouth, which will be the focus of our attention.

The **superior lip area** represents the sensitive part of the instinctive zone. An increase of its length and volume reflects the moderating influence of the intellect on the material life, whereas its dimensional reduction attests to a lack of intellectual control, inducing rapidity of action.

The philtrum, a natural connecting path between sentimental impulses and physical life, reflects the capacity for converting feelings into dynamic action. A narrow pathway indicates reserve toward the achievement of affective impulses, whereas a wide philtrum indicates the absence of a barrier between feelings and their active expressions.

The **middle part** includes the lower lip to the labiomental groove, transitional zone between the reasoned materiality and its most instinctive form, and gives a sensual and concrete mirror image of the realization of the social and affective life.

The **lower part** includes the chin and jaw, which are characteristics of the intensity of the material and physical life of the individual, focusing on the ability to realize ambitions and impulses and illustrating the potential capabilities.

When the lower facial zone presents an elective expansion relative to the others, one must identify three types of expansional designs:

1. Passive, in which the individual exhibits a round and soft lower facial relief, an absence of mandibular angle, and thick and fleshy lips, with a mouth most often maintained in a slightly opened position. This indicates the prevalence of the nutritional and sexual instinct in the form of passive pleasures (Fig 2-35).

2. Active, in which the same round relief appears, but with tighter, lightly colored cheeks and a marked lip tonicity. The nutritional and sexual instinct are still present here but result from a desire for and an active search for quality. At the same time, an instinct for material acquisitiveness begins to be perceived (Fig 2-36).

Morphopsychology

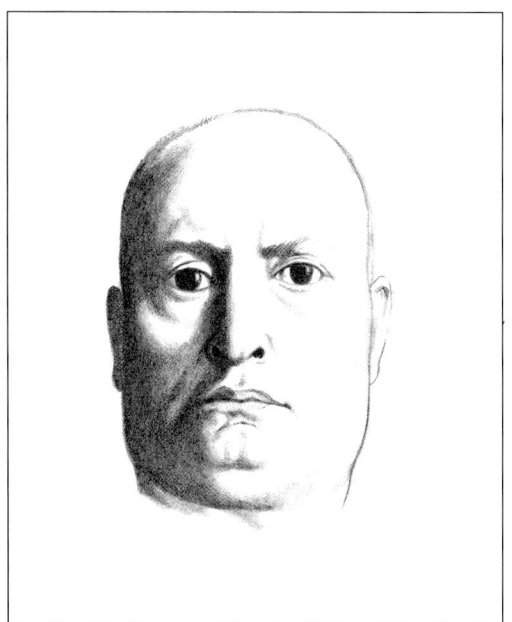

Fig 2-36 As a first impression, only a tighter nature of the tegumental relief differentiates this type of expansion from the preceding one. Closer observation evidences the projection of the chin and a will of realization stressed by the straight nasal anatomy, indicating an immediate materialization of the movements of thoughts. Note the differences in the expansion of the upper cerebral zone and the retraction of the right affective zone.

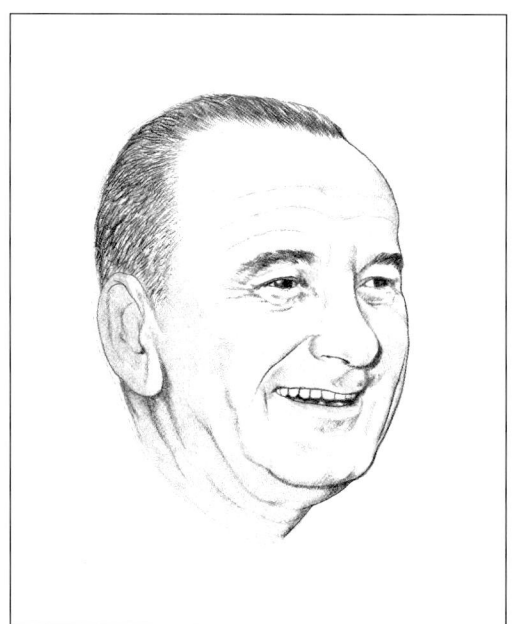

Fig 2-37 When osseous structures and tegumental cover exhibit angles and flat areas, the expansion of the lower facial zone is said to be controlled. This type of expansion is usually found in politicians, businessmen, and persons oriented to concrete action, stressing energy to realize objectives. The means to achieve these goals are differentiated and appear in the analysis of the particulars of the other facial zones and receptors.

3. Controlled, in which the relief loses its roundness, becomes roughly undulating, and lips become thinner. The need of material acquisitiveness is best realized in the controlled type, and, whatever the degree of environmental stimulation, physical activities become a necessity (Fig 2-37).

Elective expansion does not restrict itself to the expansion of one facial zone leaving the others in retraction but may involve two different facial zones. In my practice, I noted with amazement that a large number of my patients, predominantly men, presented a cerebroinstinctive type of expansion, a characteristic of qualities and preferential life activities that can best express themselves in today's society (Fig 2-38). One can observe that these traits are usually a characteristic of politicians and business people. This is not restricted to men because it can be found in a number of women, certifying their capacities for adaptation to the changes in social status that have marked these last decades; at the same time, they have maintained their femininity. The laws of adaptation to environmental conditions may favor at any given moment selective facial development. The perception of a patient's personality is a basic

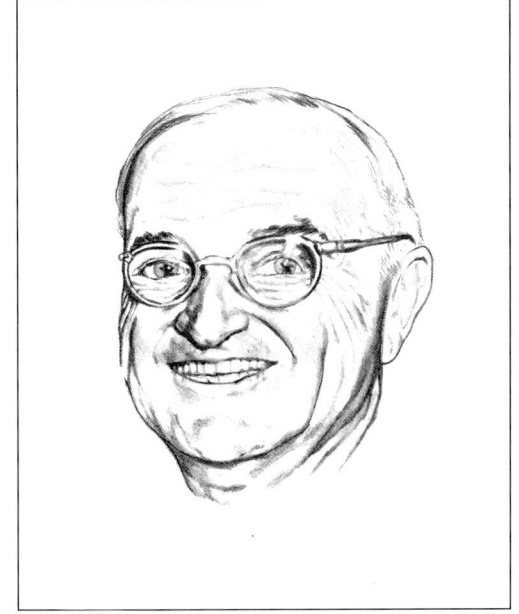

Fig 2-38 Expansion is not limited to one facial zone. Life activities can generate a double expansion, the characteristics of which can modify and alter the morphopsychologic profile. In this double-controlled expansion of upper and lower facial zones, instinctive strength linked to concrete realization is somewhat softened by the lateral development of the upper cerebral level location of imagination and abstractions, far from concrete reality.

professional requirement enabling, in all respects, a selective and individual approach easing relationships and saving time and disappointments. Considering the four basic Hippocratic types, an author, whose name remains anonymous, made this pertinent statement: "One has influence on the Bilious by firmness, on the Nervous by reasoning, on the Sanguine by feelings and on the Lymphatic by gentleness." Based on this viewpoint, the morphopsychologic science already deserves consideration, but in regard to its esthetic value it reaches another level of interest.

Morphopsychologic equilibrium reflecting individuals' impulses and potentialities is always linked to some kind of esthetic harmony. This morphopsychologic equilibrium, sometimes more difficult and subtle to analyze when it is achieved by the elective expansion of determined facial zones or sensitive receptors, is always based on the presence of the principle of dominance, a prerequisite for unity in a composition. When other esthetic principles (basically that of proportions) strongly mark facial features, the level of harmony is enhanced.

Individual desires to conform to a higher level of facial or dentofacial harmony explain the needs for esthetic improvement. This improvement can only be achieved in the respect of morphopsychologic equilibrium and esthetic harmony. Being a global concept, esthetics cannot be restricted to the oral cavity. It requires the harmonious relationship of all elements between them and between each of them related to the whole.

Mouth and lips

The study of the morphopsychologic significance of the particulars of the dentofacial composition takes a particular importance as it pertains (according to the morphopsychologic concept) to a concentrate of sensitive, affective, and instinctive expressions of life activities. By definition, a receptor is an organ assuming exchanges with the exterior. It takes with the mouth its full significance, permitting not only the intake of food, along with its gustatory appreciation, but the exteriorization of sounds, words, and mimics of expression. A definition of its anatomic design as large or small, thick or thin, does not express any valuable indication by itself, and all

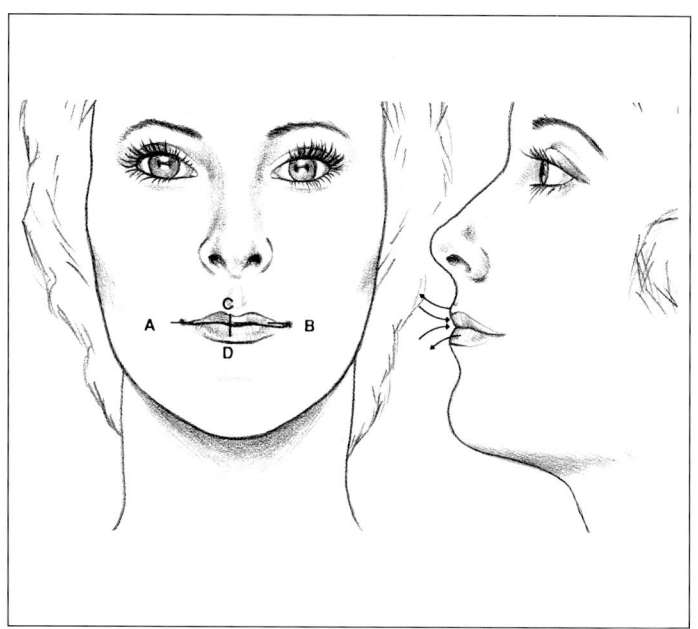

Fig 2-39 Lips, the dimensions of which conform to the mathematical formula AB = CD/4, embody an indisputable harmonious design, easing their integration into overall facial composition. The ideal would be achieved if the latter exhibited a perfect morphopsychologic equilibrium of body–feeling–soul. The morphopsychologic concept has described the lips and mouth as miniaturized elements submitted to the movements of dilatation and retraction exerted by life activities. The projection or the retraction of the dentofacial composition results from the forces exerted by the action of opposing muscles, expressing the modulation of sensitivity and sentimentality, desires and frustrations.

things considered, only the characteristic design of its normality constitutes both an esthetic ideal and a morphopsychologic feature of equilibrium (Fig 2-39).

A receptor in its size and width is proportionate to the amplitude of its exchanges with the exterior, so that a large mouth pertains to the quantitative particulars of the babbling, voracious, and impetuous, whereas its thickness testifies to capacities of apprehension or preservation of what has been received. A fleshy, thick mouth reveals large receptive potential, which, while still existing in an increase of its tonicity, introduces a perceptive element of possession and materiality. The tonic and thin lips of politicians and businessmen, which are used to keep hidden occult or secret abilities, often reflect the refusal of earthly pleasures compensated for by the need for inner cerebral satisfaction.

The laws of retraction and dilatation, both passive and active, can naturally be applied because they constitute pertinent elements of evaluation, best illustrated by means of pictures and drawings (Figs 2-40 to 2-45).

The prosthodontist must focus attention on the nature of tooth arrangement and on the type of vertical or horizontal overjet supports that are capable of restoring the original lip design—a basic requirement to ascertain a harmonious facial relationship. The design of the dentofacial composition escapes to a game of chance but results from the impulses of life manifesting themselves in a variety of muscular movements, inducing the retraction or projection of the lip-to-lip support structures. The restoration of a dental composition of a single tooth implies the simultaneous restoration or improvement of the original dentofacial composition in conformity to the morphopsychologic profile of the individual, a prerequisite to reach esthetic harmony.

Mouth and lips

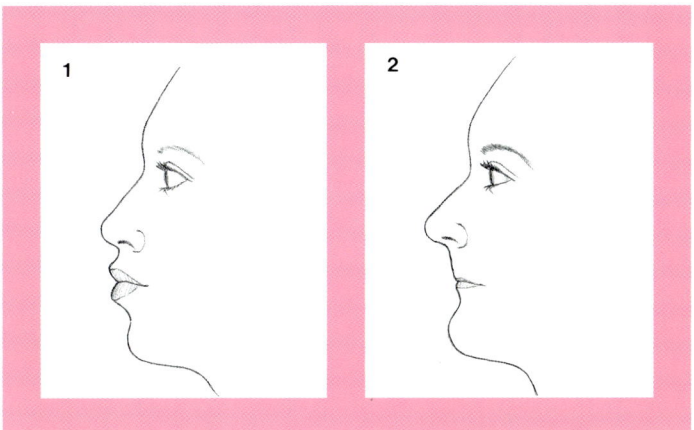

Fig 2-40 A protrusive mouth indicates strong ambition and attempts to dominate others *(1)*. A retracted mouth suggests a lack of ambition and dominance by behavioral rules *(2)*.

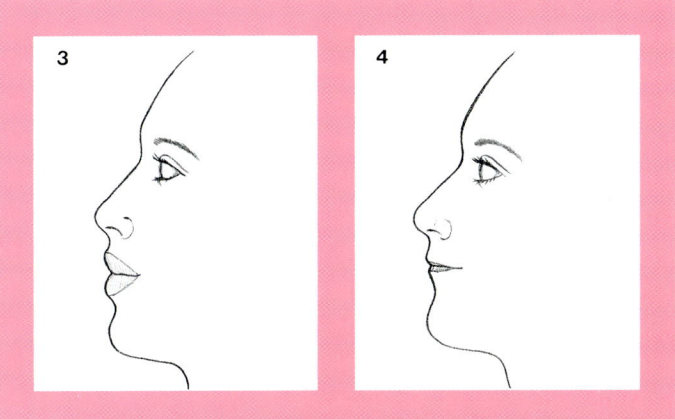

Fig 2-41 Exteriorization, subjectivity, and sometimes materialism characterize thick lips *(3)*. Interiorization, objectivity, and self-control are reflected by thin lips *(4)*.

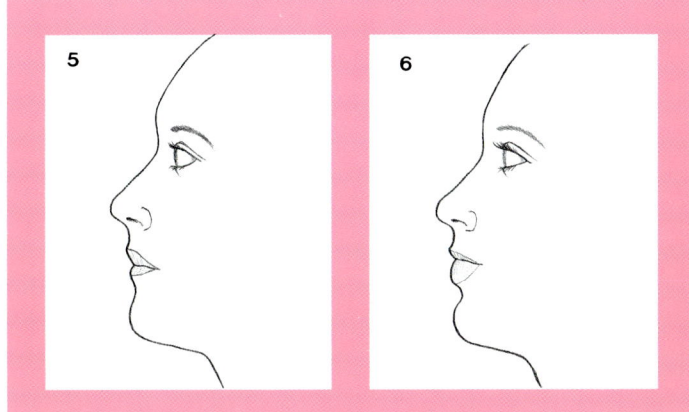

Fig 2-42 A stronger upper lip underlines ambition, goodness, and courage *(5)*. A stronger lower lip evidences ingenuousness and sensuality *(6)*.

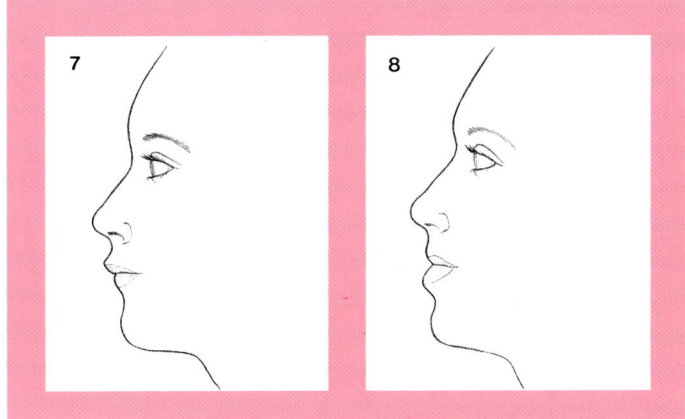

Fig 2-43 A protrusive upper lip is linked to ambition, dominating instinct, and scruples *(7)*. A protruding lower lip cannot hide disdain, obstinacy, or pride *(8)*.

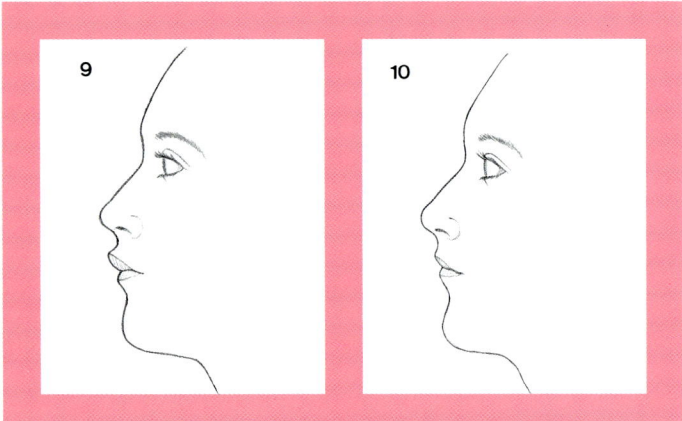

Fig 2-44 A raised upper lip cannot resist temptation *(9)*. Depressed upper lips are linked to behavioral rules *(10)*.

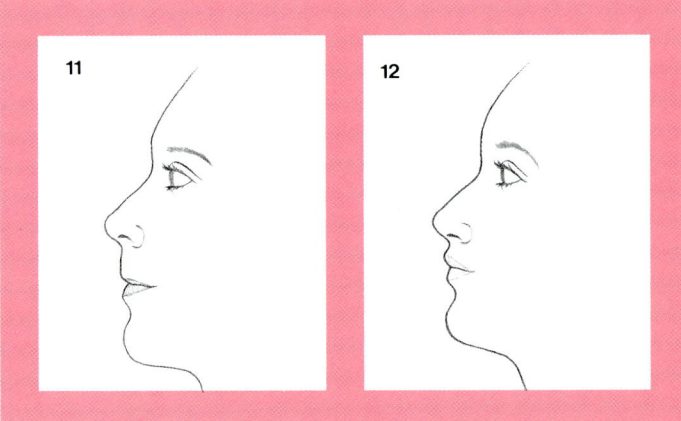

Fig 2-45 A long nasolabial space indicates caution and introspection *(11)*. A short nasolabial space reflects impulsiveness, enthusiasm, and spontaneity *(12)*.

References

Band F. Physionomie et caractère. Que sais-je? *PUF Coll.* 1947.
Binet C. In Graucher J, ed. *L'ABC de la Morphopsychologie.* 1988.
Buffard L. *Morphopsychologie, Cours de base.* Paris: Institut Français de Culture Humaine; 1982.
Buffard L. *Morphopsychologie, Cours supérieur.* Paris: Institut Français de Culture Humaine; 1982.
Carton P. In Maloine SA, ed. *Diagnostic et Conduite des Tempéraments.* Paris; 1926.
Corman L. *Nouveau Manuel de Morpho-psychologie.* Paris: Stock Plus; 1981.
Fouche S. Hommes qui êtes-vous? Essai de Morphopsychologie. *Revue des Jeunes.* 1945.
Gastin L. In Dangles, ed. *Eléments de Psychodiagnostic.* 1948.
Georges O. In Vigot, ed. *Morphologie et types humains.* 1961.
Hippocrates. *Le Corpus Hyppocratum.* Littré; 1839–1861.
Lejoyeux J. In Maloine SA, ed. *Prothèse complète.* Paris; 1979.
Lidis ed. *Vocabulaire de la Psychologie.* L'Univers de la Psychologie; 1980.
Mosher HD. The expression of the face and man's type of body as indicators of his character. *Laryngoscope.* 1951;61:1.
Mucchielli R. Caractères et visages. *PUF Coll.* 1954.
Rollet F. In Carrere, ed. *Guide pratique de Morphopsychologie.* 1987.
Sillamy N. *Dictionnaire de Psychologie: Définition.* Paris: Bordas; 1980.
Viaud G. Les instincts. *PUF Coll.* 1959.

Chapter 3

Morphopsychology and Esthetics

Claude R. Rufenacht

The evaluation of human beauty

No apparent characteristic difference exists in the esthetic appearance of the various morphologic types. Beauty is not limited to either sanguines or lymphatics, relegating the others to ugliness. The perception of beauty in the various types depends upon racial, ethnic, civilization, and individual factors. Generation, vogue, and fashion factors may contribute to actualize and favor, at any given moment, the esthetic preference for a specific directional expansion of a facial zone, but beauty basically depends upon the harmonious integration of the esthetic principles described earlier, and it is greatly influenced by the importance of psychologic factors that (radiating from individuals) may enhance or affect esthetic appearance.

"Aucune grâce extérieure n'est complète si la beauté intérieure ne la vivifie. La beauté de l'âme se répand comme une lumière mystérieuse sur la beauté du corps." (Victor Hugo)

"Physical beauty is incomplete without the animation provided by interior beauty. Like an occult light, the beauty of the soul infuses bodily beauty."

Everyone has a mental picture of his or her own appearance in space, and this self-image directly depends on a multitude of factors that influence the intellect. Magazines, media, ethnic habits, racial factors, and environment develop standards of beauty to which any individual tends to conform. In our highly conditioned Western society a considerable effort can be observed for the maintenance or perfection of appearance and well-being in adopting a personal philosophy of life where physical and psychologic factors should bring a certain equilibrium. Any individual is a collection of dynamism, and the importance that the individual gives consciously or unconsciously to the perception of esthetic problems and self-image depends on the strength of those dynamic forces and the field of interest to which they are directed. Beauty, in which utility and pleasure have been philosophically integrated as additional values, is at the center of all human aspirations. Self-satisfaction without vanity that invariably reflects on an individual's facial appearance appears as the consequence of efforts to achieve and realize goals and as the result of a favorable psychologic reaction induced by body and self-image perception (Figs 3-1 to 3-4).

The body image concept may develop progressively in young children under the protective environment of the family. Handicaps or disfigurement may take place abruptly during school years. This traumatic experience will induce a variety of character changes. An impaired self-image may be more disabling from a developmental aspect than the patient's real physical defect. The impact of facial image that cannot escape self-esthetic evaluation, through an abundance of existing comparative elements, may generate negative self-images. The more attention is focused on a particular area, the more people tend to acquire a negative self-image relative to this area. In general, the clinician is not aware of the degree of perception of dentofacial disfigurements by the patient. Its restoration in terms of its potential benefit to mental health may be underestimated. These are the reasons why it appears illusory to undertake any dentofacial restoration, no matter how "artistic" or technical it would be if we are not able to understand and interpret the reality expressed by a countenance and the form of personality manifested. A sanguine, sociable, and out-

Morphopsychology and Esthetics

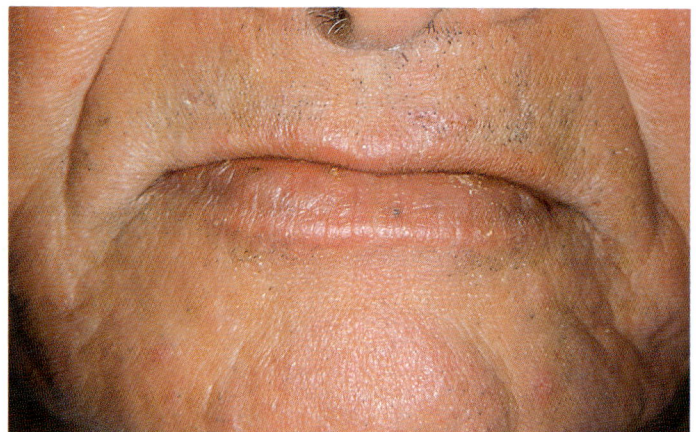

Fig 3-1 Excessive tooth wear, combined with changes affecting muscle and tegumental maintenance, have resulted in this clinical situation, illustrated by the depression of the corners of the mouth and the effacement of the upper lip.

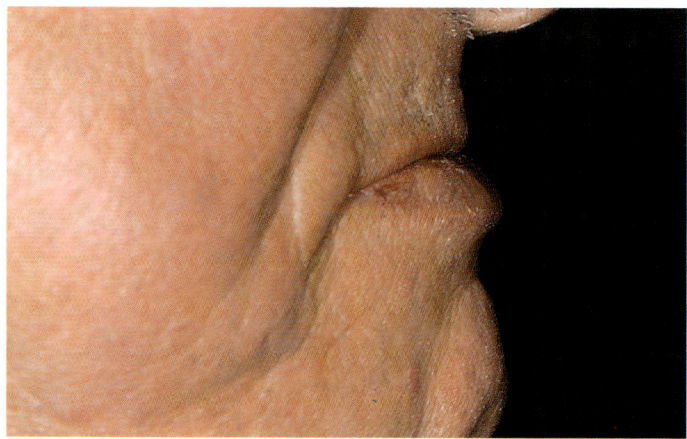

Fig 3-2 A pronounced and unesthetic nasolabial ridge surrounded by deep labial and nasolabial grooves and an unusual extension of the mentolabial groove strengthen this image of facial deterioration.

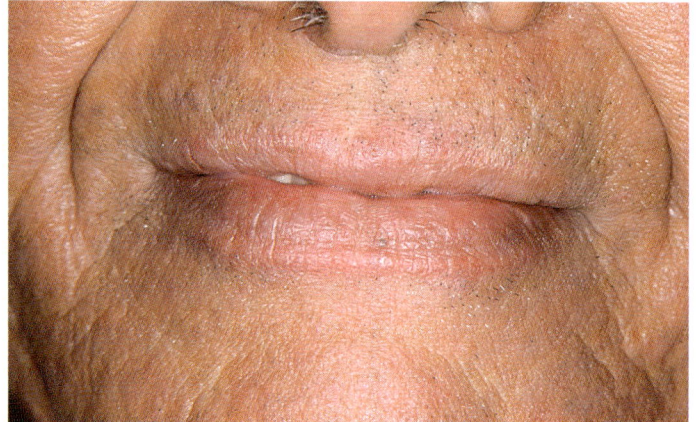

Fig 3-3 The restoration of original lip design and the restoration of the position of the corners of the mouth in the vertical plane have to be expected following oral rehabilitation.

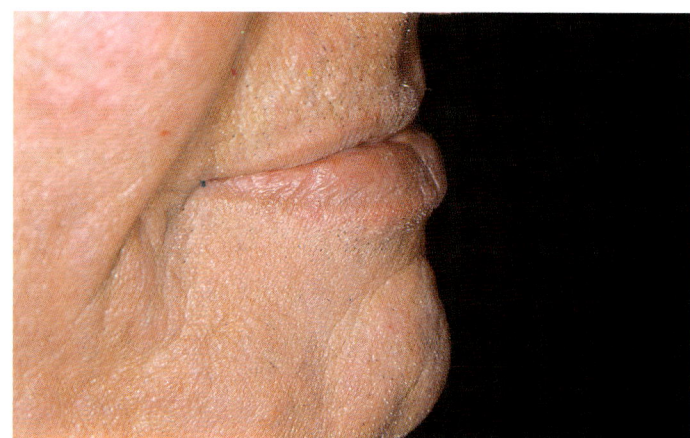

Fig 3-4 The simultaneous effacement of facial traits resulting from oral pathologies has to be achieved. Note the effacement of the nasolabial ridge and that of the labial groove. The nasolabial groove remains unaffected by intraoral therapeutic measures.

The evaluation of human beauty

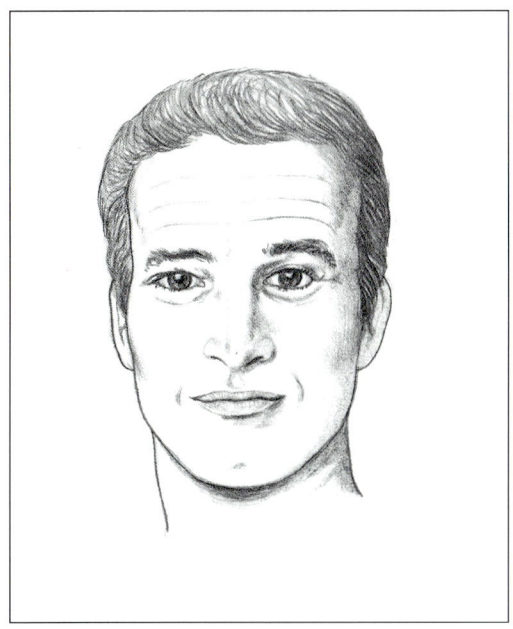

Fig 3-5 Sketch of an individual in his 30s exhibiting well-maintained facial traits, with a marked expansion of the lower third of the face, reflecting a capacity for physical activities.

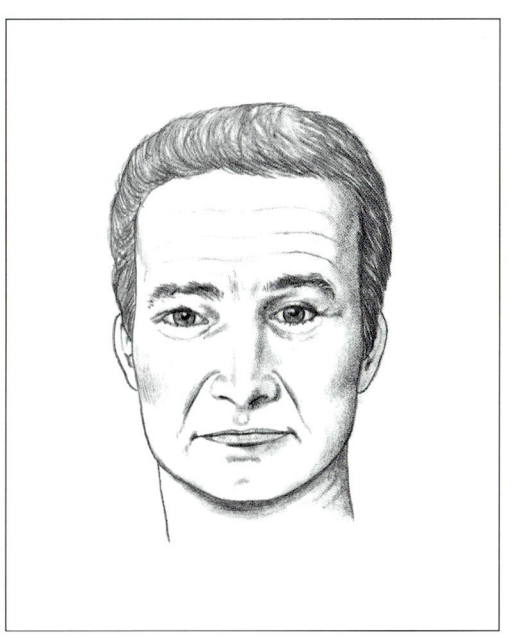

Fig 3-6 The same individual in his early 50s showing a decrease of the lower facial zone with pronounced facial traits, manifestations of oral pathologies, which alter the evaluation of his morphopsychologic profile.

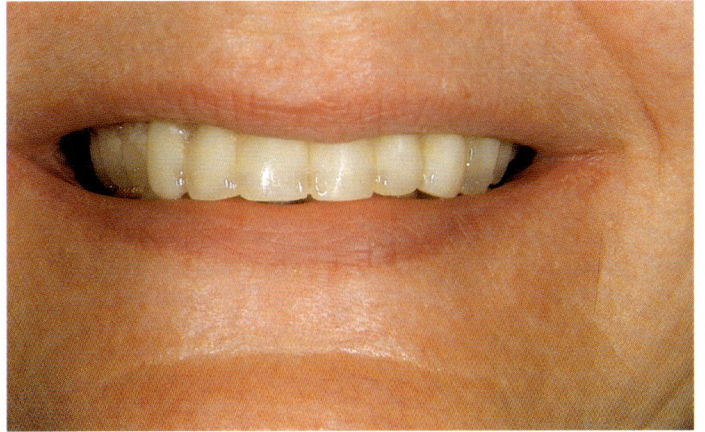

Fig 3-7 In a large number of individuals the physical appearance reflects neither the true age nor personality.

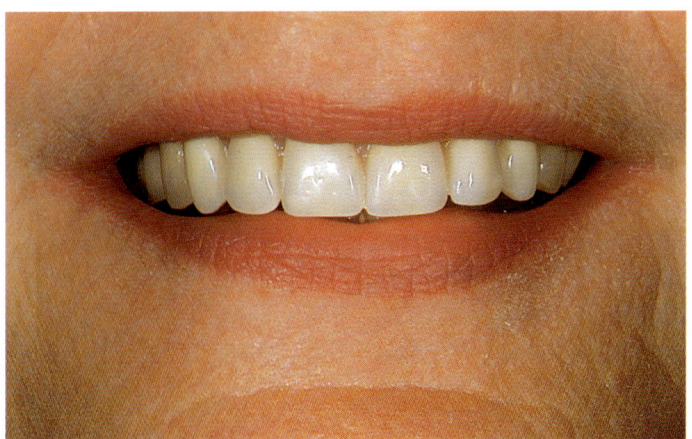

Fig 3-8 Adequate oral rehabilitation has a direct impact on the restoration of physical and psychic radiance.

Morphopsychology and Esthetics

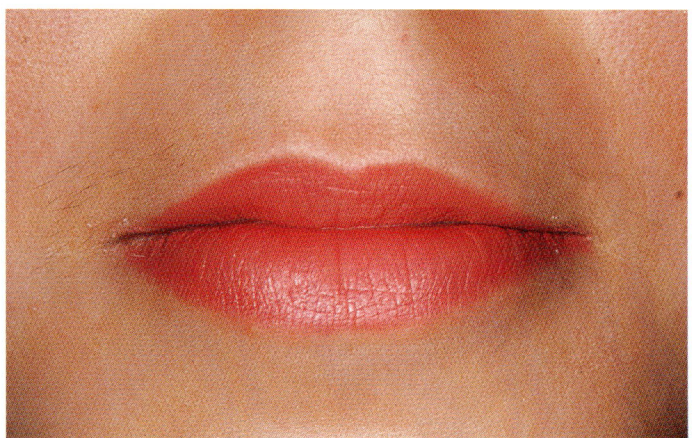

Fig 3-9 Esthetic dentistry is a multidisciplinary science, incorporating the key elements required to retard a number of manifestations of the programmed and accidental aging affecting the lower facial zone.

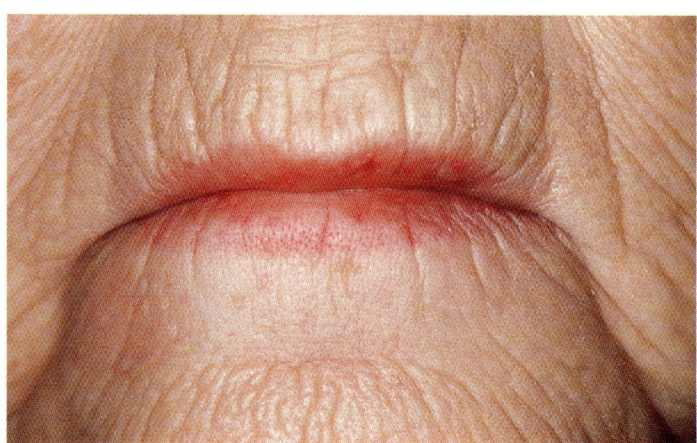

Fig 3-10 Medical care, life-style, and individual factors have contributed to this uncontrolled advancement of biologic aging. However, the major corrective factors remain in the appropriate oral restorative and maintenance measures.

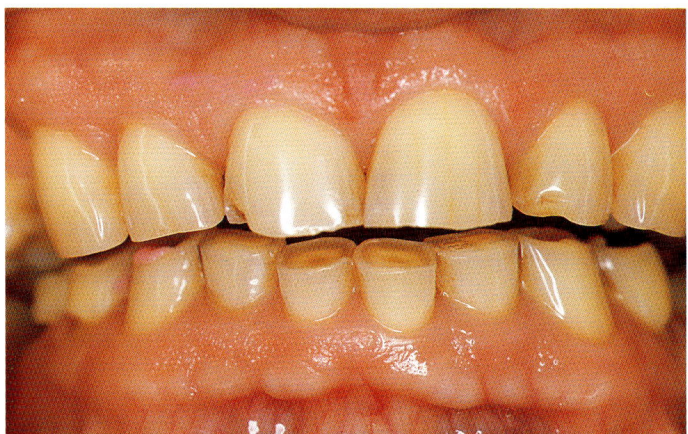

Fig 3-11 For modern humans tooth wear is not linked to the progression of age but to functional disturbances.

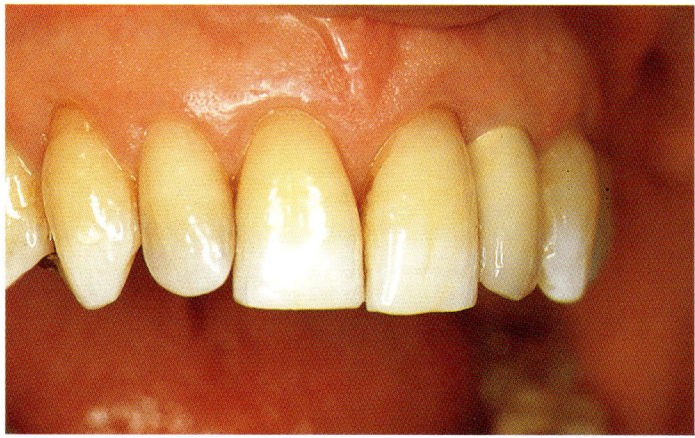

Fig 3-12 An individual in his 60s with normal anterior tooth length, indicating a vertical path of occlusion.

going individual who would be deprived of a smile by a dental composition not adapted to the psychologic profile, or a withdrawn, timid individual to whom a sparkling smile would be given, would not be models of harmonious facial composition. Such an imbalance would be perceived by the person's entourage and, above all, by the person. In turn, this could produce a profound influence on the person's psyche.

The facial map (and with it the mouth) undergoes progressive and various morphologic changes during a lifetime, indicating an individual's reactions to life events and character maturity. Clinical practice widely demonstrates that the influence of oral pathologies not only accelerates but deeply accentuates these morphologic changes, causing erroneous morphopsychologic and esthetic perception (Figs 3-5 and 3-6). This suggests our professional implication in the restoration of a facial appearance, reflecting both esthetic harmony and morphopsychologic equilibrium in conformity with the patient's needs and desires. In effacing the negative impacts of life that affect body image perception, physical and psychic radiance will be naturally restored (Figs 3-7 and 3-8).

Youth factor

Until the latter part of the nineteenth century, people were considered adults while they were teenagers, and the further back in history one looks, the earlier people were considered to be old. Over this last century, the human life span has been considerably lengthened, and in today's society, life extension is almost automatic as a result of our higher level of nutrition and medical care. As life lengthens, the period of time called youth should also be extended. In parallel, the desire to prolong youth becomes a universal preoccupation.

As a medical practice, youth extension is in its infancy, but in studying the medical aspects of cosmetic surgery, diet, exercise, and medical revitalization, it comes immediately to mind that youth extension is not only possible and practical but also available. This may sound revolutionary if we consider, as do most Western physicians, that the loss of youth is inevitable. In considering aging as a disease, careful attention must be paid so that the therapeutic approach relies on a sound medical and scientific background rather than on mysterious formula or magic drugs. During youth our body seems to be in a state of equilibrium in which the process of the replacement of cells takes place. Insidiously, with time this process slows down as the result of a programmed aging process. Trauma, stress, and diseases act as "accidental" aging and add to this degradation (Figs 3-9 and 3-10).

Although medical science has focused its attention on the determination and treatment modalities of "accidental" diseases with a large range of success, programmed aging is more frightening to consider, both philosophically and practically. Despite the accumulation of theories, the exact process that takes place in this phenomenon is not known. In the balance of negative and positive sensitivities that result from the accumulation of events marking the development of life, the time period called youth arouses the most pleasing memories, usually enhanced by a touch of nostalgia.

"Il n'existe qu'une jeunesse et l'on passe le reste de ses jours à la regretter." (Robert Brasillach)
"In life only one youth exists and we pass the rest of our days regretting it."

The association of youth with the privileges inherent in physical integrity and the plenitude of esthetic appearance are the forces that call for its maintenance, extension, or restoration.

Its loss, abruptly brought to the level of consciousness by means of accidental events, may engender a traumatic psychologic result.

"Il est des hommes qui mènent un tel deuil de la perte de leur jeunesse que leur amabilité n'y survit pas." (Sainte Beuve)
"There are men who so mourn their loss of youth that their good humor does not survive."

We know that different people age at different rates. In considering the number of people who, at an advanced age, still have a dentition characterized by its young appearance and an absence of wear, we are convinced that in dentistry most of the parameters that will allow us to keep the ineluctability of the programmed aging within normal bonds will soon be available (Figs 3-11 and 3-12). It can be stated that, based on the progress in the science of occlusion, temporomandibular joint disorders, restorative dentistry, and dental hygiene, the average patient can now be provided with real chances of maintenance. In adopting a protocol of treatment that implies the restoration of health and func-

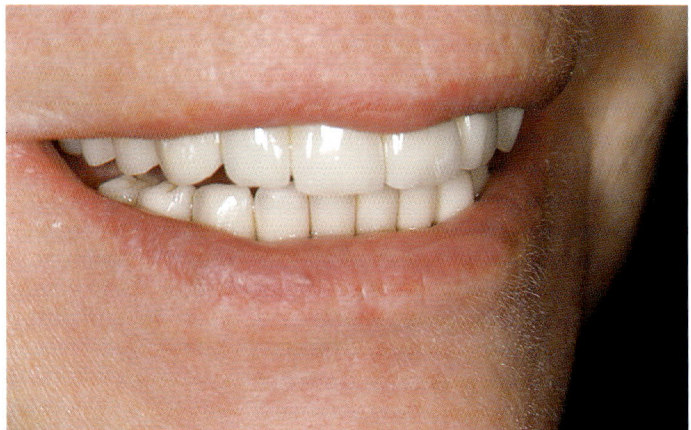

Fig 3-13 An individual in her 80s provided 20 years earlier with full mouth rehabilitation, respecting a normal anatomic design and a vertical functional pathway.

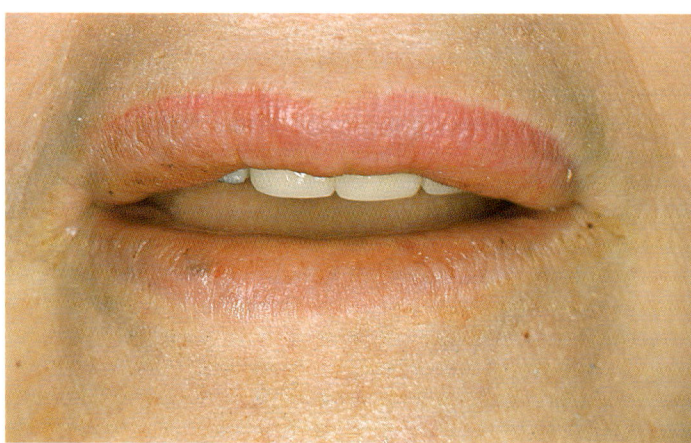

Fig 3-14 This individual, in her 90s, with well-maintained dentition, still exhibits anterior teeth by slight mouth opening. This results from daily training for the maintenance of facial muscle tonicity.

tion along with the restoration of the original natural structural beauty of the oral components, we will provide our patient with a prosthesis simulating a natural and rejuvenated dentofacial and facial composition (see Figs 3-7 and 3-8). One must, unfortunately, state that even today the profession, and with it the whole dental industry, still admits as inevitable and systematically mimics the dental particularities of programmed aging, ignoring the evolution of our life standard and our search for well-being and esthetics. We know that the overall dentofacial composition should present a harmonious psychologic dominance factor and reflect the personality of the patient. If the dominance factor is age, we have failed in our mission to fulfill our patient's most secret expectations. Those who deny this approach do not take professional responsibilities seriously. Youth is part of essential beauty, and the principles related to essential and structural beauty must be applied to the aging individual to restore esthetics (Figs 3-13 and 3-14). Following the initial reaction of surprise and disapproval that the incorporation of young and natural dental elements invariably creates, one must often face a demand for rejuvenation that is far beyond the therapeutic possibilities. This confirms that in this particular field our patients have not only been conditioned to beauty by magazines, the media, and life experience but also that this self-image of youth has been stored in their intellect and only needs to be reactivated. At the same time, the observation that the functional competence of the stomatognathic system is as well linked to maintenance as it is with the progression of age of original young dental elements takes a realistic impact.

In general, the only justification offered to the individual's legitimate aspiration to beauty is the importance of being young and looking young so that employees, business associates, and colleagues assume that they are competent. Once out of the dental office, patients have to compete in life. A youthful appearance will help them to improve their self-esteem and confidence.

Integration and sublimation

There is no real necessity to understand the principles of esthetics to be able to appreciate paintings. However, many artists, painters, sculptors, and architects made use of these principles in the same way that paintbrushes, chisels, and pencils were used. How many dental professionals whose responsibility is directly oriented toward the achievement of the individual's search for

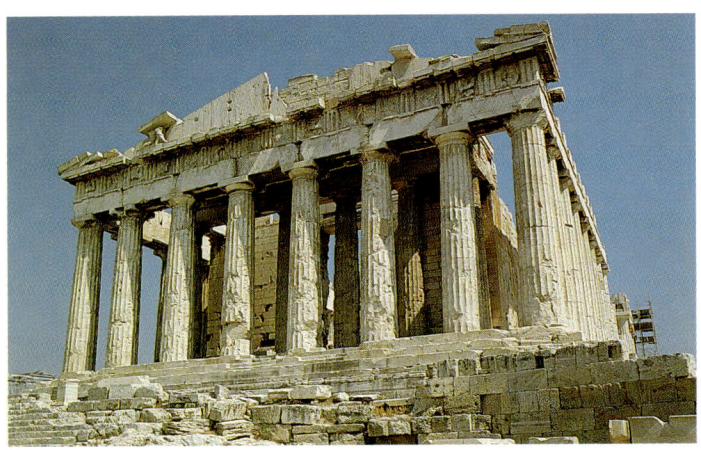

Fig 3-15 Manual disparities produce an inexplicable and repetitive visual tension, a prerequisite for intellectual sublimation.

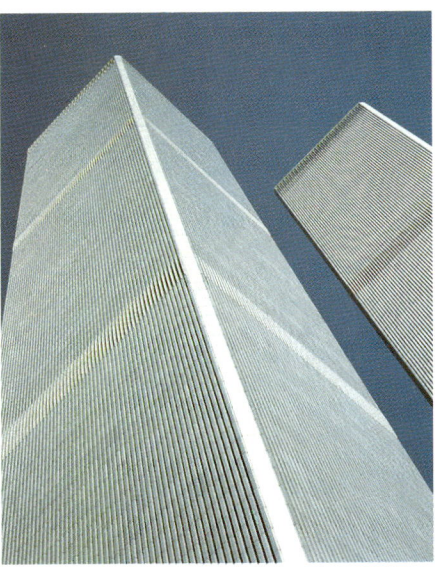

Fig 3-16 Mechanical monotony results from a strict application of rules and theories. Yet the material genius is unable to surpass the literal.

beauty have used these principles or even heard of them?

The technical orientation of our professional education has progressively dissimulated the qualities necessary to a coherent clinical practice. Scientific, artistic, and technical capabilities form a trilogy of instrumental qualities that will enable professionals to reach the largest variety of social targets. One has to understand that the unsatisfactory facial integration of a 12-unit bridge with a perfect marginal fit has no more value to the public than a beautiful restoration with poor marginal seal for the professional.

Contrary to works of art that so often exhibit a sacrifice of literal reproduction, forcing reality to compromise under the claim of imagination, a dentistry of quality requires a succession of humble microscopic or macroscopic artisan-like acts that may reach an artistic level in improving the realistic integration of all the particularities constituting the oral environment. Therefore, with this concept of esthetic dentistry, we will now focus our attention on the description of a number of facial, gingival, and dental elements, which, as part of the biologic structures, have an esthetic value that must be reproduced to assure a natural esthetic quality from which fantasy has been eliminated.

In proposing a protocol of a progressive esthetic setup designed to assure a consistent integration of these elements to oral structures and an approach to occlusion aimed at restoring functional stability and a youthful appearance, the sum of all these factors and clinical efforts may only produce a "static" esthetic quality, which appeals to the reason rather than the emotion (Figs 3-15 and 3-16). This constant training for esthetic perception and morphopsychologic evaluation, which attests to a will for perfectionism, may allow us one day to reach a degree of accomplishment in which all the parameters of rehabilitation have been integrated into the sublime. Sublimeness is the achievement of perfection in beauty and esthetics, a charismatic state of genius, a tension that originates in the hands of artists that makes the difference between mechanical monotony and manual disparities. The Parthenon has been built once and is unique. All those monuments that have been built to the same rules have never reached this state of perfection and sublimeness in which the intellect reaches the heart. No columns of the Parthenon are identical and none are different from the other. This accomplishment is the fantastic challenge offered with each case to the perfectionist professional to reach a level whereby dentistry becomes dental art.

References

Academy of Denture Prosthetics. Glossary of Prosthodontic Terms. *J Prosthet Dent.* 1968;20:447, 486.

Albino JE, Tedesco LA, Conny JD. Patient perception of dental-facial esthetics. Shared concerns in orthodontics and prosthodontics. *J Prosthet Dent.* 1984;52:9.

Aquinas, St. Thomas. *Summa Theologica.* (c. 1250).

Arnheim R. *Art and Visual Perception.* Berkeley and Los Angeles, Calif: University of California Press; 1965.

Becker, EO. Esthetics — An enigma. *J Prosthet Dent.* June, 1971.

Bercleid E, Walter E. Beauty and the best. *Psychol Today.* 1972;5:10.

Brigante RF. Patient assisted esthetics. *J Prosthet Dent.* 1981;46:14.

Brisman AS. Esthetics: A comparison of dentists and patients concepts. *J Am Dent Assoc.* 1980;100:345.

Burckett PJ, Christensen LC. Estimating age and sex by using color, form and alignment of anterior teeth. *J Prosthet Dent.* 1988;59:175–179.

Cattel RB. *The Scientific Analysis of Personality.* Chicago, Ill: Aldine Publ; 1965.

Cirici A. *Miro et son temps.* Barcelona, Spain: Ediciones Poligrafia; 1985.

Darwin ChR. *Descent of Man and Selection in Relation to Sex.* 1871.

Fechner GT. *Vorschule der Ästhetik.* Leipzig; 1876.

Fisher RD. Esthetics in denture construction. *Dent Clin North Am.* March, 1957.

Fisher S, Cleveland SE. *Body Image and Personality.* New York, NY: Dover Publications Inc; 1968.

Frush JP, Fisher RD. The age factor in dentogenics. *J Prosthet Dent.* 1957;7:5–13.

Frush JP, Fisher RD. The dynesthetic interpretation of the dentinogenic concept. *J Prosthet Dent.* 1958;8:560–681.

Frush JP, Fisher RD. Introduction to dentogenic restorations. *J Prosthet Dent.* 1955;5:586–595.

Frush JP, Fisher RD. How dentinogenic restorations interpret the sex factor. *J Prosthet Dent.* 1956;6:160–172.

Frush JP, Fisher RD. How dentinogenics interpret the personality factor. *J Prosthet Dent.* 1956;6:441–449.

Furtwangler A. *Masterpieces of Greek Sculpture.* Chicago, Ill: Argonaut; 1964.

Garret HE. *Psychology.* New York, NY: American Book Co; 1950.

Gerber, A. Creative and artistic tasks in complete prosthodontics. *Quintessence Int.* 1975;6(2):45.

Goldstein R. *Esthetics in Dentistry.* Philadelphia, Pa: JB Lippincott; 1976.

Goldstein RE, Fritz M. Esthetics in dental curriculum. *J Dent Educ.* 1981;45:355.

Graber LW, Lucker GW. Dental esthetics self evaluation and satisfaction. *Am J Orthod.* 1980;77:163.

Hambidge J. *The Elements of Dynamic Symmetry.* New York, NY: Dover Press; 1970.

Hegel GWF. In Montaigne, ed. *Vorlesungen über die Ästhetik.* Paris: 1944.

Hegel GWF. *Philosophy of History.* New York, NY: Collier; 1905.

Hershon LE, Giddon DB. Determinants of facial profile self perception. *Am J Orthod.* 1980;279–293.

Honour H, Fleming J. *Histoire Mondiale de l'Art.* Paris: Bordas; 1984.

Huyghe R. *Dialogue avec le Visible,* Flammarion. Paris; 1955.

Kant E. *Critique of Judgment,* 1790. Oxford: Clarendon Press; 1952.

Lee JH. *Dental Aesthetics.* Bristol, Conn: John Wright and Sons; 1962.

Lombardi R. Visual perception and denture esthetics. *J Prosthet Dent.* 1973;29:352–382.

Lombardi R. A method for the classification of errors in dental esthetics. *J Prosthet Dent.* 1974;11:243–248.

Lombardi R. Factors mediating against excellence in dental esthetics. *J Prosthet Dent.* 1977;9:501–513.

Meyers B. L'interprétation de l'Art. *Le Lion d'Art.* Grolier;10:1971.

Miller WH, Ratcliff F, Hartline HK. *Perception: Mechanism and Models.* San Francisco, Calif: WH Freeman and Co; 1961.

Molnar ME. *Forever Young: The Practical Handbook of Youth Extension.* West Hartford, Conn: The Withower Press Inc;

Palau J, Favre J. *Picasso en Catalogne.* Société Française du Lion, trad. française; 1979.

Peck H, Peck S. A concept of facial esthetics. *Angle Orthod.* 1970;40:284.

Plato. *Philebus.* c. 400 BC.

Plato. *Republic.* c. 400 BC.

Chapter 4

Structural Esthetic Rules

Claude R. Rufenacht

Facial components

Facial features

Although orthodontists have established a rule of sagittal norms, frontal norms do not really exist and any attempt to define frontal beauty based on biometric measurements would not be valid because of the limitations imposed by the variety of racial, ethnic, and individual types.

The combination of the numerical quantification of beauty postulated by Greek philosophers with beauty's psychophysical quantification has been advocated as being a more pertinent approach to the evaluation of human esthetics.

In introducing the presumption of the individuality of human beauty, a strict definition of frontal facial norms loses meaning because beauty depends upon esthetic and morphopsychologic principles imposed by the equilibrium existing between facial zones and the harmonious integration of the receptors.

Disturbances affecting this equilibrium as a result of our genetic heritage and environmental compulsions can be corrected or attenuated by means of dentofacial orthopedic or reconstructive surgery.

The frequency of accidental aging events and the programmed progression of age affecting facial esthetic equilibrium will also call for therapy and require the multidisciplinary approach of diverse branches of medicine and paramedicine, keeping in mind that in this field of interest morphologic changes involve skin, facial adipose tissue, aponeurosis, muscles, teeth, and facial skeleton.

The presence of grooves perpendicular to the direction of the pull of the muscles is a constant of facial anatomic features. They are more or less marked depending upon the individual, and their permanence is basically linked to the nature of the tegumental relief and the degree of advancement of biologic aging (Fig 4-1). It is interesting to note that three important facial grooves, the nasolabial groove, labial groove, and mentolabial groove, are situated along important meridians that are part of the energetic network that, according to ancient, oriental medicine, runs through the body.[1] The deepening of the nasolabial groove situated on the path of the meridian ruling vitality and opening to life testifies a loss of energy as the result of inner distress

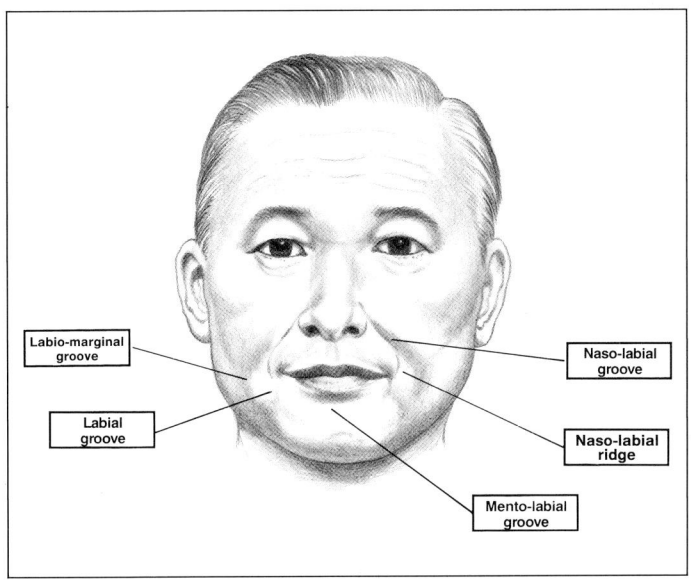

Fig 4-1 This sketch illustrates a limited number of facial grooves or sulcus surrounding the oral cavity that are associated with the nature of the individual tegumental relief or with the advancement of the biologic aging.

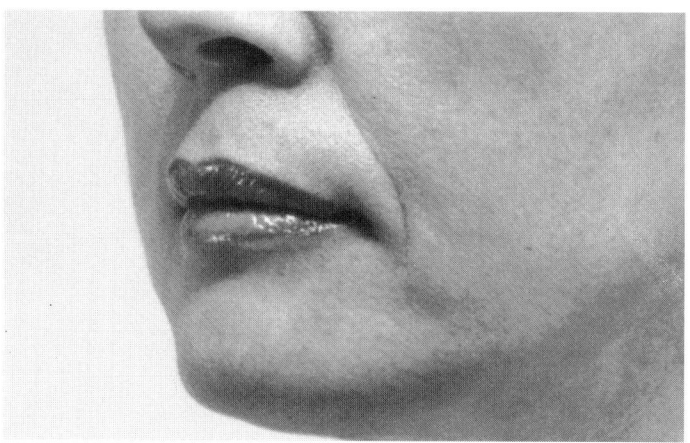

Fig 4-2 Early perception of facial aging of muscular and tegumental origin characterized by the deepening of the nasolabial groove. (Courtesy of Dr U. Bürki, Geneva.)

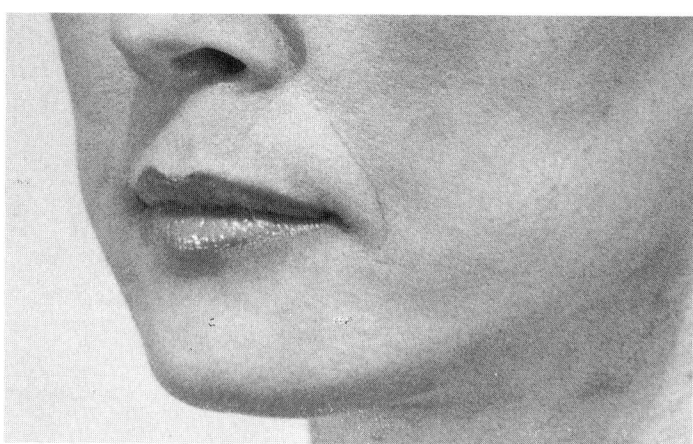

Fig 4-3 Successful effacement of the nasolabial groove and restoration of lip tonicity following rhytidectomy. (Courtesy of Dr U. Bürki, Geneva.)

originating from emotional damage. The energetic losses marking the labial lines indicate inner rebellion and supressed revolt against destiny, whereas the mentolabial groove gathers the impacts of the "vessel of tears" located under the eyes, indicating an absence of self-defense and difficulty in communicating despair. Even if few can be convinced of the poetic significance of the progressive apparition of lines and wrinkles, these considerations are valuable in that they point out that a selective muscular activity takes place under the influence of specific psychologic states having effect when the environmental conditions cause aging or decay.[2]

The anatomic changes that cause the appearance of aging take place early in life (Figs 4-2 and 4-3). Significant modifications are already apparent at the age of 25 years, with the descent of eyebrows, nasal tip, and chin vertex and the sinking of the nasal base. These movements accelerate abruptly at about 35 years of age under the influence of gravity, laxness, and thinning of the skin, which starts producing wrinkles and sulcus.[3] Thin skin textures, generally exhibiting thin epidermis, lacking elastine, and with an irregular and scarce presence of collagen, are more susceptible to wrinkling, whereas thick skin textures with thick epidermis, abundant elastine, sebaceous glands, and collagen will prove more resistant to this deterioration. These statements should be modified depending on the influence that a number of elements, such as nutritional factors, way of life, and energetic potentialities, can exert. The original skin relief evolves and an undulating relief may become roughly marked, while a plump skin relief generally droops into folds, modifying the morphopsychologic significance exhibited by an individual. In mentioning the changes that can affect the osseous structures, the loss of skin and muscle elasticity, and the diminution of muscle strength inducing the progressive appearance of wrinkles, we have a concise image of this syndrome of decadence. This will inevitably affect psychic equilibrium when some event raises it to the level of consciousness.

In focusing our attention on the localization of facial aging, it is clear that it predominantly affects the lower one third of the face. Also, the basic anatomic facial grooves surround its receptor. This not only attests to the importance of the mouth but suggests its active participation in this phenomenon of deterioration to the point at which therapeutic action may sometimes compound the problem. Being familiar with the profound morphologic changes that affect the perioral structures and the lower one third of the face in a state of edentation, one can easily imagine from this extreme situation

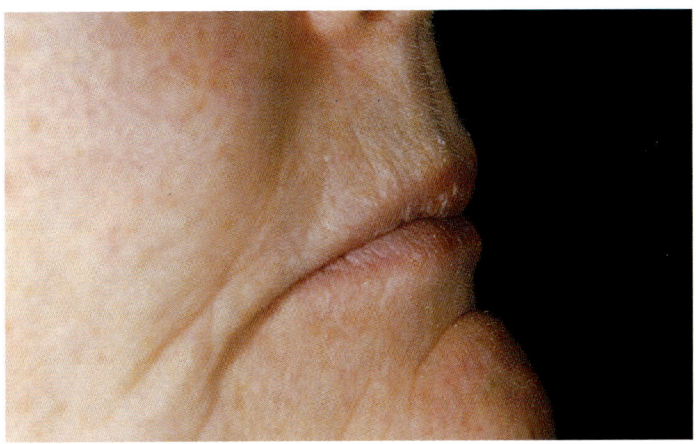 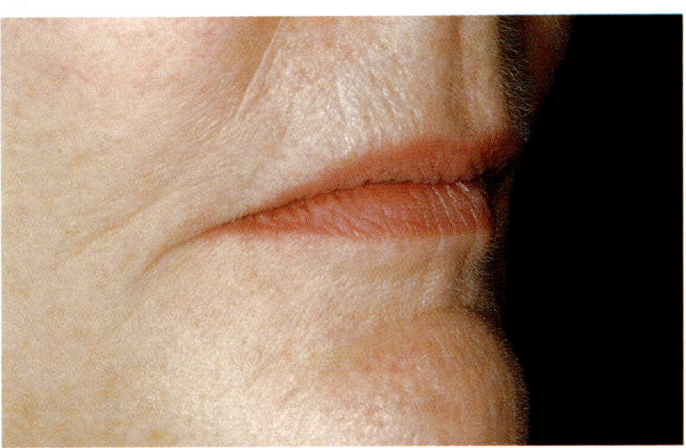

Fig 4-4 Development of the nasolabial ridge underlined by the nasolabial groove and a deep labial groove.

Fig 4-5 Effacement of the nasolabial ridge and consequent diminution of the labial groove following full mouth rehabilitation.

that the multitude and variety of intermediate states resulting from successive "accidental" traumas are capable of producing similar but attenuated consequences. Skeleton, muscle, ligaments, and teeth form a cohesive unit. Alteration to any part of it may affect regions far beyond those directly concerned.[4] Pathologic situations materialized by the loss of teeth, migrations, tooth wear, faulty restorations, or tooth arrangements not only exhibit profound local morphologic changes, but these morphologic changes directly or indirectly influence the surrounding structures. This influence systematically affects facial muscles. Muscle collapse following tooth loss not only affects those muscles that have benefitted from this tooth support but also involves the collapse of associated muscles, which are connected by means of a network of fiber intrication (Figs 4-4 and 4-5).

Considering the alterations that can have an effect on the elements of the orofacial unit and their consequences, it seems that we are in the presence of a chain of reactions confirming the links existing between its constitutive elements.[5,6] The diagrammatic representation of head posture maintenance demonstrates the close interdependence existing between these constitutive elements and reveals the collapse that may result from any accidental event (Figs 4-6 and 4-7).

Abnormal facial equilibrium, either morphologic or esthetic, can be ascribed to two major causes: *(1)* physiologic or programmed aging, generating changes in muscle and skin tonicity, and *(2)* pathologic aging, generated by accidental traumas affecting the oral cavity.

The difficulty consists of determining what in the facial appearance are the elements that result from oral pathologies and those that are a consequence of physiologic, programmed aging. This difficulty is greatly increased when it concerns individuals reaching an age at which this sequence of events may be considered normal.

The restoration of health and function of the oral organ will shed some light on these differences, with the restriction that there does not exist from one individual to another a chronology in the apparition of lines, sulcus, and wrinkles. A similarity of the effects resulting from a specific oral clinical situation, as a result of the variety of muscle fiber intrication and the nature of the original tegumental relief, is highly unusual.

The differential diagnosis seems somewhat easier when lip design comes into consideration. Lip design, which according to the morphopsychologic concept, results from the influence stemming from cerebral, sentimental, and instinctive action, depends upon its den-

Structural Esthetic Rules

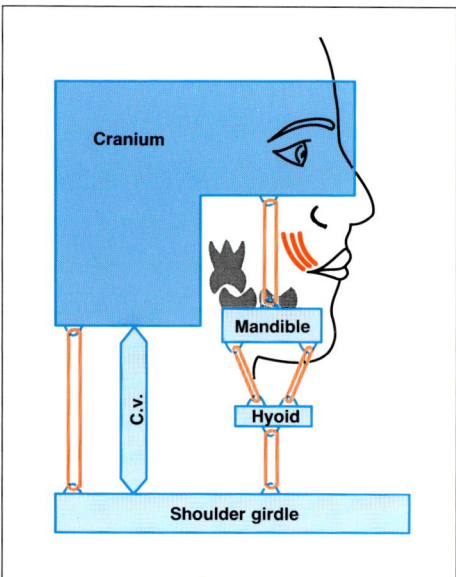
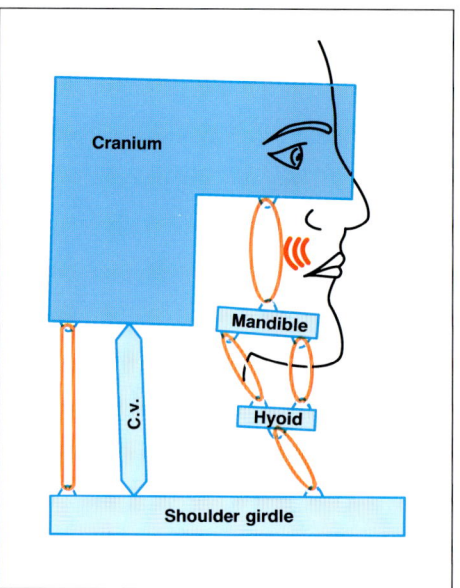

Fig 4-6 Diagrammatic representation of head posture maintenance and balance of craniomandibular muscles. The relaxation of facial muscles does not affect this equilibrium. (According to Sarnat.[5])

Fig 4-7 This diagram, simulating the loss of dental support, underlines its direct impact on the maintenance of facial musculature and the imbalance created on the whole craniomandibular system. (According to Sarnat.[5])

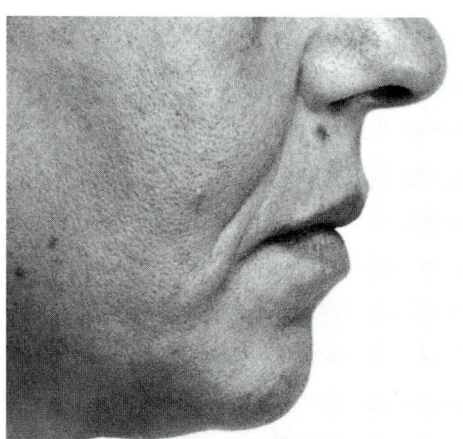
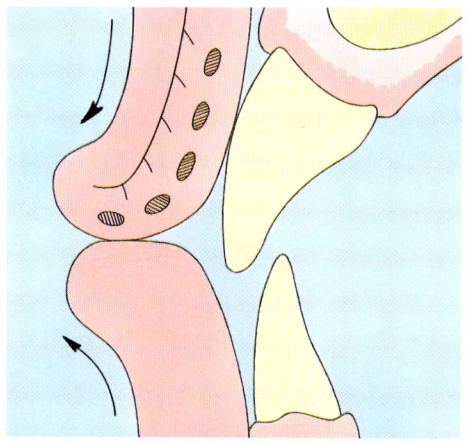
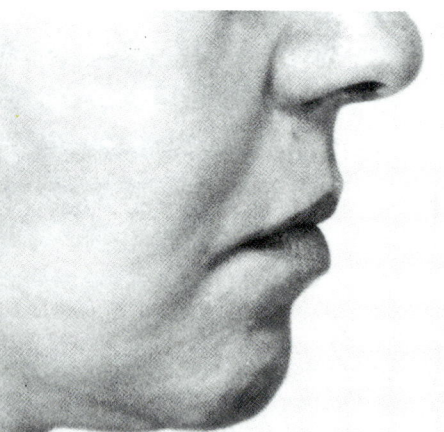

Fig 4-8 Muscle and tegumental laxness affecting the oral environment, producing a characteristic outward roll or redundancy of the upper and lower lips and deepening the nasolabial groove. (Courtesy of Dr U. Bürki, Geneva.)

Fig 4-9 Schematic illustration of the outward roll of the lip. Its muscular and tegumental origin can be determined when tooth support is unaffected.

Fig 4-10 Restoration of tegumental and muscle tonicity and the restoration of lip design after rhytidectomy. (Courtesy of Dr U. Bürki, Geneva.)

Facial components

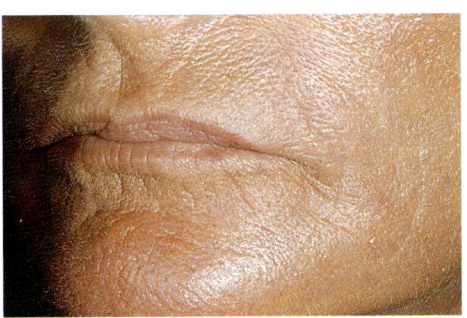

Fig 4-11 Effacement of lip design with marked inward roll of the lip margin toward the corners. Deepening of the mentolabial groove. Vertical wrinkles underline the lower lip.

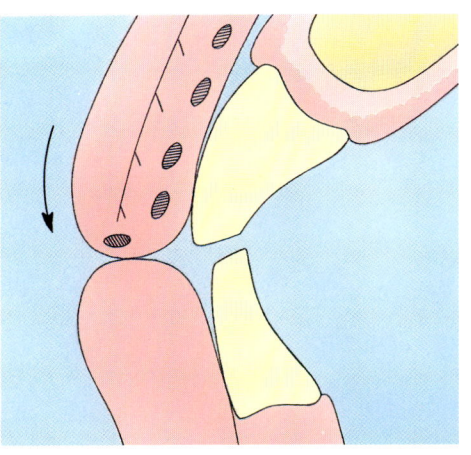

Fig 4-12 Schematic illustration of the inward roll of lip margin whenever a vertical reduction of tooth support takes place.

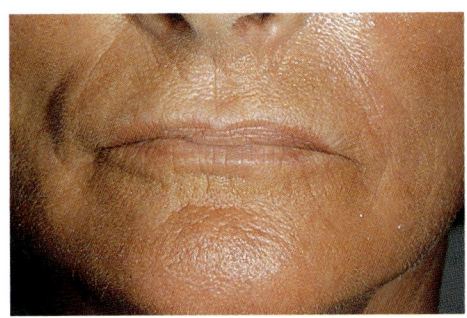

Fig 4-13 A frontal view illustrates the pathology affecting lip design and evidences the presence of a nasolabial ridge, predominantly on the right side, underlined by a labial groove.

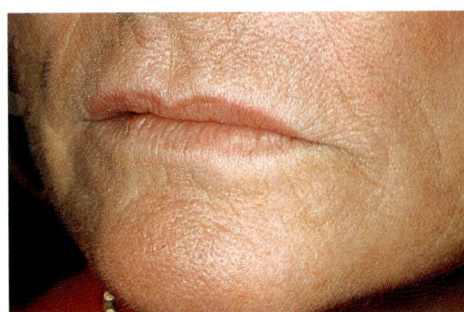

Fig 4-14 Following rehabilitation, restoration of lip design with diminution of the mentolabial groove. Perioral structures regained strength as confirmed by the diminution of the vertical wrinkles surrounding the lower lip.

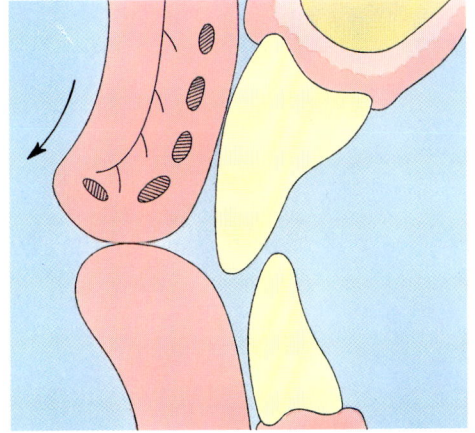

Fig 4-15 Schematic illustration of the closed lip posture when normal occlusal, muscular, and tegumental conditions exist. Typically, the incisal third of the maxillary incisor does not contact the inner part of the upper lip.

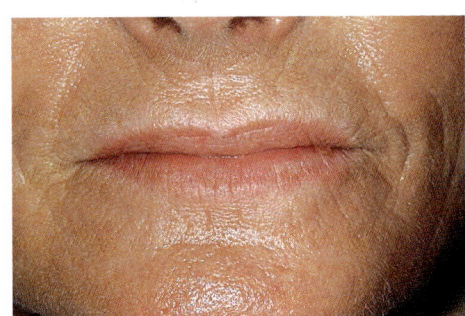

Fig 4-16 Restoration by means of fixed partial denture ending at the second premolar favoring abnormal contraction of the buccinator did not permit the total effacement of the nasolabial ridge, but this frontal view confirms the restoration of lip design.

Structural Esthetic Rules

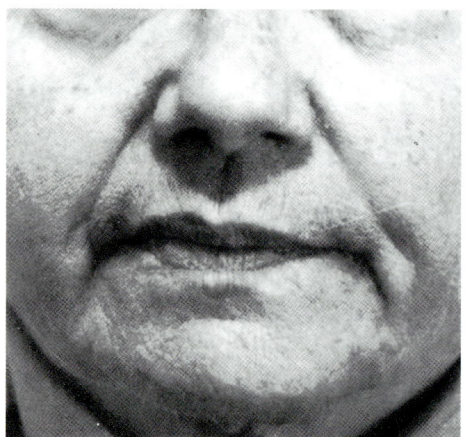

Fig 4-17 Impressive image of facial decadence, exhibiting an important nasolabial ridge surrounded by unesthetic labial and nasolabial grooves. Lip design is distorted and the corners of the mouth depressed. (Courtesy of Dr U. Bürki, Geneva.)

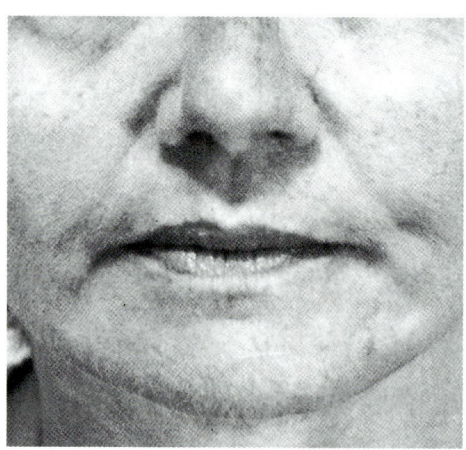

Fig 4-18 After rhytidectomy the mouth design still looks unattractive and unnatural. An upper lip design presenting an inward roll toward the corners of the mouth can be considered a specific manifestation of oral pathologies. In this case, the competence of the surgeon has fortunately resulted in an avoidance of excessive tegumental pull. (Courtesy of Dr U. Bürki, Geneva.)

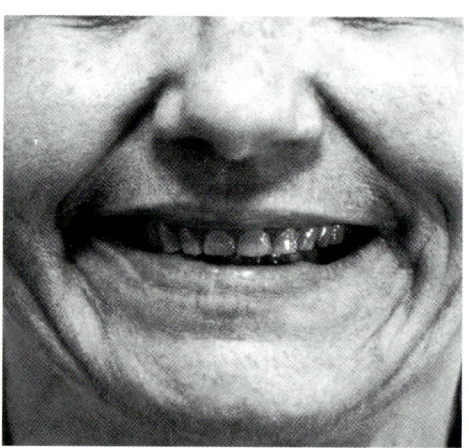

Fig 4-19 The picture of the smile showing a marked reduction of the tooth length confirms the expected pathologic oral situation. It indicates that the correction of specific facial deformities are within the competence of the dental profession. (Courtesy of Dr U. Bürki, Geneva.)

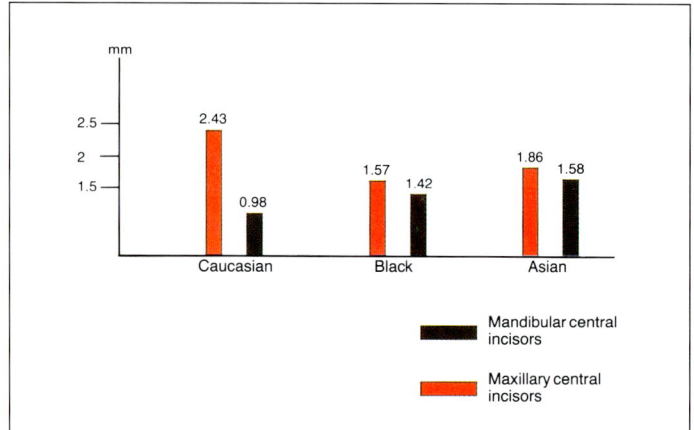

Fig 4-20 Diagram of exposure of maxillary and mandibular central incisors related to racial factor. (From Vig and Brundo.[7])

toalveolar support with which it is ultimately connected. It is also linked with the strength and tonicity of its muscular support. Any alteration affecting the dentoalveolar support will have a direct influence on facial musculature. From clinical practice we have observed that a protrusive outward roll of the upper and lower lip originating in a loss of skin and muscle tonicity takes part in the development of facial sagging (Figs 4-8 to 4-10). A loss of the vertical dimension of the lower facial one third affecting the strength and the extent of the working length of the infraorbital musculature, predominantly the quadratus labii superioris and zygomaticus, induces a muscle collapse. When this loss is illustrated by anterior tooth wear or lack of dentoalveolar support, an inward roll of the upper lip margin toward the corners can be observed. In case of anterior tooth migration affecting lip movements, a large variety of lip postures can take place (Figs 4-11 to 4-16). Functional disturbances naturally reflect on facial appearance, attesting to the link existing between function and esthetics. Although esthetic dentistry must take into consideration the interdependence existing among the elements constituting the oral environment, clinicians in esthetic dentistry and esthetic medicine should be aware of the effects of oral pathologies on premature aging of the face. This clearly calls for closer cooperation between these two specialties (Figs 4-17 to 4-19).

Tooth visibility

The amount of tooth exposure when lips and lower jaw are at rest is, like body posture, a muscle-determined position. This has been generally disregarded as an element of esthetic appraisal, if not totally ignored by the restorative dentist. For the prosthodontist, the determination of the incisal edge–lip length relationship was mainly based on clinical experience or on phonetic values, assuming that this should automatically achieve the correct position of the maxillary anterior incisor in the vertical plane.

An interesting study related to tooth exposure according to gender, racial factors, age, and lip length[7] elucidated the extreme variability of this factor.

Tooth exposure showed an increase from blacks to Asians and whites for the maxillary central incisor and a decrease for the mandibular central incisor from Asians to blacks and whites (Fig 4-20).

Tooth exposure according to gender appeared to be significantly more important for females than for males because an average exposure of 1.91 mm was stated for males, whereas females had nearly twice as much tooth exposure (3.40 mm) of the maxillary central incisor, yet a minimal amount of 0.5 mm of mandibular incisor exposure. This suggests that treating patients using the same therapeutic values in this matter is an error that increases in importance when considering the parameters of lip length and age.

Age

The study evidenced a significant decrease of maxillary tooth length exposure relative to age, predominantly between the age of 30 and 40 years and a proportionate increase of mandibular incisor exposure, a situation that is esthetically, unanimously rejected (Figs 4-21 to 4-25).

Table 4-1 Lip length

Lip length (mm)	Exposure of maxillary vertical incisor	Exposure of mandibular central incisor
10–15	3.92	0.64
16–20	3.44	0.77
21–25	2.18	0.98
26–30	0.93	1.95
31–36	0.25	2.25

Table 4-1 shows that people with short upper lips expose the maximum maxillary incisor texture, whereas people with long upper lips expose predominantly lower anterior incisors.

The assumption that tooth exposure is mainly of muscular origin influenced our decision to adopt the muscle retraining techniques as part of a maintenance program, preventing the sagging of the face at as early an age as possible.

Maxillary incisor visibility is an important parameter in esthetic appraisal because its decrease contributes to the early perception of aging of individuals in their 40s.

In selected clinical situations in which face sagging has proceeded too far and muscle retraining techniques become illusory, tooth anatomy must be elongated to fulfill rejuvenation's requirements. This approach is only possible when it does not conflict with either functional problems or esthetic factors (Figs 4-26 to 4-28).

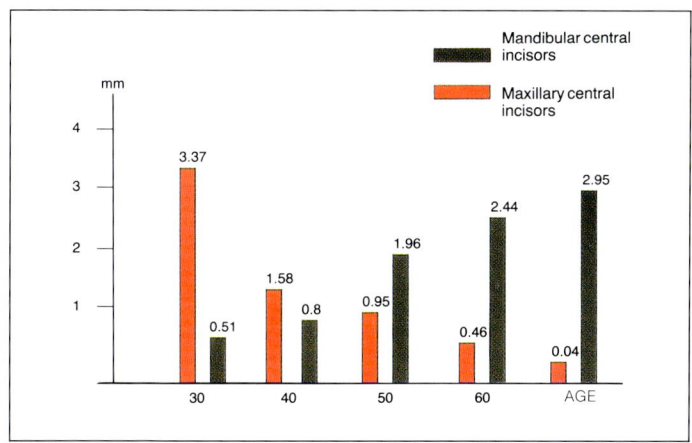

Fig 4-21 Diagram of exposure of maxillary and mandibular central incisors related to age. (From Vig and Brundo.[7])

Structural Esthetic Rules

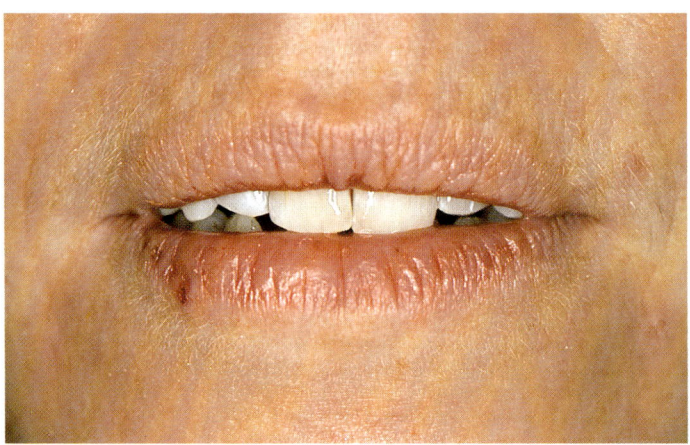

Fig 4-22 Average tooth exposure of a man in his 20s with natural dentition in slight mouth opening.

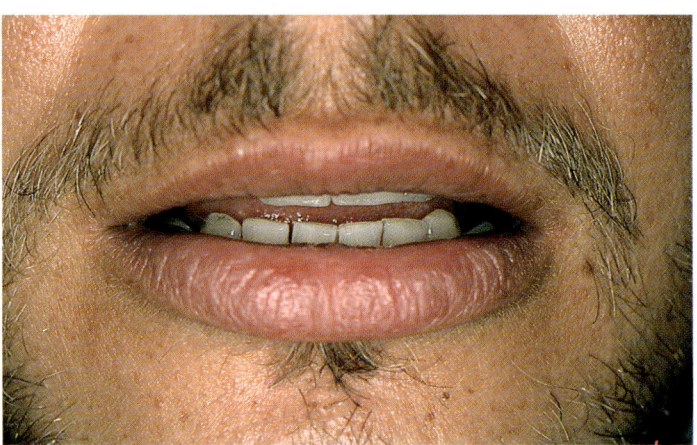

Fig 4-23 Facial sagging starts to proceed insidiously between 35 and 40 years of age. Slight mouth opening begins to display mandibular dentition as well.

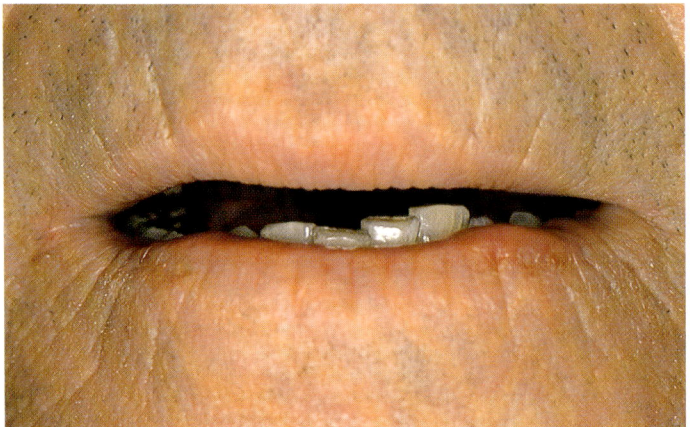

Fig 4-24 In the 60s the maintenance of a healthy dentition does not assure the esthetic appearance of the dentofacial composition when facial muscle tonicity has not been maintained over the years.

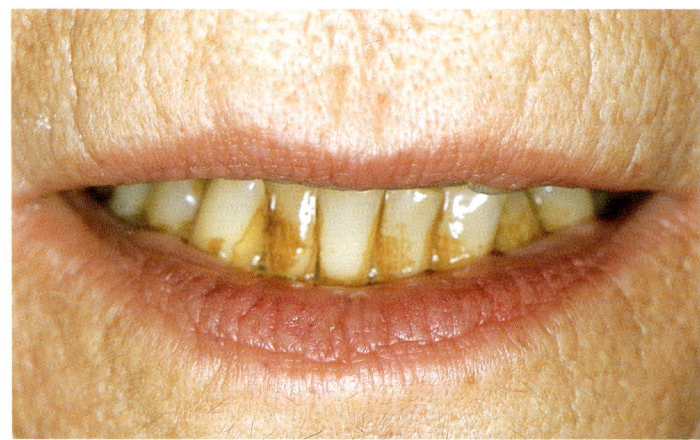

Fig 4-25 At 70 years of age and in absence of oral pathologies, face sagging has proceeded so far that the restoration of an esthetic appearance is not affected by dental therapies and muscle retraining techniqes.

Facial components

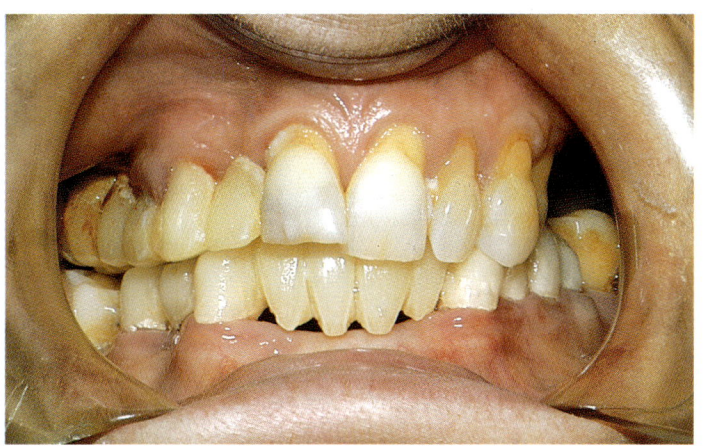

Fig 4-26 Pathologic clinical situation affecting an individual in her 70s, exhibiting periodontal and occlusal breakdown.

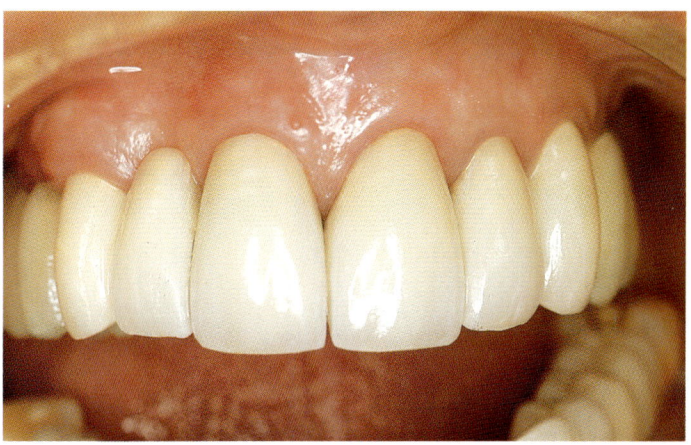

Fig 4-27 Whenever tolerated by the length of the lip line, the restoration of health, function, and esthetics implies a drastic increase of tooth length, such as that illustrated by this long-term provisional acrylic resin stabilization, following initial periodontal treatment.

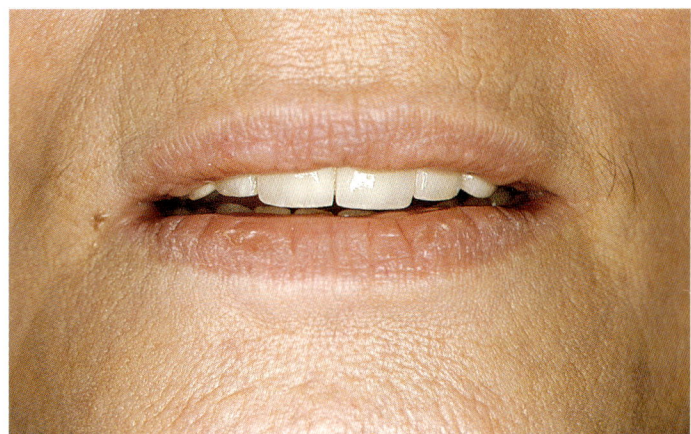

Fig 4-28 As a result, tooth display masks chronologic age but conforms to the advancement of the biologic age illustrated by the quality of skin texture. The nature of the tegumental relief enhances this rejuvenated image.

Structural Esthetic Rules

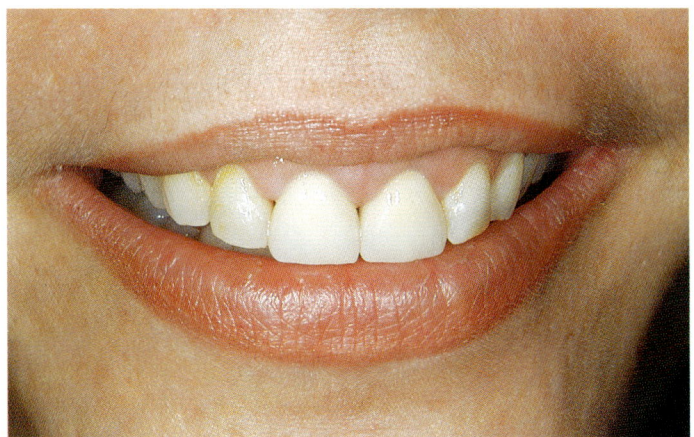

Fig 4-29 High lip line in smiling displays teeth and gingiva.

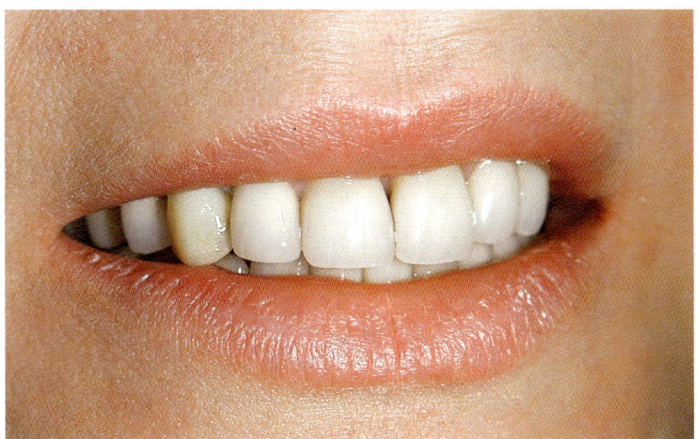

Fig 4-30 Middle lip line displaying teeth and marginal interdental papillae when smiling.

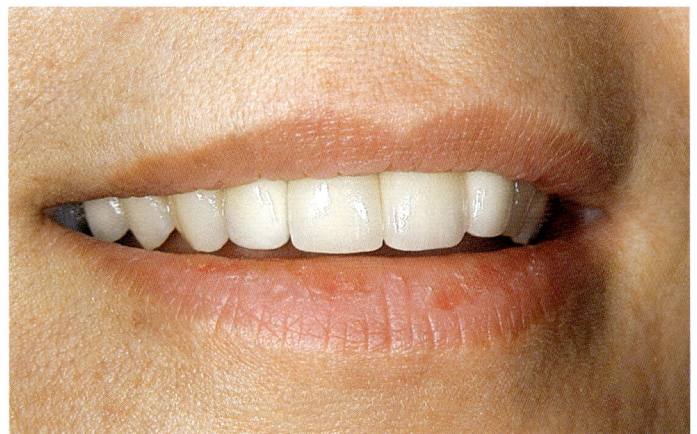

Fig 4-31 Low lip line displaying a limited part of tooth anatomy when smiling.

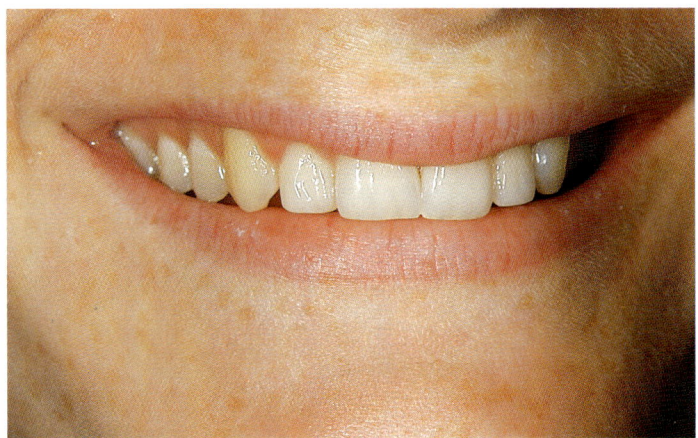

Fig 4-32 Anterior low lip line with gingival posterior display.

Components of the smile

The smile, which represents the most primitive form and the essence of human communicative ability, appears early in life in young children. Smiles and later facial expressions express transient feelings and emotions. A pleasant smile may produce an aura that enhances the beauty of the face as it pertains to the qualities and virtues of the human personality.

The perception of these qualities engenders the "attractive power," a necessary vector to success in today's world.

The individual's ability to exhibit a pleasing smile directly depends upon the quality of the dental and gingival elements that it contains, their conformity to the rules of structural beauty, the relations existing between teeth and lips during smile, and its harmonious integration in the facial composition.

While the modalities of the development of facial expressions have been focused on by some authors,[2,8-10] the esthetic lip–tooth relationships existing when smiling have been the object of surprisingly little investigation,[11-15] as if the elements determining a favorable or negative connotation were unanimously recognized.

Rather than assuming what is of esthetic importance in the lip–tooth relationship during a smile, one should focus attention on the elements that receive esthetic approval[16] and analyze them in the light of fundamental esthetic principles.

Lip line

The amount of tooth exposure during a smile depends on a variety of factors, such as the degree of contraction of the muscles of expression, soft tissue level, skeletal particularities, and the design of restorative elements, tooth shape, or tooth wear. Dentistry has arbitrarily classified three types of smiles that, relating the height of the upper lip relative to the maxillary anterior central incisors, are referred to as presenting a low lip line, middle lip line, or high lip line (Figs 4-29 to 4-32). While low lip line can sometimes become a cover for poor dentistry, the high lip line displaying a large amount of gingival tissue, reflecting aggressivity, affects those individuals exhibiting some type of maxillary protrusion or having a strong infraorbital facial musculature. The modalities for treatment of the high lip line are limited. Orthognathic surgery is disproportionate to the clinical situation. Orthodontic intrusion or surgical tooth lengthening with subsequent crown length reduction that may appeal to the esthetically concerned dentist could be of real help when the indications for this type of treatment really do exist. Muscle retraining techniques are often illusory as they are not able to provide a diminution of the strength of contraction of the infraorbital musculature. Surgical procedures carried out on the implicated facial muscles are most disappointing in their results. The ideal lip line seems to be obtained when the upper lip in reference to the maxillary incisors reaches the interdental gingival margin when smiling, a situation that is common to a large number of people.

Smile line

The smile line appears to be one of the most important factors contributing to a pleasant connotation of a smile. The smile line can be defined as a hypothetical curved line drawn along the edges of the four anterior maxillary teeth that has to coincide or run parallel with the curvature of the inner border of the lower lip. This situation, always favorably regarded, confirms the effect that cohesive forces can exert in any type of composition.

Observations may show that the degree of curvature of the incisal line is more pronounced for women than for men (Figs 4-33 and 4-34). A reverse incisal line or an abnormal lower lip posture, in effacing the elements that enable the perception of these cohesive forces, deeply affects the degree of attractiveness of the smile.

Structural Esthetic Rules

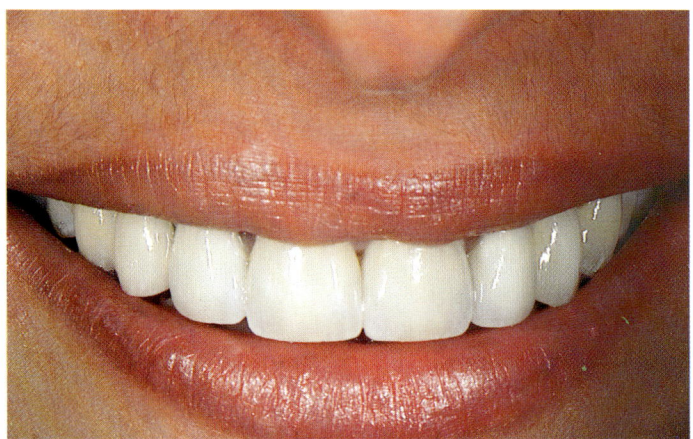

Fig 4-33 Feminine type of smile line characterized by the curvature of the incisal line that coincides with that of the lower lip.

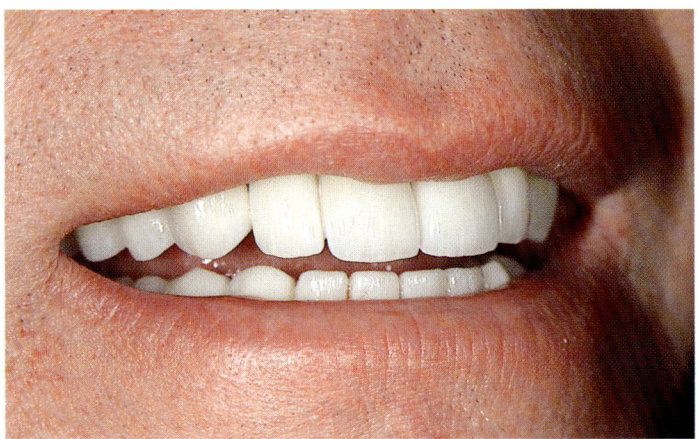

Fig 4-34 Masculine type of smile line showing a straighter incisal line and producing a stronger morphopsychologic impact.

Upper lip curvature

In smiling, the position of the upper lip height relative to the teeth has been ideally located at the gingival margin of the maxillary central incisors and appears as an important factor of attractiveness (Figs 4-35 to 4-38).

The upper lip curvature that is expected to run upward from this central position to the corners of the mouth, depending on the sequence and degree of implication of facial muscles in the development of smile, has been found to be straight and even downward in a certain number of people, affecting the attractiveness of these smiles. In this type of situation some improvement can be obtained using muscle retraining techniques when the other components of smile do not compensate for this deficiency.

Facial components

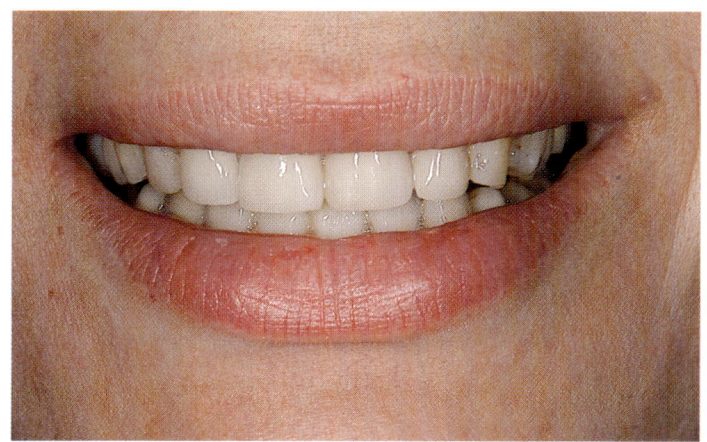

Fig 4-35 In smiling, the curvature of the upper lip may be directed upward.

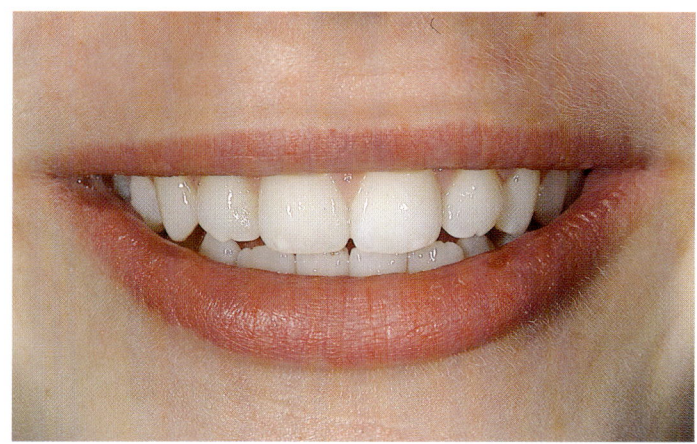

Fig 4-36 The specific strength of the muscles involved in the smile may produce a lateral stretch of the corners of the mouth.

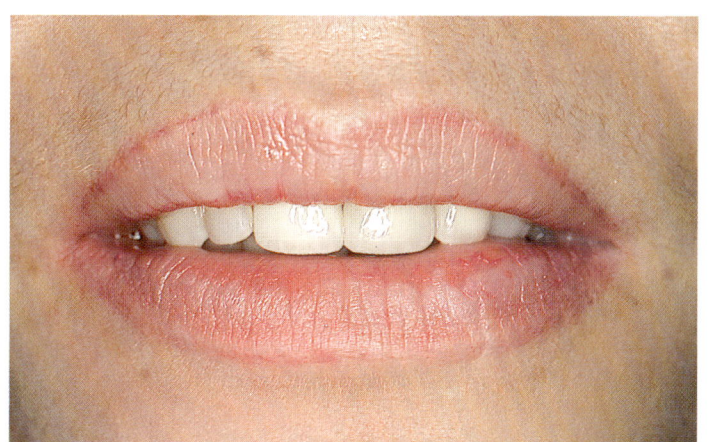

Fig 4-37 A slightly downward curvature of the upper lip may occasionally be seen.

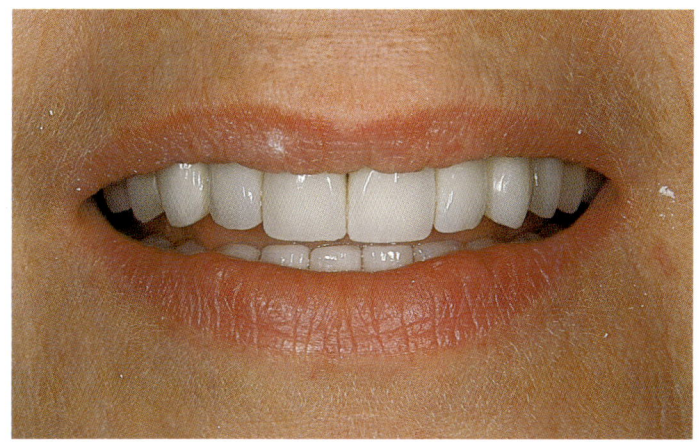

Fig 4-38 A pronounced downward curvature of the upper lip in smiling is not unusual.

Structural Esthetic Rules

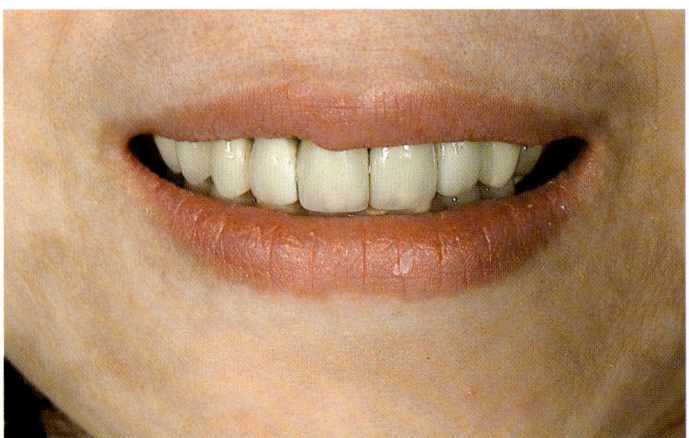

Fig 4-39 The presence of a lateral negative space may be considered a prerequisite of dentofacial esthetics, giving depth and mystery to the smile.

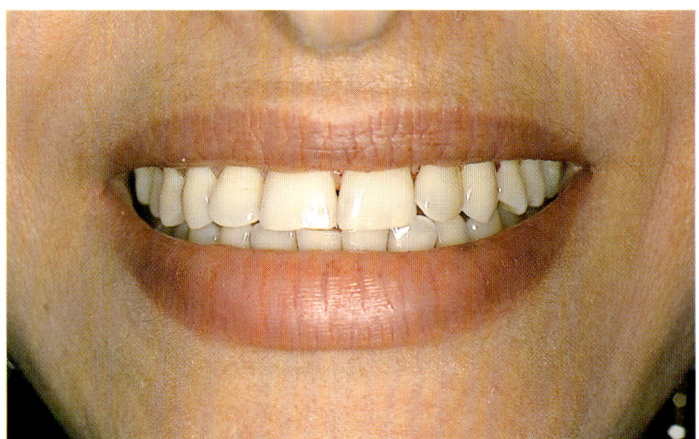

Fig 4-40 The absence of a negative space usually appraised by the public reflects exuberance and brilliance but indicates occlusal disturbances or inadequate restorative dentistry.

Negative space

Negative space can be described as the dark space that appears between the jaws during laughter and mouth opening. This dark space contributes to the individualization of the dental composition that is projected by color contrast. A similar dark space appears between the outer surface of the maxillary teeth and the corner of the mouth in smiling (Figs 4-39 and 4-40). These lateral negative spaces that result from the difference existing between the width of the maxillary arch and the breadth of the smile have been described to be in golden proportion with the anterior smiling segment.[15] An adequate restoration of the lateral negative spaces will permit the characterization of the smile in conformity with the individual's personality.

The importance of this space must be stressed even if it escapes the attention of the public because it not only represents a key factor in the harmony of the smile itself but also a factor of the harmonious proportionate relationship between the smile and other facial features. This indicates that some fundamental esthetic principles or their distortion are more easily perceived than others.

Smile symmetry

The implication of this important esthetic element in a pleasant connotation of smile refers to the relative symmetric placement of the corners of the mouth in the vertical plane (Figs 4-41 and 4-42). Symmetry can only be perceived in reference to a hypothetical central point or central midline. A close look at the nature of the symmetry of the dental composition determines the placement of this midline. A radiating type of dental symmetry draws this line automatically between the central incisors and contributes to the identification of the central contact line, whereas in a horizontal type of symmetry, the eye fixes on a central midline, the coincidence of which with the central interdental space does not assume any importance. When viewed from a distance the dental composition progressively loses its details and is perceived as a specific dental shape mimicking a horizontal type of symmetry on which the mind fixes a hypothetical midline in reference to facial parameters. Smile symmetry may be appreciated in the frame of the dentofacial or facial composition, depending upon the distance from which it is evaluated. In turn, facial midline or dental midline assumes the function of the central point.

Facial components

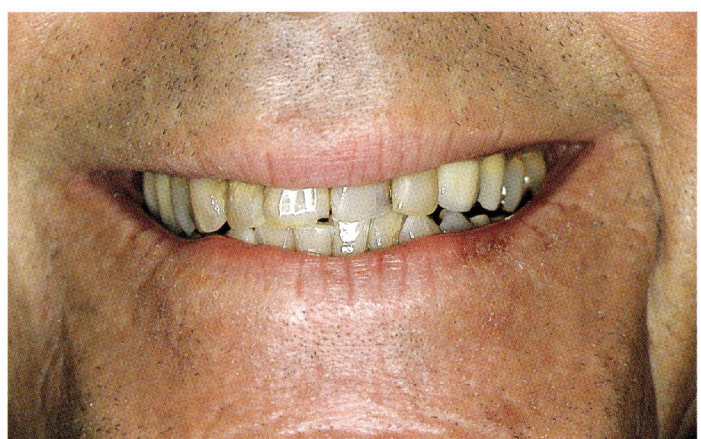

Fig 4-41 Smile symmetry refers to an identical placement of the corners of the mouth in the vertical plane of the face. It can hardly be evaluated at this distance of focus.

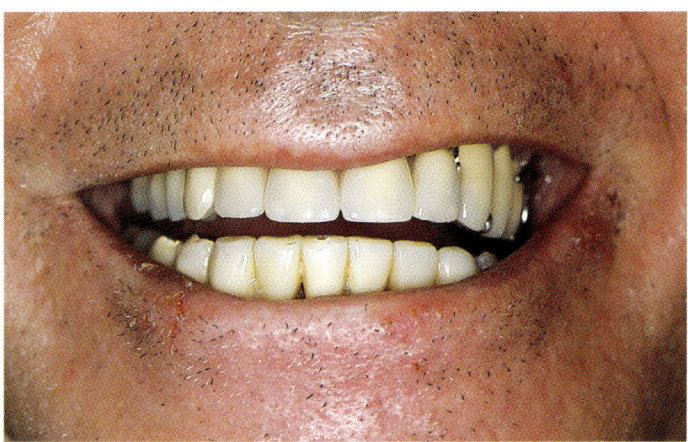

Fig 4-42 Smile asymmetry implies differences in the placement of the corners of the mouth in the vertical plane of the face. It is barely perceptible at this distance.

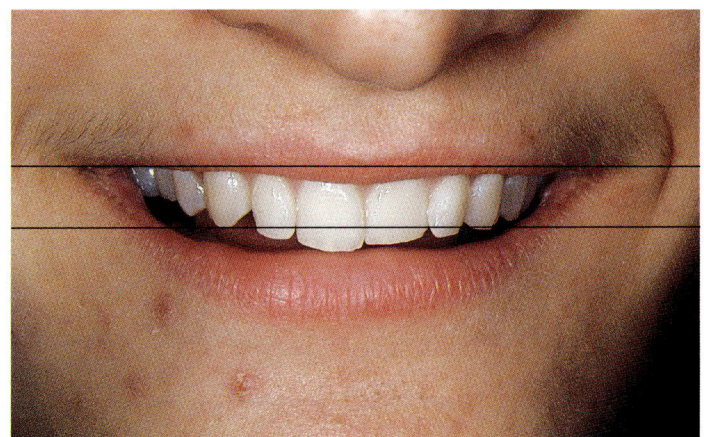

Fig 4-43 In this dentofacial composition, the evaluation of the symmetric placement of the corners of the mouth in the vertical plane can only be done with reference to the coincidence of the commissural and occlusal lines. Note that asymmetric right and left anterior dental segments around the central midline can be observed (see Fig 4-56).

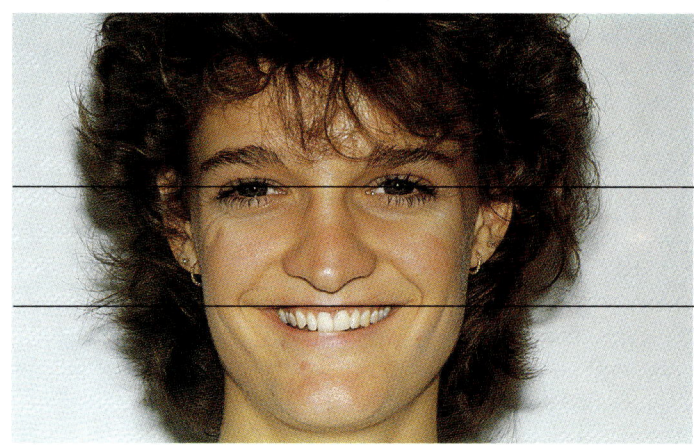

Fig 4-44 When attention is focused on the facial composition, the coincidence of commissural and pupillary lines becomes a prerequisite for the esthetic appraisal of the smile that seems unaffected by the asymmetry exhibited by the right and left anterior dental segments in the horizontal plane.

Structural Esthetic Rules

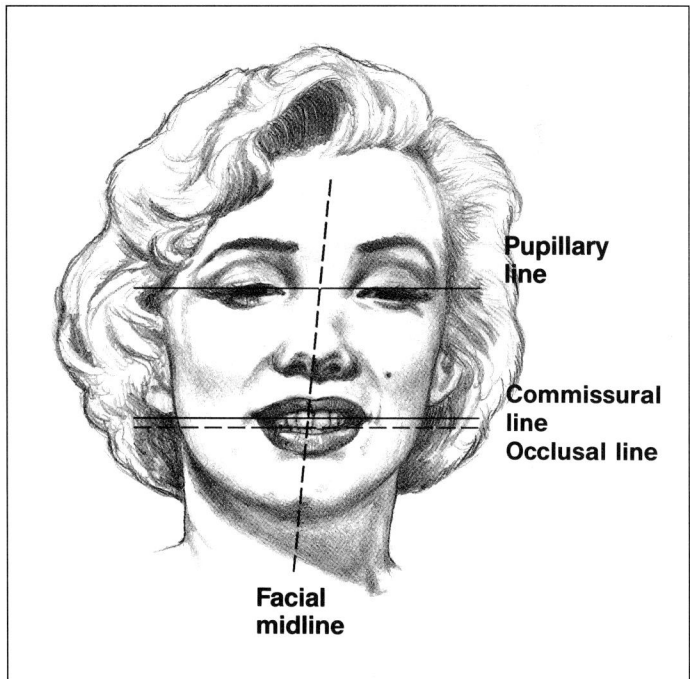

Fig 4-45 Illustration of the coincidence of pupillary and commissural lines, prerequisite requirements of smile attractiveness at this distance of focus. Smile and facial components must be evaluated by reference to facial factors.

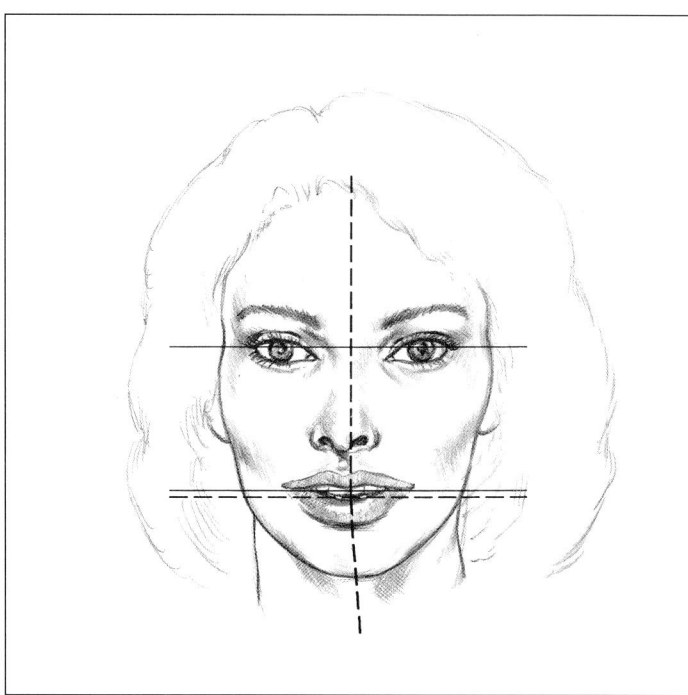

Fig 4-46 The esthetic integration of the smile in the facial composition appears unaffected by the directional variation of the facial midline but requires the presence of cohesive forces, illustrated by the coincidence of pupillary and commissural lines and subsequently by that of the occlusal line.

In viewing the dentofacial composition, the need for a coincidence between the commissural line and the line running from the tip of a cuspid to the other, which will be named occlusal line or occlusal plane, can be demonstrated (Fig 4-43). From a distance enabling the perception of the facial composition, observation will show the progressive importance of the parallelism of lines that must exist between the corners of the mouth or commissural line and the occlusal line (Fig 4-44). This infers that in smiling the placement of the corners of the mouth should conform to a succession of parallel lines, cohesive forces assuring the esthetic strength of the facial or dentofacial composition (Figs 4-45 to 4-48). The central midline, hypothetical or imposed by the nature of the elements constituting the facial or dentofacial composition, crosses this succession of lines, ensuring the presence of segregative forces, a prerequisite for esthetic appraisal. The esthetic evaluation of smile symmetry relies on the unconscious perception of the involved crossing joint.

Occlusal line or occlusal frontal plane

In today's dentistry our field of vision is restricted by the miniaturization of restorative procedures and is hampered by the use of protective material and by the constraints of our working position. For the majority of professionals the perception of lines is limited to those that are part of the dental composition (Figs 4-49 and

Facial components

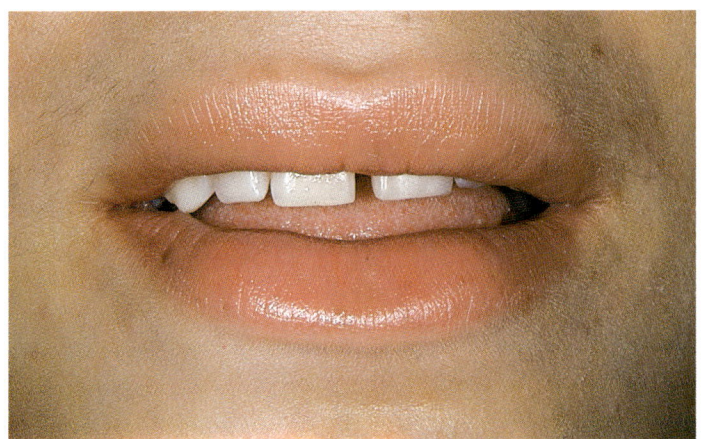

Fig 4-47 At first glance this noncoincidence of commissural and occlusal lines results from tongue parafunctional interference. A more precise examination of the facial composition evidences noncoordinate retraction and elevation of the mouth corners during the smile process, leaving the left side of the mouth in a lower position. The dental composition illustrates a type of individual dominance. (See Figs 1-53 and 1-54.)

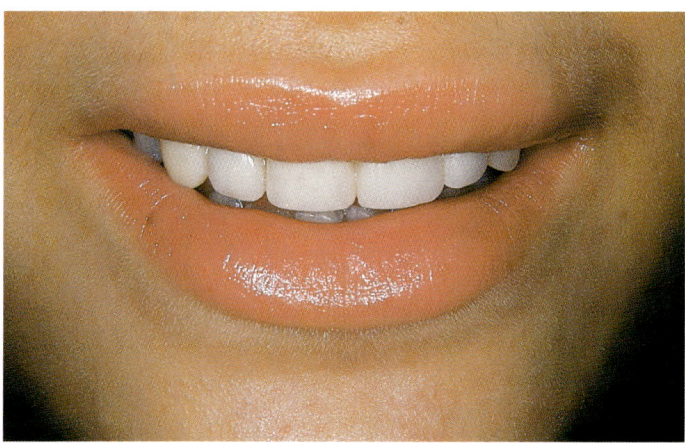

Fig 4-48 Treatment techniques have focused on the control of the parafunctional tongue habits and on a coordinated muscular development of the smile. Restoration was carried out taking into consideration the restoration of line coincidence to ensure esthetic strength of the composition. After restoration, the dental composition exhibits a segmental dominance, stressed by the color change, reflecting segregative forces that approach a level of interference even if it conforms to the patient's desires.

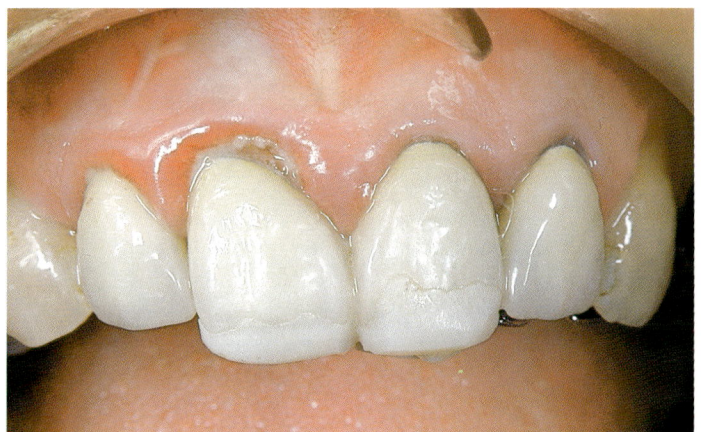

Fig 4-49 At a usual working distance, visual perception evaluates the coincidence or noncoincidence that may exist between the occlusal line and other hypothetical lines drawn in the oral cavity, cohesive forces assuring the esthetic strength of the composition. Attracted by segregative forces beyond the level of tolerance, this evaluation does not take place.

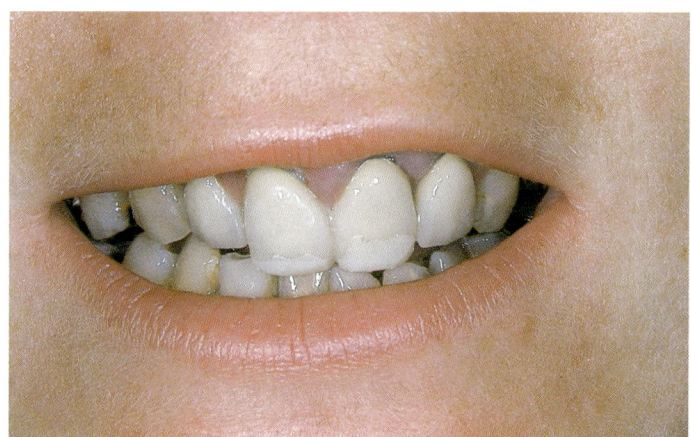

Fig 4-50 The visualization of the dentofacial composition reinforces the necessary coincidence of the occlusal and commissural lines. By reason of the substitution of the incisal line for the occlusal line this coincidence of lines is not perceived.

Structural Esthetic Rules

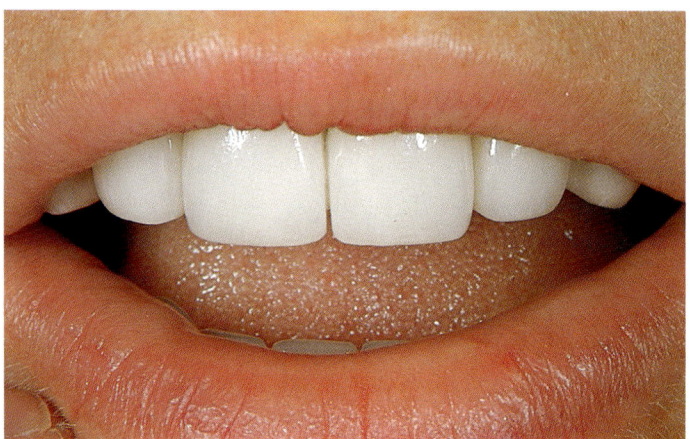

Fig 4-51 The restoration of the coincidence of the commissural and occlusal lines, cohesive forces of a composition, strengthens the composition. At any level of mouth opening or smile, this coincidence should be extended to the lower dental composition. Here muscle retraining techniques should help correct the still existing deficiencies.

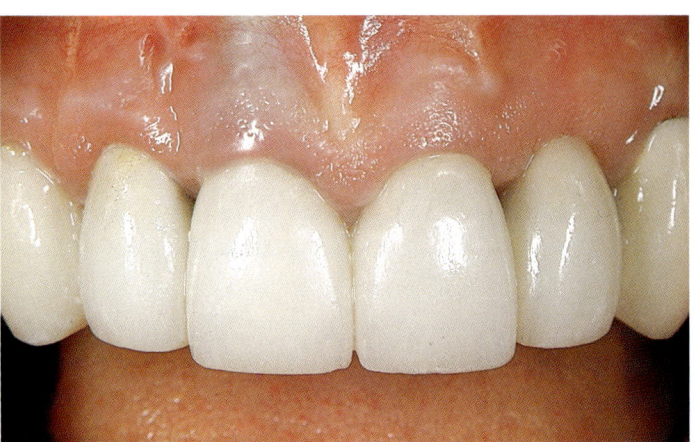

Fig 4-52 Restoration of the coincidence of the occlusal and gingival lines, running along the zenith of the canine and lateral incisors. (Root bleaching has been limited to the marginal area.)

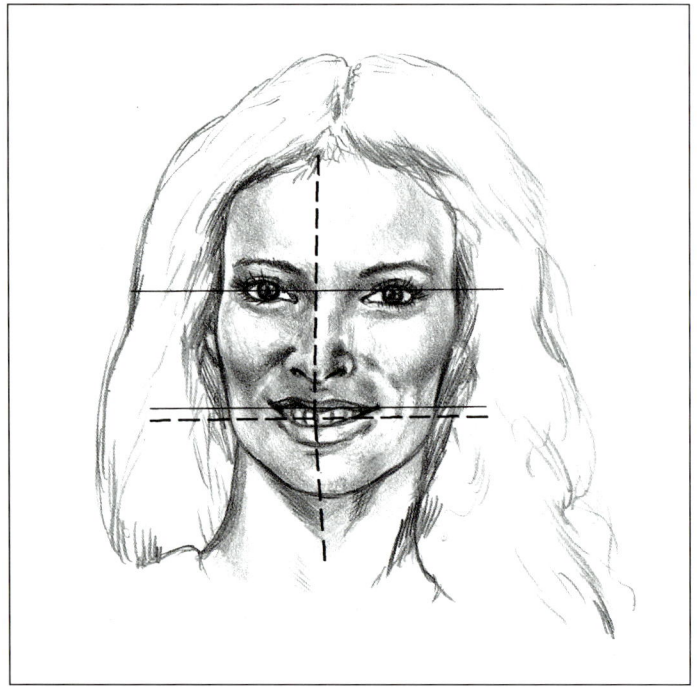

Fig 4-53 The esthetic connotation of a smile is usually seen as a succession of coincidental lines, cohesive forces characterizing the dental, dentofacial, and facial composition.

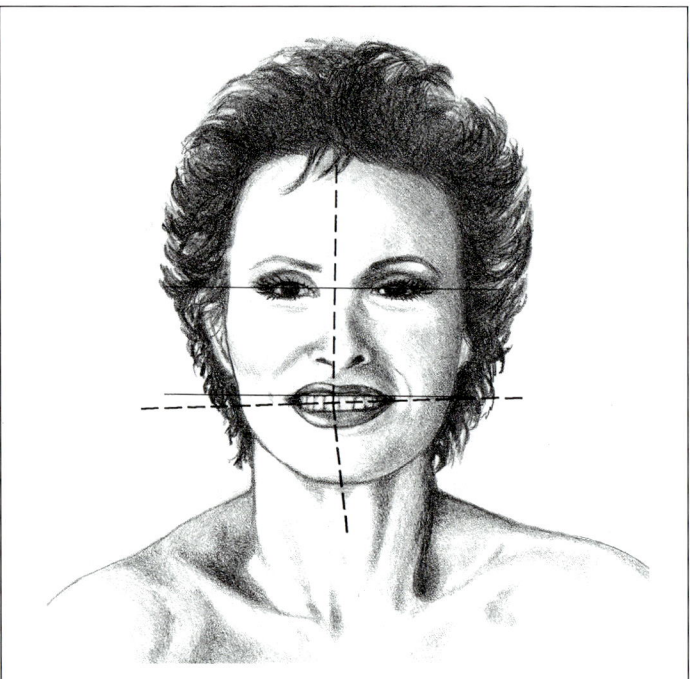

Fig 4-54 Whenever a divergence can be stated, not only is the esthetic strength of these cohesive forces greatly reduced but there is also evidence of a facial muscle or functional disturbance.

4-50). A noncoincidence of lines between the occlusal frontal line and the hypothetical gingival line running from the zenith of anterior teeth, usually from the right to the left canine, exhibiting an imbalance of shapes, should be perceived, but usually, the attention is focused on the occlusal line, delimiting the incisal silhouette and perceived by color contrast with the anterior negative space. This characteristic has been widely reproduced by magazines and underlined by caricaturists to the point that this image of a straight incisal line has been adopted by the public as a standard of dental esthetics. This stresses the differences existing between professional and public perception of the particularities of dental composition.

Instead of fighting against this distortion of reality, when restoring details of the anterior dental segment, one must understand and make understood that these differences of perception simply originate from different distances of focus. The observation will stress the fact that this occlusal line can be visualized as being part of the dental, dentofacial, and facial composition, which tends to explain the importance attributed to it. From the viewpoint of esthetic analysis, this occlusal line, underlined by the segregative forces of the negative space, takes part in a system of coinciding lines, cohesive forces, the multiplicity of which assures the esthetic strength of the composition (Figs 4-51 to 4-53). Whenever this system loses cohesion, careful examination may often evidence disturbances or pathologies showing the link between function and esthetic (Fig 4-54).

The perfect smile

According to these statements a perfect smile is characterized by a middle tooth–lip line relationship, an incisal line running against the upper border of the lower lip, and an upper lip presenting an upward curvature. The mouth corners are symmetrically aligned to the pupillary line and leave a proportionate bilateral negative space. When it contains and is surrounded by dental and facial elements that conform to fundamental esthetic principles, it may reach another level of appreciation if their harmonious integration into the individual's morphopsychologic profile generates an emotional psychologic reaction.

Dental components

Dental midline

The problem of the placement of the dental midline, an imaginary vertical line that separates the two central incisors and a prerequisite for the restoration of the anterior edentulous area, has been mentioned when dealing with smile symmetry. Nevertheless, some clarification seems necessary because the literature that deals with this question reveals a real division of thought. Recommendations include the following:

1. Place this midline precisely in the facial midline or in the middle of the mouth using the lingual papilla or the labial frenum as landmarks.[17]
2. Never establish it in the precise midline because it may contribute to an artificial appearance.[18]

Research has statistically demonstrated, using the lip philtrum as a reference guide, that the maxillary midline coincided precisely with the facial midline in 70% of cases and that esthetics was not compromised by a slight deviation from the central midline. The same study revealed that maxillary and mandibular midlines failed to coincide in 75% of cases. This definitely means that the lower midline should not be regarded as a reference for the placement of the maxillary midline[19] when dealing with the restoration of the anterior edentulous areas.

Although a facial composition may give the general feeling of symmetry, it is well known that variations between both sides of the face exist, and when mirror images of one side are placed together, an entirely new face is created that tends to look artificial[20] because the subtle differences in shape, lines, and color have been eliminated and with them the basic elements of sublimation that nature most often engenders. This may give credit to those who believe that a precise midline placement may contribute to an artificial appearance.

The use of anatomic landmarks, or more specifically, the incisive papilla can contribute to an initial evaluation of the placement of the dental midline, and the observation confirms the reliability of this initial placement. One should keep in mind that both facial and dental midlines are the necessary vectors that enable esthetic appraisal through the perception of the parameters of symmetry and balance. By reason of the differences existing between the right and left side of the face, the

Structural Esthetic Rules

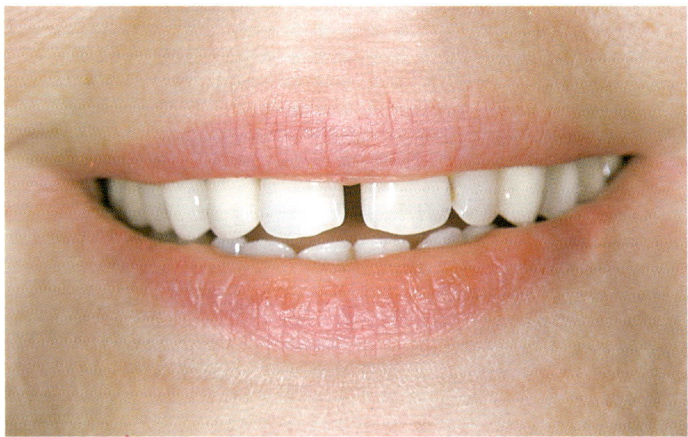

Fig 4-55 A large diastema establishes a strong central midline, the location of which in the center of the smile is needed to avoid visual tension. Esthetic appraisal is evaluated according to the principle of symmetry.

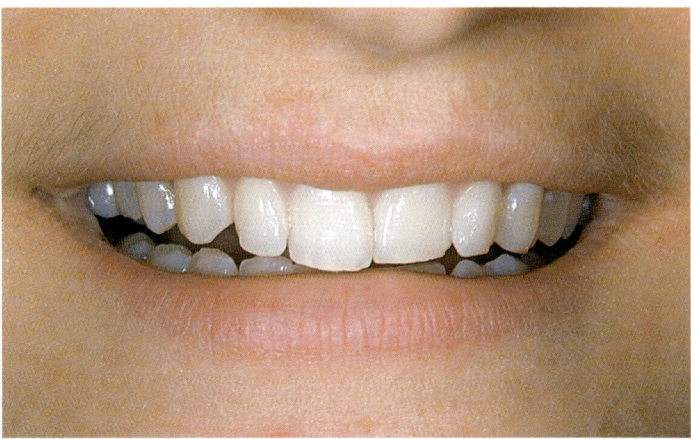

Fig 4-56 When the central midline does not coincide with the center of the smile, esthetic equilibrium may be achieved by the balance of lines, of size and the amount of light reflecting from the right and left anterior segments. It can be observed how the lower lip stresses the position of the hypothetical midline.

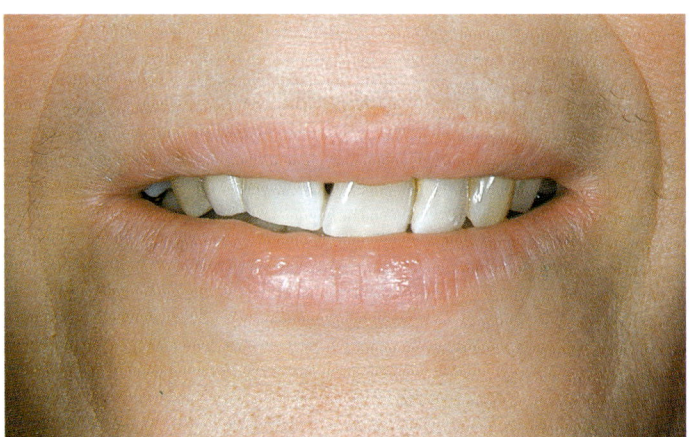

Fig 4-57 Both central incisors diverge from hypothetical midline drawn perpendicular to the commissural line, inducing imbalance of the lines. This factor generates esthetic reproval.

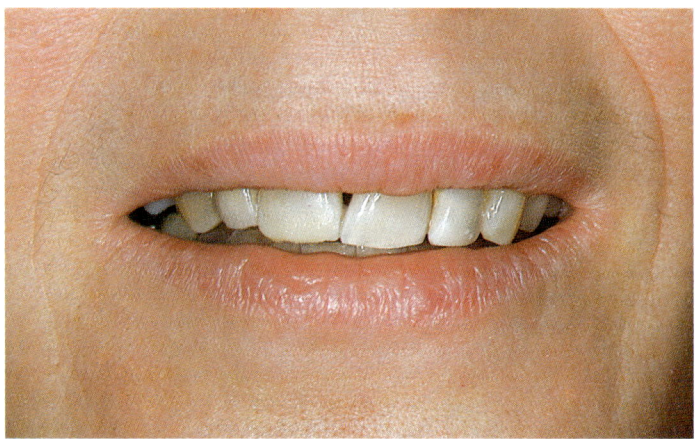

Fig 4-58 This improvement of axial line equilibrium, by shortening the left lateral incisor and lengthening the right central incisor, took place during esthetic evaluation. It restored the axial direction of the central midline.

facial midline is far from providing a precise geometrical division.

This may explain the variables stated in the definition of this parameter:

1. Vertical line drawn through the forehead, nose columella, dental midline, and chin.[21]
2. Imaginary line that runs vertically from the nasion, subnasal point, interincisal point, and pogonion.[22]

Although both definitions include the coincidence of dental and facial midlines, the relationships of which have been suggested as having a definite influence on the harmony of the dental composition,[23] one should point out that the visualization of this coincidence, requiring various degrees of smile or mouth opening, is only hypothetical, keeping in mind that the dental midline can hardly be perceived at the distance from which facial composition can be evaluated.

Part of the dentofacial composition, the dental midline, is best visualized in the dynamics of the smile. It should logically be placed in its center. It is important that the coincidence of the dental midline with the precise midline of the smile be determined by the nature of the symmetry exhibited by the dental composition. An anterior diastema or a marked radiating symmetry determines the placement of this midline, tending to induce visual tension when placed off the center of the smile unless equilibrium required by the phenomenon of balance is affected by the visualization of equal right and left dental segments (Figs 4-55 and 4-56). This explains why when placed off the precise center of the philtrum, the dental midline does not often induce visual tension.

What becomes important is the fact that the predominant cohesive forces, commissural, occlusal, and pupillary lines determine the perpendicular direction of segregative forces, precisely illustrated by the dental midline and the dental elements related to it. Deviations affecting these elements can hardly be compensated for by the phenomenon of balance and will create strong visual tension (Figs 4-57 and 4-58).

Golden rules

The definition of the laws of beauty and harmony has been a constant preoccupation of Greek philosophers and mathematicians. The connection of beauty with numerical values conforms to the philosophy that beauty always appears as fundamentally exact. The finding of an intriguing relationship in the harmony between two parts, which can be described as follows, has been attributed to Pythagoras: The smaller to the larger is equal to the sum of the whole related to the larger (Fig 4-59).

$$\frac{S}{L} = \frac{L}{S+L} = \frac{2}{1+\sqrt{5}} = 0.618$$

Fig 4-59 Mathematical formula of the golden proportion.

Ever since its formulation in antiquity, this number, called the "golden number" or "golden section," has attracted the attention of mystics, artists, and scientists. Johannes Keppler (1611) saw in this golden section "an idea used by the Creator to generate the similar from the similar," and its esthetical value was stressed by Luca Pacioli[24] in his book *Divine Proportione* (1509) illustrated by Leonardo da Vinci. The extension of the study of the golden number from its linear form to the surface form is attributed to Hambridge,[25] and more recently Le Corbusier[26] developed a scale based on the golden proportions of the human body that he intended to integrate in a dimensional living space in accordance with its movements and positions. Harmony in proportion has been defined as an esthetic principle, part of the essential beauty. When considering the size and design of natural elements,[27] we must always keep proportion in mind because this golden relationship has been demonstrated in organic forms of nature and in animal and human forms.[28,29]

The reason that elements perceived through the division of this golden number are different from any other

Structural Esthetic Rules

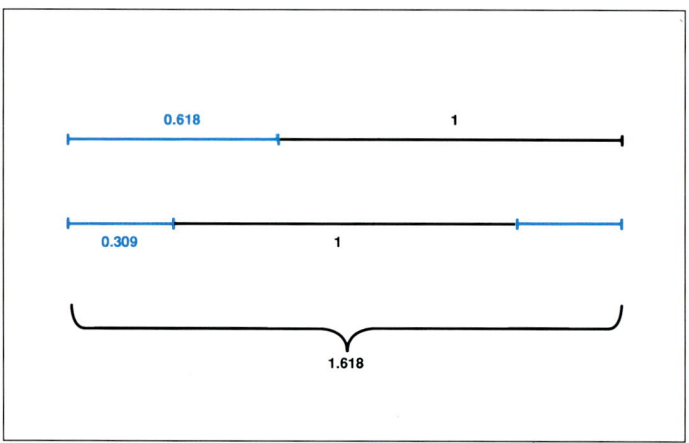

Fig 4-60 Linear golden section and golden bilateral form.

Fig 4-61 Angular representation of the golden proportion.

proportion, and what these differences are, have been demonstrated mathematically.

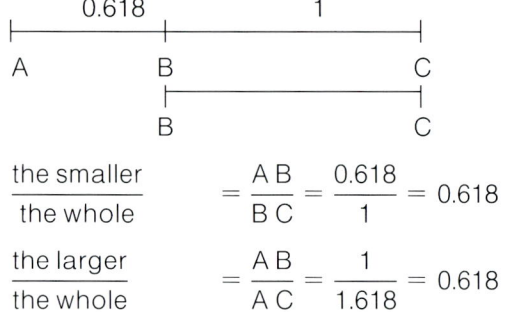

if AC is divided by B into two inequal parts

$$\frac{\text{the smaller}}{\text{the larger}} = \frac{AB}{BC} = \frac{2}{5} = 0.4$$

$$\frac{\text{the larger}}{\text{the whole}} = \frac{BC}{AC} = \frac{5}{7} = 0.71$$

The results of these equations are different, whereas the results of the equations that use the golden number as surface or line division are equal.

$$\frac{\text{the smaller}}{\text{the whole}} = \frac{AB}{BC} = \frac{0.618}{1} = 0.618$$

$$\frac{\text{the larger}}{\text{the whole}} = \frac{AB}{AC} = \frac{1}{1.618} = 0.618$$

This tends to prove mathematically that any line divided in the golden proportion is in equilibrium around the point of division.

Linear progressions and surface division by this same number are common in nature[30] both geometrically and arithmetically.

Geometric progressions can be obtained by multiplying each term by 1.618 or dividing by 0.618:

1.000 × 1.618 = 1.618   1.000/0.618 = 1.618
1.618 × 1.618 = 2.618   1.618/0.618 = 2.618
2.618 × 1.618 = 4.236   2.618/0.618 = 4.236

In the arithmetic progression each term is the sum of the preceding two terms:

0.618 + 1.000 = 1.618
1.000 + 1.618 = 2.618
1.618 + 2.618 = 4.236

It can therefore be stated that the progression using the golden number is unique because three different methods produced the same result.

This mathematical concept can be applied to geometrical calculations with real satisfaction. However, its strict and unsophisticated application to organic figures is not evident and the concurrence is never perfect. This explains why some considered it necessary to distinguish

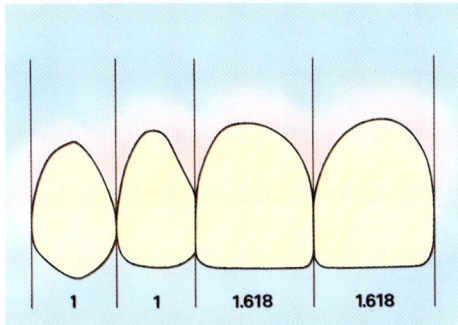 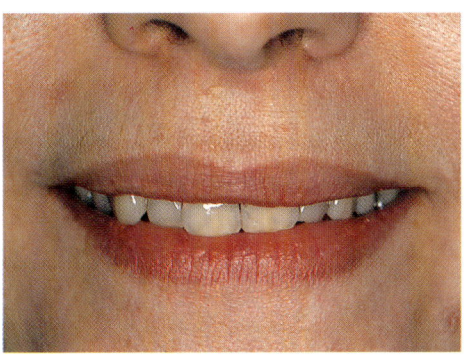 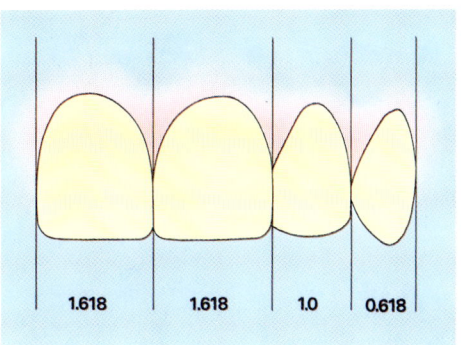

Fig 4-62 Although a golden relationship between central and lateral incisors can be observed, the type of proportion existing between lateral incisor and canine disturbs the anterior dental arrangement.

Fig 4-63 Clinical illustration of the adjacent diagrams. The equilibrium of this tooth arrangement is disturbed by the poor relationship existing between the right lateral incisor and the canine visualized in its full width.

Fig 4-64 The golden proportional relationship existing between the elements of the anterior segment produces a steady impression of harmony.

between "constructive systems" acting in graphic designs and "objective systems" in regard to living forms.[31] Philosophically, it seems easier to consider that this numerical value simply tends to point out a quality of information for esthetic appraisal. Yet, studies and experiments[32] have amply demonstrated that this surface division, sensed by the eye, independently from ethnic or civilization factors, creates an esthetic appeal.

Our attention must be focused not only on the simple manifestations of this golden section but on the subtle and fascinating variations that nature exhibits (Figs 4-60 and 4-61). Among them the most common, the bilateral form, can be easily described.

The application of the golden number to dentistry was first mentioned by Lombardi[33] and developed by Levin,[34] and today a number of parameters that conform to this golden number can be considered elements that participate in the structural or biologic beauty of the dentofacial composition and can be systematically applied in rehabilitations.

Using calipers that invariably open at a constant golden proportion between the larger and the smaller parts, Levin[34] observed that in esthetically pleasing dentitions, viewed from the front, the width of the central incisor is in the golden proportion to the width of the lateral incisor, which in its turn is in the golden proportion to the anterior part of the canine. "The width of the incisors is in the golden proportion to the others as seen from the front"[34] (Figs 4-62 to 4-64). He further demonstrated that the lateral negative space, the area of darkness that appears between the anterior segment of the teeth and the corner of the mouth in smiling, is in the golden proportion to one half the width of this anterior segment.

From these observations he developed a grid to test the validity of this statement. In this grid, central incisors are quoted within a large range of widths (between 7 and 10 mm) and the outer part of the esthetic segment has been fixed according to the most prominent tooth that outlines the corner of the mouth, either the canine or the first premolar (Figs 4-65 and 4-66).

The use of this grid is designed to help the prosthodontist detect what is esthetically wrong in the anterior proportional relationship (Figs 4-67 and 4-68) and to serve as a training aid for visual appreciation.

In considering the number of biometric studies predominantly aimed at finding numerical correlations among dental and facial elements, the low rate of satisfactory results is clear. It suggests that in this matter, qualitative and quantitative relationships specific to any individual can induce esthetic evaluation (Fig 4-69). Their determination is based on the "esthetic sense" and result from constant, conscious, or unconscious training and relies heavily on proportions. The challenge is the esthetic integration of the dental element and dental composition in its environment, whatever the distance focused on by the viewer (Figs 4-70 to 4-72).

Structural Esthetic Rules

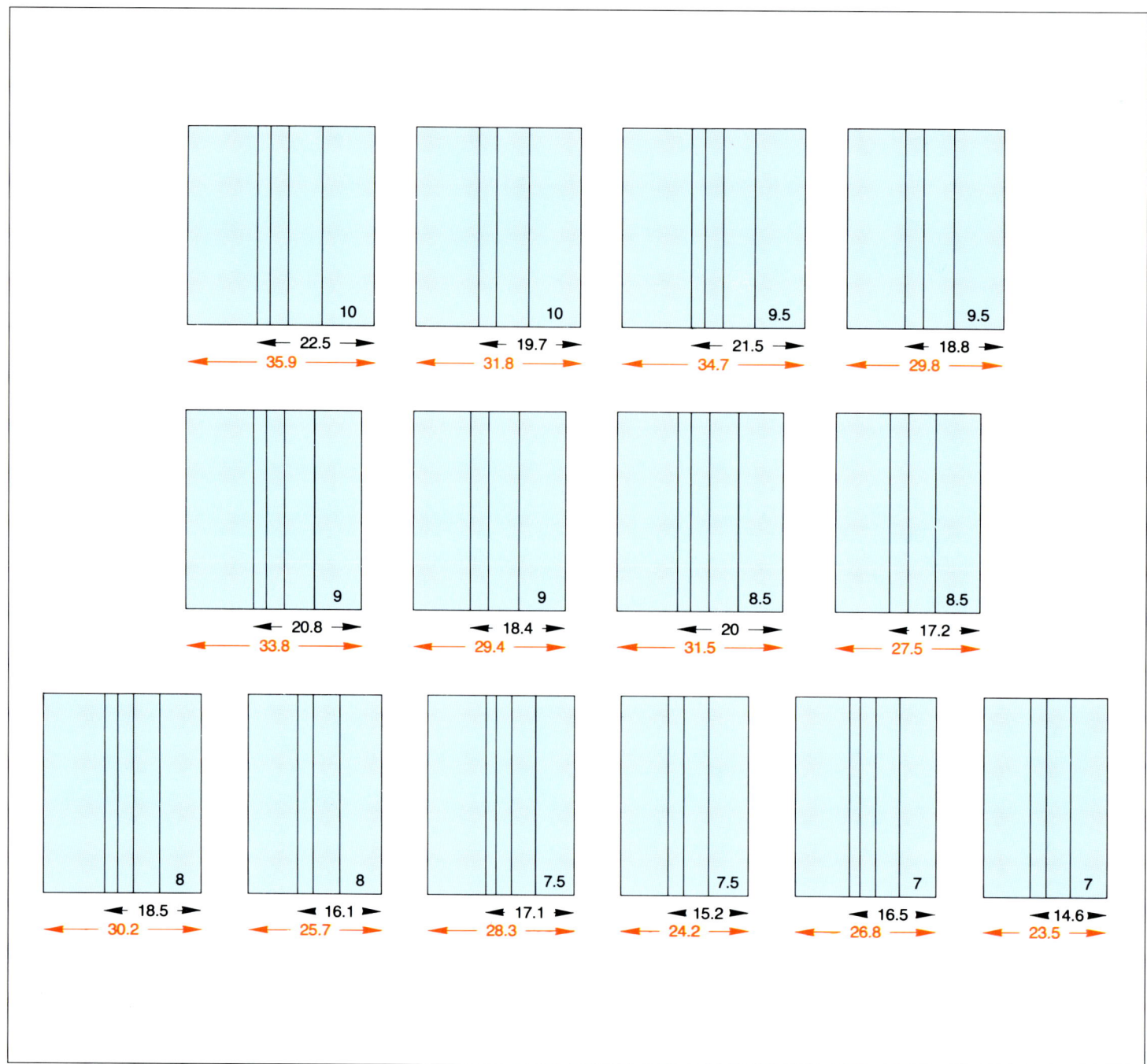

Fig 4-65 Grid of the golden proportional relationships existing among the elements of the anterior dental segment showing three or four teeth when smiling by reference to a determined width of the maxillary central incisor. (Courtesy of E. Levin.)

Width of half the anterior segment showing four teeth	Half width of smile (four teeth)	Width of maxillary central incisor	Half width of smile (three teeth)	Width of half the anterior segment showing three teeth
16.5	26.8	7	23.5	14.6
17.1	28.3	7.5	24.2	12.2
18.5	30.2	8	25.7	16.1
20	31.5	8.5	27.5	17.2
10.8	33.8	9	29.5	18.4
21.5	34.7	9.5	29.8	18.8
22.5	35.9	10	31.8	19.7

Fig 4-66 Method of application of the grid. With a determined width of the maxillary central incisor, the width of the visible part of the anterior segment showing either three or four teeth has been calculated according to the proportional relationships that have to exist with one half the width of the smile. (Courtesy of E. Levin.)

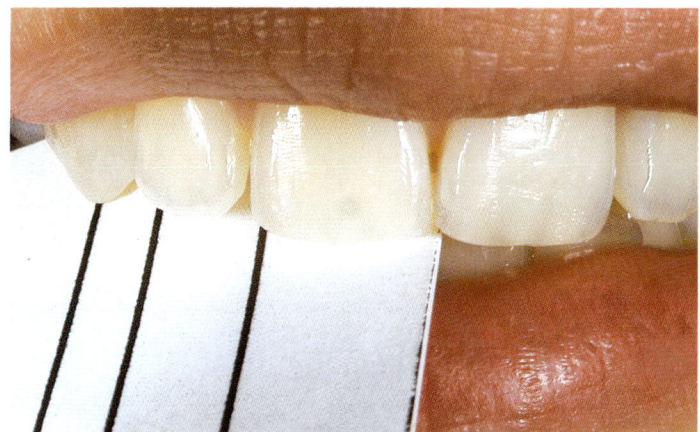

Fig 4-67 Demonstration of the clinical application of the grid. The anterior teeth are in a golden relationship.

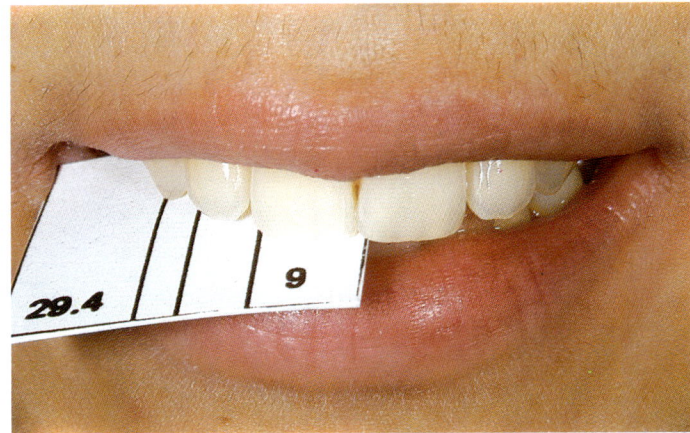

Fig 4-68 Demonstration of the clinical application of the grid. The lateral negative space is in a golden relationship with one half the width of the anterior segment.

Structural Esthetic Rules

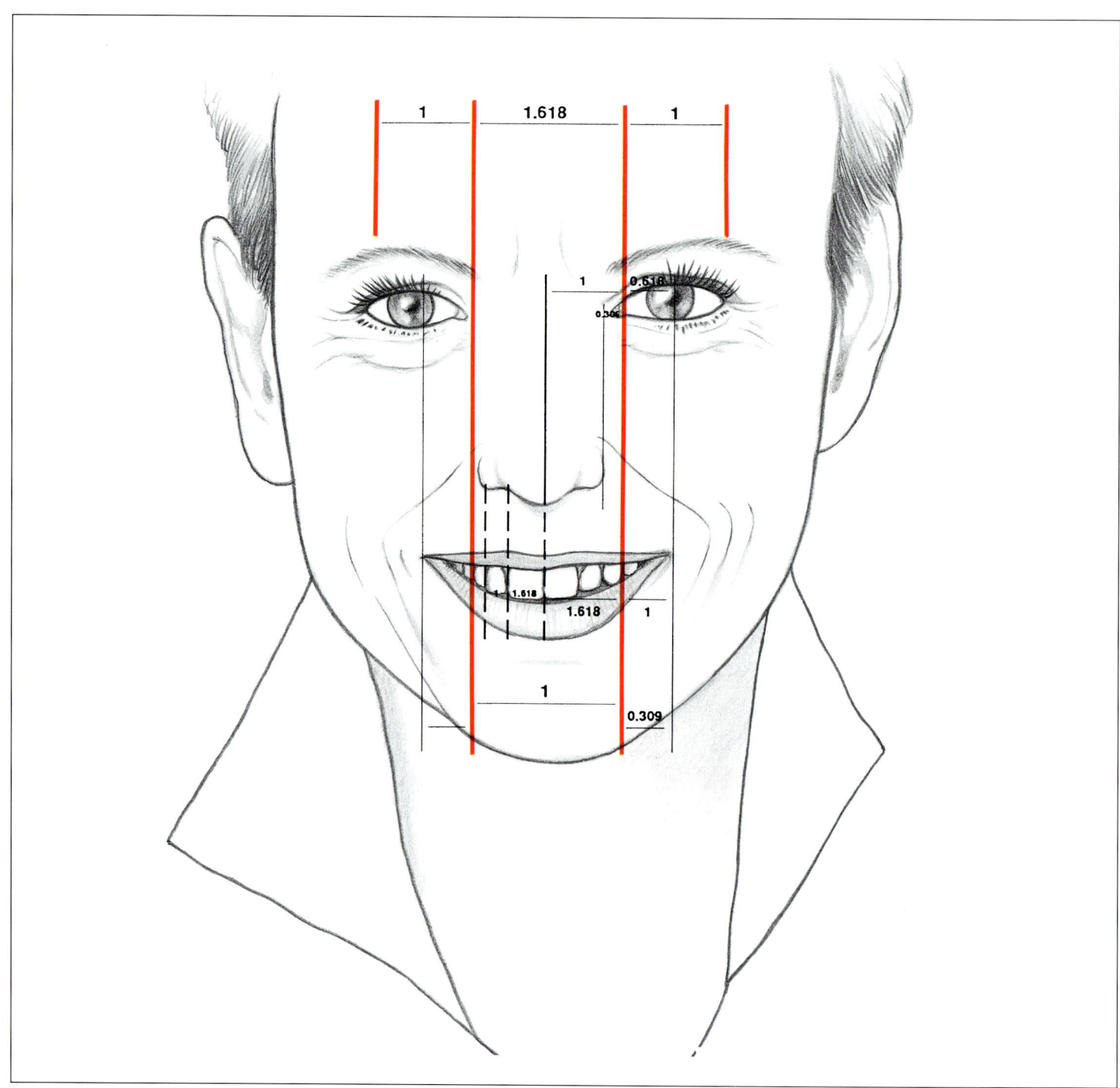

Fig 4-69 Dental, dentofacial, and facial compositions contain a variety of relationships that can be evaluated according to the golden proportion in its linear and bilateral values and the variety of geometric forms. Facial proportions can be different from one individual to another. Proportionate relationships provide a qualitative value of esthetic appraisal.

Dental components

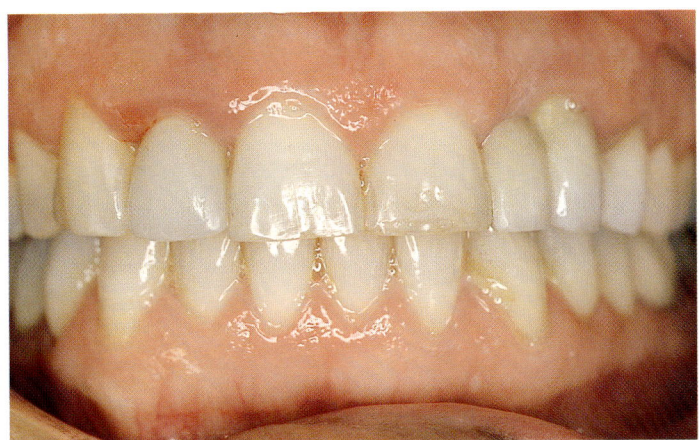

Fig 4-70 A wide right lateral incisor and a narrow left lateral pontic wedged between adjacent teeth have resulted in this inharmonious anterior relationship. Treatment will consist in restoring harmonious proportions.

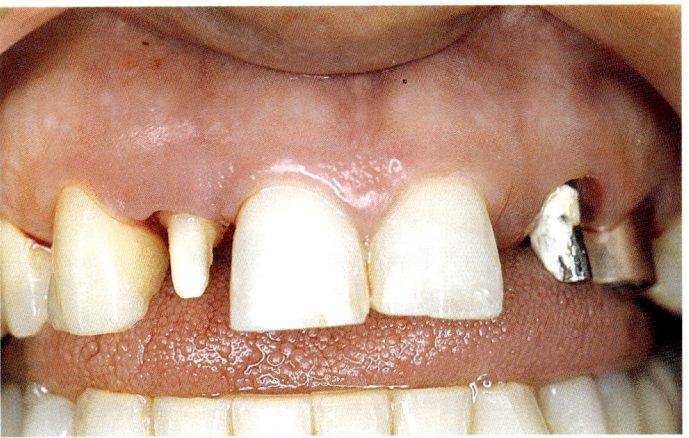

Fig 4-71 The central incisors have been moved orthodontically to the right, permitting a reduction in the size of the right lateral incisor and an increase in the size of the left lateral pontic.

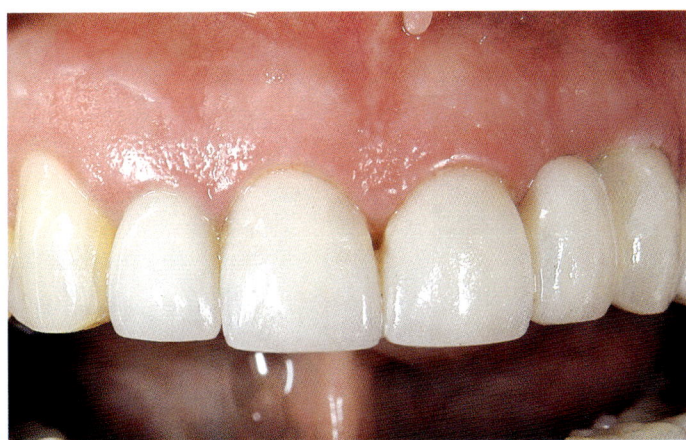

Fig 4-72 As a result of the patient's requests to save as much tooth structure as possible, the central incisors received veneer facets of a metal-free porcelain fixed partial denture. Optical illusive effects have been used to compensate for the still existing proportional discrepancies.

Structural Esthetic Rules

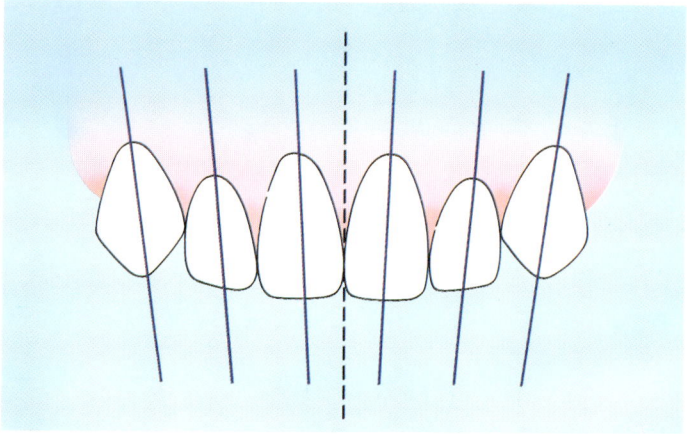

Fig 4-73 Axial alignment of the anterior segment. The general mesial inclination tends to be more pronounced from the central incisors to the canines. Equilibrium is realized around the central fulcrum.

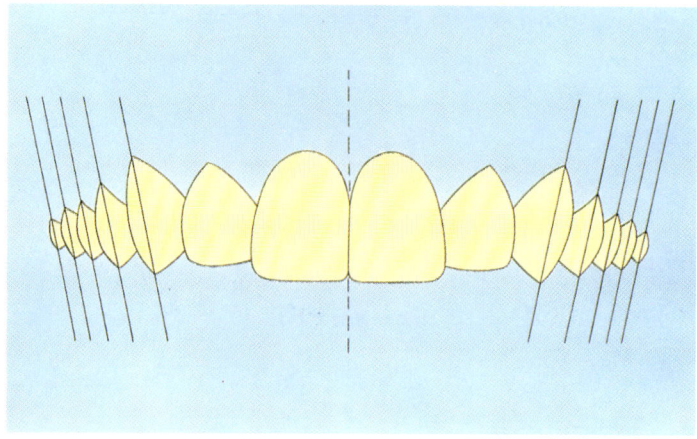

Fig 4-74 The bilateral axial alignment of the teeth of the posterior segment responds to the phenomenon of balance of lines around a central fulcrum.

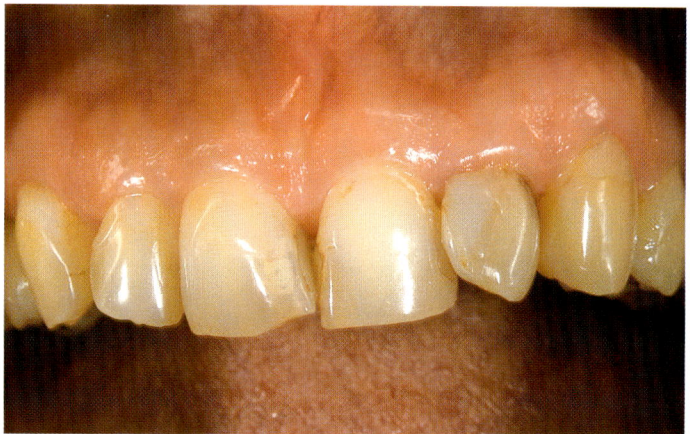

Fig 4-75 The mesial axial inclination of anterior teeth is not respected and a balance of axial lines can hardly be realized around the central fulcrum. Visual tension is increased by an imbalance of shape, affecting the left lateral incisor.

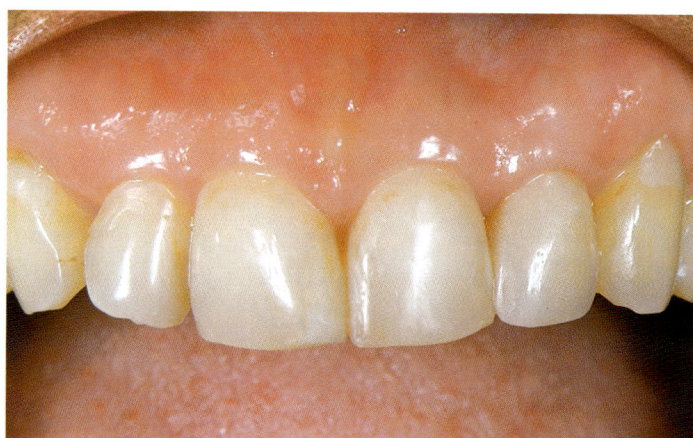

Fig 4-76 An improvement of the equilibrium of axial tooth inclination, achieved with limited restorative procedures and the correction of the imbalance of shape of the left lateral incisor, has produced an interesting and personalized dental composition.

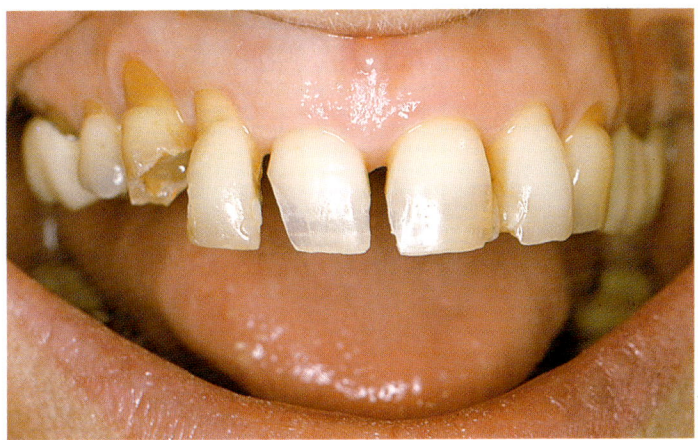

Fig 4-77 Occlusal disturbances have produced the progressive flare of anterior teeth with sufficient stress to break an existing acrylic resin splint.

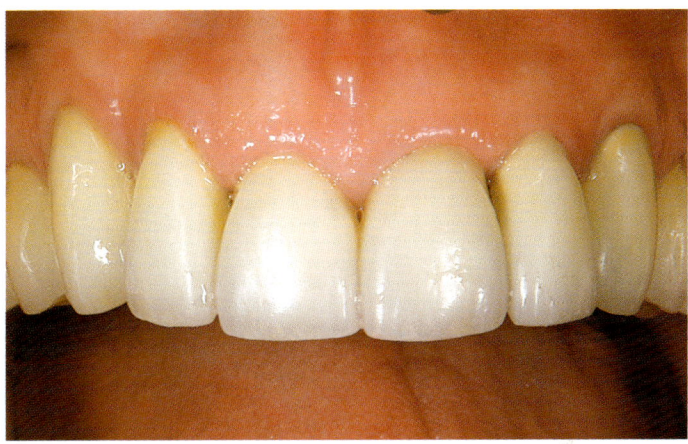

Fig 4-78 The restoration of the anterior segment still reflects esthetic instability. The imbalance of axial lines due to the position of the left lateral incisor suggests the necessity for splinting. Esthetic and function may be submitted to the same requirements.

Axial alignment

The direction of anterior teeth in relation to the central vertical midline has been determined by the observation of photographs and study models. It is generally accepted and acknowledged that superior anterior teeth present (or should present to the frontal perception) an incisal inclination that becomes progressively more pronounced from the central incisors to the canine[35–37] (Fig 4-73). The canine's inclination can be explained by the fact that canines are perceived through their mesial surface outlined by the curvature of the buccal middle and incisal outer inclines and the apically directed mesioincisal edge, which invariably gives to this tooth a greater or lesser mesial inclination.

Posterior teeth from the first premolar to the first or second molar are perceived in a similar fashion. This perception is not affected by the decrease in visibility, so that smiling elements of both posterior segments, right and left, exhibit a general mesial inclination (Fig 4-74). In this frontal perception, the central vertical midline serves as a fulcrum in a phenomenon of a balance of lines, materialized by the perception of tooth inclination. If we refer to the observation of natural dentition, we notice a wide range of deviation from this standard axial incisal inclination (Fig 4-75). In the presence of moderate and pleasing axial deviation, these inclinations most often singularize and enhance the personality, provided an equilibrium or a balance of lines has been achieved around the central fulcrum (Fig 4-76). There is a direct relationship between the pleasing effect that these smiles can generate and the equilibrium in the balance of lines of tooth inclination. A distally inclined lateral incisor should be compensated by a slight increase in the inclination of the canine or premolars on the opposite side. In the principle of balance, the "weight" of elements far away from the fulcrum grows in importance. Deviations beyond a certain degree of equilibrium are invariably rated as unattractive and must be corrected accordingly. Also, when equilibrium of axial tooth inclination has not been achieved in the dental composition, the resulting visual tension may also point out a possible factor of occlusal instability[38] (Figs 4-77 and 4-78). Even if the exact surface upon which the field of forces relative to this fundamental esthetic principle takes place has yet to be drawn, its determination should certainly throw light on the obscure reasons why divergent teeth invariably create visual tension (Figs 4-79 and 4-80) and psychologic refusal.

Structural Esthetic Rules

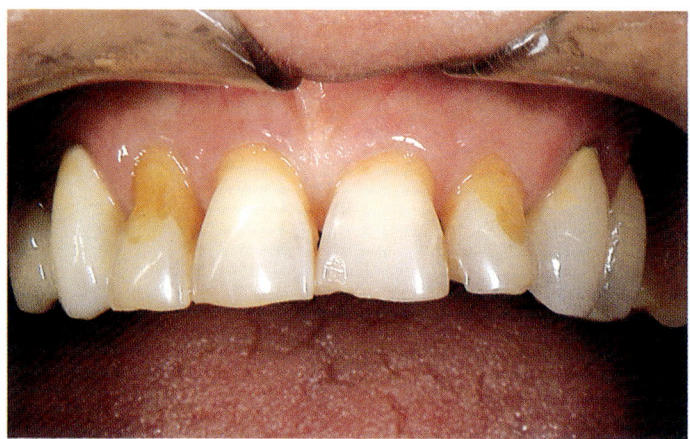

Fig 4-79 Although flaring or divergent teeth may well reach an equilibrium according to the principle of balance of lines, they still generate visual tension. This type of composition looks instable, interfering with the field of forces that are present in the structure of the mouth.

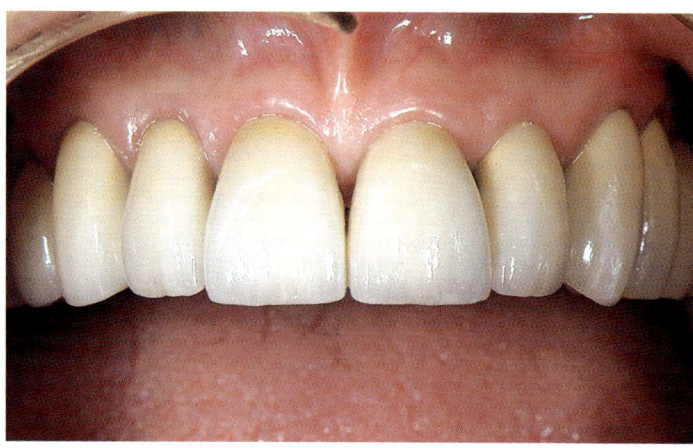

Fig 4-80 The restoration of proper axial alignment of anterior teeth and posterior teeth is prerequisite to providing esthetic equilibrium and occlusal stability.

Tooth arrangement

Anterior teeth, in achieving lip and associated muscle support, enable the fulfillment of esthetic, phonetic, and functional requirements. Following extraction, the choice for the correct placement of anterior teeth presents a number of difficulties that increase with the degree of edentulousness and crest resorption and create a number of problems for even the most experienced clinicians.

Tooth placement is usually obtained by three different methods: empirical, phonetic, and according to anatomic landmarks. The empirical approach can certainly be cited as the most commonly used. How many practitioners simply refer cases to the laboratory without any specific information, with the exception of reference to the shade guide, expecting the systematic placement of denture teeth on the existing crest according to the principles of dentistry and ignoring the principles of nature.

Phonetic methods have proved to be important means of determining vertical dimension[6,39] and provide an indication as to the placement of the central incisors, assuring naturalness in the dynamics of speech. Therefore, their use as a functional reference of the maxillary–mandibular anterior tooth relationship should be carried out throughout the entire process of any type of rehabilitation. However, anterior tooth placement, based on this method, needs appropriate refinement to reach esthetic satisfaction.

In an attempt to determine the original anterior tooth placement on the alveolar crest, most authors rely on anatomic landmarks, and there is general acknowledgment to refer to the position of the incisive papilla,[40] assuming that this could be a solid reference point, because its position has been observed to be little affected by bone resorption.[41]

It has been demonstrated that a line drawn from the tip of the canines invariably bisects the middle of the incisive papilla in 92% of the cases[42] (Fig 4-81) and, with the exception of some discordant voices, that the distance from the middle of the incisive papilla to the outer labial surface of the central incisor averages 10.2 mm.[43,44] Ortman et al[45] stated that from the posterior border of the incisive papilla this distance averages 12.454 mm (Fig 4-82) with a standard deviation of 3.867 mm. A similar statement was made in reference to

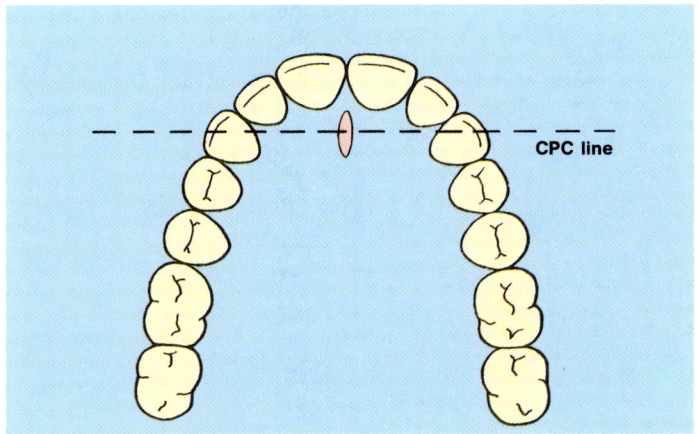 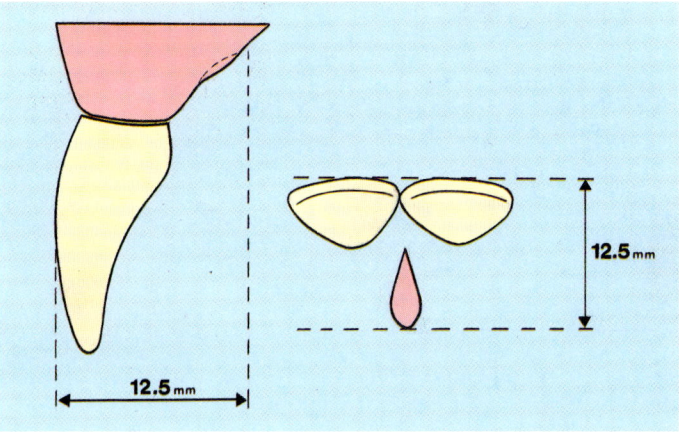

Fig 4-81 A line drawn from cusp tip to cusp tip of maxillary canines crosses the middle of the incisal papilla in 92% of the cases. Called the CPC line, it may serve to detect migrations or malpositions. The average distance from this line to the outer labial surface of the maxillary incisors has been evaluated at 10.2 mm.

Fig 4-82 The average distance from the posterior part of the incisal papilla to the outer labial surface of maxillary incisor averages 12.5 mm, with a standard deviation of 3.8 mm. The range of deviation assessed by other studies indicates the variability of the position of the maxillary central incisors.

the first palatal ruga, the end of which is located 1.5 to 2 mm from the lingual surface of the canine.[46]

These different statements, which can be considered reliable initial indications for anterior tooth placement, demonstrate that using average measurements as constant reference values is an error that, when ignored by technically oriented practitioners, violates the laws of nature. In using anatomic landmarks for initial tooth placement, we must constantly keep in mind these restrictions and be prepared to accommodate the requirements imposed by esthetic reevaluation.

Assuming that these anatomic landmarks can be considered as relatively stable points of reference, clinicians have evaluated the arch of circle on which the teeth lie.[44,47] They have even proposed devices for predicting the parabolic dimension of the anterior arch, adopting a predetermined concept of arch form.

If one visits any dental laboratory specialized in prosthodontics, one will notice that dentures invariably exhibit an ovoid or parabolic anterior arch form, which corresponds to a general acknowledgment of the ideal in anterior arch form, both by professionals and nonprofessionals. However, the methodical and unconscious application of this approach and the blind alignment of anterior teeth along this parabolic line may generate disappointment in the esthetic results of rehabilitations.[6]

It is true that a curved line can be traced from the labial outline of anterior teeth, but the invariability of its ideal parabolic shape should be adapted to precisely conform to nature or reality. The individual variations of the arch form have been arbitrarily classified into square, ovoid, and tapered, with the multitude of intermediate combinations that nature endows.[48] The study related to the CPC line[45] was done in reference to 507 models and concluded that two thirds of the models could be considered square, followed by the tapered and ovoid arch forms. This again strongly contrasts with the universality given to the ovoid arch form. It appears that tooth placement on a hypothetical preexisting or restored dental arch is the basis for restoration of dentofacial harmony and that each type of arch form assumes a certain type of tooth position. This implies that anterior teeth must be positioned according to the degree of tolerance permitted by the arch form to assure the integration of the dental composition (Figs 4-83 to 4-85).

Structural Esthetic Rules

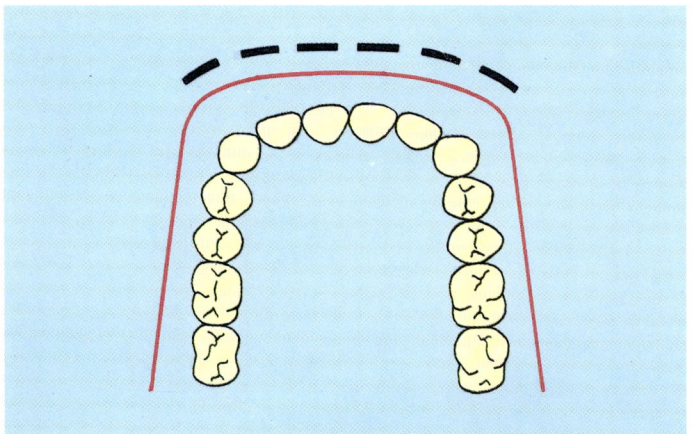

Fig 4-83 Square dental arch. In the square dental arch, the maxillary incisors assume a position almost in line with the canines. The four maxillary incisors are usually positioned without rotation or overlap. This tooth position ensures excellent light reflection and the dental arch appears wider and lighter in color.

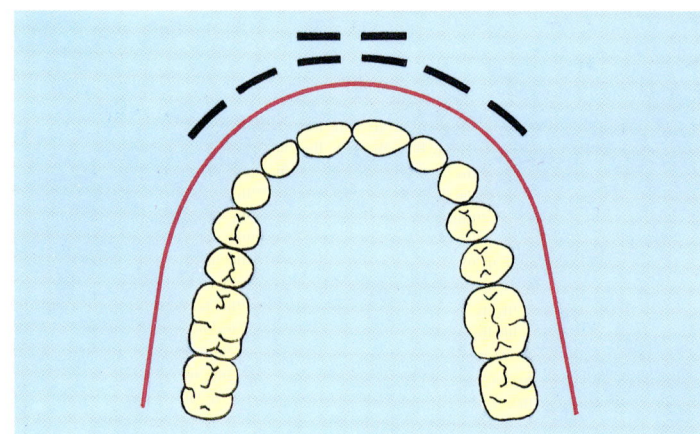

Fig 4-84 Ovoid dental arch. In this type of arch form, central incisors appear along or across the curvature of the arch, whereas lateral incisors and canines are aligned along the curvature. Rotations are unusual.

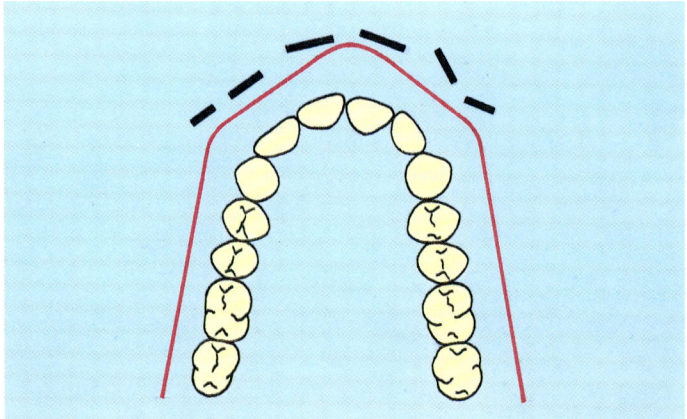

Fig 4-85 Tapered dental arch. This type of arch form shows the greatest variety in tooth position, from the central incisors that are generally found in a V-shape to the other anterior teeth that exhibit marked rotations or overlaps.

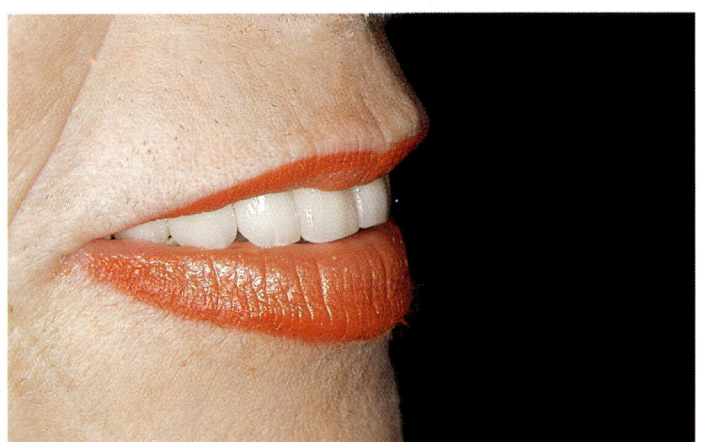 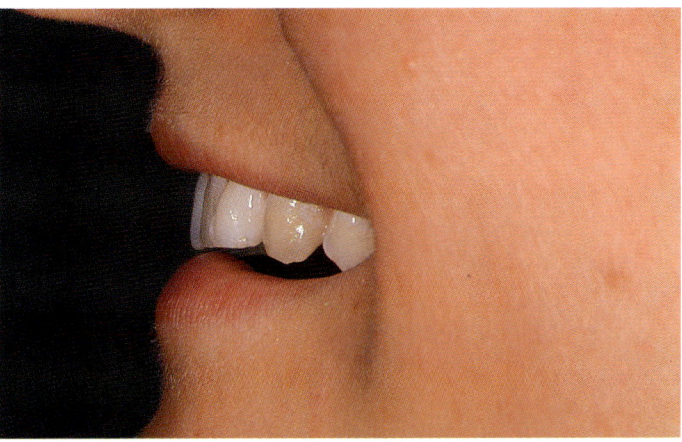

Fig 4-86　Individual exhibiting a bimaxillary protraction[51] and an anterior tooth inclination that conforms to this mouth shape. Note the position of the incisal edges of the maxillary central incisors relative to the lip in the dynamics of the development of the smile.

Fig 4-87　The retraction of both upper and lower maxillaries is accompanied by a less pronounced tooth inclination. Irrespective of this inclination, the tooth–lower lip relationship does not apparently differ from the preceding case.

Perfect tooth alignment without overlap or rotation on a tapered type of arch form will look unnatural, as will badly placed teeth on an ovoid type of arch form. It must be stressed that the beauty of dentofacial composition is totally independent of the type of arch form. Even though the media and the public seem to favor the ovoid type of arch form as an ideal, particularly the female arch form,[6] this could be illusory because the evaluation of the type of arch form is impossible without the visualization provided by laboratory models.

According to the Academy of Dental Prosthesis, anterior teeth should maintain some of the irregularities observed in nature. This recommendation is better achieved by tooth placement according to an arch form that assures a natural variety, rather than by inappropriate tooth rotation or malposition, or by the introduction of a pathology best illustrated by tooth wear, fractures, or colored deposits.

Although the restoration of the original arch form by means of adequate fashioning of denture or partial base materials and by surgical procedures is not restricted, the extreme difficulty in predicting this original arch shape should be strongly stressed.

A harmonious interrelationship between the shape of face, the dental arch form, and the teeth, or Nelson triade, has been advocated by many prosthodontists. Unfortunately, the demonstration of the absence of correlation between the shape of the face and the shape of the teeth[49,50] destroyed this hypothesis but has not kept practitioners from using this attractive approach in the absence of any other scientific or technical alternative.

One has to consider that proper placement of the tooth base in its alveolar support without taking into consideration that both maxillary and mandibular anterior tooth inclination and the nature of vertical arrangement do not assure optimum relation to achieve facial harmony.

Investigations done according to a specific facial classification[51] based on readily located facial landmarks have evidenced closed relationships between tooth inclination and facial types.[52] Correlating tooth arrangement with facial types would certainly constitute a better esthetic approach than imposing a systematic application of average norms, erroneous in regard to the variety exhibited by facial profiles (Figs 4-86 and 4-87).

The initial statement that anterior teeth had to achieve lip support opens the hypothesis that improper tooth placement should affect facial muscle equilibrium by reason of the connections of these muscles with the orbicularis oris (Figs 4-88 to 4-94).

Structural Esthetic Rules

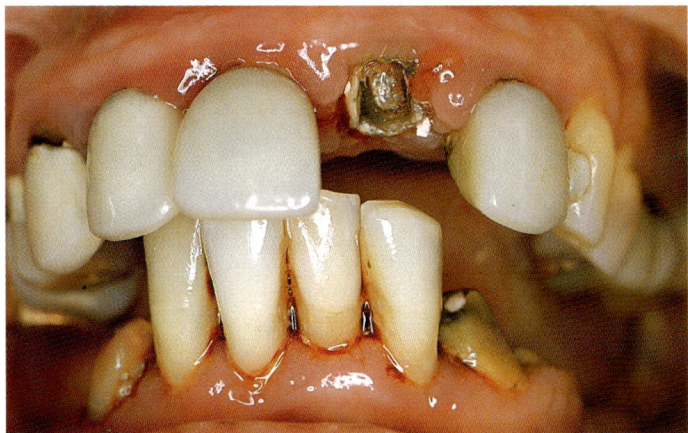

Fig 4-88 Clinical situation of a periodontally and occlusally severely involved case. The results of the initial and surgical periodontal therapies have opened the possibilities to fulfill the patient's desire to receive a fixed maxillary restoration.

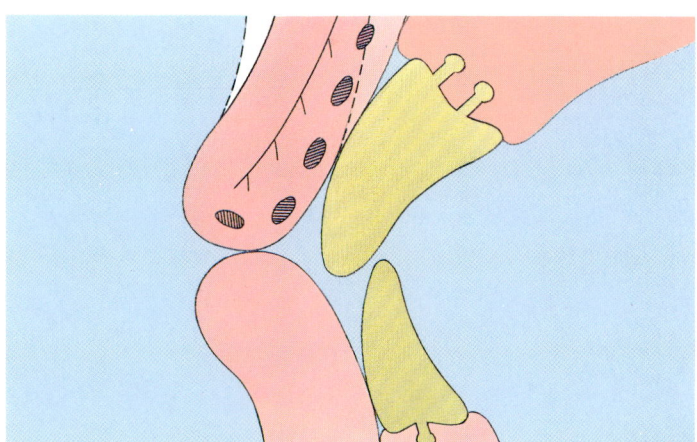

Fig 4-89 Changes in tooth arrangement modify lip posture and perioral muscular activity. The restoration of these elements relies on the correct restoration of tooth position. Unlike removable dentures, fixed restorations are not dislodged by unnatural muscular activity that most often remains unobserved.

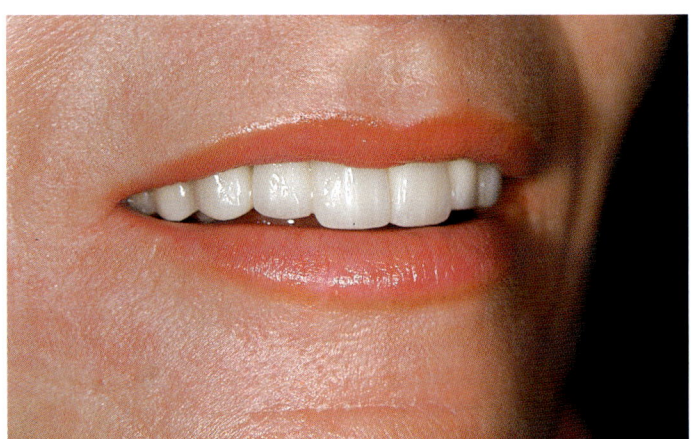

Fig 4-90 Considering the state of the initial situation that required the extraction of the two maxillary central incisors, the new dentofacial composition is impressive. However, this feeling must be attenuated by the fact that the patient complained that she never "regained her original physical appearance."

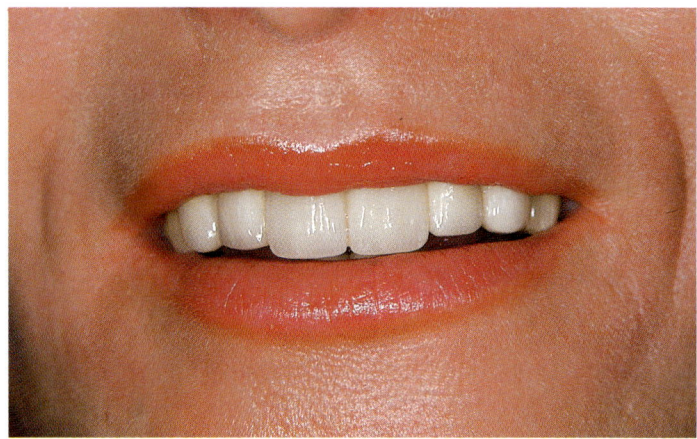

Fig 4-91 This frontal view of the dentofacial composition stresses a clear esthetic error. Irrespective of the reduction of the canine tip in an attempt to determine the origin of this problem, careful observation reveals both an absence of negative space and the presence of a nasolabial ridge and sulcus on the lateral aspect of the corners of the mouth, indicative of excessive activity of the outer muscular belt.

Dental components

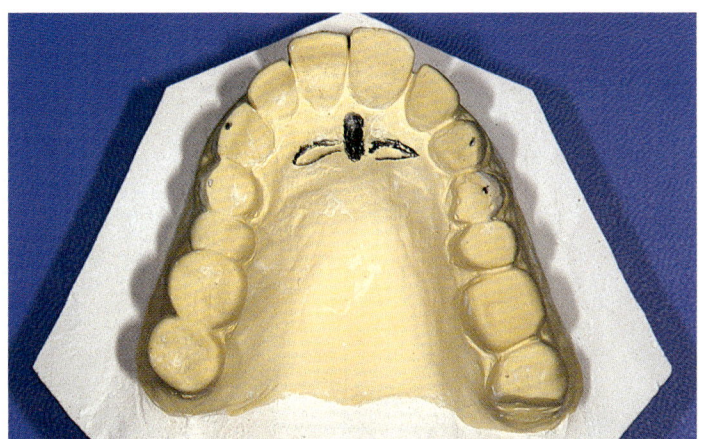

Fig 4-92 The examination of the initial model shows a horizontal migration of the maxillary incisors. This is indicated by the position of the cingulum relative to the anterior part of the incisal papilla. Taking into account this factor, the original arch shape could be described as tapered or tapered-ovoid.

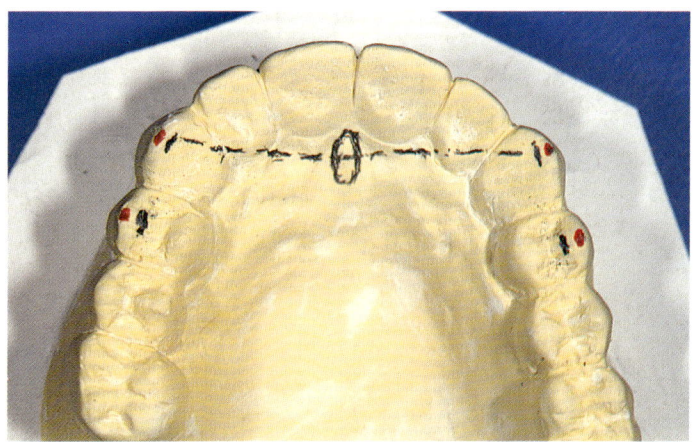

Fig 4-93 This type of arch form has not been reproduced in the final restoration, the tooth position of which conforms to a beautiful ovoid type of arch form. The right and the left canines are correctly placed along the CPC line. Note the black points indicating the original position of canines and first premolars, and those in red of the final restoration.

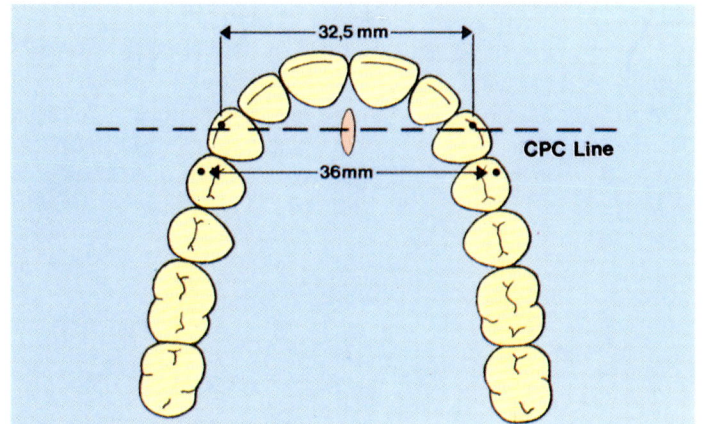

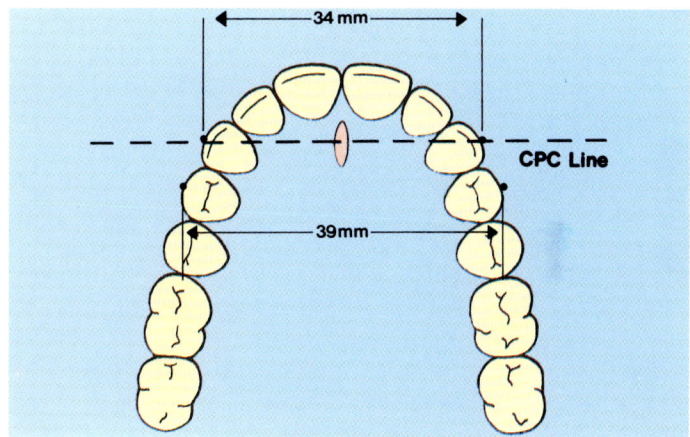

Figs 4-94a and b Although the position of the tip of the canines along the CPC line has been correctly achieved, it shows an increase of 1.5 mm. This expansion is even more pronounced in the first premolar area where it reaches 3 mm. This has totally modified the initial natural arch form and explains the diminution of quasi-absence of negative space, the muscle disturbance in the area of the modiolus, and the resulting imbalance of the perioral muscles.

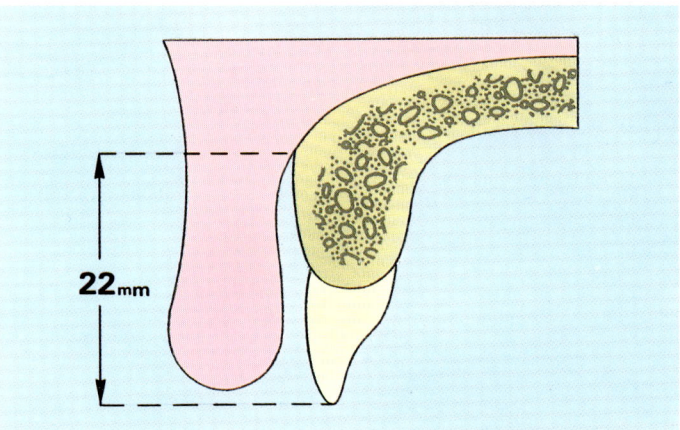

Fig 4-95 A number of clinicians (Turbyfill WF, Dourdakis J. Personal communications, May 1989) have observed a constant in the distance measured from the base of the sulcus to the tip of the maxillary incisor. This observation appears to provide a good reference to the placement of this tooth in the vertical plane.

Although this equilibrium is probably more affected by variations in the vertical dimension that first has to be ascertained, the impact of tooth arrangement is far from being negligible.

In a normal dentate state the tooth position is determined by a functional equilibrium existing between the forces of the tongue and the compensatory action of the cheek musculature and lips. This means that the tooth support is effective in the dynamic of oral movements. Investigations have suggested that there exists a relaxed lip posture that is independent of tooth and alveolar process.[53] This gives some credit to the hypothesis that modifications of tooth arrangement can affect the range and extent of lip and facial musculature movements, inducing atrophic tissue changes unless adaptative potentialities compensate for these deficiencies.

Superficial observations have shown that retrusively relaxed lips produce retrusive dentitions. At the same time the relaxed lip posture of the lower lip has been discussed as a possible guide for positioning the maxillary incisor.[53] This confirms our observations of the close relationships existing between lower lip and maxillary incisor, or more precisely, between the varieties of lip design and the particulars of tooth arrangement (Figs 4-95 to 4-98).

More information and scientific confirmation of these observations would be needed to advance the problem of tooth arrangement that appears to have a variety of impacts and to be a key factor in maintaining the soft tissue mass of the lip along with the progression of age.

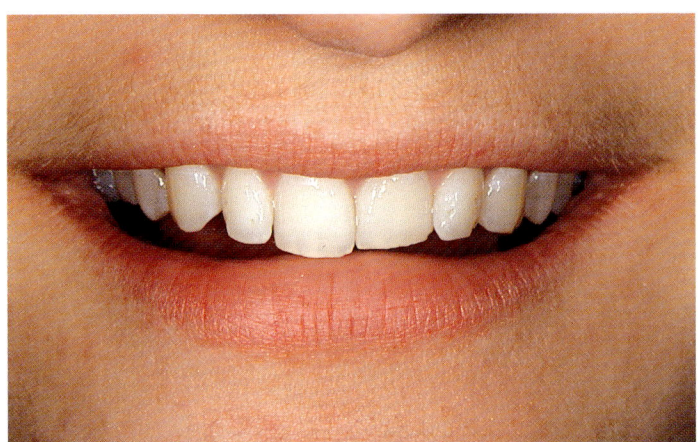

Fig 4-96 The presence of a tubercle on the lower lip is associated with the elongation of the maxillary right incisor, showing that careful observation of lip morphology should provide information about a specific arrangement of the dental elements of the anterior segment.

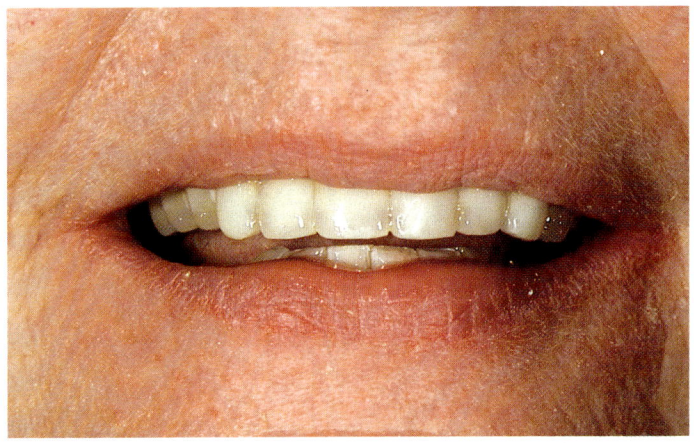

Fig 4-97 The two central tubercles of the lower lip are not associated with the individualization and elongation of the central elements of the dental composition. This evidences a mistake in the vertical arrangement of the anterior segment.

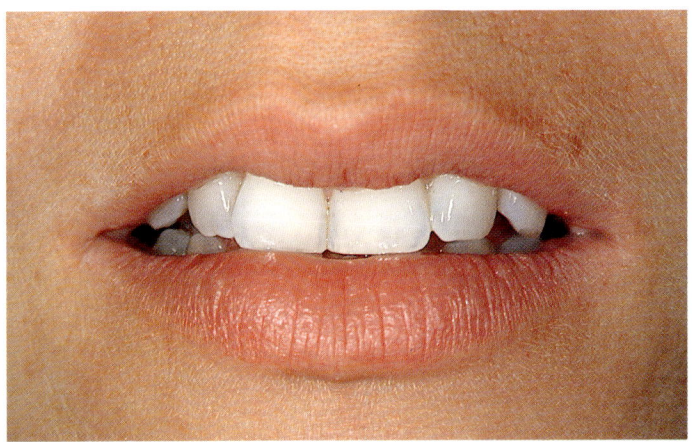

Fig 4-98 A strongly reversed and thick lower lip in its median and left part underlines the tissue stimulation that takes place in the dynamic of oral movements. Note the thinness of the right part of the lower lip associated with the retraction of the maxillary right lateral incisor.

Structural Esthetic Rules

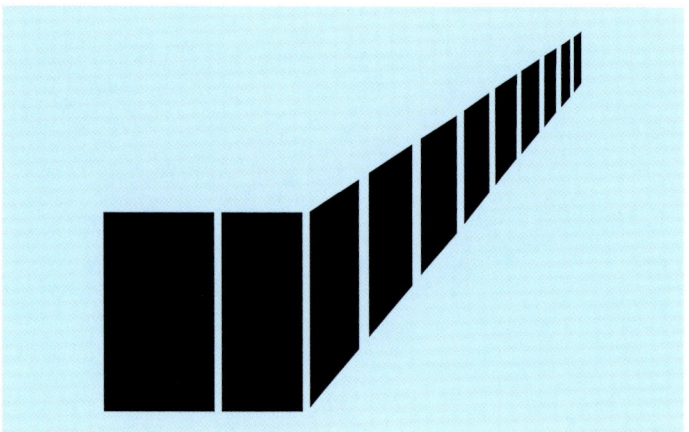

Fig 4-99 When similar structures are aligned one after the other, they undergo a progressive visual reduction of size from the nearest to the farthest.

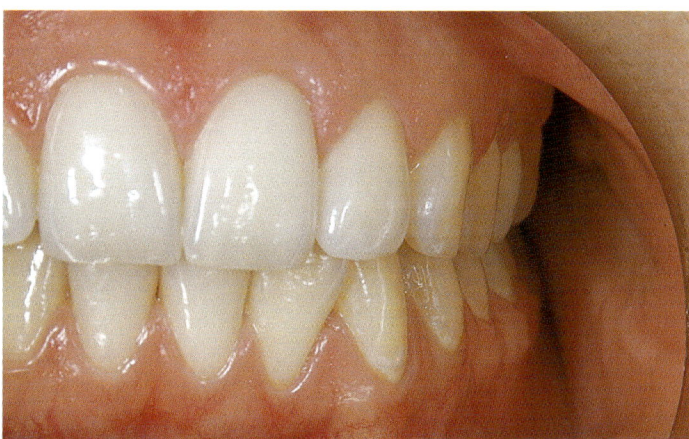

Fig 4-100 Clinical illustration of the gradation effect, accentuated by the natural reduction of light affecting the most posterior elements.

Gradation

When two similar structures are placed at different distances from the viewer, the closest will appear the largest. Should one introduce and align other similar structures between these two, a gradual reduction of size from the closer to the farther will be experienced (Fig 4-99).

This phenomenon of front–back progression is commonly used in architecture to give an illusion of infinite depth and has been mastered in Greek monuments and mosques in creating a perception of mystery and permanence.

The smile is the most effective means by which people convey their emotions. Usually, the smile is viewed from the front, rather than in profile. To introduce into the smile the subtle changes of individual feeling as well as the mystery that it implies, it requires the knowledge and the control of the principle of gradation, which involves the perception of a progressive reduction of size from the most anterior to the most posterior teeth (Fig 4-100).

The prerequisite of the front–back progression is the alignment of the outline or contour of the buccal surface, incisal third, median third and, at a lower rate, gingival third, as well as the alignment of the incisal mesiobuccal inclines (Figs 4-101 and 4-102).

The presence of a poorly placed tooth, differences in tooth length, gingival disharmonies and colored restorations create problems with respect to the gradation effect. These elements can be perceived and have a negative effect, depending upon the magnitude of the deviation from what would be considered a normal front-back progression.

The buccal corridor or lateral negative space between the buccal outline of posterior teeth and the corner of the mouth helps in achieving the gradation effect in progressively altering tooth illumination. While it diminishes the perception of detail, it increases the illusion of distance and depth. Attention must be paid to variations of shades that contrast with the progressive diminution of illumination, so that they do not conflict with the gradation effect.

The width of the smile is outlined by the handsome curvature of the upper and lower lip and the position of the angle of the mouth, which determines the degree of exposure of both anterior and posterior teeth and gingival tissue as well as the width of the buccal corridor.

Dental components

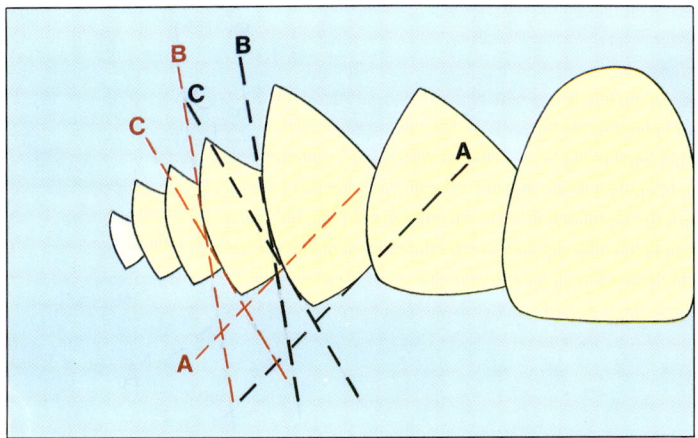

Fig 4-101 The perception of the front–back progression requires the alignment of the central and incisal outlines as well as that of the incisal edges.

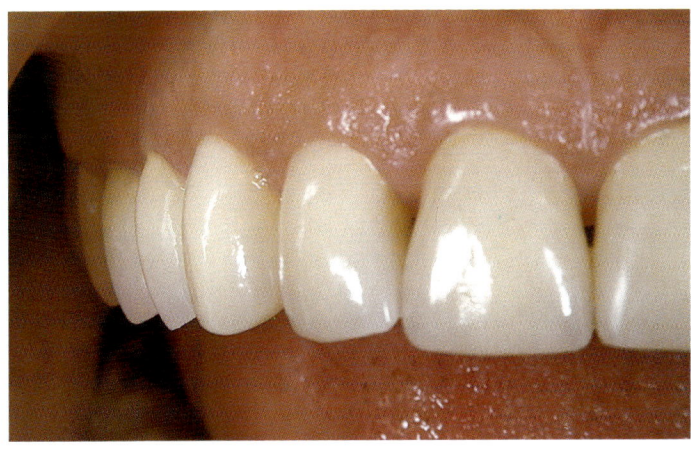

Fig 4-102 Clinical illustration of the alignment of tooth outlines and incisal edges.

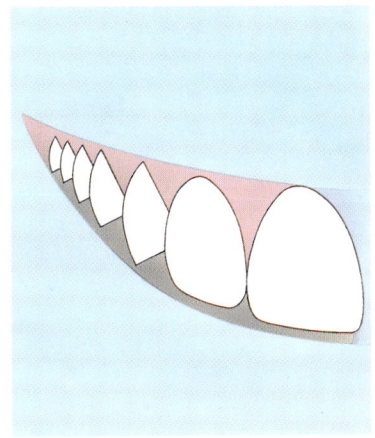

Fig 4-103 Idealized picture of the front–back progression of the dental composition.

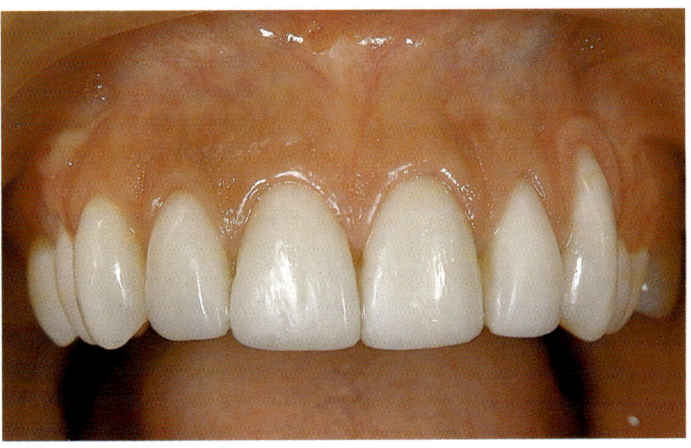

Fig 4-104 Mimicking the adjacent drawings, an incisogingivally elongated canine and a shortened premolar displaying gingiva disturb the front–back progression of the left posterior segment, as does a malposed first premolar on the right side.

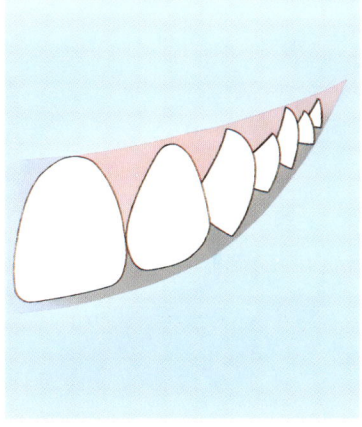

Fig 4-105 A short and a malposed tooth are the most frequent clinical situations in which the front–back progression of teeth is disturbed.

Structural Esthetic Rules

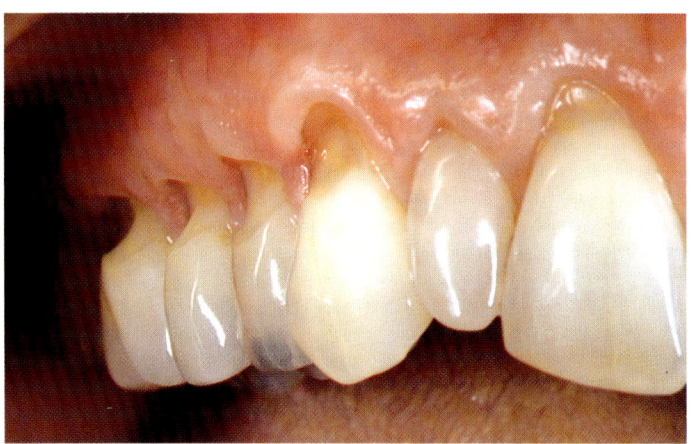

Fig 4-106 Ideal but unnatural front–back progression.

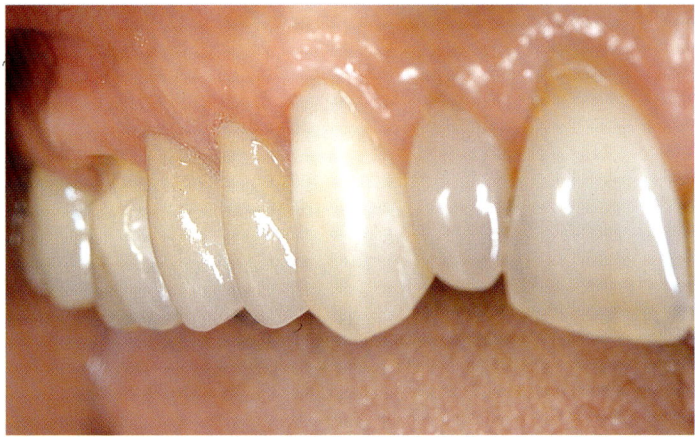

Fig 4-107 Creation of an unsatisfactory front–back progression with maintenance of the cervical defect on the first molar.

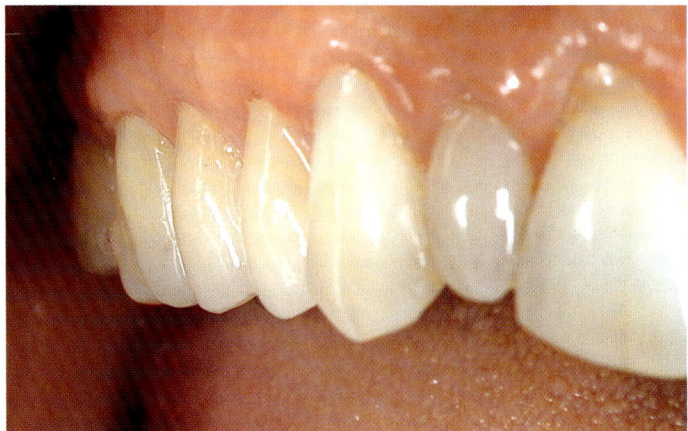

Fig 4-108 Satisfactory restoration of a natural front–back progression.

Dental components

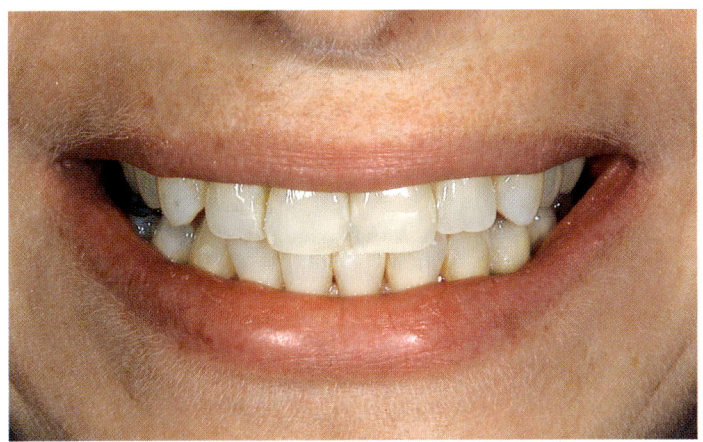

Fig 4-109 A key element or key tooth, usually the canine or premolar, is prerequisite for ensuring the visualization of the gradation effect.

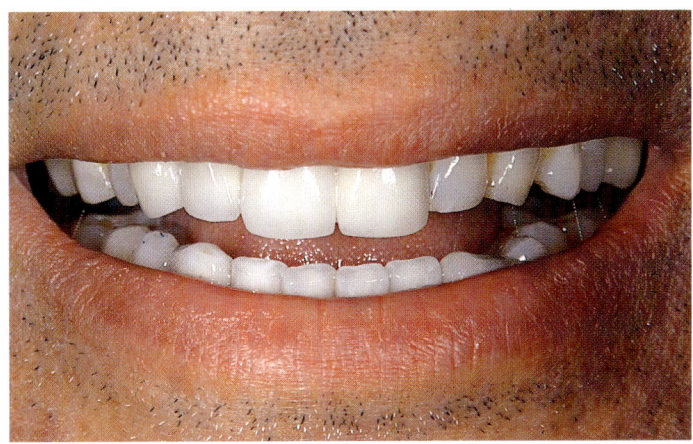

Fig 4-110 In the absence of a key tooth, the gradation effect is not ensured. This may introduce an element of artificiality.

This front–back perception is determined by the arch form and the key tooth that assesses this natural transition (Figs 4-109 and 4-110).

In prosthodontics and in natural dentition, the perception of this transitional element is an important factor in the harmony of the dentofacial composition. Failure to perceive this, which is a common mistake in dentistry, eliminates the gradation effect and invariably creates a dull or strange dentofacial composition.

The positioning of this key element, most frequently the canine or first premolar, evidences the materialization of the buccal corridor and the gradation effect, the manipulation of which is an important factor that allows the prosthodontist to enhance a patient's personality.

Dental morphology

The anatomy of those dental elements that have esthetic importance must be appreciated within the framework of their relationship to the surrounding structures, mainly the gingiva and the lips.[54,55]

Teeth have been generally defined according to their two-dimensional outline, which can be easily objectivized,[56–58] but their successful characterization depends on the evaluation and reproduction of three-dimensional characteristics, a situation that appears more complex and is affected by the parameters of texture, color, shape, and contour.

Texture

We are not only able to feel a surface texture, but we are able to evaluate it optically through the amount of light that is reflected or deflected, so that a tooth surface may be easily perceived as being smooth or rough.

The characterization of the tooth surface is a function of two types of convexities and concavities:

1. The anatomic grooves, facets, and prominences that

Structural Esthetic Rules

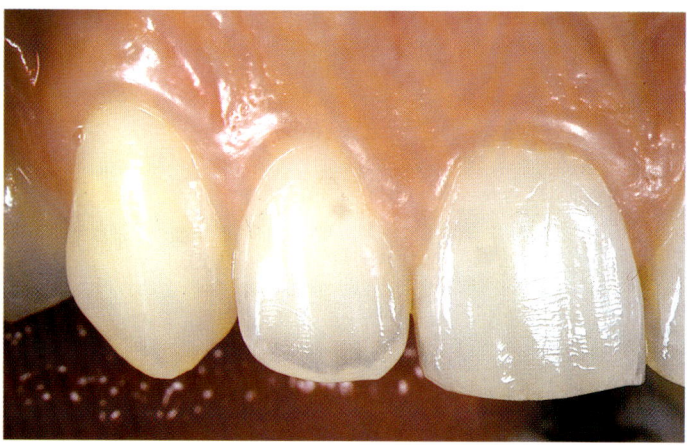

Fig 4-111 More or less pronounced anatomic grooves and prominences characterize tooth structure.

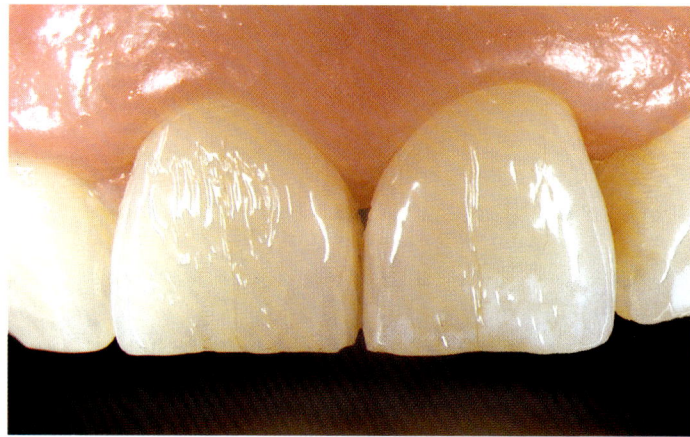

Fig 4-112 Nonanatomic stippling and rippling of tooth texture may also be observed.

exist in various degrees on any tooth surface (Fig 4-111).
2. The perikymatae, stippling, and rippling that may affect the enamel surface (Fig 4-112).

The quality of an artificial tooth directly depends on the blending of light effects that produce a result similar to that produced by a natural tooth. It also explains why the excessive use of lines, grooves, and glaze does not provide the expected esthetic results.

The observation of nature shows no evidence of a proportionate relationship between tooth surface texture and the texture of the skin. Criteria used to roughen or not to roughen the artificial tooth depend on the texture of the adjacent teeth and in edentulous states on the esthetic sense of the operator who may or may not decide to identify and harmonize tooth and skin texture.

Shape of the teeth

The average tooth outline and dimensional values must be interpreted according to the infinite variety of tooth contour that nature provides and arbitrarily have been classified into square, ovoid, tapered, and mixed because of the influence of the laws of harmony proposed in 1914 by Williams.[59] Williams established a relationship that was supposed to exist between the contour of the face and the contour of the maxillary incisor. This statement, accepted by the dental profession, imposed itself on the industry even though it has been invalidated by various studies[49,50,60] and subjected to criticism.[61] The advice of Williams to beware of any excess in the systematization did not prevent a number of researchers from attempting to demonstrate the existence of a number of numerical dentofacial relationships between the following:

A. Osseous and dental landmarks.
   1. Bizygomatic width and maxillary central incisor width.
   2. Bizygomatic width and maxillary incisor width.
   3. Skull length and maxillary incisor length.
   4. Skull circumference and width of maxillary incisors.
   5. Nasal width and maxillary incisors width[62,63] and many others.
B. Soft tissue facial contour and tooth contour.
C. Color of the face and tooth contour.

These studies and findings motivated dentists and the dental industry to commercialize infallible methods or devices for proper tooth selection. Attracted by the "frame harmony method"[64] or the *Automatic Instant Selection Guide*,[65] dentists plunged into the ocean of instantly ready products from which they still have not emerged, depriving them of the necessary time to train and develop their sense of harmony and appreciation.

Without denying the relationship between some of the aforementioned factors that merit attention, such as the nose–tooth relationship, it must be pointed out that, once again, they introduce elements of numerical quantification that do not blend with elements of esthetic interpretation.

The topographic integration of the embryogenic processes that are at the base of the constitution of the face may create similarities in specific skeletal and tooth arrangement that appear as the result of the action of forces of life exerted on each individual (Corman, see Chapter 2, reference number 15). The direct impact of vital forces on tooth anatomy has yet to be demonstrated, including the correlation that may exist between facial shape and tooth contour.

The location of the dental elements framed by the lips, within the oral receptor and in the lower one third of the face, should logically develop harmonious relationships, both morphopsychologic and esthetic with these elements.

The criticisms that can be made of William's concept do not really depend upon an invalidation resulting from scientific investigations that have no esthetical value. Rather, they rely on the simple fact that the proper distance required for the evaluation of each of the parameters involved (ie, tooth and skull) is totally different and their concordance or nonconcordance is relatively unimportant.

Considering the morphopsychologic equilibrium and esthetic harmony that should reflect from the lower one third of the face, what seems to be important does not depend on tooth contour but on the particularities of tooth arrangement providing harmonious relationships with the variety of lip designs (Figs 4-113 to 4-124).

The four faces in Figs 4-113, 4-116, 4-119, and 4-122 can only be differentiated by the particularities of lip design, producing differences in their morphopsychologic interpretation. According to the concepts developed in dentistry, each of these individuals should receive or exhibit the same type of tooth contour. Although careful examination leads to a possible variety of tooth contours it also progressively stresses the fact, based on previous observations (see Figs 4-96 to 4-98), that adequate tooth arrangement could be the key factor for realizing a harmonious dentofacial composition. The maintenance of the particularities of lip structure in its degree of retraction or dilatation requires a constant stimulation by the dento-osseous support.

Dental arrangements of maxillary teeth, affected by the modulations of arch form, should take into account the necessary stimulation of the antagonist lip structure and requiring the selected projection of specific dental elements or that of the whole anterior segment.

There exists an intimate connection among the particularities of the lip's mucous cover, the thickness of its connective tissue, and the frequency and nature of the contacts produced by the incisal edges. Repeated and localized contacts stimulating the underlying tissues will induce the formation of labial tubercles, whereas a thick and sensual lower lip requires a constant stimulation of its inner wall by the incisor's incisal edges. The realities of the lip and lip support connections, necessary elements of esthetic appraisal of the lower one third of the face, always take care of the dispute that the determination of tooth contour may generate. These realities, determined by the observation of anatomic landmarks, arch shape, and lip morphology, will suggest the nature of the alignment and the retraction or projection of the whole anterior segment, that of specific dental elements. However, the predominant importance of the lip and lip support connections will not prevent the restorative dentist from the obligation to characterize the natural shape and contour of the elements that belong to it.

Unfortunately, at the present time, information concerning the definition of an individual's tooth contour does not exist. Therefore, in the absence of documentation, such as old models or photographs, tooth shape, predominantly maxillary central incisors, not subject to rigid rules, must be selected according to a basic tooth design and evaluated and corrected in regard to its integration with the facial environment.

Structural Esthetic Rules

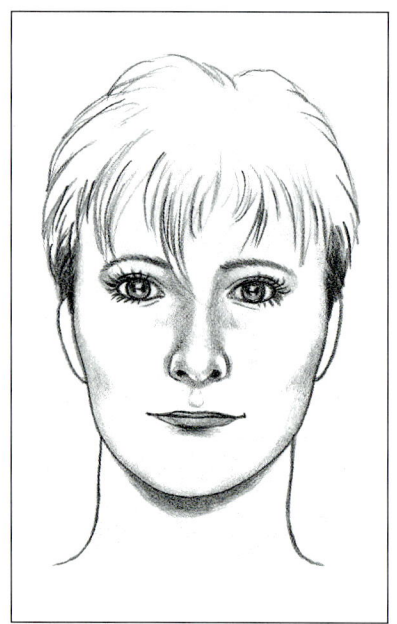

Fig 4-113 Face sketch A. Thin upper and lower lips.

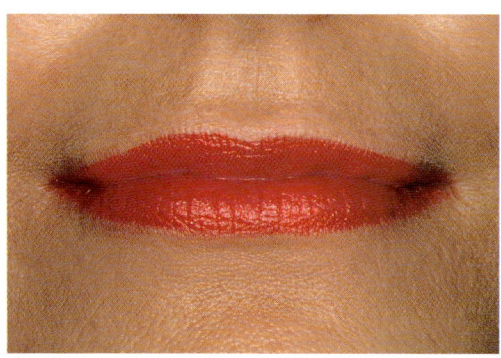

Fig 4-114 Thin upper and lower lips, reflecting self-control and satisfaction.

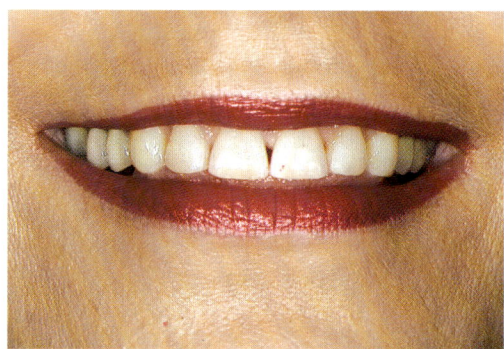

Fig 4-115 Weak dominance of the anterior segment with horizontal symmetry.

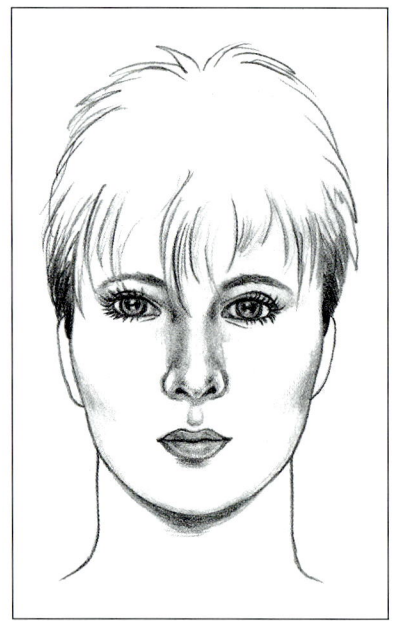

Fig 4-116 Face sketch B. Dominance of the lower lip.

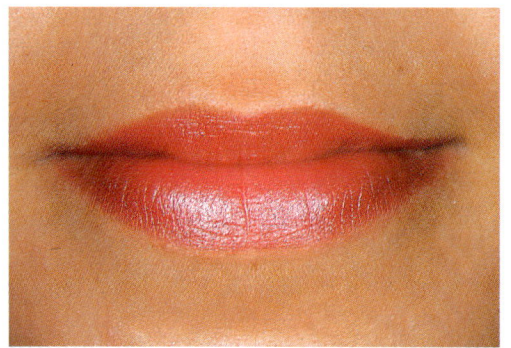

Fig 4-117 Dominance of size of the lower lip, irradiating controlled and sensual ingeniousness.

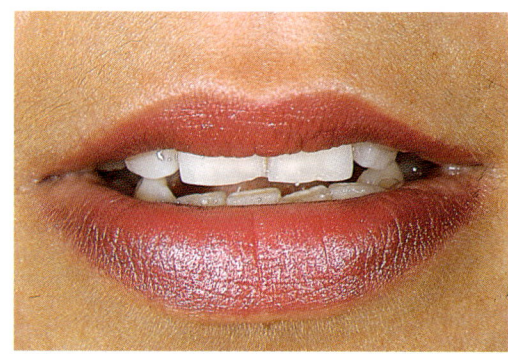

Fig 4-118 Strong individual dominance of the central incisors.

Dental components

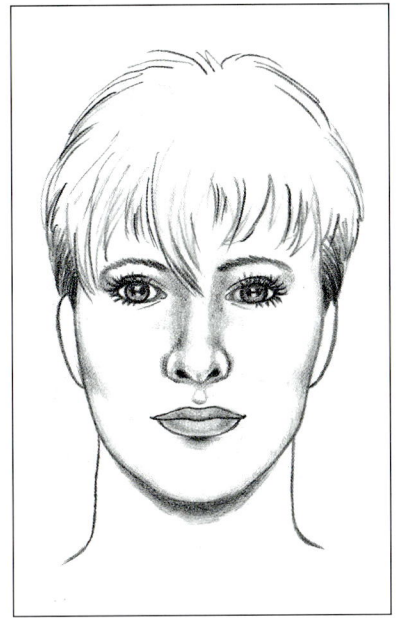

Fig 4-119 Face sketch C. Equilibrium of upper and lower lips.

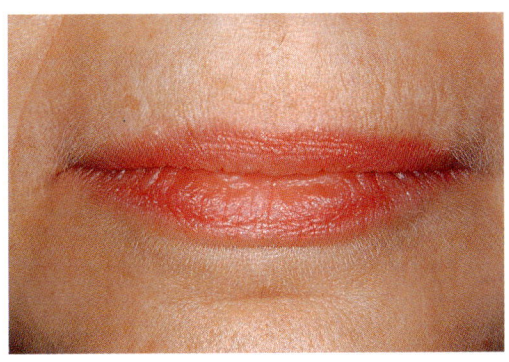

Fig 4-120 Relative equilibrium of upper and lower lips, expressing characteristic harmony, will, and kindness.

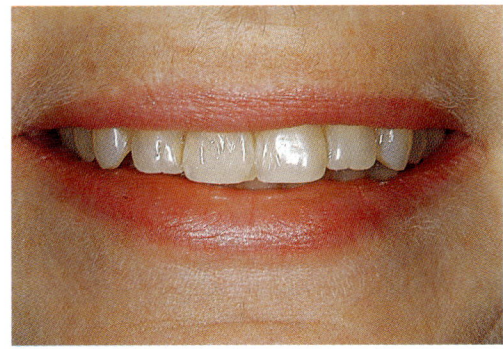

Fig 4-121 Dominance of the anterior segment with radiating symmetry.

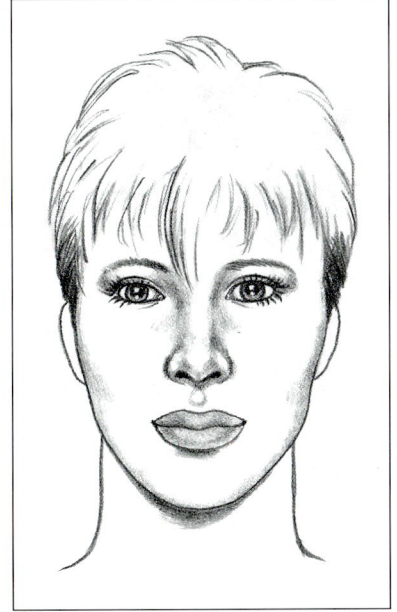

Fig 4-122 Face sketch D. Thick upper and lower lips.

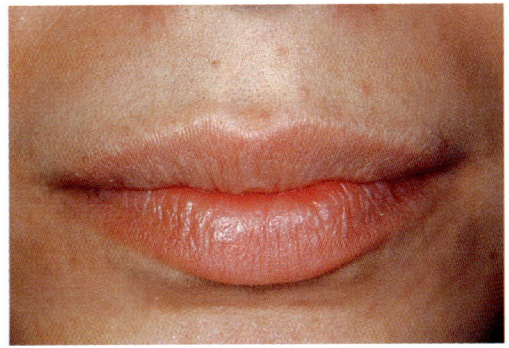

Fig 4-123 Thick upper and lower lips suggest an extrovert and easygoing personality.

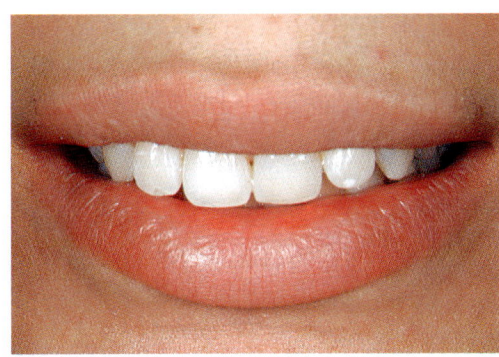

Fig 4-124 Individual dominance of the dental elements.

111

Structural Esthetic Rules

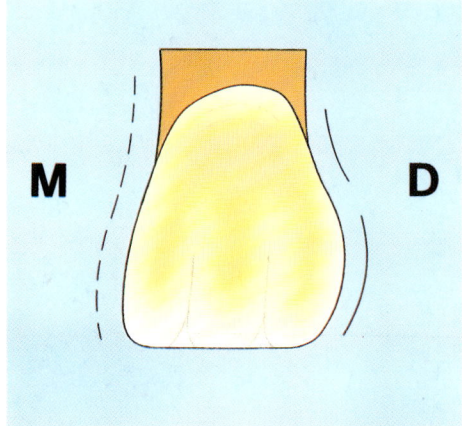

Fig 4-125 Maxillary central incisor. Its mesial outline, either slightly convex or concave on the cervical one third, goes slightly convex or straight along the contact line. The distal outline has a more pronounced convexity and its cervical one third is concave. The labial surface presents three prominences of equal size, separated by two depressions.

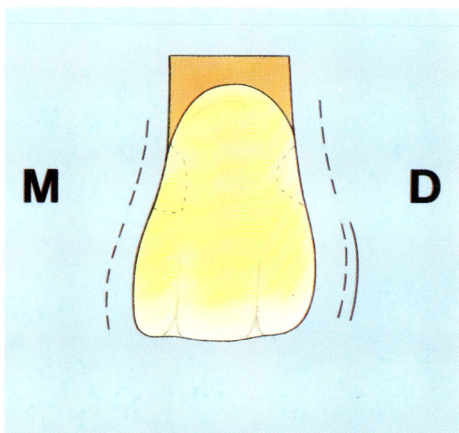

Fig 4-126 Maxillary lateral incisor. It presents an outline identical to the central incisor but less pronounced convexities of the distal and mesial outlines. The mesial and distal angles are rounder and the labial surface shows a barely marked wide central prominence. Slight convexities on the cervical labioproximal angles can sometimes be observed. The lateral incisor can exhibit a large variety of shapes.

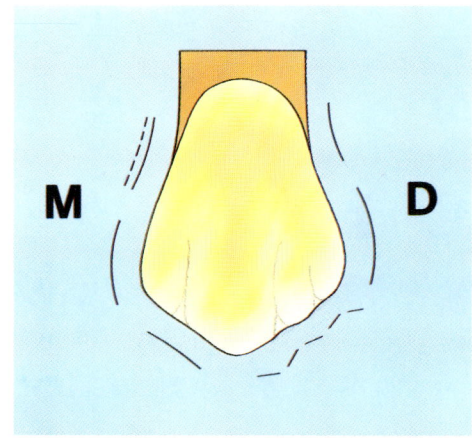

Fig 4-127 Maxillary canine. The mesial outline runs straight or slightly concave to the contact point, whereas the distal outline shows a greater concavity on the cervical area. The incisocervical labial surface is characterized by two bulges: one at the cervical area and the other located at its incisal one third.

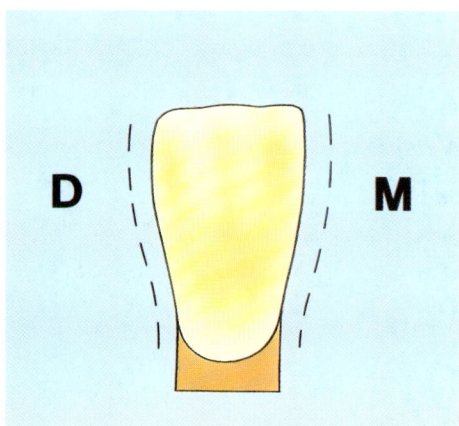

Fig 4-128 Mandibular incisor. It exhibits a symmetric straight or slightly convex mesial and distal outline. The buccal surface looks flat and dull, which surprisingly creates problems in fabricating a satisfactory design. The functional importance of this tooth is stressed in Chapter 5.

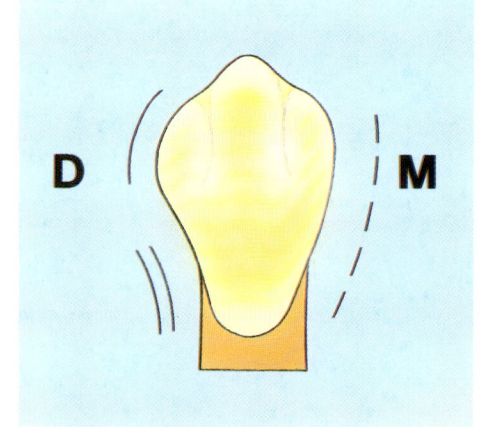

Fig 4-129 Mandibular canine. The mesial outline is always slightly convex, whereas the distal angle and outline form a large convexity, ending with a pronounced concavity in the distocervical area. The maintenance of a sharp cusp tip testifies of functional normality.

```
- - - -   slight curvature
———        normal curvature
════       pronounced curvature
```

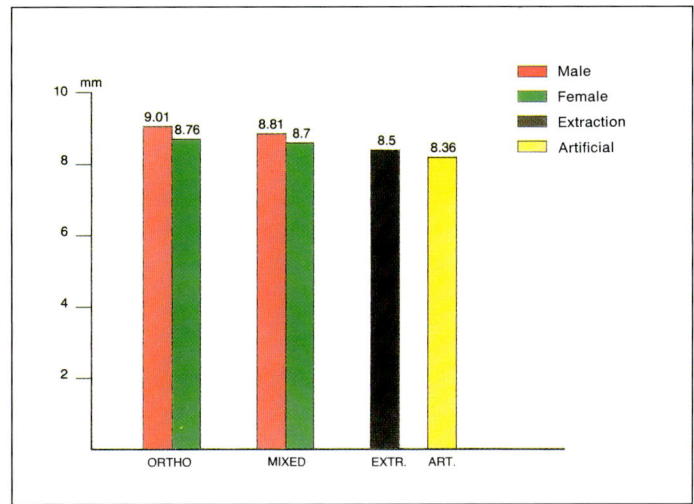

Fig 4-130 Comparative tooth width. The comparison of orthodontic samples to manufactured teeth underlines that the latter teeth are undersized. (From MacArthur.[72])

Diagrammatic tooth contour

Description of the average anatomic features of anterior teeth may be important because it will provide the esthetic dentist with basic geometric norms that, without restricting the esthetic sense, will, on the contrary, allow the dentist to introduce the most characteristic elements of appreciation and to detect suspicious disharmonies, achieving a final result from which error has been eliminated.

The influence of a number of authors[48,56,57,66,67] greatly contributed to the design of the following diagrams, which should be interpreted, keeping in mind that in the matter of human esthetics, final beauty is achieved more easily by the respect of norms in which variety has been adequately introduced (Figs 4-125 to 4-129).

Mesiodistal width

It would not be possible to correctly interpret this diagrammatic tooth presentation without appropriate information about average dimensional values. Both in fixed prosthodontics and denture prosthesis, edentulous anterior areas must be restored with teeth exhibiting normality in their mesiodistal width independent from other esthetic criteria. This dimension, probably a much more critical dimension than the incisogingival for anterior tooth replacement, has been widely investigated,[68–72] and different studies have reported similar values. It was also found that the mean sex-specific incisor diameter was larger in men than women as well as for black people than for whites.[73–76]

Proximal tooth wear that seems to affect the aging population[77] was confirmed by the differences stated in the mesiodistal width of the central incisors between subjects of varying age groups,[72] orthodontic, adult subjects, and edentulous samples idéntified as the most senior segment of the population (Fig 4-130). This last result was compared with the mesiodistal width of artificial teeth of edentulous patients. The degree of difference was consistent with the other results, and it was stated that artificial replacement teeth are not significantly undersized. This statement must be refuted. Indeed, when artificial teeth are compared with orthodontic samples, the difference stated should reinforce the feeling that the reduction of tooth width is another factor of perception of facial aging.

Thirty years after Frush and Fisher[78] rediscovered the relationship between teeth and the trilogy of sex, age, and personality, it can be observed that the profession,

Structural Esthetic Rules

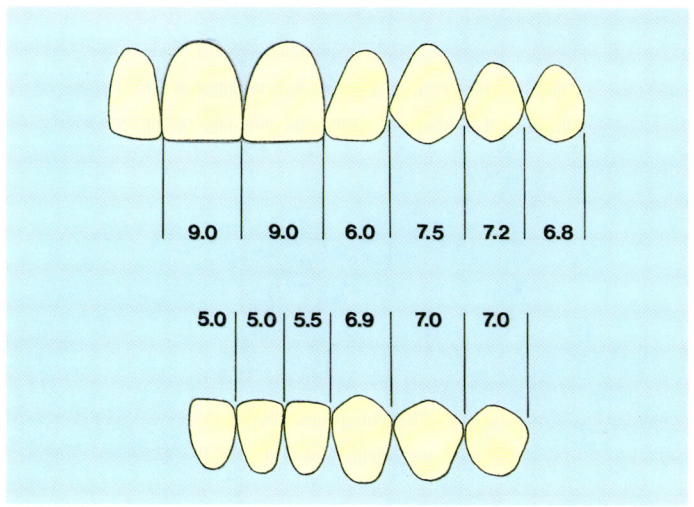

Fig 4-131 Average mesiodistal width of anterior teeth, which can be adapted to conform to current requirements. (From Reynolds.[68])

and with it the entire industry, has maintained rigid rules reluctant to changes and ignoring the constant evolution of the standards of living and the level of medical care. Most importantly, the individual desire to maintain a youthful appearance in the search for well-being has not been taken into account.

There will not be any future in esthetic dentistry if a more dynamic approach is not taken. One should not consider the adjustment of teeth to age but should strongly recommended that patients be provided with young orthodontic dental elements. In giving back full youth, disharmonies will seldom originate from tooth width or length but rather from inappropriate color selection, which increases in saturation with the advancement of age. Tooth width, both for dentate and edentulous patients, should exhibit similar mesiodistal diameters (Fig 4-131). The postextraction tissue loss in edentulous patients naturally implies the setting of teeth off the ridge in a position that favors phonetics and esthetics, without jeopardizing denture stability or increasing ridge resorption.[79] The sexual factor in its strict sense and racial factors will be the only significant variables.

Incisogingival height

This dimensional value has been regarded as much less critical than the mesiodistal width because it seems highly dependent on clinical situations. In restoring teeth that have undergone periodontal surgery of excessive wear, the clinician is left with the task of filling the space available and adapting the amount of vertical overbite to assure phonetics and functional validity (Figs 4-132 to 4-135). Attention will only be focused on tooth length when it passes a certain degree of esthetic tolerance.

The simulation of natural appearance[80] that is advocated by specialists of denture prosthetics is clouded by the rule that teeth in their length and width should be related to the patient's age. As a consequence, progressive anterior tooth wear that affects a large percentage of the population familiar with usual dental care is considered normal, until temporomandibular joint problems make both dentist and patient aware of a pathology, well present during the years but not recognized as such and left untreated.

In considering a number of cases that, despite aging, still exhibit teeth with normal occlusal design and gingivo-incisal length and with it a young and attractive

Dental components

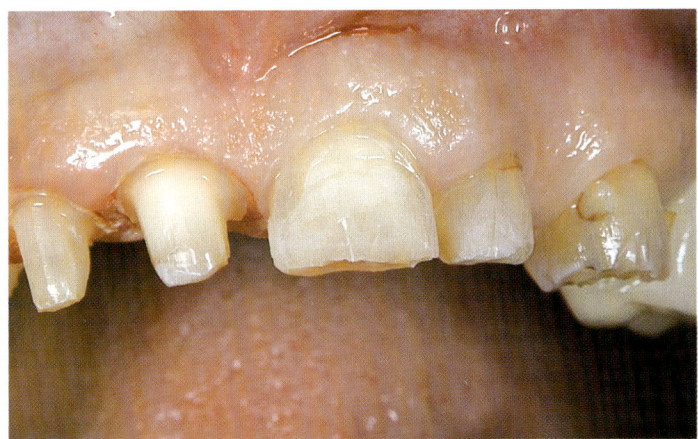

Fig 4-132 Because teeth always exhibit some type of tapered design, incisal wear produces a reduction of their mesiodistal width.

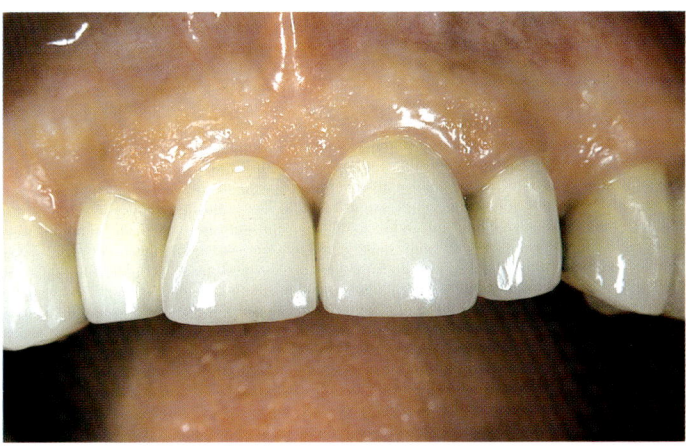

Fig 4-133 Conversely, the increase of tooth length promotes an increase of the incisal width, a prerequisite for rejuvenation, best accomplished in the restoration of the original tooth morphology.

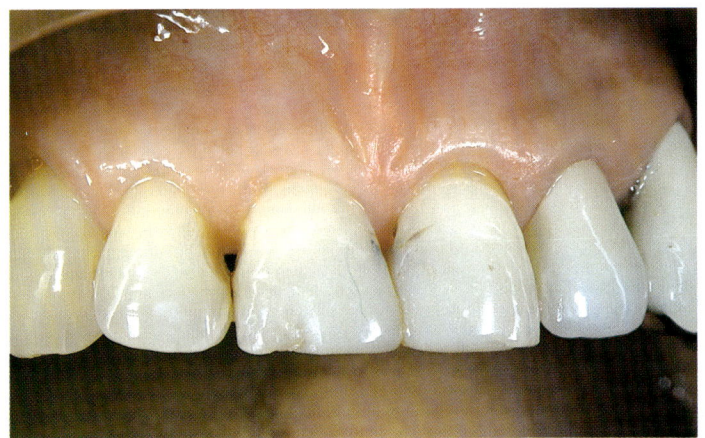

Fig 4-134 Anterior dental composition exhibiting limited anterior wear.

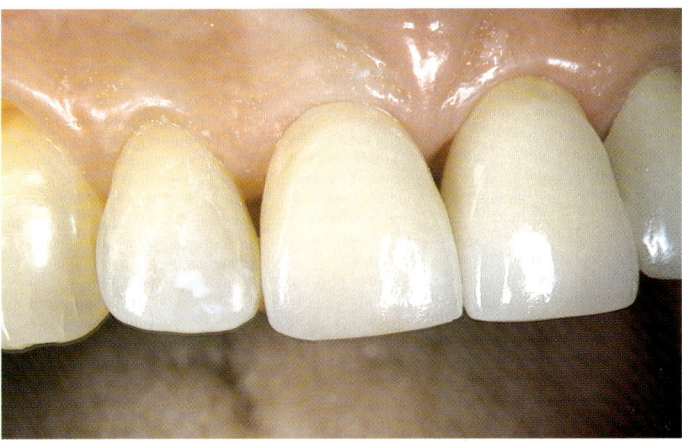

Fig 4-135 The restoration of the original tooth length is a prerequisite for the achievement of esthetic requirements.

Structural Esthetic Rules

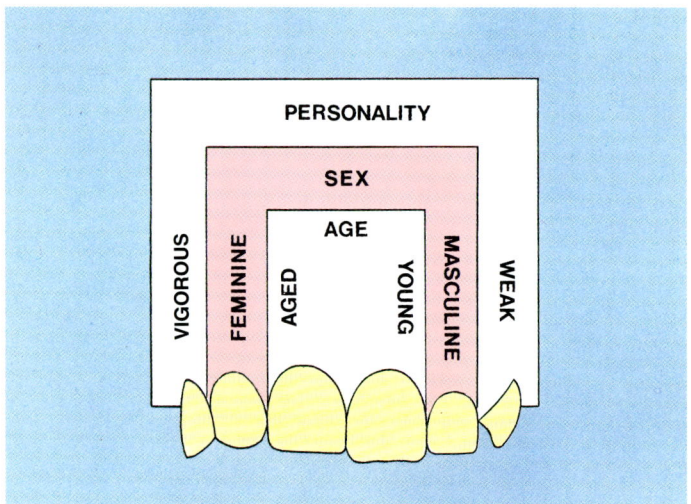 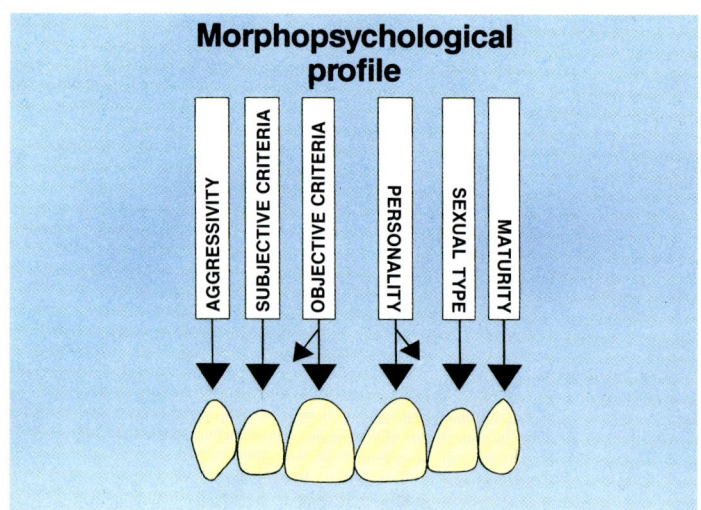

Figs 4-136 and 4-137 SAP concepts: sex, age, and personality (from Frush and Fisher[78]) and SAP concepts: sexual type, aggressivity, and personality (Rufenacht). Both concepts are aimed at characterizing the dental elements of the anterior segment. The differences between the two concepts are mainly evidenced by the significance and evolution of the maxillary central incisor. Submitted to progressive wear with the advancement of age, for Frush and Fisher (see Fig 4-136) the length of the maxillary central incisor should be considered as a constant throughout life. Tooth wear only stresses functional disturbances (Rufenacht) (see Fig 4-137).

appearance, we assumed that function and esthetics should be intimately linked. From this statement the restoration of anterior teeth in their youthful normality becomes a prerequisite for the restoration of function. Similarly, the importance of the dimensional value of anterior tooth length was revived. Because of the limited number of studies relating measurements of human teeth at the desired age period, a number of additional measurements of orthodontic models were performed that revealed similar mean values. Consequently, a basic value of 12 mm for the length of the maxillary central incisor was fixed, keeping in mind the larger range of variation of this value according to sex, racial, and individual parameters but convinced by clinical experience of its importance to assure functional maintenance.

Characterization of the anterior segment

The anterior dental segment is anatomically integrated into the instinctive facial zone and in turn covered, involved in, or representative of the various actions of the mouth. The morphopsychologic concept has characterized the oral organ as concentrating the impulses of life working within each individual. Movements of retraction or dilatation have naturally shaped a morphologic mouth design, reflecting an individual's personality. The idea of introducing different aspects of the personality into dental elements to permit a more precise characterization of the dental composition is at the origin of the sex, age, and personality concept (SAP) proposed by Frush and Fisher[78,81,82] (Fig 4-136).

In the light of the evolution of a number of factors, this concept needs to be reevaluated (Fig 4-137). The ineluctability of anterior tooth wear, along with the age progression, is no longer compatible with the general desire for youth extension and the therapeutic possibilities of functional maintenance. Therefore, tooth length should be considered a constant value throughout the progression of age. From a morphopsychologic point of view, the maxillary central incisors, the most prominent elements of the dental composition, strongly reflect the individual's personality, modulating or confirming the significance produced by the characteristics of lip design. The central incisors focalize the concrete features of personality, strength, energy, authority, magnetism, apathy, or retraction.

In substituting the sexual type for the sex factor, one introduces a more pertinent personality trait because one cannot identify specific particularities or qualities restricted to either men or women. The sexual type should not be considered negatively by either men or women. It concentrates on the lateral incisors the abstracts: artistic, emotional, or intellectual elements of personality. When these elements are not preponderant, they may be submerged by the objective qualities contained in the central incisors to the point where the four anterior teeth exhibit an identical contour. Canines are definitely related to the popular significance, expressing animal aggressivity and danger, directed by ambition and obstination. Age most often attenuates this character trait, introducing into tooth shape a "certain maturity."

Characterization of the maxillary central incisor

Reflecting personality, the shape of the maxillary central incisor will focus attention, permitting the individualization of the basic diagrammatic tooth contour. For this purpose the following protocol has been adopted:

1. Evaluation of the different facial zones and determination of the relative importance of the lower instinctive zone.
2. Introduction of this factor into the mesiodistal cervical width of maxillary central incisors. The more strength that reflects from the instinctive zone, the larger the incisor cervical width. This observation-based statement not only permits the determination of the nature of tooth base but suggests the type of contour that the tooth will exhibit.
3. The introduction of character factors into tooth outline can then be achieved by means of two geometric shapes, ie, curves and angles. Curves imply plasticity, affability, adaptability, and regularity. Angles imply strength, will, and action.

Attempts to introduce the type of expansion of the different facial zones in tooth length or width has proved to be unsuccessful. It appears that the infinite variation of tooth design exhibited by natural teeth will invariably invalidate all theories relative to this problem. These are the reasons why this protocol of tooth design restricts its pretensions to the integration of teeth into their environment in conformity with esthetic principles and morphopsychologic equilibrium.

Contact points

The influence of contact points between the teeth in preventing food impaction is obvious. Marginal ridges, marginal fossa, and spillways seem to be helpful aids in maintaining food away from contact areas. Contact points or surfaces of contact between teeth are generally located in the occlusal one third[83,84] of the proximal walls, slightly buccal to the central fossa[83,85,86] in the molar and premolar area with the exception of the maxillary first and second molars. On the anterior segment and from a frontal view, the contacts are situated in a position that seems to go from incisal to cervical and from maxillary central incisors to canines (Fig 4-138). It is generally accepted to locate the contact between central in-

Structural Esthetic Rules

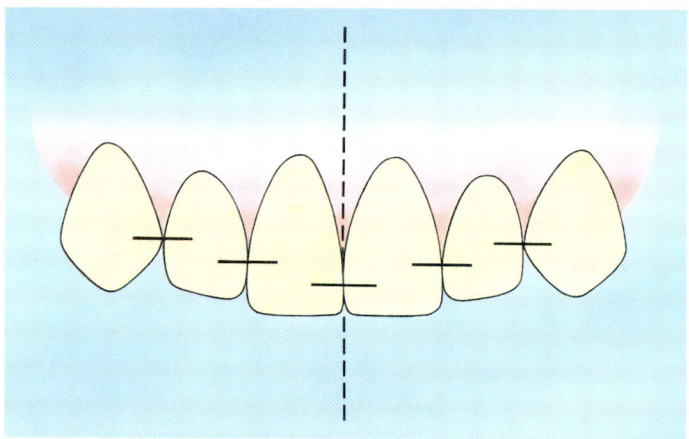

Fig 4-138 Position of anterior contact points, progressing from incisal to cervical and from the central incisors to the canine.

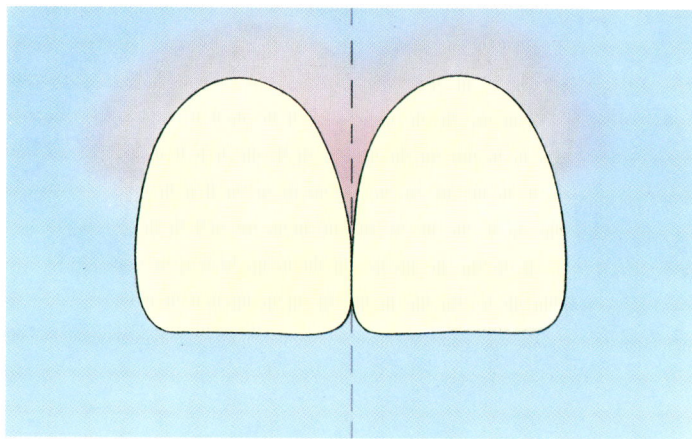

Fig 4-139 The perception of the maxillary central contact point is that of a vertical line.

cisors at the most incisal one third, a point that terminates a long vertical interincisal line of contact. This line serves as a reference line from which symmetry and balance between the two parts of the dental composition can be appraised (Fig 4-139). If we draw an imaginary line between the anterior contact points, we have a curvature that greatly reinforces the curvature of the outline of the incisal edges as well as that of the lower lips. We know that a line does not need to be drawn to be unconsciously perceived because the mind organizes and simplifies its perception in terms of forms it recognizes.

The lip line, incisal line, and contact line represent an ideal in the cohesive forces of the dentofacial composition, the harmony of which is realized by their connection with the segregative forces materialized by the nature of their curvature. When occlusal disturbances and stress-inducing tooth wear have brought tooth contacts to the incisal edge, morphopsychologic hardness is reflected in these individuals. In losing cohesive forces, the esthetics of the dentofacial composition is disturbed (Figs 4-140 to 4-143). Therefore, an adequate manipulation of this factor is recommended.

Anatomy of the contact point

The form of the contact point, or rather the contact area in its orobuccal and coronoapical extension, is directly influenced by the morphology of the teeth, their width, and arrangements. It influences the width and depth of the depression or col marking the interdental papilla. This depression covered with squamous epithelium is difficult to detect clinically. The absence of tooth contact brings an absence of col or depression, and in diastema the orobuccal shape of the interdental papilla is invariably convex[87,88] (Figs 4-144 and 4-145).

Dental components

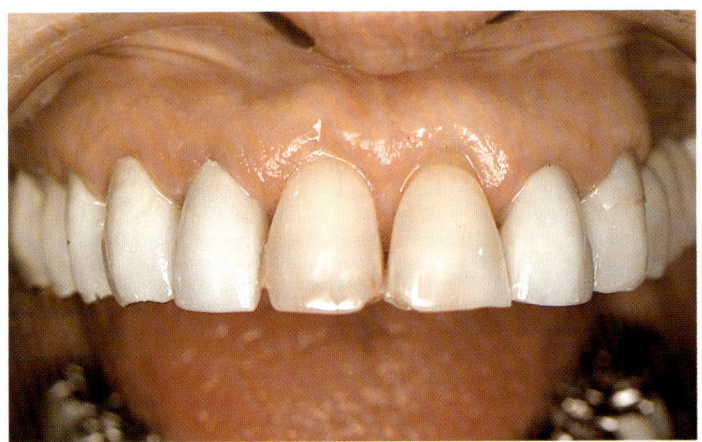

Fig 4-140 The incisal location of anterior contact points is a characteristic of anterior tooth wear. The dental composition reflects a loss of esthetic cohesion.

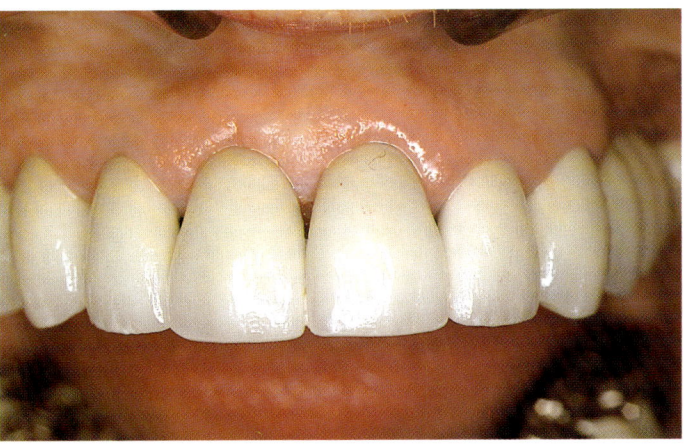

Fig 4-141 The restoration of contact points and the perception of the incisal curvature increase the esthetic strength of the composition.

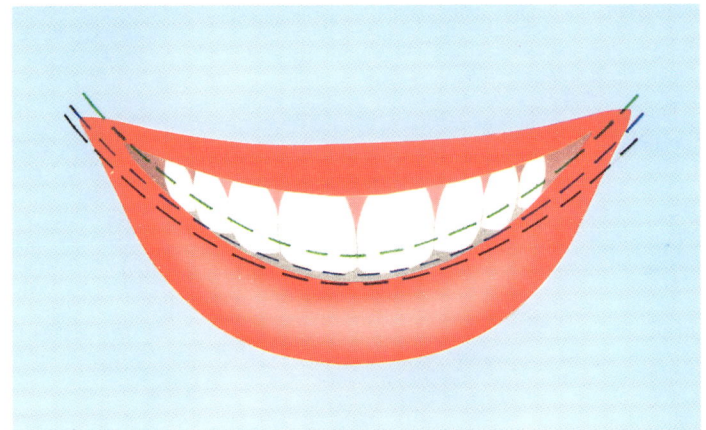

Fig 4-142 The directional coincidence of contact, incisal, and lower lip lines provides cohesive forces to the dentofacial composition. At the same time the degree of curvature introduces segregative forces in the composition.

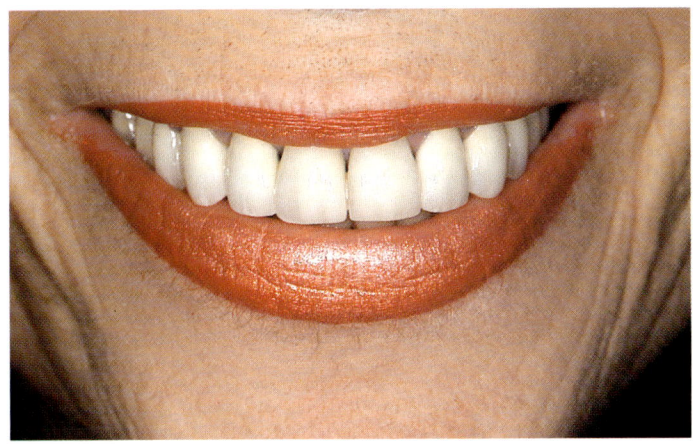

Fig 4-143 Final restoration of the dentofacial composition underlining the directional coincidence of contact, incisal, and lower lip lines, enhanced by their degree of curvature.

Structural Esthetic Rules

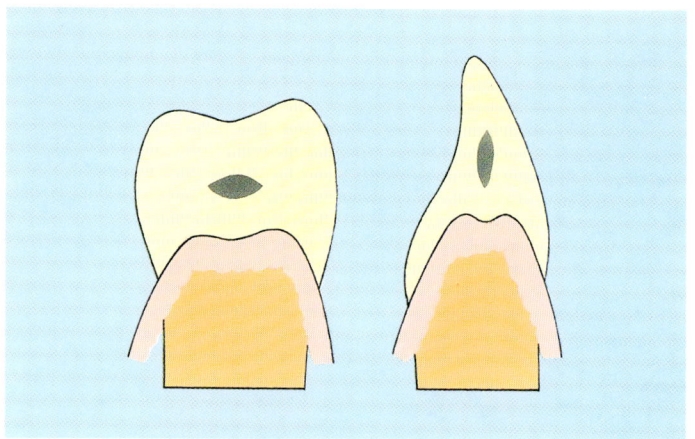

Fig 4-144 The orobuccal shape of tooth contact directly determines the shape of the gingival col, a microscopic depression situated in the interdental papilla.

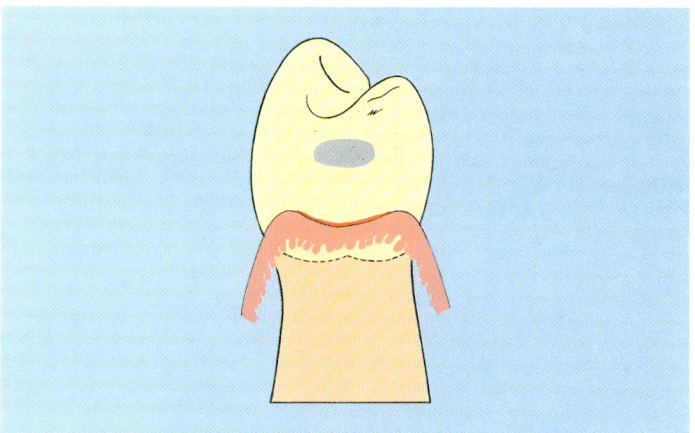

Fig 4-145 The gingiva of the col differs from the marginal gingiva in that it is covered by squamous epithelium less resistant to inflammation.

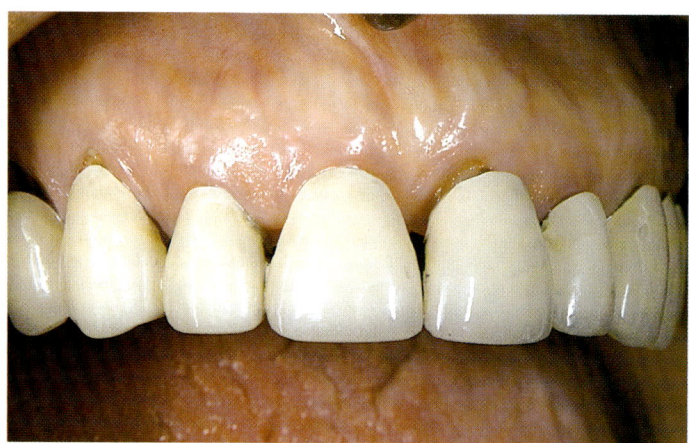

Fig 4-146 Whatever the reasons, wide open interdental embrasures (segregative forces beyond the limit of tolerance of nature), are an offense to esthetics. Even if gingival recession after periodontal surgery is not taken into consideration, the location of the contact points at the incisal tooth edge has already diminished the strength of this composition and its esthetic value.

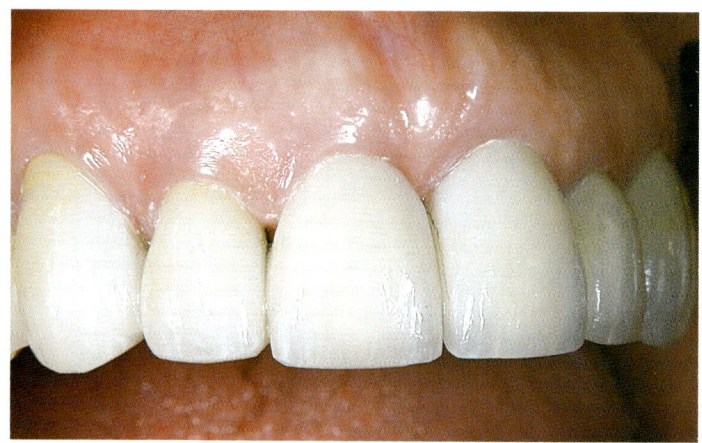

Fig 4-147 The restoration and maintenance of normal embrasures are made possible whenever adequate interdental anatomy, margin placement, and fit of restoration respect the biologic normality. The restoration of the incisal line distinct from the line of contact points introduces more cohesive forces in the composition.

Embrasures or interdental spaces

The cervical portion of the contact area, the interproximal wall of the adjacent teeth, and the interdental papilla form the interdental embrasure, a segregative esthetic factor assuring harmony in the dental composition. This space, or virtual space, is of primary importance in dentistry because caries and inflammatory tissue problems frequently originate in this area, which seems to be a favored location for microorganisms. The vulnerability of the interdental tissue is evidenced in daily practice. The spread of the inflammatory process to the interdental papilla, extending through the transeptal fibers and following the course of the blood vessels directly into the interdental canals of the osseous septum has been demonstrated.

Consequently, understanding the anatomy of the interproximal embrasures must be stressed because we know that most of our restorative procedures deal with the restoration of one or two of the basic elements that form the canopy housing the interdental papilla.

Whereas the shape of the col depends on the location and orobuccal shape of tooth contact, the interdental gingiva follows the shape of the bone. This shape varies following its location. On the anterior area it appears convex, reduced in width, and producing a pyramidal or knife-edge shape, and it becomes more flat in the posterior region. It is a well-established principle that the closer the roots, the higher and more convex the interproximal tissues between them are. Conversely, the more separated the roots, the flatter the interdental tissues will be.

Restorative procedures

In restorative treatment, sufficient tooth preparation is required to allow maintenance of the embrasure space. We know that exact restoration of enamel reduction is impossible. To prevent any overcontouring, some overpreparation of the tooth is indicated, assuming that the potential endodontic problems may be solved.

If the maintenance requirements cannot be fulfilled following inadequate interproximal width, then orthodontic therapy, root amputation, or total tooth removal should be envisaged.

In parallel to the slight overpreparation of the tooth, a systematic opening of the contact area both in the mesiodistal or orobuccal direction has been advocated, dictated by the statement that a slight inflammation is always possible when restorations are present, leading to an enlargement of the papilla whatever the material used. This statement loses validity when a systematic and accurate approach to tooth preparation and tissue protection is observed. The amount of enlargement of the embrasure space initiated with tooth preparation and finalized by the design of the restorations is dictated by cosmetic considerations and accessibility for oral hygiene. The same requirements have to be applied in the restoration of cases in which a reduction of the gingival level following periodontal disease or periodontal surgery has taken place (Figs 4-146 and 4-147). The decrease in esthetics is proportional to the increase in accessibility for oral hygiene. In the posterior area, wide open embrasures favor accessibility for oral hygiene and sufficient room for the gingiva[87–93] but do not allow for lateral food impaction, provided tooth contact is maintained.[94,95] However, the maintenance of wide open embrasures in the front–back progression of the arch is not compatible with esthetic or phonetic requirements. This militates in favor of a reduction of these embrasures, accomplished both in increasing the apicocoronal length of the contact area and in redesigning the direction of the interproximal walls. An orobuccal broadening of the contact area, favoring the formation of an oversized col, is contraindicated.

In all circumstances when a normal tooth structure exists as well as an adequate interproximal root proximity and a sound periodontal state, maintenance of the embrasure space depends directly on the amount of preparation, margin placement, fitness of restoration, emergence profile, interproximal tooth design, and location and width of the contact area. Consequently, it can be stated that, independently of the patient's oral hygiene, maintenance of a healthy embrasure is totally dependent on the ability and capability of the restorative dentist.

Gingival components

Gingival morphology

The gingiva belongs to the oral mucous membrane that covers the marginal part of the teeth and the alveolar process. It begins at the mucogingival junction (linea girlandiformis) and finishes at the tooth collar. Labial and lingual healthy gingiva have a matt and pink color

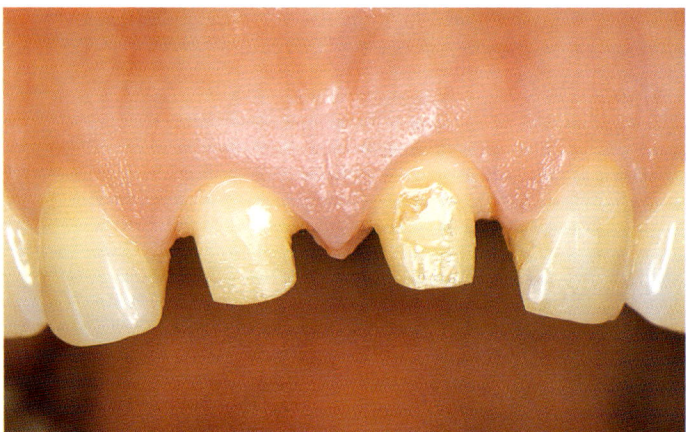

Fig 4-148 Clinical situation after tooth preparation respecting the integrity of the interdental and marginal gingiva.

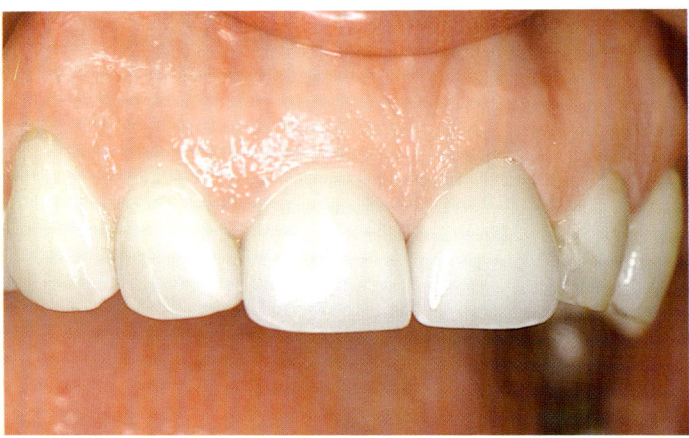

Fig 4-149 The tolerance of marginal tissue is proportionate to the respect of biologic parameters (see Chapter 10).

and are firmly attached to one another around the neck of the teeth with the exception of the free marginal gingiva. This firm attachment of the gingival tissue by way of the epithelial basement membrane to the underlying collagen fibers gives this tissue an orange peel appearance through minute depressions and elevations. This stippling varies with age, being less conspicuous in childhood that in adulthood. It is more common on the facial than the lingual surface. The gingiva is divided into the free and the attached gingiva. From the free gingiva we may distinguish the marginal gingiva that surrounds the teeth on the buccal and palatal side in an average width of 0.5 to 2 mm and the interdental gingiva or interdental papilla. The free gingiva describes a wavy course around the four surfaces of the tooth, with its margin on the interproximal surfaces constituting the most incisally located part of the gingiva (Figs 4-148 and 4-149).

The interdental papilla is the extension of the free marginal gingiva. Its form and size are determined by the contact relationship of the adjacent teeth and the width of the proximal surfaces. Apically, from the contact point between facial and oral papilla, we can find a small depression or col clinically invisible, wide, or deep, according to the width or shape of the contact point and covered by sulcular epithelium.

In case of large open contacts, the gingiva goes to a convex shape from oral to labial without any depression, and its outer surface is covered with a normal keratinized gingival epithelium. The attached gingiva extends from the bottom of the marginal gingiva to the mucogingival junction. Its width varies from one individual to the other and from specific locations to others. It generally appears wide in the maxillary and mandibular incisors and shows a decrease in width toward canine and premolar (Fig 4-150).

An increase in width of the attached gingiva proportionate to the increase in age has been recently stated. The maintenance of a good, healthy marginal periodontal tissue, providing a pleasing esthetic appearance, requires a minimal width of 2 mm of attached gingiva. According to some authors this width may not be sufficient. From a clinical point of view, it may be advisable to increase this minimal width and, above all, to eliminate the invading dense connective tissue frenulae before any restorative procedure because no professional can guarantee constant perfection in tooth preparation, casting adaptation, or accuracy following cementation.

Gingival components

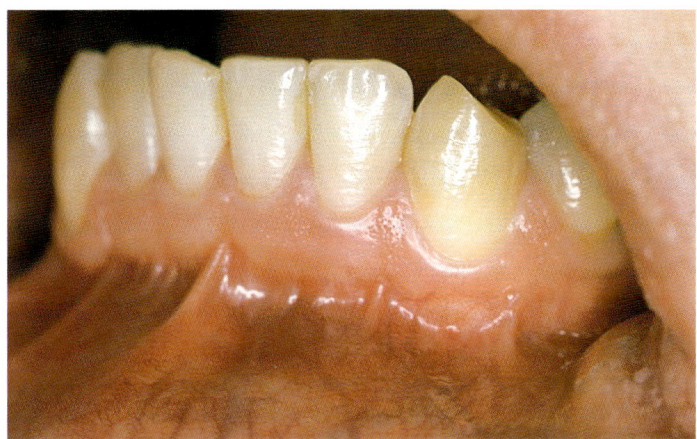

Fig 4-150 Clinical illustration of the attached gingiva and its precise delimitation from the alveolar mucosa, ie, Linea girlandiformis.

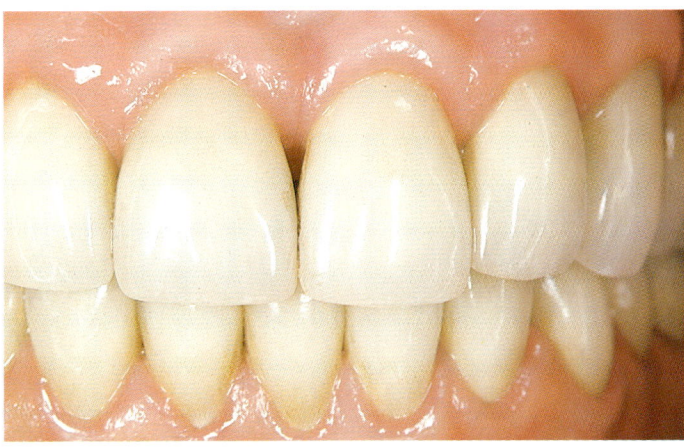

Fig 4-151 The gingival groove can be described as a shallow groove running parallel to the gingival margin, influenced by the arrangement of collagenous fibers.

The gingival groove can be described as a marked, shallow, V-shaped groove, which runs parallel to the margin of the gingiva at a distance of 0.5 to 2 mm. It may be found on the facial or buccal aspects of the gingiva. Measurements indicate that the distance from gingival margin to the gingival groove roughly corresponds to the depth of the sulcus (Fig 4-151).

The presence or absence of the groove is dependent on the arrangements of the supra-alveolar collagen fibers running from the cementum into the free and attached gingiva.

Gingival tissue and racial factor

If healthy gingiva exhibits minor differences in its pink matt coloration, blacks exhibit various degrees of dark brown pigmentation. Histologic examination reveals the presence of melanocytes located in the squamous stratified epithelium. These pigmentations are confined to the attached gingival tissue, which appears firm and keratinized and can also exhibit the typical orange peel stippled appearance. The free marginal gingiva and buccal mucosa do not contain these organic granules (Fig 4-152).

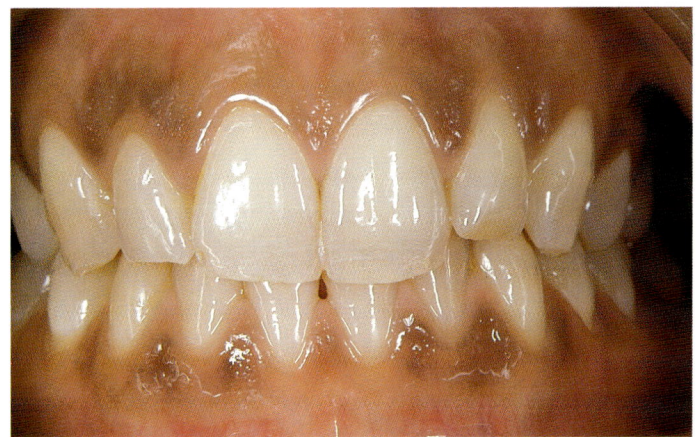

Fig 4-152 Gingival pigmentation is limited to the attached gingiva. Neither the free gingival nor the alveolar mucosa shows this peculiarity, a characteristic of blacks.

Structural Esthetic Rules

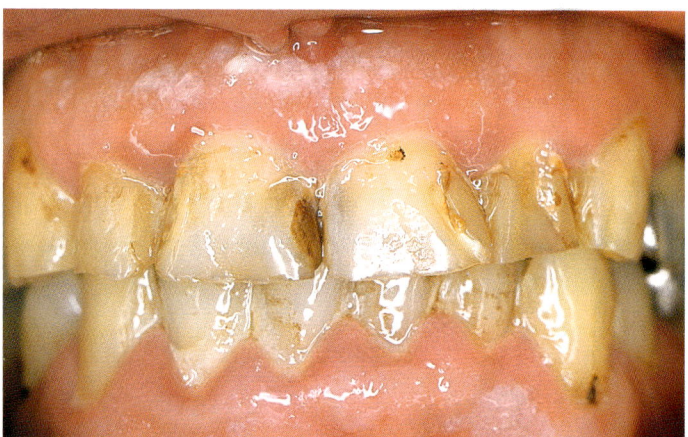

Fig 4-153 An absence of hygiene has favored an accumulation of deposits and dental plaque and produced periodontal inflammation and decay.

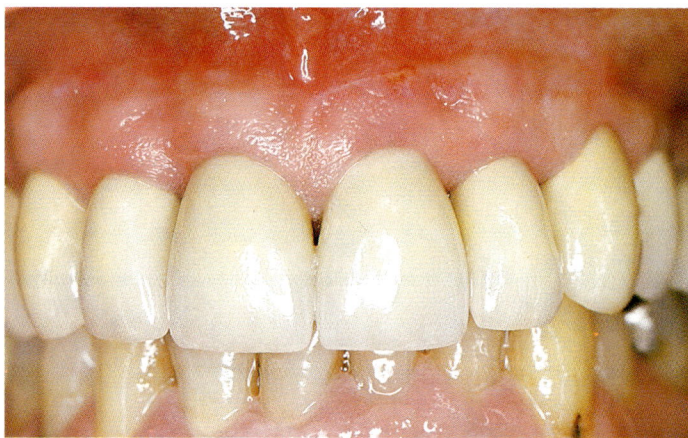

Fig 4-154 The patient's motivation, initial periodontal therapy, and provisional stabilization have contributed to the restoration of tissue health. The undertaking of necessary restorative procedures can be envisaged.

Alveolar mucosa

The alveolar mucosa is relatively sharply delimited from the attached gingiva at the mucogingival junction. This junction is usually more pronounced on the labial than the lingual aspect where the alveolar mucosa blends imperceptibly with the mucous membrane covering the palate. The alveolar mucosa covers the basal part of the alveolar process and continues into the vestibulum or the floor of the mouth. In contrast to the attached gingiva, the alveolar mucosa is loosely attached to the periosteum and therefore movable. The surface is smooth and nonkeratinized and has a more reddish appearance.

Gingival health

Healthy gingival tissue, as part of biologic structural beauty, is an important factor of esthetic perception. Health and its maintenance, or its evolution into disease restricted to the gingiva, or including the supporting structures is caused by microorganisms that produce inflammation and are influenced by a variety of factors. The severity of gingival inflammation is dependent on the intensity, frequency, and duration of the local irritants and the systemic resistance of the patient. The predictable reversibility of the disease is restricted to acute or chronic gingivitis. In periodontitis, which exhibits various types and degrees of bone destruction, the reversibility of the disease is limited to situations in which new bone formation, new attachment, or reattachment can be observed. However, in most situations, even if the disease can be controlled and healing occurs, the duplication of the previous healthy situation is not to be expected (Figs 4-153 and 4-154).

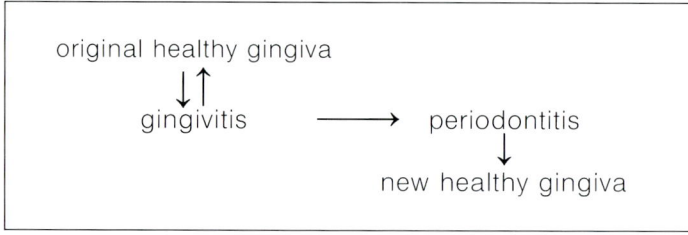

Gingival contour

Depending upon the individual's anatomic features and according to the lip line, the gingival tissues are usually

Gingival components

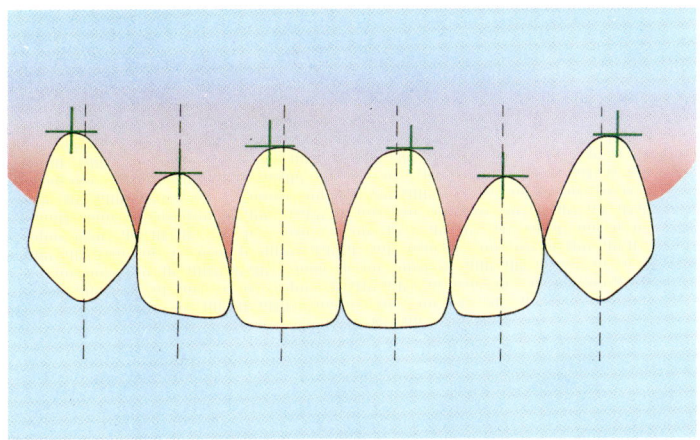

Fig 4-155 The location of gingival zenith in reference to tooth axis is distal on the maxillary central incisors and canines and coincidental on lateral incisors.

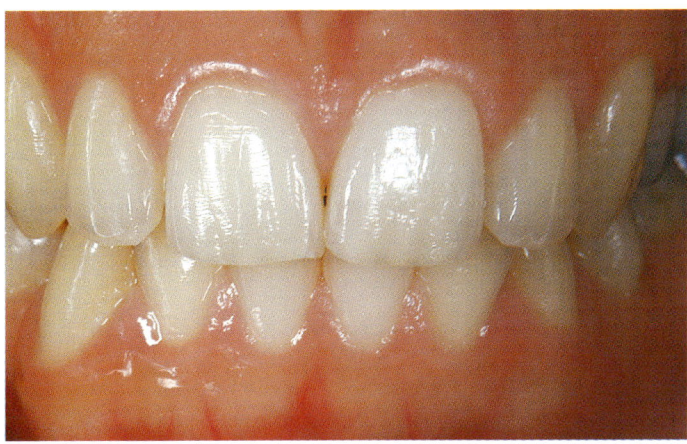

Fig 4-156 Clinical illustration of the natural location of the gingival zenith more or less marked according to tooth anatomy.

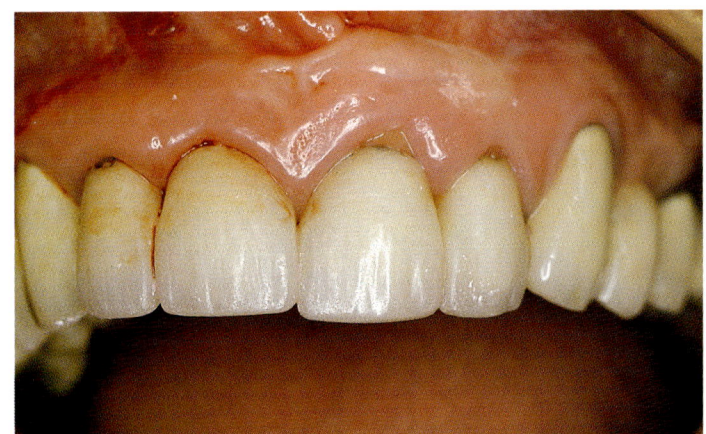

Fig 4-157 Loss of marginal gingival contour, attributed to localized presence of poor crown margin and muscular pull, corrected by means of free gingival graft.

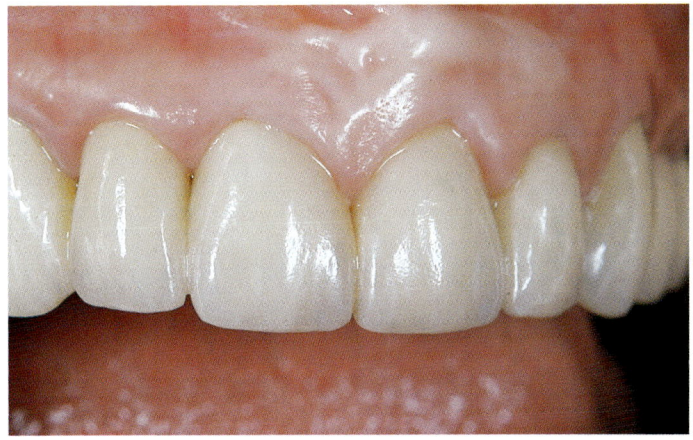

Fig 4-158 Restoration of the natural location of the gingival zenith with subsequent correction of the posterior front–back progression.

Structural Esthetic Rules

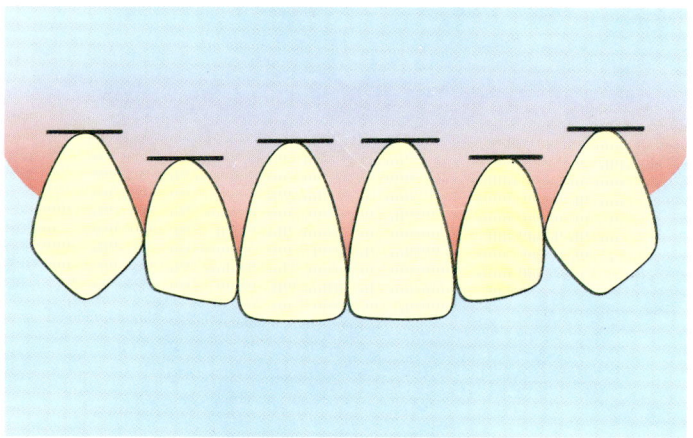

Fig 4-159 The average location of the gingiva in Class I shows a symmetric level on the maxillary central incisors, a lower location of the lateral incisors, and again a higher and ideally symmetric level on the canines.

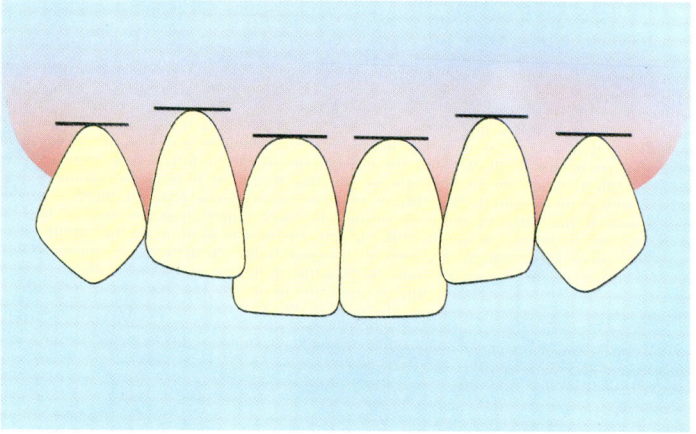

Fig 4-160 Average location of the gingiva and coordinate tooth position in Class II or pseudo-Class II, exhibiting a higher location of the gingival height on the lateral incisors relative to the central incisors.

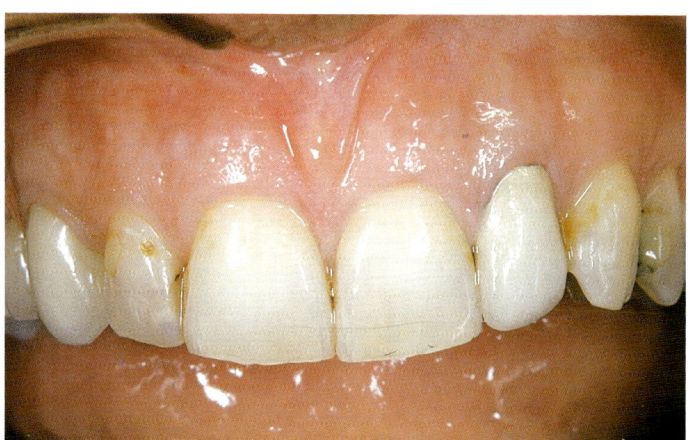

Fig 4-161 Original situation requiring esthetic improvement. Class I on the right and Class II on the left side, underlined by an imbalanced position of the left lateral incisor.

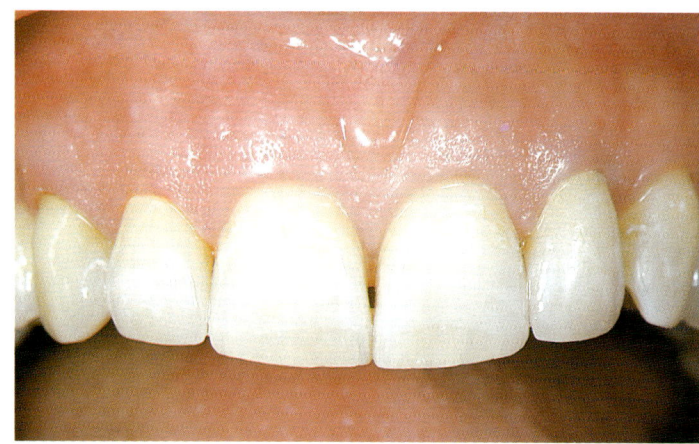

Fig 4-162 Final restoration respecting the natural position of the lateral incisors, relative to Class I and Class II, with a slight overlap of the left lateral on the central incisor to restore equilibrium.

exposed during smile, laughter, and even during normal speech. The evaluation of normal gingival color and contour is not limited to professionals but can be appreciated by nonprofessionals during daily social contacts. Any strange gingival contour will immediately be perceived and interpreted according to its degree of deviation from normality. This normality will also be judged according to four subsidiary factors.

1. *Embrasures.* In healthy individuals, the gingival tissue blends into tooth embrasure, which is totally filled from buccal to lingual. This embrasure is esthetically ideal. Unfortunately, it tends to appear, usually following gingival recession or periodontal therapy, by the development of a black interdental triangle. Whenever restoration procedures are accomplished, esthetic dentistry has to take into consideration restoration of the embrasure.

2. *Gingival zenith.* Clinical and study model observations have revealed that the most apical point of gingival tissue is located distal to the long axis of the tooth on both maxillary central incisors and canine (Figs 4-155 to 4-158). In the lateral maxillary incisor and the mandibular incisors the highest or lowest point of the gingival tissue is located along the tooth axis.

3. *Gingival height Class I.* In Class I occlusal tooth position, the marginal gingival tissue must be perceived by the observer at a parallel level on both central incisors (Figs 4-159 to 4-161). The same symmetric, parallel, and horizontal alignment of gingival tissue is apparent on lateral incisors and canines but at different levels, lower to the centrals for the lateral incisors and slightly higher for the canines. The pleasing symmetry of horizontal lines is enhanced by the perception of an attractive undulating line produced by the rise and fall of marginal gingival tissue.

4. *Gingival height Class II.* In Class II, division 2 or in pseudo-Class II, the horizontal level of the gingival margin of lateral incisors is located higher in reference to the central incisors. Concomitantly, the lateral incisor tends to slightly overlap the central (Figs 4-160 to 4-162). The dominance of the central incisor, which is exhibited in Class I and reflected by the differing lengths of exposed anatomic crown, is diminished in this tooth arrangement to the benefit of another characterization of the dental composition. The attractive perception of the undulating line of marginal tissue is maintained. This characteristic gingival margin placement and the slight overlap of lateral incisors that goes along with it is most often neglected by dentists or technicians who miss an opportunity to provide natural variety in dental compositions whenever this possibility is offered.

Physical components

Illusions

The size and shape of artificial teeth, particularly their length and width, as the end result of a situation created by surgical procedures or the existing morphology, may appear offensive with reference to normality. The ideal treatment techniques to correct deformities or to provide adequate availability of space for dental elements may prove disproportionate to the problem involved, contraindicated, or simply unrealistic.

Where nature would have answered with tooth rotation, malposition, or diastema, the restorative dentist has either to face the extreme difficulty of mimicking natural deformities, which may prove adventurous when dealing with pontic elements, or building teeth in line and using optical illusive procedures. The use of optical concepts to create optical illusions of size and shape that are different from reality may turn out to be the best way to solve or hide an esthetically difficult situation.

Visual perception is possible only if objects contrast in color, shape, and lines. The perception of the contour of objects is dependent upon the deflection or reflection of the light that reaches them because the surface form of these objects is responsible for light reflection (Fig 4-163). The control of the phenomenon of light reflection and the control of color contrast will provide us with the means of creating illusion and thereby reestablish proportions because "our vision is often fooled by optical illusive effects"[23] (Figs 4-164 and 4-165). However, the use of illusive optical procedures (Figs 4-166 to 4-183) should only be carried out taking into account all the morphologic characteristics of the dental units within the limits of the patient's visual tolerance, keeping in mind that illusions will be accepted until some event proves they are just illusions. The understanding of these principles must be shared by the dental technician and the dentist because only a combined coordination of both operators in the laboratory and in the dental chair will allow for an optimal result.

Structural Esthetic Rules

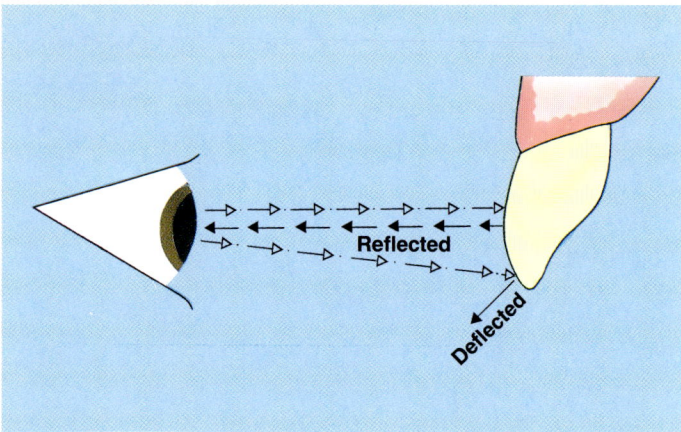

Fig 4-163 The modification of the amount of light that is deflected or reflected from objects and affects the sharpness of perception will be used to create the phenomenon of illusion.

These principles can be summarized as follows:

1. Increased contrast increases visibility.
2. Increased light reflection increases visibility.
3. Increased light deflection diminishes visibility.

These principles are best illustrated by the observation of the following points:

1. Shadows create depth.
2. Light creates prominences.
3. Vertical lines accent length.
4. Horizontal lines accent width.

In dentistry these optical principles should be applied by means of tooth contouring and color manipulation. Tooth contouring must be limited to angles, natural grooves and prominences, incisal or gingival inclines, and incisal edges. However, the manipulation of color is best applied in their natural locations: gingival inclines, interdental areas, and selected tooth surfaces.

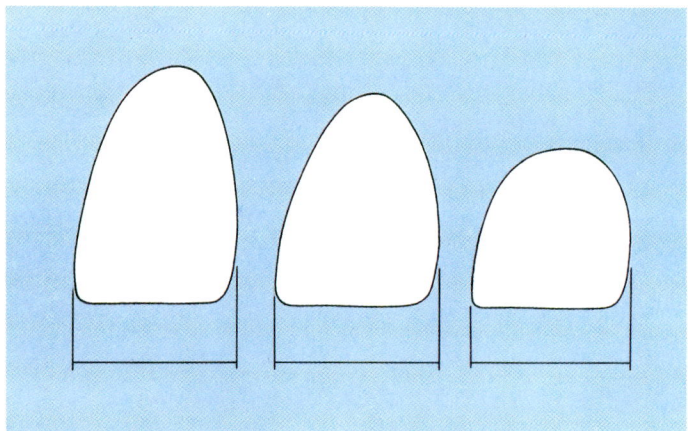

Fig 4-164 Standard illustration of optical illusive differences of width of teeth having different lengths.

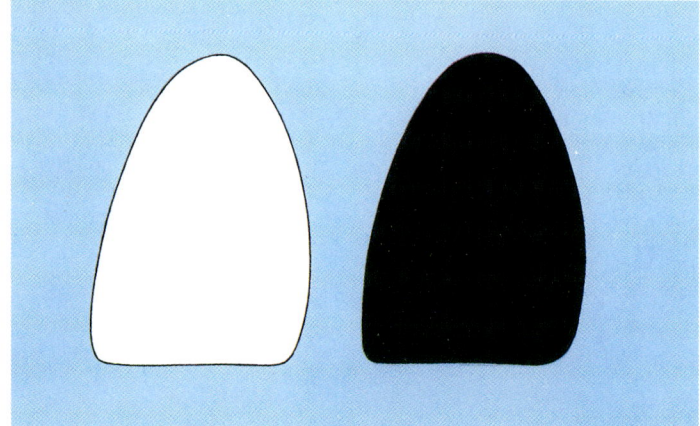

Fig 4-165 Illustration of illusive differences of size of two identical teeth due to differences in the color value.

Physical components

Initial situation

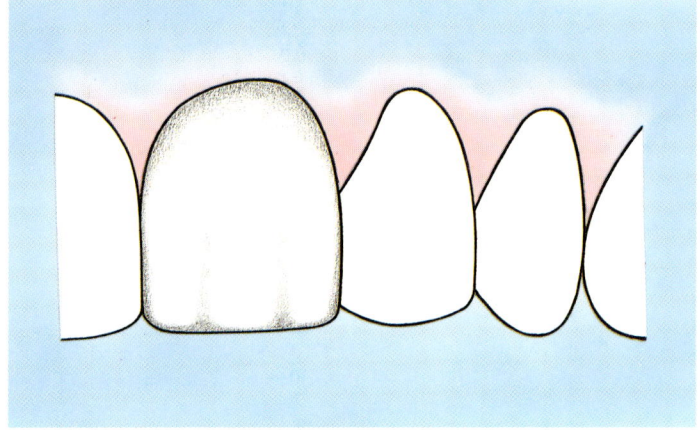

Fig 4-166 The labial surface of the maxillary central incisor is characterized by three labial prominences.

Initial situation

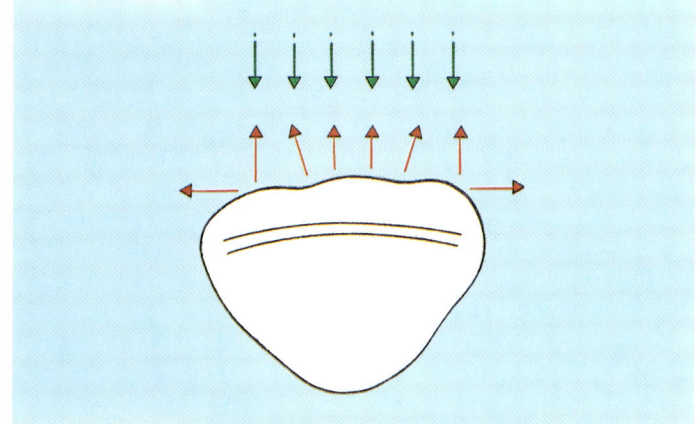

Fig 4-167 Schematic evaluation of the amount of light reflected or deflected from the tooth surface.

Narrowing illusion

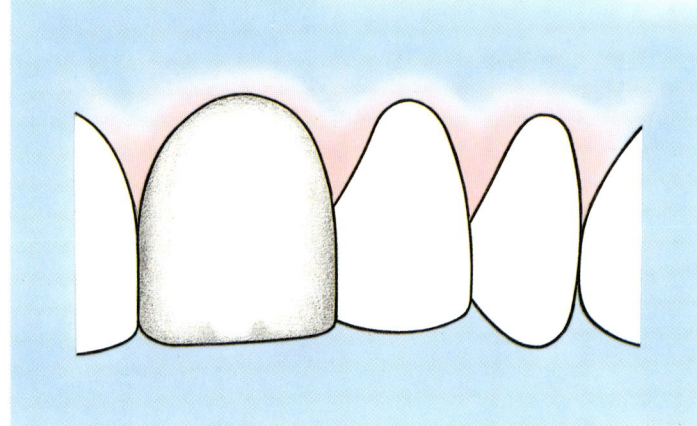

Fig 4-168

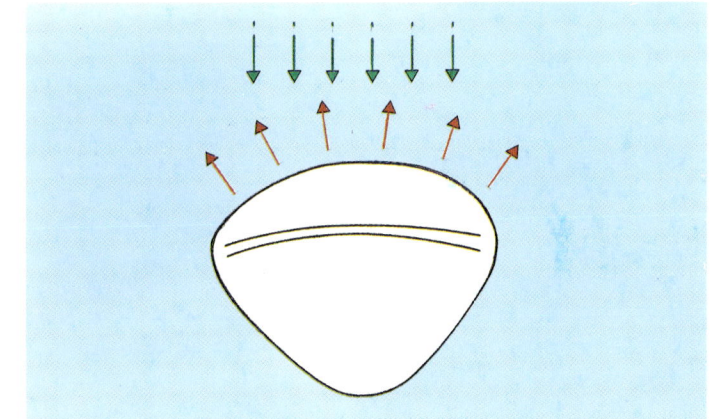

Fig 4-169

Tooth contour modification: Adjust the lateral prominences toward the center; increase the curvature of the central prominence mesiodistally; increase moderately the length of the central prominence.

Tooth color modification: Increase the staining of the interproximal areas.

129

Structural Esthetic Rules

Widening illusion

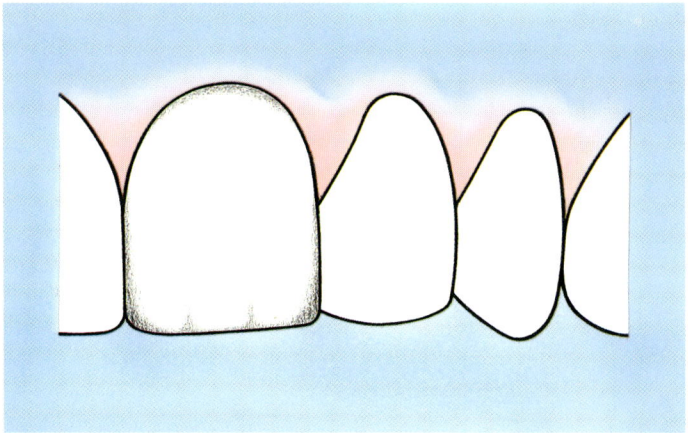

Fig 4-170

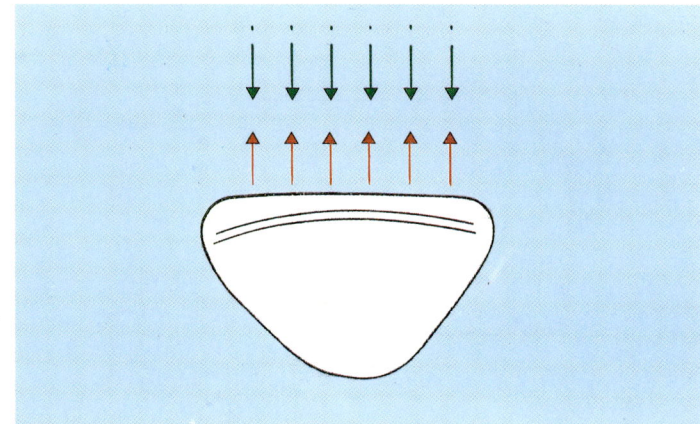

Fig 4-171

Tooth contour modification: Adjust the lateral prominences proximally; diminish the curvature of the central prominence mesiodistally; diminish moderately the length of the central prominence.

Tooth color modification: Diminish the staining of the interproximal area.

Initial situation

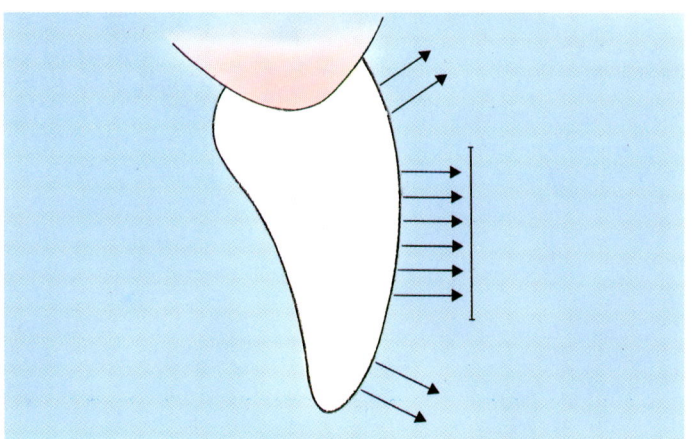

Fig 4-172   Cross section of the maxillary central incisor.

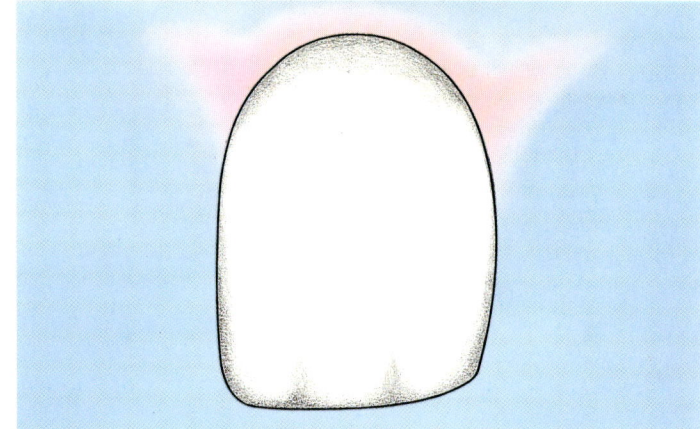

Fig 4-173   Illustration of the labial surface.

Physical components

Shortening illusion

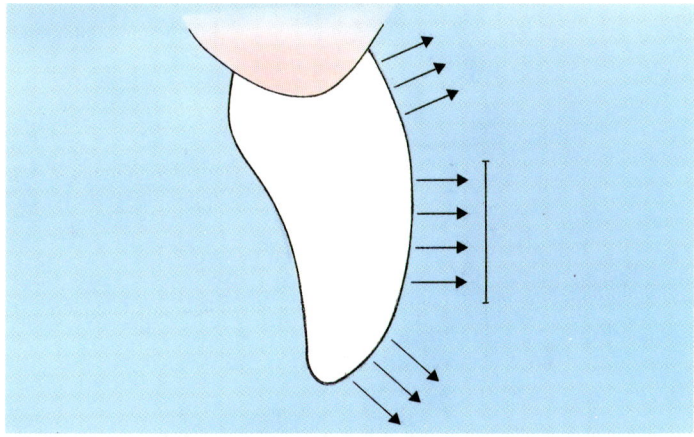

Fig 4-174

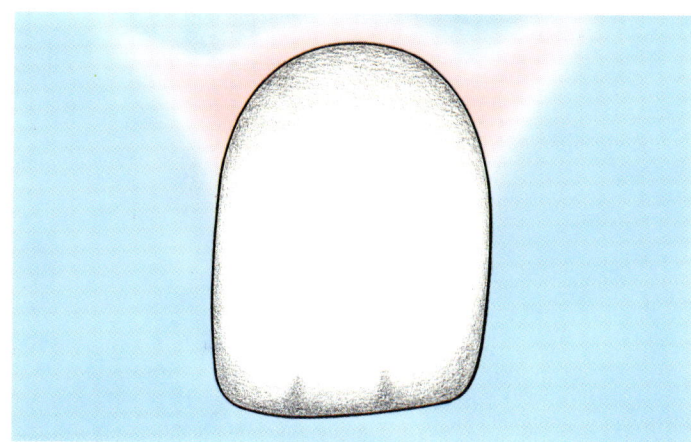

Fig 4-175

Tooth contour modification: Adjust the incisal incline lingually; diminish the length of the central prominence; accentuate the horizontal characterizations of surface; flatten the middle third of labial surface to broaden the surface of light reflection.

Tooth color modification: Darken the gingival third and diminish the interproximal staining.

Lengthening illusion

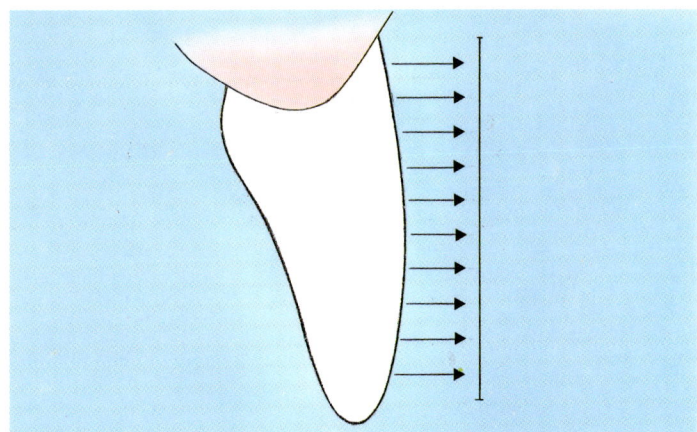

Fig 4-176

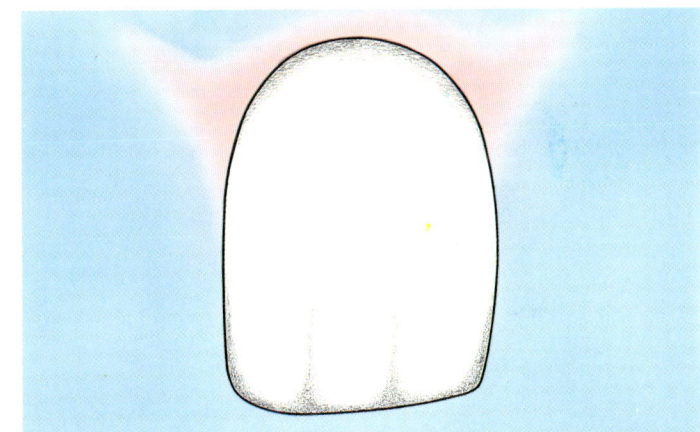

Fig 4-177

Tooth contour modification: Flatten the labial surface gingivoincisally; increase the length of the central prominence; round the labial surface mesiodistally; accentuate the vertical characterizations surface.

Tooth color modification: Lighten the gingival third and increase the interproximal staining.

Structural Esthetic Rules

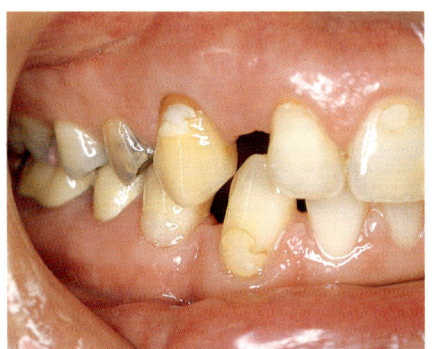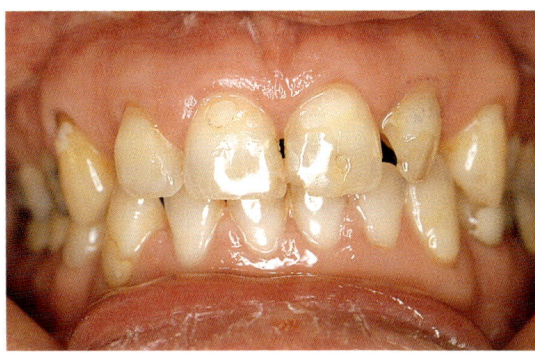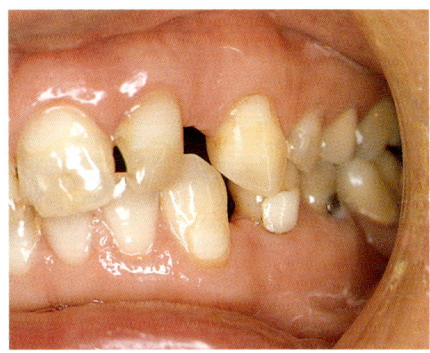

Figs 4-178 to 4-180 Attracted by the spiral cavity restoration, this meticulous individual has maintained his dentition throughout the years until the migration of the left lateral incisor and the progressive enlargement of the existing unesthetic lateral diastemas brought him to the orthodontist's office. Unwilling to undergo the duration of such type of a treatment, it was stated after occlusal analysis and waxing that future stability of this case could be obtained using prosthetic measures. Major restrictions were imposed on the esthetic appearance as the width left for both maxillary canines did not exceed 4.5 to 5 mm.

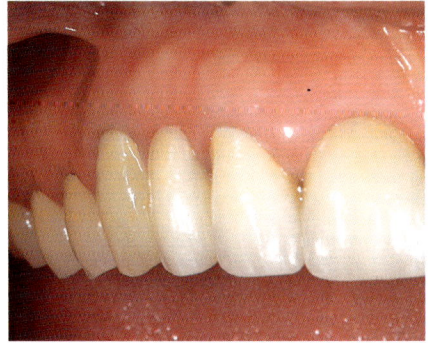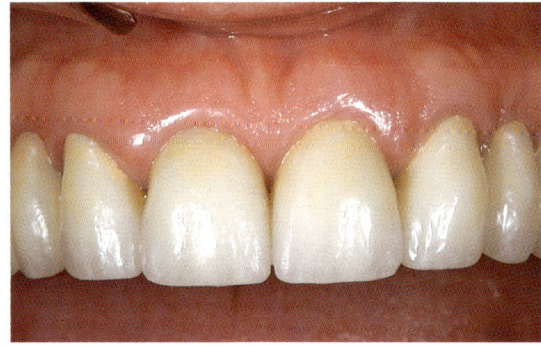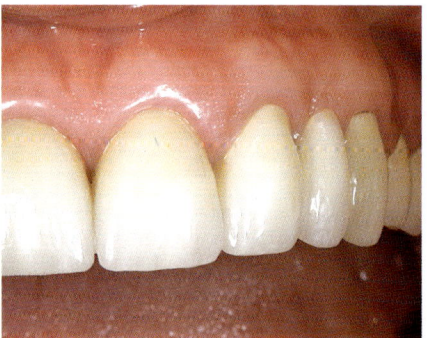

Figs 4-181 to 4-183 The decision to use optical illusive procedures to hide the existing anatomic deficiencies appealed to both dentist and dental technician. Restricted to the introduction of widening illusions by modification of tooth contour and color, the procedure was performed without significant complication. The try-in, however, showed that typical canine anatomic design for such a narrow tooth (regardless of the results of the illusive procedure) was inadequate. A compromise canine lateral incisor was adopted and finalized the ultimate effect.

References

1. Rollet F; Carrere ed. *Guide Pratique de Morphopsychologie*. Paris: 1987.
2. Martone AC. Anatomy of facial expressions and its prosthodontic significance. *J Prosthet Dent*. 1962;12:1020–1041.
3. Gonzales-Uhloa M, Meyer R, Smith JW, Zaoli G. *Esthetic Surgery*. Padova: Piccin; 1988.
4. Brodie A. Anatomy and physiology of head and neck musculature. *Am J Orthod*. 1950;11:831.
5. Sarnat BG. *The temporo-mandibular joint*. Springfield, Ill: Charles C Thomas, Publisher; 1951.
6. Silverman MM. *Occlusion*. Washington, DC: Mutual Publishing Co; 1962.
7. Vig RG, Brundo GC. The kinetics of anterior tooth display. *J Prosthet Dent*. 1972;39:502.
8. McKenzie RT. Human facial types: Facial expressions. *Dent Cosmos*. 1935;77:639.
9. Huber E. *Evolution of Facial Musculature and Facial Expressions*. Baltimore, Md: Johns Hopkins Press; 1931.
10. Lightholler GS. The action of the M. mentalis in the expression of emotion of distress. *J Anat*. 1927;62:319.
11. Matthews TG. The anatomy of smile. *J Prosthet Dent*. 1978;39:128.
12. Lombardi RE. A method for the classification of errors in dental esthetics. *J Prosthet Dent*. 1974;32:501.
13. Lombardi RE. The principles of visual perception and their clinical application to denture esthetics. *J Prosthet Dent*. 1973;9:358.
14. Frush JP, Fisher RD. The dynesthetic interpretation of the dentogenic concept. *J Prosthet Dent*. 1965;8:558.
15. Levin EI. Dental esthetics and the golden proportion. *J Prosthet Dent*. 1978;40:244.
16. Hulsey CM. An esthetic evaluation of lip–teeth relationships present in smile. *Am J Orthod*. 1970;57:132.
17. Heartwell CM. *Syllabus of Complete Dentures*. Philadelphia, Pa: Lea & Febiger; 1968.
18. Frush J. *Swissdent Technique and Procedure Manual*. Los Angeles, Calif: Swissdent Corp; 1971.
19. Miller EC, Bodden WR, Jamison HC. A study of the relationship of the dental midline to the facial median line. *J Prosthet Dent*. 1979;41:657–660.
20. Renner RP. *An Introduction to Dental Anatomy and Esthetics*. Chicago, Ill: Quintessence Publ Co; 1985.
21. AAOMS. Dento-facial deformities: Evaluation guide. 1986;2:9.
22. Lejoyeux J; Maloine SA, ed. *Prothèse Complète*. Paris: 1979.
23. Goldstein RE. *Esthetics in Dentistry*. Philadelphia, Pa: JB Lippincott Co; 1976.
24. Pacioli L. *Divine Proportione*. Wien Graser: C. Winterberg; 1896.
25. Hambridge J. *The Parthenon and Other Greek Temples, Their Dynamic Symmetry*. London; 1920.
26. Le Corbusier. *Le Modular*. Paris; 1950.
27. Meyers B. *Le Livre d'Art. L'Interprétation de l'Art*. New York, NY: Grolier; 10:1971.
28. Glyka PC. *Esthétique des Proportions dans la Nature et dans les Arts*. Paris; 1927.
29. Coxeter HSM. *The golden section. Phyllotaxis and Wythoff's Game*. New York, NY: Scripta Mathematica; 1953.
30. D'Arch WT. *Growth and Form*. Oxford: Cambridge University Press; 1952.
31. Panotsky E. L'évolution d'un schéma structural. *Meaning in the Visual Art*. 1955.
32. Fechner GT. *Vorschule der Ästhetik*. Leipzig; 1876.
33. Lombardi RE. The principles of visual perception and their clinical application to dental esthetics. *J Prosthet Dent*. 1973;29:358–381.
34. Levin EI. Dental esthetics and the golden proportion. *J Prosthet Dent*. 1978;40:244–252.
35. Goldstein RE. Esthetic principles for ceramo-metal restorations. *Dent Clin North Am*. 1977;21:803.
36. Zeisz RC, Nuckolls J. *Dental Anatomy*. London: Henry Kimpton; 1949.
37. Lee JH. *Dental Esthetics*. Bristol, Conn: Wright and Sons Ltd; 1962.
38. Silverman MM. Accurate measurement of the vertical dimension by phonetics and the speaking centric space. *Dent Digest*. 1951;57:261–265, 308–311.
39. Morrison LM. Phonetics as a method of determining vertical dimension and centric relation. *J Am Dent Assoc*. 1959;59:680–695.
40. Lynn BD. The significance of anatomic landmarks in complete denture service. *J Prosthet Dent*. 1964;14:456.
41. Harper RN. The incisive papilla. The basis of a technique to reproduce the positions of key teeth in prosthodontic. *J Dent Res*. 1948;27:661.
42. Schiffman P. Relation to the maxillary canine and the incisive papilla. *J Prosthet Dent*. 1984;14:469.
43. Watt MD. *Designing Complete Dentures*. Philadelphia, Pa: WB Saunders; 1967.
44. Mavroskoufis MD, Ritchie GM. Nasal width and incisive papilla as guides for the selection and arrangement of maxillary anterior teeth. *J Prosthet Dent*. 1981;45:592–597.
45. Ortman HR, Tsao Ding H. Relationship of the incisive papilla to the maxillary central incisors. *J Prosthet Dent*. 1979;42:492–496.
46. Marxkors R. Die Aufstellung der Frontzähne. *ZWR*. 1975;11:522–527.
47. Preti G, Pera P, Bassi F. Prediction of the shape and size of the maxillary anterior arch in edentulous patients. *J Oral Rehabil*. 1986;13:115–125.
48. Gysi A. Unregelmässige Stellung der Frontzähne für prothetische Arbeiten. *Schweiz Monatsschr Zahnheilkd*. 1936;46:58.
49. Mavroskoufis F, Ritchie GM. The face form as a guide for the selection of central incisors. *J Prosthet Dent*. 1980;43:301–505.
50. Bell RA. The geometric theory of selection of artificial teeth: Is it valid? *J Am Dent Assoc*. 1978;97:637–640.
51. Simon PW. *Fundamental Principles of a Systematic Diagnosis of Dental Anomalies*. Boston, Ma: Statford Co; 1926.
52. Hughes GH. Facial types and tooth arrangements. *J Prosthet Dent*. 1951;1:82–95.
53. Burstone CJ. Lip posture and its significance in treatment planning. *Am J Orthod*. 1967;53:262–284.
54. Shelby DS. Esthetics and fixed restorations. *Dent Clin North Am*. 1967.
55. Weinberg LA. Esthetics and the gingivae in full coverage. *J Prosthet Dent*. 1960;10:737.
56. Stein RS. *Fortbildungskurs*. Zürich, Switzerland: 1978.
57. Wheeler RC. *Dental Anatomy and Physiology*. Philadelphia, Pa: WB Saunders; 1969.

58. Kraus BS, Jordan RE, Abrams L. *Dental Anatomy and Occlusion: A Study of the Masticatory System.* Baltimore, Md: Williams & Wilkins; 1969.
59. Williams JL. A new classification of human tooth forms with special reference to a new system of artificial teeth. *Dent Cosmos.* 1914;56:627.
60. Seluck LW, Brodbelt RHW, Walker GF. A biometric comparison of face shape with denture tooth form. *J Oral Rehabil.* 1987;14:139–145.
61. Lehman W. Tooth form and face form: A comedy of errors. *South Calif State Dent J.* 1950;17:29.
62. Gerber A. *Proportionen und Stellung der Frontzähne im natürlichen und künstlichen Zahnbogen.* Berlin: Quintessenz Verlags-GmbH; 1965.
63. Kern BE. Anthropometric parameter of tooth selection. *J Prosthet Dent.* 1967;17:431.
64. *A Manual for Plastic Teeth.* Philadelphia, Pa: HD Justi Co; 1949.
65. *Automatic Instant Selector Guide.* Chicago, Ill: Austenal Dental, Inc; 1951.
66. Dawson P. Personal communication, 1983.
67. Schärer P. *Aesthetische Richtlinien für die Reconstructive Zahnheilkunde.* Berlin: Quintessenz Verlags-GmbH; 1980.
68. Reynolds JM. Abutment selection for fixed prosthodontics. *J Prosthet Dent.* 1968;19:483.
69. Bjorndol AM, Henderson WG. Anatomic measurements of human teeth extracted from males between ages of 17 and 21 years. *Oral Surg.* 1979;38:791–803.
70. Shillingburg HT, Kaplan MJ, Grace CS. Tooth dimensions: A comparative study. *J South Calif Dent Assoc.* 1972;40:830–839.
71. MacArthur DR. Determination of the approximate size of maxillary anterior denture teeth when mandibular anterior teeth are present. Part III: Relationship of maxillary to mandibular central incisor widths. *J Prosthet Dent.* 1985;53:540–542.
72. MacArthur DR. Are anterior replacement teeth too small? *J Prosthet Dent.* 1987;57:462–465.
73. Garn SM, Lewis AB, Walenga AJ. Maximum confidence values for the human mesio-distal crown dimension. *Arch Oral Biol.* 1968;13:841–849.
74. Garn SM, Lewis AB, Kerawsky RS. Sexual dimorphism in the buccolingual tooth diameters. *J Dent Res.* 1966;45:1819.
75. Lavelle CLB. Maxillary and mandibular tooth size in different racial groups and in different occlusal categories. *Am J Orthod.* 1972;61:29–37.
76. Mack PJ. Maxillary arch and central incisor dimension in a Nigerian and British population sample. *J Dent.* 1981;9:67–70.
77. Lammie GA, Posselt U. Progression changes in the dentition of adults. *J Periodontol.* 1965;36:443–454.
78. Frush JP, Fisher RD. The age factor in dentogenics. *J Prosthet Dent.* 1957;7:5.
79. Pound E. Esthetic dentures and their phonetic values. *J Prosthet Dent.* 1951;2:98–112.
80. Krajicek OD. Simulation of natural appearance. *J Prosthet Dent.* 1962;12:28–32.
81. Frush JP, Fisher RD. How dentinogenics integrate the sex factor. *J Prosthet Dent.* 1956;6:160–172.
82. Frush JP, Fisher RD. How dentinogenics integrate the personality factor. *J Prosthet Dent.* 1956;6:441–449.
83. Goldman HM, Cohen DW. *Periodontal Therapy.* 4th ed. St. Louis, Mo: CV Mosby; 1968.
84. Wheeler RC. *Dental Anatomy: Physiology and Occlusion.* Philadelphia, Pa: WB Saunders Co; 1940.
85. Okeson J, Lawell H. Periodontal health through restorative contour. *J Indiana Dent Assoc.* 1976;55:17.
86. Graver H. Restorative dentistry must be preventative dentistry. *J Prev Dent.* 1976;3:17.
87. Rateitschak KH, Rateitschak EM, Wolf HF. *Parodontologie.* Stuttgart: Thieme; 1984.
88. Takei HH. The interdental space. *Dent Clin North Am.* 1980;24:169.
89. Ramfjord S. Periodontal aspects of restorative dentistry. *J Oral Rehabil.* 1974;1:107.
90. Hazen S, Osborne J. Relationship of operative dentistry to periodontal health. *Dent Clin North Am.* 1967;2:45.
91. Weinberg LA. Esthetic and the gingiva in full coverage. *J Prosthet Dent.* 1960;10:737.
92. Hirshberg SM. The relationship of hygiene to embrasure and pontic design: A preliminary study. *J Prosthet Dent.* 1972;27:26.
93. Burch J. Ten rules for developing tooth contour in dental restorations. *Dent Clin North Am.* 1971;15:611.
94. Glickman I. *Clinical Periodontology.* Philadelphia, Pa: WB Saunders.
95. Beaudreau D. Procedures in general dentistry that affect the periodontium. In Goldman H, Cohen DW (eds). *Periodontal Therapy.* St. Louis, Mo: CV Mosby; 1968:956–958.

Part II
Intraoral and Extraoral Means to Rejuvenation

Chapter 5

Esthetics and Its Relationship to Function

Robert Lee

Introduction

However pleasing a dental restoration may appear, if it is destructive to the biologic system, it is "ugly." Many dentists and laboratory technicians lack knowledge concerning natural tooth morphology and tooth positions that help create beautiful teeth and smiles and good function. Dentists who have devoted much of their lives studying and practicing occlusal rehabilitation have generally ignored esthetics while concentrating on improved function, joint stability, and comfort for their patients. On the other hand, dentists who have concentrated their efforts on esthetics have often paid little attention to function. If we understand the functions of teeth, it is easier to reproduce them in natural-like artificial forms because form follows function. Today's challenge is to give patients the best of both worlds: good function and good esthetics.

In modern humans the primary functions of the teeth are for (1) mastication, (2) swallowing, (3) speech, (4) expression (eg, smiling), (5) psychologic, (6) esthetics, and (7) craniomandibular stabilization.

Bioesthetics is the study or theory of the beauty of living things in their natural forms and functions. This chapter presents bioesthetic relationships of natural unworn tooth forms to (1) rest position, (2) centric relation position, (3) vertical dimension of occlusion, (4) vertical and horizontal overbite, (5) condyle positions during rest and function, (6) plane of occlusion, and (7) mastication. The role of anterior crown morphology and tooth position and their importance for both esthetics and function will be covered in particular.

Esthetics involves more than the six anterior maxillary teeth, however. In most people it goes at least back to the first molars during a large smile or laugh (Fig 5-1). Consideration will also be given to the form and function of posterior crowns. Because occlusal loading affects the longevity of the teeth, periodontium, joints, and dental restorations, this chapter discusses how tooth morphology relates to occlusal loading of the gnathic system. Some important aspects of clinical treatments for bioesthetic occlusion will be presented in the latter part of this chapter.

Natural unworn permanent crown morphology

The following discussion of the crowns of teeth is not intended to be a complete anatomic description but rather highlights some significant morphologic factors

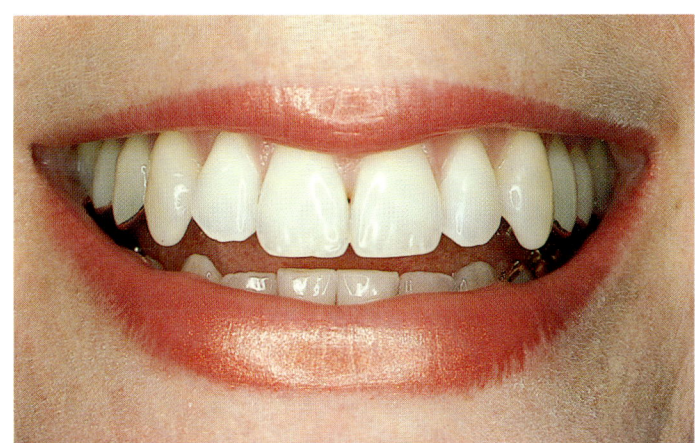

Fig 5-1 Smile of a 27-year-old woman showing mesial of maxillary first molars.

Esthetics and Its Relationship to Function

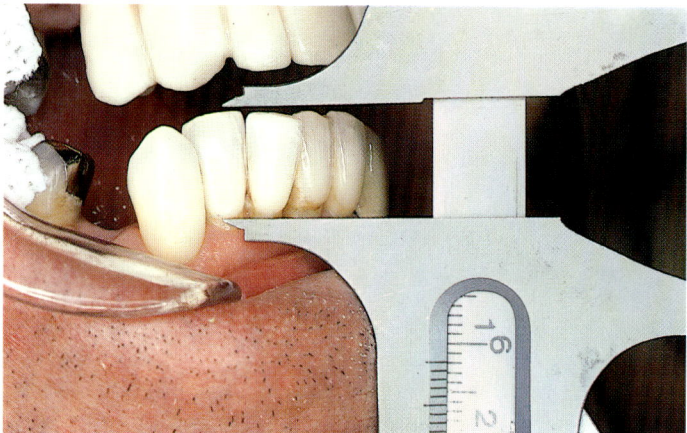

Fig 5-2 A 12-mm mandibular incisor.

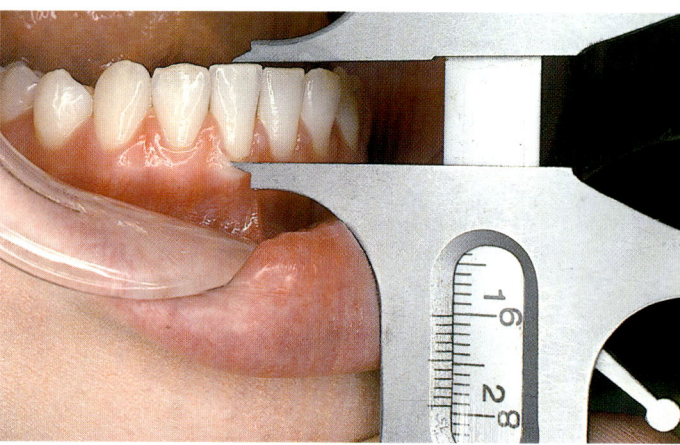

Fig 5-3 A 10-mm (average length) mandibular incisor.

relating to oral functions and esthetics, which perhaps have been overlooked. Dental morphology and anatomy books often show average tooth lengths skewed to the low end because they include worn teeth.[1-4] It is necessary to have unworn crown morphology for good esthetics as well as function. Nature produces sharp tooth morphology on both anterior and posterior occlusal surfaces. However, to protect the extremely hard prismatic hydroxyapatite enamel from fracturing the sharp incisal edges, cusp points, and ridges, nature has provided convexity at the crests and apexes of these tooth structures.

Mandibular incisors

Although the mandibular incisors are the smallest teeth in the mouth, they are a physiologic cornerstone for good occlusion. It is almost impossible to have long-lasting nontraumatic functional occlusion without adequate clinical crown lengths of these teeth. Unworn natural mandibular central and lateral incisors range from 9 to 12 mm from the cementoenamel junction to the incisal edge (Fig 5-2) with an average length of 10 mm (Fig 5-3). The central incisors are slightly narrower than the laterals. The incisal edges from labial to lingual are about 0.5 mm (Fig 5-4). The actual incisal edges are even sharper because of their convexity (Fig 5-5). The mandibular incisors have a labial angulation in the dental arch.

Maxillary incisors

A facial view of maxillary unworn natural anterior teeth in the mouth generally show relatively large, long central incisor crowns (see Fig 5-1). Mesial and distal incisal edges of unworn central incisors are rounded. The straight incisal edges often observed on central incisors are usually caused by wear patterns. Labial to lingual incisal edge contours are convex but sharp (about 0.7 mm). The lateral incisors are smaller and shorter, with more rounded mesiodistal incisal edges than the central incisors. The crown length of maxillary unworn central incisors ranges from 11 to 13 mm, with an average of 12 mm from the cementoenamel junction to the incisal edge (Fig 5-6). The lateral incisors are about 10 mm long with the incisal edge about 1 to 2 mm shorter than the central incisors. The gingival height of the lateral incisor is about 1 mm below the central incisor (Fig 5-7). The maxillary incisors have a labial incisal angulation in the dental arch. The concave lingual fossa of the maxillary incisors is designed for phonetics and

Natural unworn permanent crown morphology

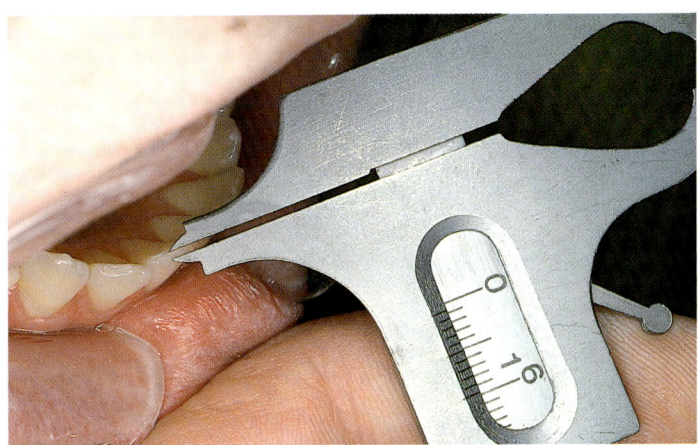

Fig 5-4 Cutting edges of unworn mandibular incisors are 0.5 to 0.75 mm.

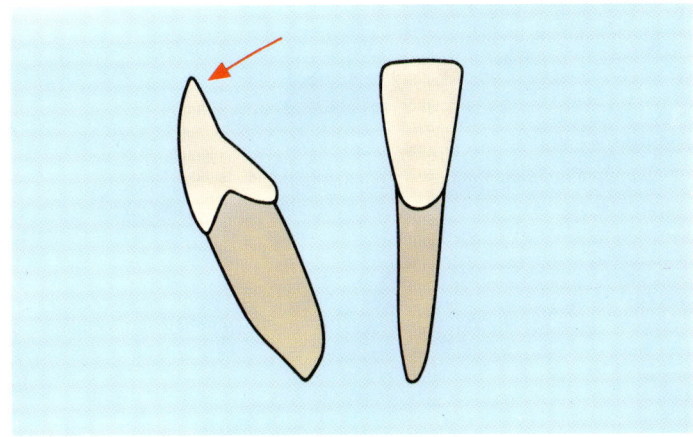

Fig 5-5 Profile tracing of actual mandibular incisor. The arrow indicates sharp convex cutting edge.

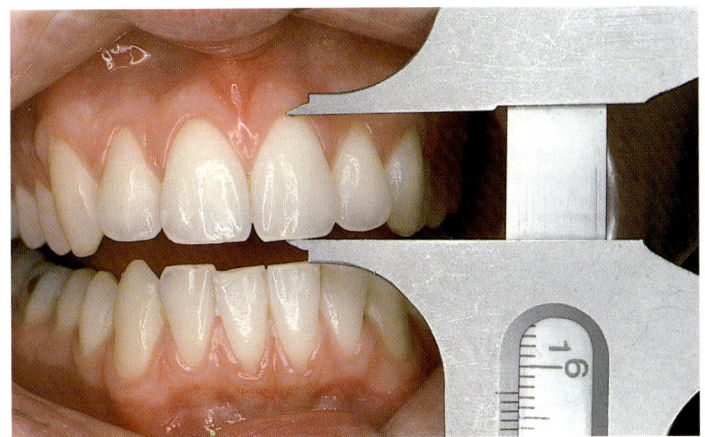

Fig 5-6 A 12.5-mm maxillary central incisor with slightly worn incisal edge.

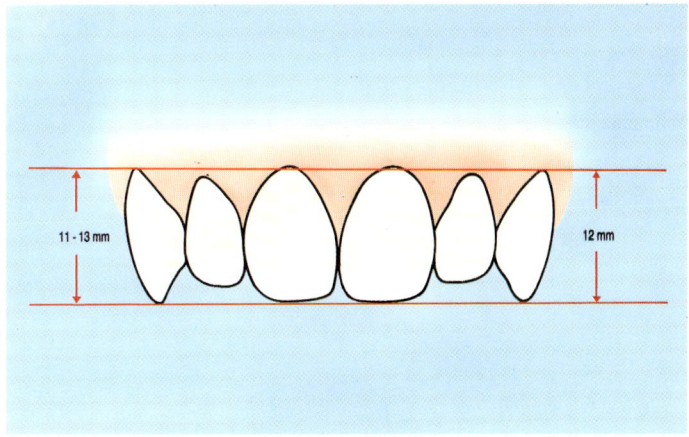

Fig 5-7 In good occluding dentitions the maxillary central incisors and canines are positioned about the same vertically and the lateral incisors are shorter both cervically and incisally.

139

Esthetics and Its Relationship to Function

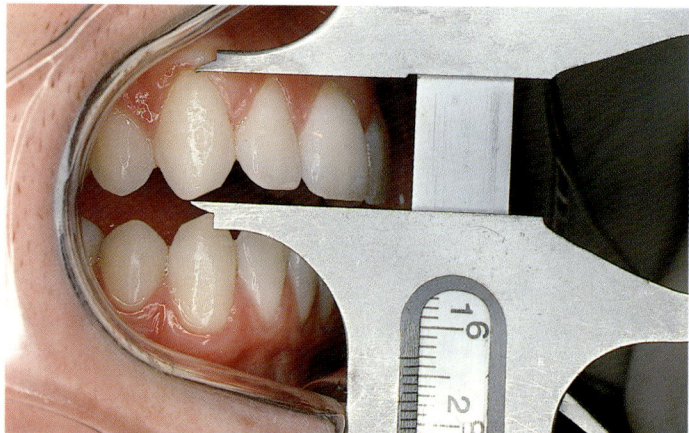

Fig 5-8 A 13-mm right maxillary canine with slight attrition.

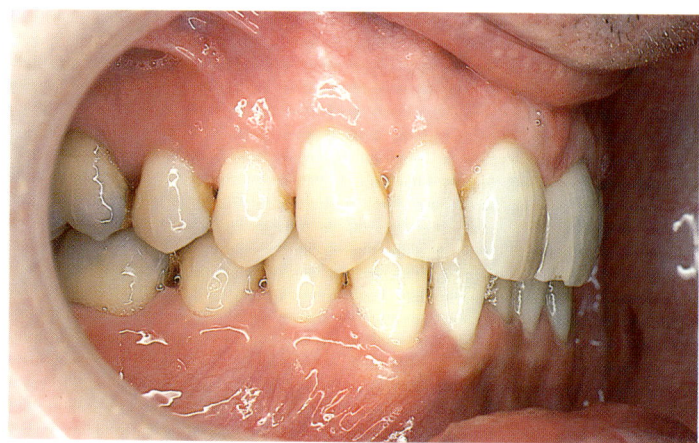

Fig 5-9 Dentition of a 55-year-old man showing the gradation effect of the "first canine," "second canine" (first premolar), and "third canine" (second premolar).

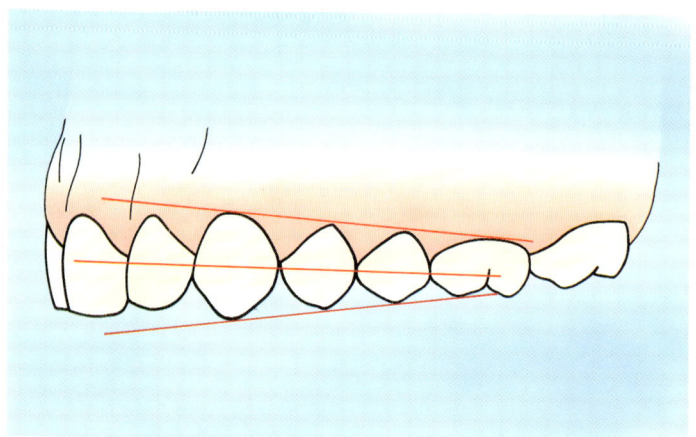

Fig 5-10 Distally converging lines (gradation effect) show height of cementoenamel junctions, interproximal contact points, and buccal cusp tips.

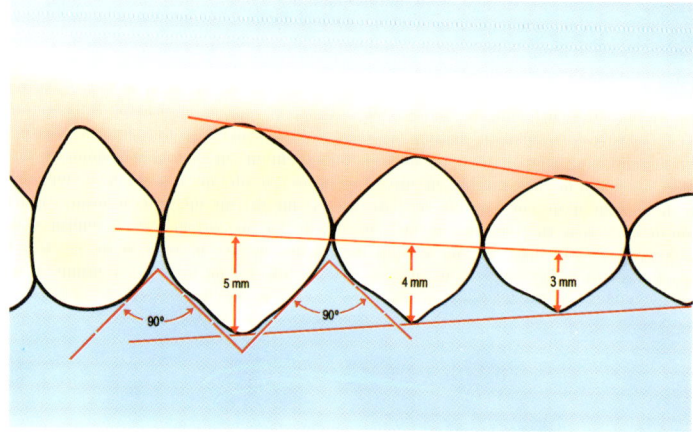

Fig 5-11 The length of the buccal cusps of the "first, second, and third" canines (measured from the interproximal contact points) are about 5, 4, and 3 mm, respectively. The mesial and distal embrasures of the "first canine" are about 90° generally.

Natural unworn permanent crown morphology

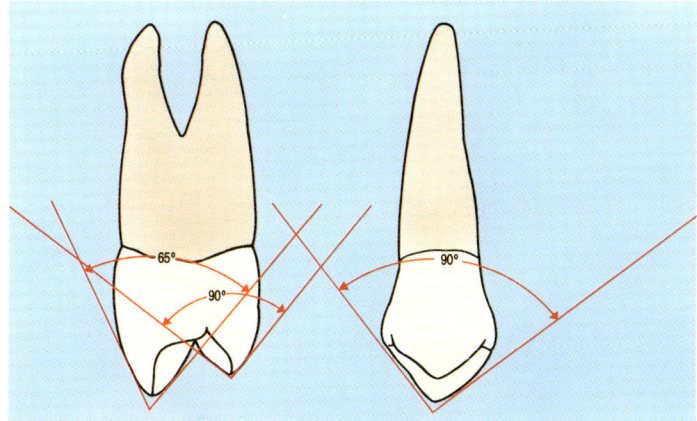

Fig 5-12 The buccal cusp of the maxillary "second canine" is about 65° buccolingually and about 90° mesiodistally, whereas the lingual cusp is about 90° buccolingually and 65° mesiodistally.

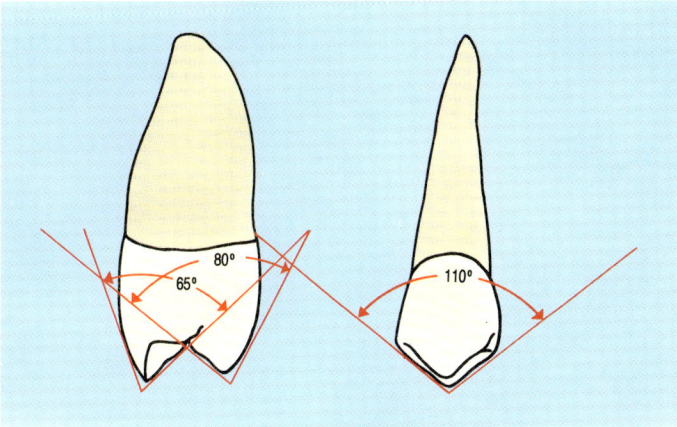

Fig 5-13 The buccal cusp of the "third canine" (second premolar) is about the same as the "second canine" (first premolar) buccolingually but is more obtuse (110°) mesiodistally. The lingual cusp of the second premolar is at least as sharp (80°) as the first premolar buccolingually. The lingual cusp of the second premolar is about 90° mesiodistally.

forward posturing of the mandibular incisors in speaking and rest positions. The lingual fossae of the maxillary incisors also allow space for protrusive and lateral cyclic movements of the mandibular incisors during mastication.

Maxillary "canine area"

It may be helpful to think of the canine and premolar teeth as the "canine area." Viewing the buccal aspects of the maxillary teeth, the canine (first canine) cusp tip is the longest and sharpest. Maxillary canines range from 11 to 13 mm with an average length of about 12 mm (Fig 5-8). The cusp tips of the canines are nearly as long as the central incisors in the plane of occlusion. The cervical height of the maxillary canines is at least as high as that of the central incisors. The buccal cusp of the "second canine" (first premolar) is slightly shorter than the first canine. The "third canine" (second premolar) buccal cusp is slightly shorter than the "second canine." In the canine area the buccal cusp tips of the first, second, and third "canines" form a straight line (Fig 5-9). This straight line includes the mesiobuccal cusp of the first molar. The contact areas of these teeth also form a straight line (Fig 5-10). The buccal cervical heights of the first, second, and third "canines" and back to the cervical line of the first molar form a straight line (Fig 5-10). These three straight lines created by the cusp tips, cementoenamel junctions, and contact areas are not parallel but are distally converging lines, which help produce better functional tooth morphology while also producing good natural esthetics. The arrangement of these teeth to form these converging lines has been referred to as the graduation effect. The large buccal cusps of these teeth are important in medial guidance by the chewing side (ipsilateral) teeth. They guide the lateral mandibular movements in a more vertical manner in the coronal (frontal) plane and are the major factors in preventing harmful posterior contacts of the non-chewing side (contralateral) teeth.

In a good unworn natural dentition the buccal embrasures mesial and distal to the first canine are generally about 90° (Fig 5-11). The mesial and distal marginal ridges of the first, second, and third canines are located gingivally. These gingivally placed marginal ridges create generous, beautiful, natural buccal cusp forms, which are also compatible both functionally and

141

Esthetics and Its Relationship to Function

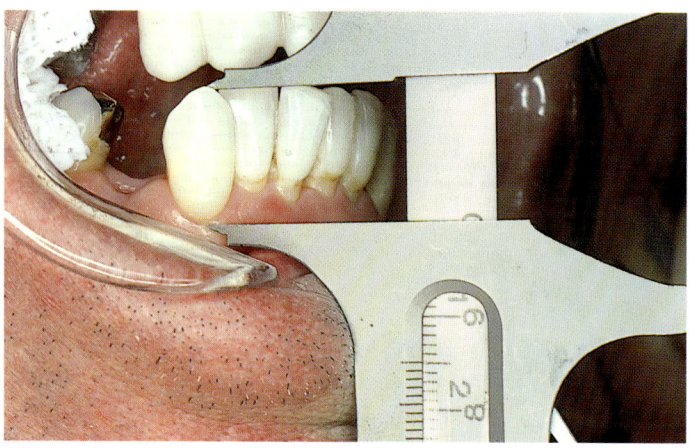

Fig 5-14 Mandibular canine teeth usually have the longest clinical crowns in the mouth; this mandibular canine measures 15 mm.

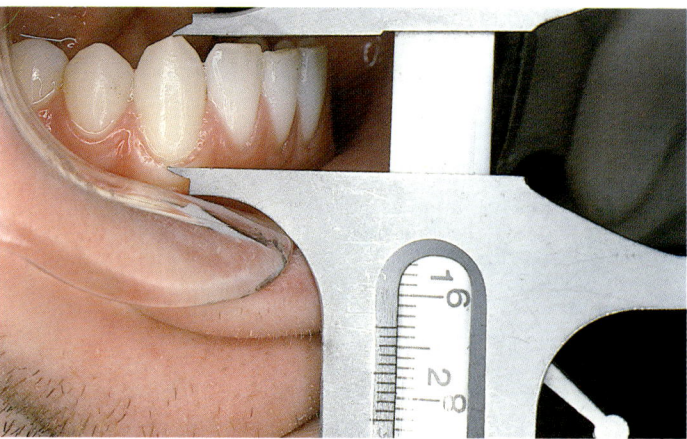

Fig 5-15 Mandibular canines average 12 to 13 mm from the cementoenamel junction to the cusp tip.

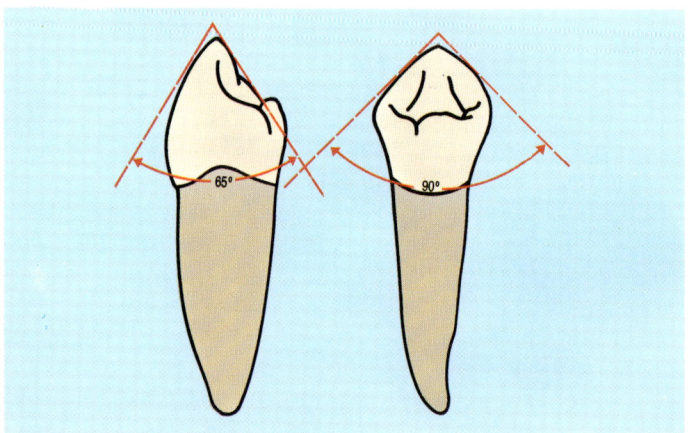

Fig 5-16 The buccal cusp of the mandibular "second canine" (first premolar) is about 65° buccolingually and 90° mesiodistally.

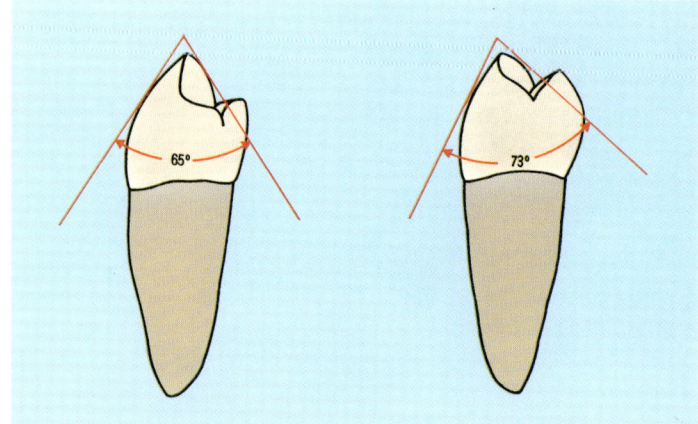

Fig 5-17 The buccolingual angle of the mandibular "third canine" (second premolar) is about 75°, which is about 10° less than the first premolar.

Natural unworn permanent crown morphology

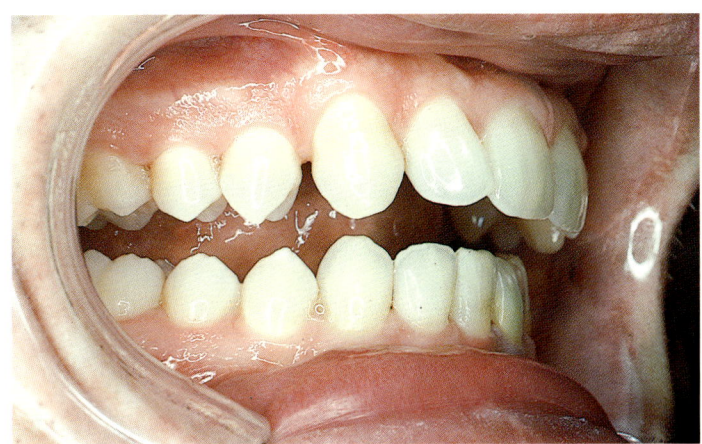

Fig 5-18 Mandibular canine area teeth in natural dentition of a 32-year-old man showing large, steep embrasures.

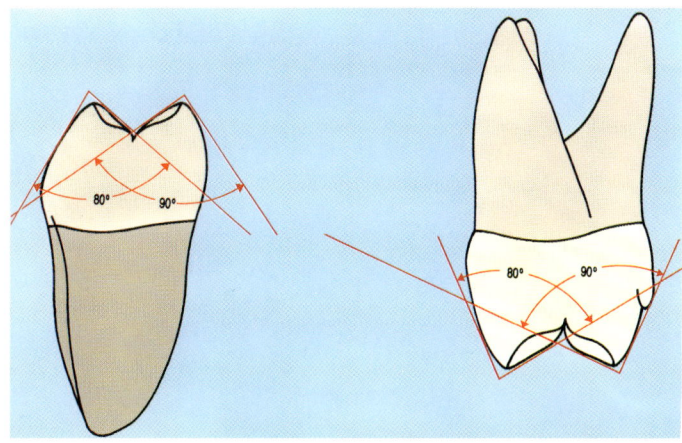

Fig 5-19 The buccal angles of maxillary and mandibular first molars are sharp, averaging generally between 80° and 90° buccolingually.

esthetically with the good anterior lengths and positions of the incisors. On the first premolar the buccolingual angle of the buccal cusps is about 65° and the lingual cusp about 90° (Fig 5-12). The triangular ridge height to groove depth is often 90° or steeper. The cusp tip-to-fossa depth is about 4 mm in the first premolar. The maxillary second premolar cusps are not quite as sharp and long as the first premolar (Fig 5-13).

Grooves of premolar teeth are naturally deep for function and to allow the pressure of food to dissipate during mastication. The deep grooves of the teeth add immensely to natural esthetics when the patient is laughing and the occlusal surfaces are showing. The functioning of sharp premolar teeth are important during mastication of tough or hard foods, such as meat, carrots, apples, bread crusts, and nuts, as well as vertical guidance of the mandible.

Mandibular "canine area"

Unworn mandibular canines have the longest crowns in the mouth (Fig 5-14). Mandibular canine crown lengths range from 11 to 15 mm with an average length of about 12 mm (Fig 5-15). The canine tips are sharp and pointed. The mandibular canines and premolars also have gingivally placed marginal ridges that produce large buccal cusps. The buccal cusp of the first premolar is exceptionally large and sharp. The buccolingual angle of the buccal cusp of the first premolar is about 65° (Fig 5-16). The buccolingual cusp angle of the mandibular second premolar is about 75°, which also makes it sharp (Fig 5-17). The mesial and distal embrasures on the mandibular canines and first premolars are steep (about 90°) (Fig 5-18).

Molars

Although cusp angles of molars are not as steep as those in the canine area teeth, it is usually a surprise to realize just how long and sharp the cusps are on unworn molars. The mesiodistal cusp angles average about 100° and the buccolingual cusp angles average about 90° (Fig 5-19). The triangular ridge height to groove depth often exceeds 90°. Unworn molar cusp heights to fossa depths range from 3 to 4 mm. The cusp ridges are angular to about 90° buccolingually. The cusp triangular

Esthetics and Its Relationship to Function

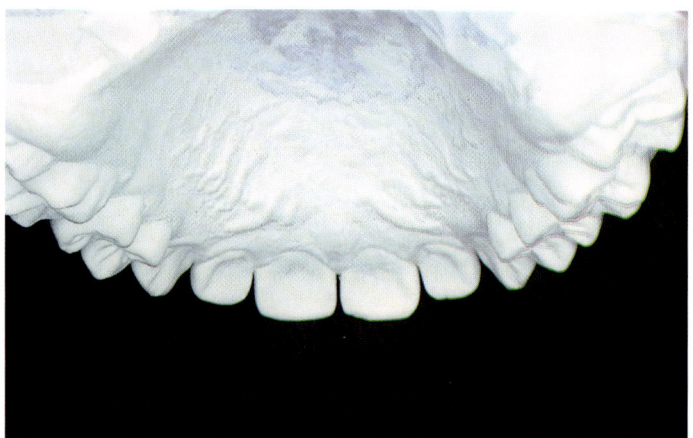

Fig 5-20 Casts of a young teenage girl representing the low end of cusp height range.

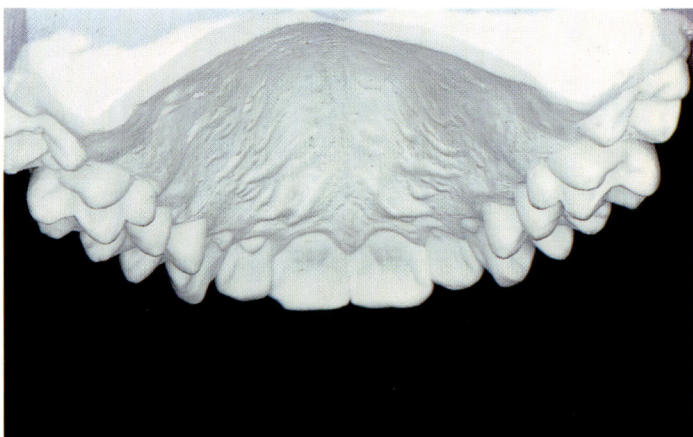

Fig 5-21 Casts of a young teenage girl representing the steep end of cusp height range.

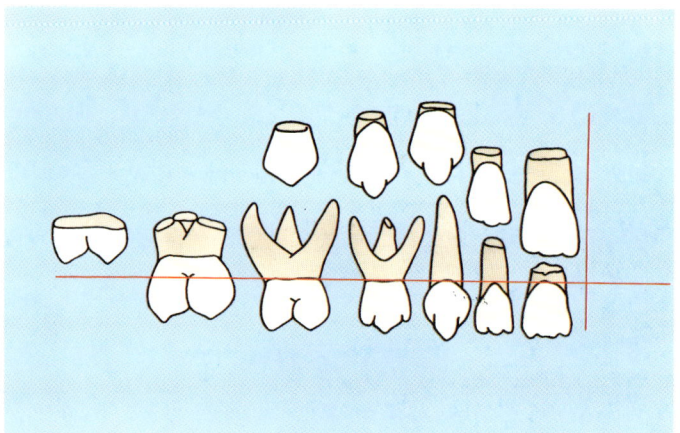

Fig 5-22 The genetic morphology of young unworn permanent crowns is sharp and complete in every detail before eruption into the oral cavity.

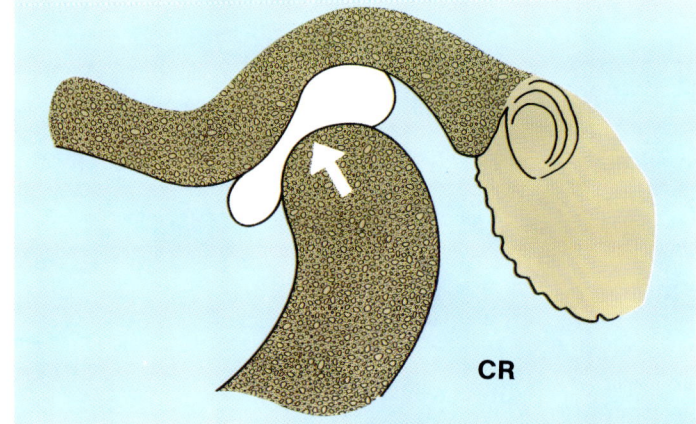

Fig 5-23 The normal physiologic position of the condyles in CR is in their most superior position in intimate contact to the thinnest portion of the biconcave discs at the most posterior slope of the articular eminences.

ridges are also basically about 90°. The buccal cusps of the maxillary molars are for protection of the cheek and mucosa, proprioceptive against the cheek and mucosa, and for holding food on the occlusal table. The lingual cusps of mandibular molars are for protection of the tongue, proprioceptive against the tongue, and for holding food on the occlusal table. The lingual cusps of maxillary molars and the buccal cusps of mandibular molars are for piercing food followed by the cusp ridges, which split, shear, and crush the food (see Fig 5-19). The steep triangular ridges are designed for vertical shearing and crushing of food. The grooves and embrasures are for the escape and extrusion of food and to reduce the load of mastication on the teeth and other components of the gnathic system.

It is important that molar crown morphology be in a naturally sharp, unworn form to be compatible with the bioesthetics and naturally steep occlusal function of the incisors, canines, and premolars. The cusp of Carabelli often seen on maxillary molars may be of benefit in protection of the tongue and for proprioceptive guidance against the tongue. The cusp of Carabelli can also help to create a sharper buccolingual profile to the mesiolingual cusp of maxillary molars (see Fig 5-19).

Tooth genetics

Tooth morphology is totally genetic and is not specific to race or gender. Unerupted permanent teeth of young people of all races, including primitive people, such as aborigines, have sharp cusps. One cannot tell a young unworn Australian aborigine's tooth form from that of a young unworn white's. Anatomists and physiologists agree that tooth morphology is not specific to individuals any more than other organs of the body. There is a biologic spectrum or range of cusp lengths in natural tooth morphology (Figs 5-20 and 5-21). In any case, however, nature always produces sharp teeth genetically.

Natural crown morphology of both anterior and posterior teeth develops early in life and is complete in every detail prior to tooth eruption into the oral cavity (Fig 5-22). However, the other components of the gnathostomatic system, including the joints, ligaments, muscles, maxilla, mandible, and other cranial facial bones, continue to change significantly long after the occlusal morphology of the teeth is complete. These changing components, such as the temporomandibular joints, maxilla and mandible, are predetermined by genetics. The skeletal components, however, are subject to environmental modification by factors such as abnormal posturing of the mandible due to poor occlusion, face sleeping, abnormal swallowing, thumb-sucking, and other abnormal habits. It seems that nature intends the protective covering of teeth (enamel) to last a lifetime (100 years) because there are no provisions for healing or regeneration.

Physiology of occlusion

Occlusion refers to the act of closure or the state of being closed. We will first consider the state of being closed.

Centric relation (CR) = intercuspal position (IP)

Normal physiologic CR position of the jaws may be defined as the stable, comfortable, functional craniomandibular relationship in which the condyles are in their most superior position in intimate contact with the thinnest central bearing area of their respective discs against the distal surface of the articular eminences at any vertical rotational position of the mandible (Fig 5-23).

CR is a comfortable physiologic work position during mastication and swallowing, provided there are no deflective interferences from the teeth. CR is not a rest position; therefore, considerable electromyographic activity may be observed when the mandible is in the CR position. In dentitions in which IP = CR, CR is used during mastication and swallowing (and other random contacts of the teeth, including occasional clenching) about 5,000 times each day (Fig 5-24). The CR position has been found clinically to be the best location for maximum intercuspation of the teeth.[5-7] Whenever IP does not occur at CR (centric occlusion or habitual occlusion) there are always posterior occlusal interferences in lateral border jaw movements with subsequent avoidance patterns.[8]

Clinical CR position may be simply defined as the completely retruded position of the mandible with the condyles in their most superior anterior position at any ver-

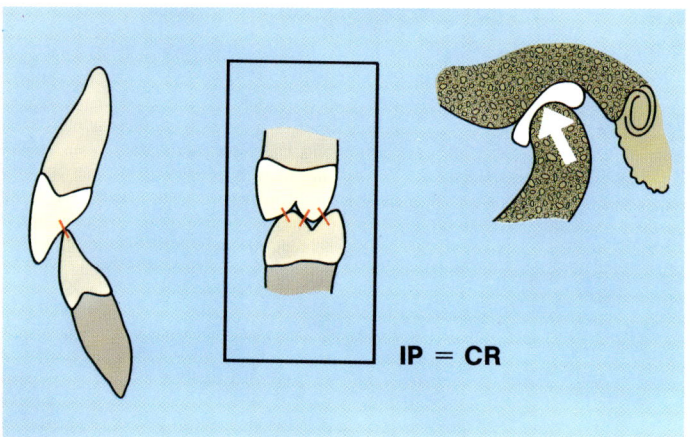

Fig 5-24 All of the teeth in the mouth should occlude evenly (IP) when the condyles are in CR position.

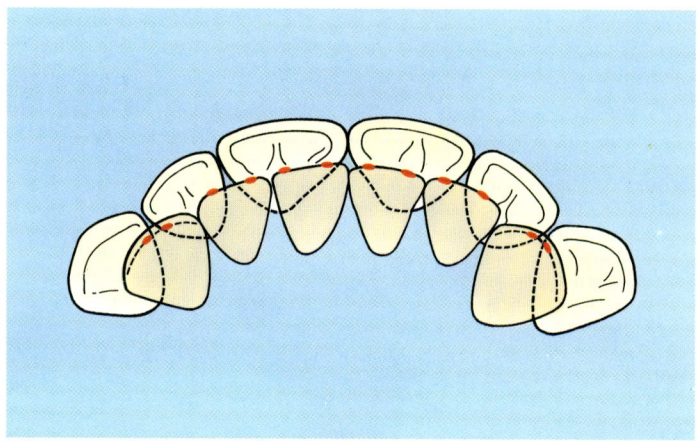

Fig 5-25 IP contacts on the anterior teeth should average about two for each tooth.

tical rotational position of the mandible. Clinical CR does not require normal disc or condyle morphology or position. Clinical CR can be used as a treatment position when it has proven to be a stable, comfortable, repeatable position for the patient.

In good occlusion all of the teeth in the mouth make simultaneous contacts (IP) in CR including the anterior teeth (see Fig 5-24). However, the anterior teeth should never contact harder than the posteriors or fremitus may be produced with possible endodontic and periodontal trauma and/or interproximal separation of the teeth. Good posterior crown morphology and proper anterior overbite reinforces the integrity of the bi-concave discs of the temporomandibular joints each time the teeth are brought together in full occlusion in CR (about 5,000 times a day). This IP–CR relationship not only helps stabilize the condyle disc complex in CR position in the fossae but also helps maintain total craniomandibular stability.

Normally, occlusal contacts on the anterior teeth in CR are not broad, but rather two or three spots per tooth on the incisors and one on each canine (Fig 5-25).

In good natural dentitions one rarely observes the actual cusp tips of posterior teeth making occlusal contacts. Instead, the contacts are usually found on cusp ridges and mesial and distal marginal ridges (Fig 5-26). Occlusal contact spots are small in good natural dentitions. The total tooth contact area has been estimated to be about 4 mm^2 for the entire mouth, including all of the anterior and posterior teeth.[9] The ideal contact location for the buccal cusps of the lower premolar is on the mesial and distal marginal ridges of the opposing premolars (cusp to marginal ridge).[10] The contacts are just anterior and posterior to the point of the cusp on as they touch the marginal ridges of the upper premolars (Fig 5-27). This location allows for the maxillary canine to be in the embrasure distal to the mandibular canine (Class I) for maximum vertical guidance in lateral chewing. There is seldom, if ever, an occlusal contact with the rudimentary lingual cusp of the lower "second canine" (first premolar). Tripodization of mandibular buccal cusps and maxillary lingual cusps is rarely seen in natural occlusions. Tripodization is permissible in artificial crown occlusion provided the naturally sharp anatomic vertical profiles of the teeth are not violated. Cusp–fossa (moderate Class II) relationship is sometimes necessary for posterior artificial crowns (Fig 5-28). With cusp fossa relationship there is a tendency to produce flatter arti-

Physiology of occlusion

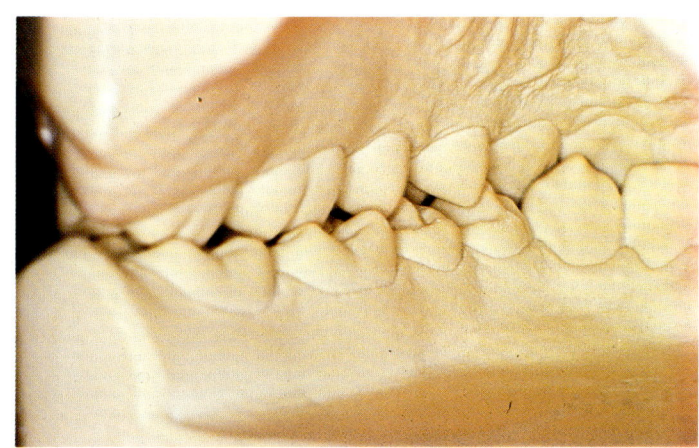

Fig 5-26 A lingual view of casts with normal posterior occlusal relation. Note the large embrasures and spaces. Also note that the rudimentary lingual cusps of the mandibular first premolar has no occlusal contact.

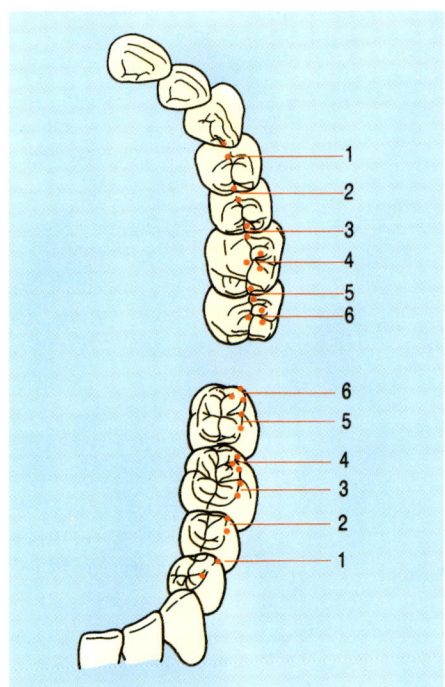

Fig 5-27a In a normal Class I relationship, the buccal cusps of the mandibular premolars contact the marginal ridge of the maxillary premolars (cusp to marginal ridge). The mesiobuccal cusp of the first mandibular molar occludes on the adjacent marginal ridges between the maxillary first molar and second premolars while the distobuccal cusp of the mandibular first molar occludes in the central fossa of the maxillary first molar.

Fig 5-27b In a normal Class I relationship, the lingual cusps of the maxillary premolars occlude on the marginal ridges or in the distal fossae of the mandibular premolars. There is usually no occlusal contact with the rudimentary lingual cusp of the mandibular first premolar. The mesiolingual cusp of the maxillary first molar occludes in the central fossa of its mandibular mate while the distolingual cusp occludes on the adjacent marginal ridges between the mandibular first and second molars.

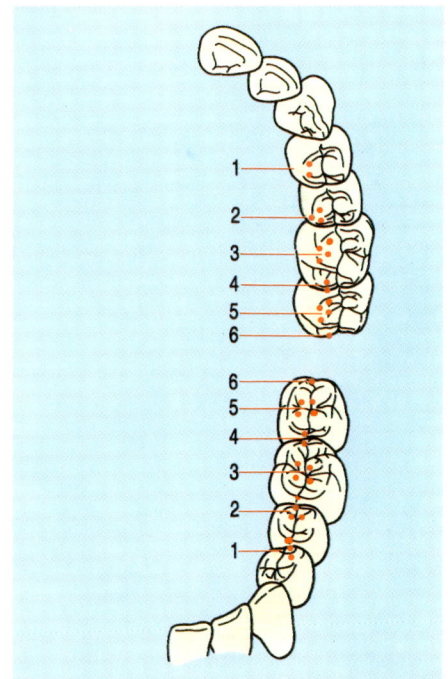

Figure 5-27a

Figure 5-27b

Esthetics and Its Relationship to Function

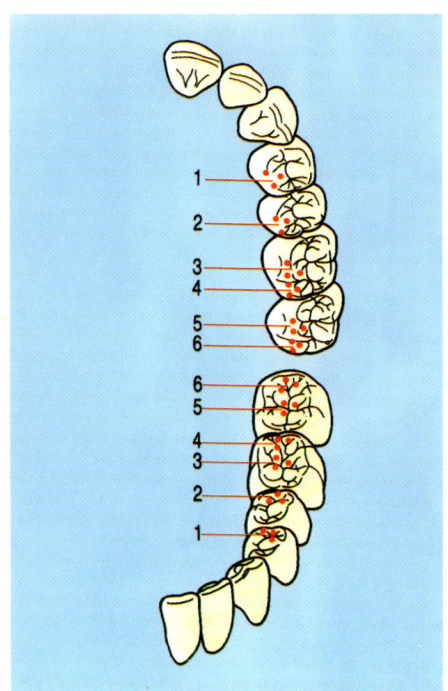

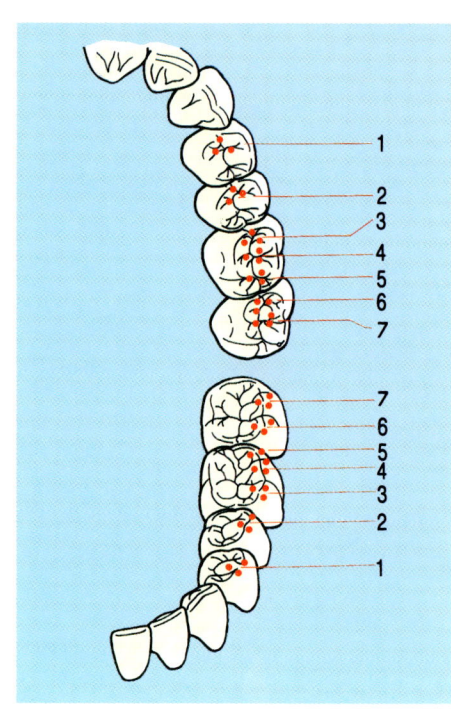

Fig 5-28 Cusp-fossa occlusal arrangement (moderate Class II) is sometimes necessary. However, care should be taken not to sacrifice natural tooth morphology in these cases. *(left)* The contacts of the maxillary lingual cusps shown against the mandibular teeth; *(right)* the contacts of the mandibular buccal cusps against the maxillary teeth.

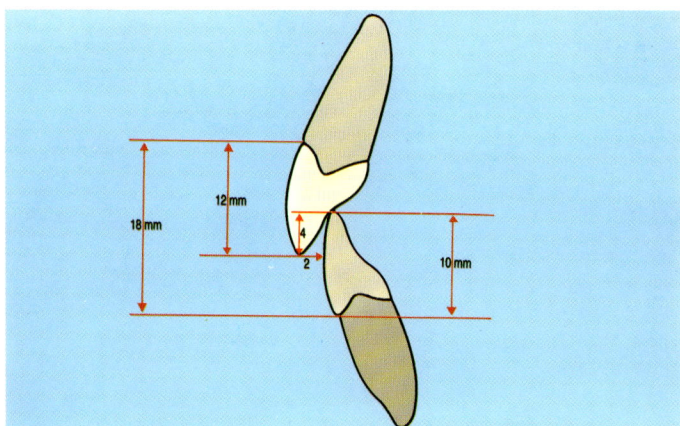

Fig 5-29 Central incisor vertical overbite averages about 4 mm with a 2- to 3-mm horizontal overbite. With an average maxillary incisor length of 12 mm and an average mandibular incisor length of 10 mm, there will be approximately 18 mm from upper cementoenamel to lower cementoenamel junction.

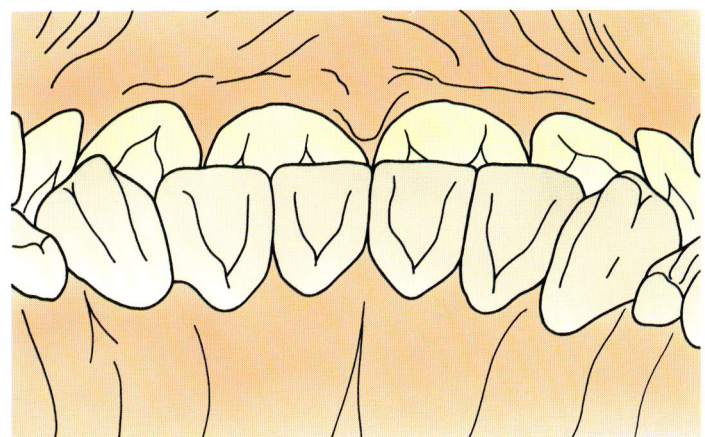

Fig 5-30 In full occlusion the incisal edges of the mandibular teeth touch the deepest portion of the lingual fossae of the maxillary incisors near the cingulum.

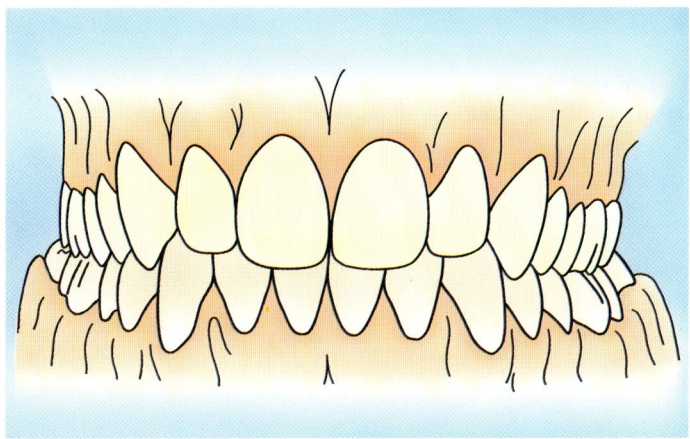

Fig 5-31 Horizontal overbite of the canines is minimal.

ficial cusp forms than in cusp–marginal ridge relationship because of poor tooth position and lack of interocclusal space. In any event, the common denominator in the posterior region in good natural dentitions seems to be: unworn (sharp) posterior tooth forms that occlude evenly in CR with small contact points (16 to 32 per side). The maxillary lingual cusps and mandibular buccal cusps occlude in opposing fossae or on mesial and distal marginal ridges or on cusp ridges.

Complete occlusion of the teeth (IP) is a specialized articulation of the craniomandibular system and can have a profound effect on the alignment and stability of the total craniomandibular articulation complex, including the maxillary and temporal bones as well as the temporomandibular joints. Full contact of all the teeth in the CR position of the condyles approximately 5,000 times per day helps to realign and stabilize the craniomandibular relationship into a state of biological equilibrium. This stabilization includes not only the teeth and temporomandibular joints but also affects other cranial articulations (sutures) in the skeletal system through the muscles. Stabilization of the craniomandibular relation in CR is important to the comfort, function, and longevity of dental restorations. The use of a properly constructed, adjusted, and maintained maxillary, anterior guided occlusal splint is probably the best way to align and stabilize the craniomandibular relationship prior to treating the occlusion and articulation of the teeth.

Anterior overbite
In well-related teeth the vertical overbite of the maxillary central incisors ranges from 4 to 5 mm when the teeth are in full occlusion (Fig 5-29). The horizontal overbite of the maxillary incisors is between 2 and 3 mm in full occlusion (see Fig 5-29). The incisal edges of the mandibular incisors contact the deepest portion of the lingual fossae of the maxillary incisors where the cingulum begins (Fig 5-30). The distobuccal convexity of the mandibular canine fits into the mesial lingual concavity of the maxillary canine. There is about 4 to 5 mm of vertical overbite of the canines. The natural convexity of the mandibular canine as it fits into the lingual concavity of the maxillary canine causes a rapid diminishing of the horizontal overbite (Fig 5-31). The horizontal overbite of the maxillary canines is much less than the incisors (about 1 mm) from the tip of the cusp to the labial surface of the mandibular canine (Fig 5-32).

Esthetics and Its Relationship to Function

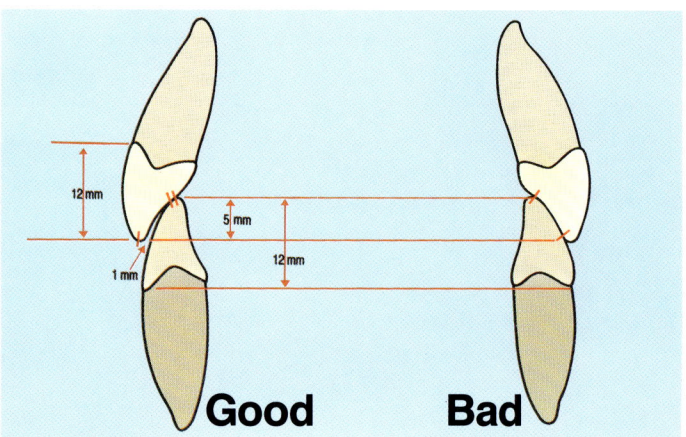

Fig 5-32 Horizontal overbite of the canines is usually less than 1 mm. However, there should not be large, flat surface contacts of the canines in IP.

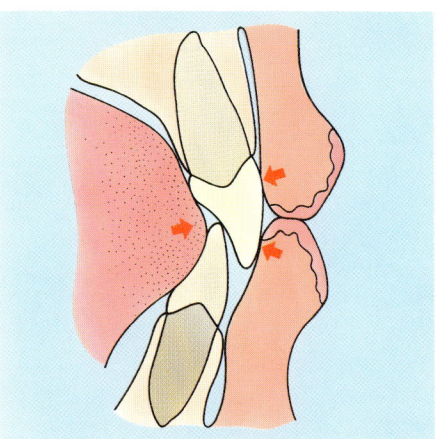

Fig 5-33 The lower lip as well as the upper lip should both be supported by the maxillary teeth when the teeth are in IP. During swallowing the pressure of the lips and the counter-pressure from the tongue help to stabilize the positions of the anterior teeth (arrows).

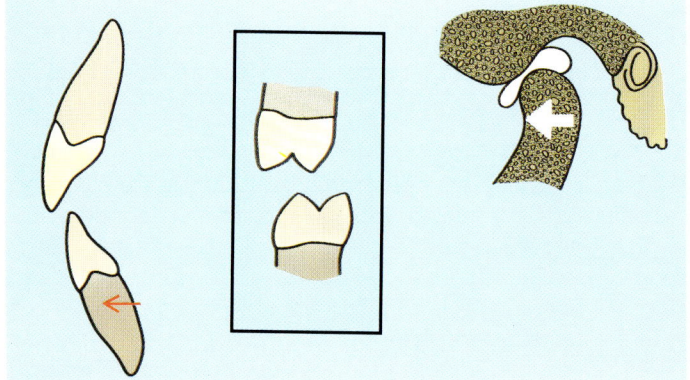

Fig 5-34 In rest positions the condyles do not remain in the CR position but are forward and the teeth are separated.

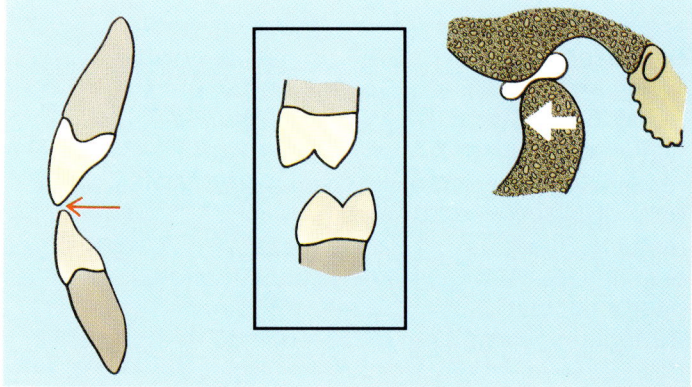

Fig 5-35 In normal speaking positions of the "S" sounds, the condyles are forward to CR and there is a very close position of the incisal edges of the anterior teeth with a larger space between the posterior teeth.

Physiology of occlusion

In full occlusion the lower lip and upper lip rest against the labial surface of the maxillary incisors. The lower lip helps retain the maxillary teeth against the mandibular anterior teeth while the tongue holds the mandibular incisors against the maxillary incisors in a state of equilibrium, sometimes referred to as the neutral zone (Fig 5-33). This lip–tooth–tongue relationship helps produce a negative pressure seal during mastication and swallowing as well as stabilization of teeth positions.

Maxillary and mandibular arch forms should be of adequate size to conform to each other and support normal size teeth without crowding. It is best if the arch midlines be coincidental with each other as well as the midsagittal plane of the patient's head so that proper incisive and canine guidance and esthetics can better be achieved (see Fig 5-31). If any compromise with the midline is to be made in dental treatments, it should be with the mandibular midline rather than the maxillary midline.

"Rest position" and "free way space"

Most of the time (22 hours per day) the mandible is not in the CR position but is in a rest or semirest position with the anterior teeth separated anywhere from 1 mm to as much as 10 mm. The condyles do not remain in the deep portion of the fossae (CR) when the mandible is in various relaxation postures but are usually 1 to 2 mm forward on the eminentia (Fig 5-34). During enunciation of certain words (eg, S sounds), the condyles are usually forward down the eminentia about 2 to 3 mm from CR, depending on the amount of anterior horizontal overbite (Fig 5-35). The incisor horizontal overbite of 2 to 3 mm is important because it allows for this forward posturing of the mandible to take place comfortably without the feeling of mandibular confinement. However, the 2- to 3-mm horizontal overbite required in the incisors is not needed in the canines because normally the jaw does not move laterally during the periods of relaxation or speaking. If the incisor horizontal overbite exceeds 3 mm, there is a chance that the lower lip may be pulled up under the maxillary incisors, causing labial tooth migration and poor esthetics with the lips. The free way space used during speaking averages about 1.7 mm. Free way space is learned and, if anterior tooth relationships are changed, requires new learning but usually returns to about 1.7 mm in a short period of time.

Vertical dimension of occlusion

It has been commonly believed and taught in prosthodontics for many years that vertical dimension of occlusion is critical. It was considered that, because of muscle length, free way space, and rest position, one should never increase occlusal vertical dimension (OVD). It was also believed that passive eruption of the teeth kept the OVD at its original level in worn dentitions and that if OVD was increased it would gradually return to the worn-down position.[11]

The author, however, has been increasing OVD for more than 30 years with restorative dentistry, orthodontics, and orthognathic surgery, and has had no problems with rest position or free way space.[12] The free way space returns to about 1.7 mm following the increase of OVD in these patients. Cephalometric radiographs 5 and 10 years posttreatment show that the increased distance between nasion and menton is not being lost.

Garnick and Ramfjord[13] found that the interocclusal distance (free way space) averaged 1.7 mm in the clinically determined rest position, whereas the average distance was 3.29 mm with an additional resting range of 11 mm when determined electromyographically on the basis of minimal muscle activity. He stated that determining clinical rest position also involves the influence of emotional and exteroceptive and proprioceptive inputs to the neuromuscular system. Such input from joints, muscles, lips, tongue, cheeks, mucosa, teeth, and periodontal membrane undoubtedly contribute to the learning of rest position or conditioning of reflexes. Concepts regarding rest position of the mandible should be reevaluated and revised in light of the recent research and clinical experiences. When changing OVD in restorative dentistry, excellent anterior guidance and posterior crown morphology should be established to CR position of the condyles. The improved anterior and posterior guidance helps the patient form learned ingrams in the cerebral cortex for the new chewing patterns at the restored OVD.

There is a limit to the amount one can increase OVD. It appears, however, that the range is large (up to 10 mm on some people) and that OVD is one of the least critical factors in rehabilitating the occlusion. In restorative dentistry there is no advantage in increasing OVD more than is necessary to obtain good crown morphology on anterior and posterior teeth. If the anterior teeth are unworn and OVD is increased, it usually requires orthodontics

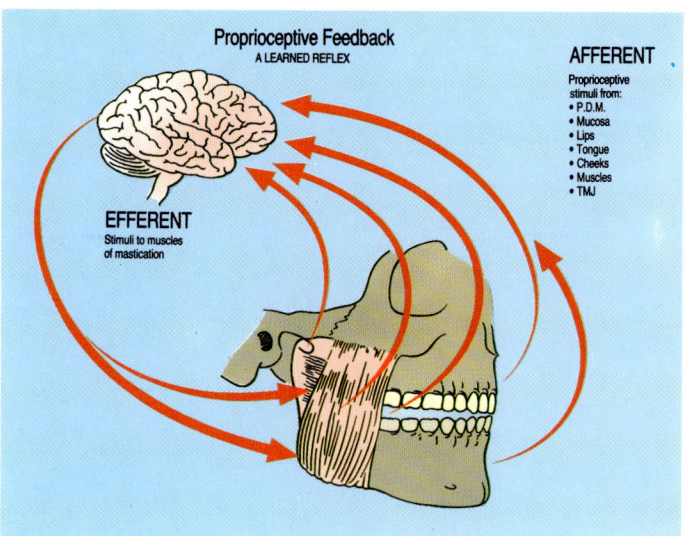

Fig 5-36 In addition to the pressoreceptors in the periodontal ligaments, there are many other components of the gnathic system, including the lips, tongue, cheeks, mucosa, skin, muscles, and temporomandibular joints, which contain proprioceptive bodies. These proprioceptors continuously monitor the position of the mandible and feed the information to the brain. The brain, in turn, tells the muscles how to move the mandible. Good chewing patterns are placed on a learned reflex level provided the teeth have good morphology and proper positions.

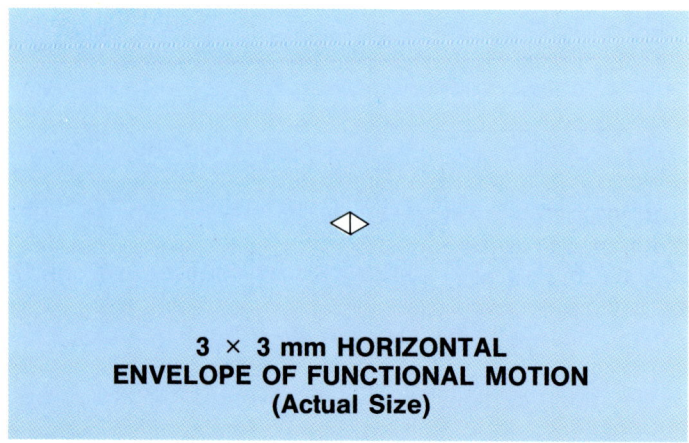

Fig 5-37 Actual size of functional mandibular movement in the horizontal plane takes place within a small diamond-shaped area only 3 mm to the right and to the left and forward.

or orthognathic surgery to obtain good anterior relations.

Development of occlusion

With the growth of the infant and the eruption of the teeth into the oral cavity, afferent stimuli from receptors in the periodontal membrane, lips, tongue, cheeks, mucosa, and temporomandibular joint influence the central nervous system and, reflexively, the position of the mandible (Fig 5-36). With the eruption of the teeth the process of mastication is learned, and learning depends upon the cerebral cortex.[14] In other words, mastication is not part of the autonomic nervous system, similar to swallowing. Wickwire and Gibbs[15] reported that the chewing patterns of young children with primary dentitions are generally wide. When the permanent teeth erupt into the oral cavity they begin establishing the ingrams for more vertical chewing patterns. The 6-year molars are the first guide teeth in establishing adult lateral chewing patterns. If the child (6 to 12 years) is fortunate enough to develop good relationships of the teeth, learned reflexes develop by which the mandible functions more vertically as the mandibular teeth approach the maxillary teeth in the final portion of the chewing cycles. When tooth morphology and/or tooth position is restored or changed, new ingrams for occlusion must be developed in the central nervous system. These new learned reflexes are not always immediate and may take longer for some people. There are five guidance factors involved in occluding the teeth: *(1)* anterior teeth, *(2)* posterior teeth, *(3)* right condyle path, *(4)* left condyle path, and *(5)* neuromuscular mechanism (cerebral cortex). Research shows that the teeth are the primary factors in jaw closing patterns and that teeth frequently make contact during mastication and swallowing.[16-19] However, if tooth relationships do not allow for proper condylar positioning with the disc or if the teeth inhibit condylar movements, they can cause traumatic occlusion. Traumatic occlusion may be defined as any closures of the teeth that produce visible or invisible unphysiologic stress, damage, or overload to the teeth, joints, muscles, bones, periodontium, or nervous system.

Traumatic occlusion is evidenced by the following: *(1)* abrasion and fracturing of teeth, dental restorations, and prostheses; *(2)* craniofacial pain (myalgia); *(3)* craniomandibular dysfunction (temporomandibular joint, TMJ); *(4)* tooth migration; *(5)* tooth mobility; *(6)* overload on the periodontium; and *(7)* exostoses (overload).

There are several basic identifiable interferences that can cause traumatic occlusion:

1. Centric relation: slide (anterior, lateral) and fulcrum.
2. Protrusive–retrusive, incisive.
3. Lateral border: nonworking side and working side.

Of the centric interferences, the fulcrum type is probably the more traumatic because the condyle is continually distracted from the disc during mastication and swallowing, often leading to disc derangements because the disc is unsupported, whereas with a slide the condyle is engaged with the concave portion of the disc during mastication and swallowing. Of the border interferences, those on the nonworking side are usually most disturbing to the neuromuscular system, often resulting in excessive wear on anterior teeth due to avoidance patterns. In addition to occlusal interferences, the presence of flat (unnatural) occlusal morphology in artificial crowns and natural teeth is also a cause of traumatic occlusion through overload.

Original natural tooth morphology per se is not the cause of traumatic occlusion (except perhaps in connection with microdentia, enamel aplasia). It is the relationship of the mandibular teeth to the maxillary teeth as the jaws close (in function and nonfunction) that creates the majority of problems in occlusion. Some of the poor relationships of the teeth are due to skeletal disharmonies connected with growth and development, poor posturing, abnormal habits, and so on. Other bad relationships of the teeth may be caused by lost teeth and subsequent tooth drift, worn teeth, or iatrogenic causes, such as flat artificial crowns, poorly carved restorations, high crowns and fillings, and improper orthodontic treatment.

Considering the fact that normal chewing function and parafunction (when viewed in the horizontal plane) take place within a small diamond-shaped area, only 3 mm to the right, 3 mm to the left, and 3 mm forward to intercuspal position, it should be no surprise that small changes or discrepancies (0.1 mm or less) in the occlusion can have serious effects (Fig 5-37).

Anterior tooth guidance

Anterior guidance is generally recognized as an important aspect in present-day concepts of occlusion.[20-22] This guidance is of two types: *(1)* incisal guidance in protrusive–retrusive movements and *(2)* canine guidance in mediotrusive lateral movements. The primary importance of protrusive guidance is for proper incising as well as rest positions and speaking function. The primary importance of canine guidance is to help prevent lateral eccentric posterior tooth interferences and allow the condyles to move uninhibitedly along their border pathways in the fossae as well as guiding jaw closures more vertically to load the posterior teeth in their long axis.

Scientific guidelines have not been established as to how much the anterior overbite should be. Orthodontics has generally advocated an arbitrary amount of about 1.5 mm of vertical overbite. The term "cuspid disclusion" has been used by some dentists to describe canine function that separates the posterior teeth in lateral movements of the mandible. The word "disclusion," however, is quantitatively ambiguous and can be used to mean as little as a few hundredths of a millimeter (Fig 5-38). Minimal "lift" on the canines usually disappears in a relatively short period of time (crowns at best acquire some wear in time). Minimal canine disclusion does not allow for in vivo functional physiologic factors, such as

Esthetics and Its Relationship to Function

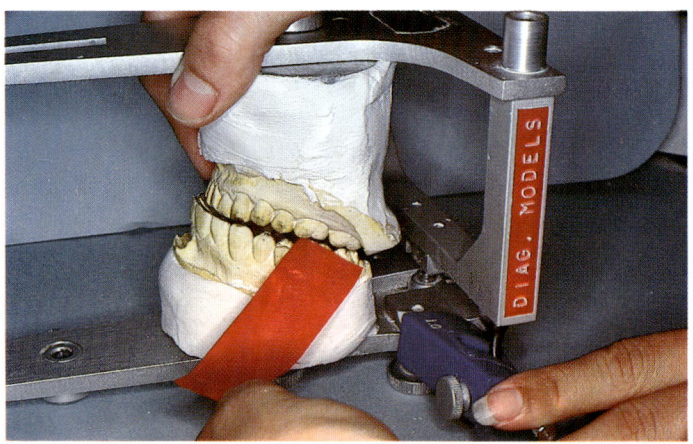

Fig 5-38 In the laboratory, "posterior disclusion" in lateral movement of the articulator can be accomplished with as little as a few hundredths of a millimeter of space between the teeth. This small space may not be adequate to keep the posterior teeth separated under functional loading (see Figs 5-80 to 5-83).

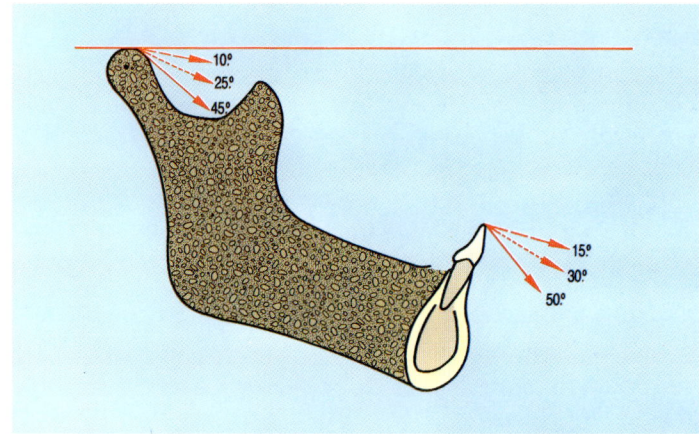

Fig 5-39 There is no scientific or clinical rationale for making incisal overbite with a minimal relation to the condylar path, as some suggest. If the notion that anterior overbite should be only 5° steeper than the condylar path, then one would have to make abnormally flat posterior teeth in the case of more horizontal condyle paths.

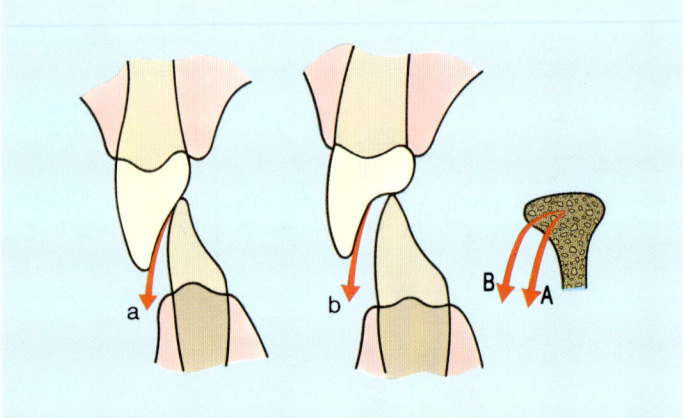

Fig 5-40 If one follows the notion of increasing the lingual fossa of a patient's canines (b) to correspond to large amounts of condylar Bennett movement (B), then there would have to be abnormal (flat) posterior crown morphology to avoid lateral interferences. Flat occlusal morphology produces functional overload.

Physiology of occlusion

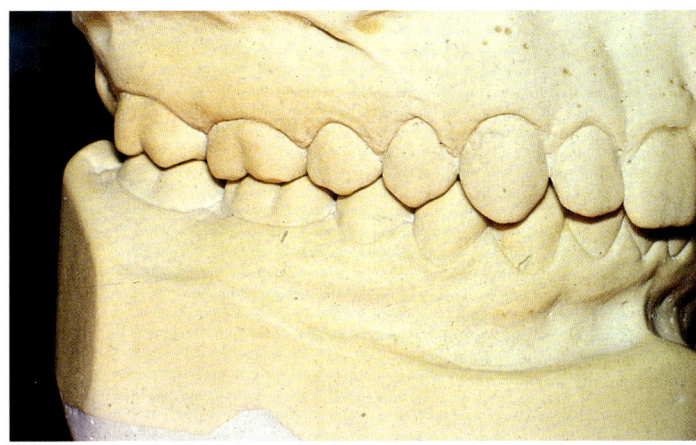

Fig 5-41a Compare the natural crown morphology to the unnatural morphology in Fig 5-41b.

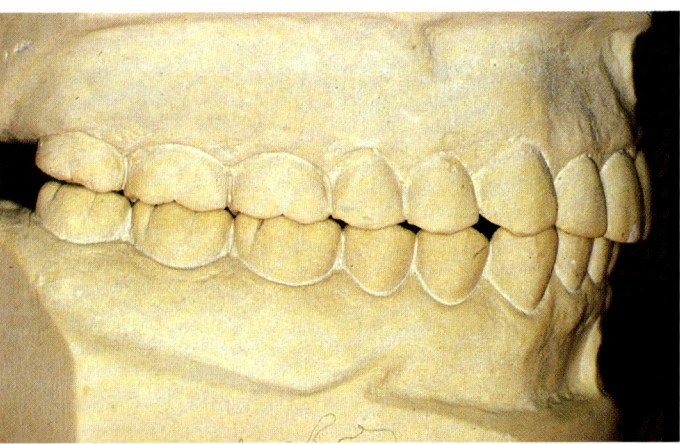

Fig 5-41b Note the abnormal flattening (low vertical profile) of the posterior artificial crowns because of the unnatural (poor) overbite of the canine.

flexions and compressions of certain components of the gnathic system that result in posterior teeth coming into early premature lateral contact. The term also seems to imply that it is "normal" for the mandible to move from centric to eccentric positions with the teeth in contact. The term "cuspid disclusion" is inadequate to describe the potential physiologic guiding function of the canines. (It seems that the most physiologic way to "disclude" one's teeth is to simply open the mouth.) "Canine guidance" is probably a more preferable term because it implies normal physiologic jaw functions.

Some dentists have tried to relate the overbite of the anterior teeth to condyle movements on a direct basis. Some advocate the notion of making the incisal guidance 5° steeper than the condylar path (Fig 5-39) or contouring the lingual of canines to "harmonize" with the Bennett path of the condyles (Fig 5-40). This practice is not supported by observations of natural teeth and, if done, increases the chance of posterior eccentric interferences or requires the dentist to flatten the posterior crown morphology from its original natural form (Figs 5-41a and b). Flattened occlusal posterior crown morphology causes more overload on the teeth and supporting structures.

Posterior tooth guidance

There has been a great deal of emphasis placed on canine guidance or disclusion since it was first postulated by D'Amico[17] in the late 1950s. According to some authorities, the canine teeth should receive all eccentric tooth contacts in lateral border movements of the mandible.[17,18,20] However, canine guidance is not the only factor of importance in medial guidance of the mandible. Young children in the most formative years of their lives (ages 6 to 12) have no canine guidance. It seems that if canines were the only teeth of vital importance in medial guidance of the jaw, nature would have placed these teeth early in the mouth. If the teeth are the primary guidance factors for occluding the teeth (which research shows), it is obvious that at age 6 it is the cusps of the 6-year molars that guide the lateral closures, followed later by the premolars (Fig 5-42). Finally, at about 12 years of age, the canines erupt into guiding function. Kawamura reported that even though the incisors are the most sensitive teeth to presoreception in the periodontal ligament, the posterior teeth are also extremely sensitive.[23] This posterior exquisite sensitivity can be demonstrated clinically on some patients with mylar occlusal ribbons that are only 0.01 mm thick.

Esthetics and Its Relationship to Function

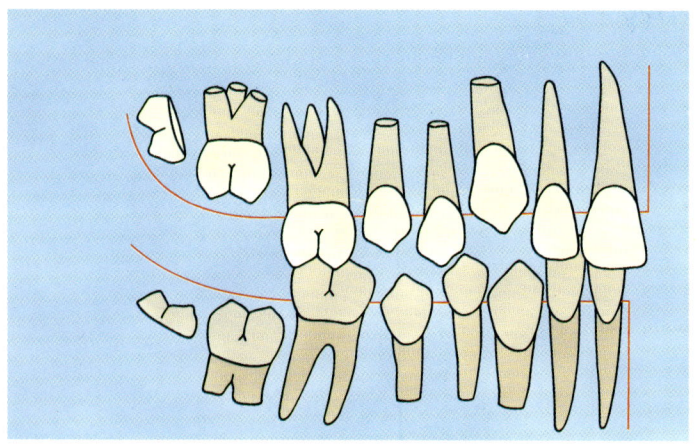

Fig 5-42 In the most formative years of life (6 to 12 years), nature provides only posterior tooth guidance in lateral movements.

Perhaps the best rule to follow in treating patients is to simulate the tooth relationships found in untreated, nontraumatic, long-lasting natural dentitions. Observations of these people show the following:

1. Good masticating and swallowing function.
2. Minimal wear on the teeth.
3. Minimal stress on the TMJ.
4. Minimal stress on the periodontium.
5. Comfortable muscle activity.
6. Good esthetics.

These people have anterior teeth with similar characteristics. The crowns of maxillary central incisors are relatively large and long, the lateral incisors are shorter and rounded mesiodistally on the incisal edges, and the canines are long and pointed (Figs 5-43a, 5-44a, and 5-45a). The vertical anterior overbite ranges from 3 to 5 mm and the horizontal overbite of the incisors ranges from 2 to 3 mm. The horizontal overbite of the canine teeth is less than 1 mm. These patients also have relatively unworn posterior teeth with sharp occlusal morphology, which is compatible with their naturally steep canine guidance (65° to 70°). The IP of the teeth is less than 0.5 mm from the CR position of the condyles. They usually have few dental restorations, especially artificial crowns. These patients show 2- to 3-mm spaces between their posterior teeth when they touch the incisal edges of their mandibular incisors or canines against the maxillary anterior teeth (Figs 5-43b and c, 5-44b and c, and 5-45b and c).

Physiology of occlusion

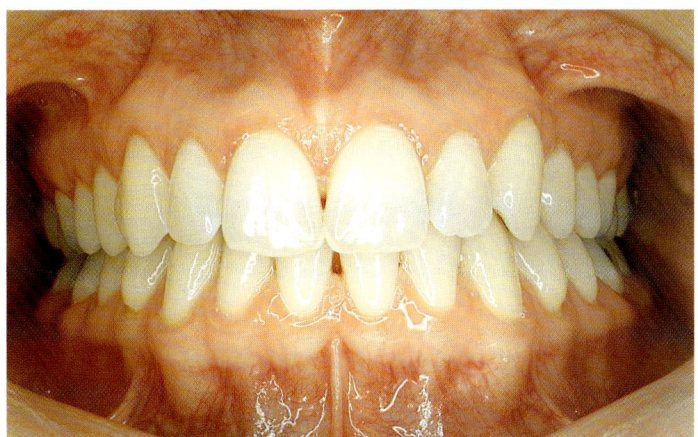

Fig 5-43a A 36-year-old woman with nontraumatic natural occlusion showing large central incisors, short rounded lateral incisors, and long pointed canines.

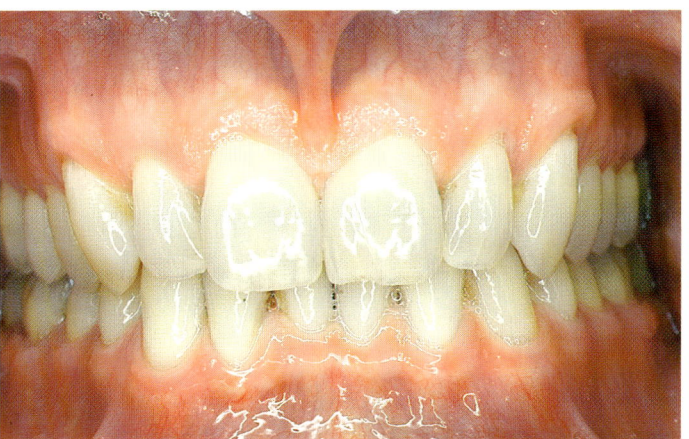

Fig 5-43b A 55-year-old man with nontraumatic natural occlusion showing large central incisors, short rounded lateral incisors, and long pointed canines.

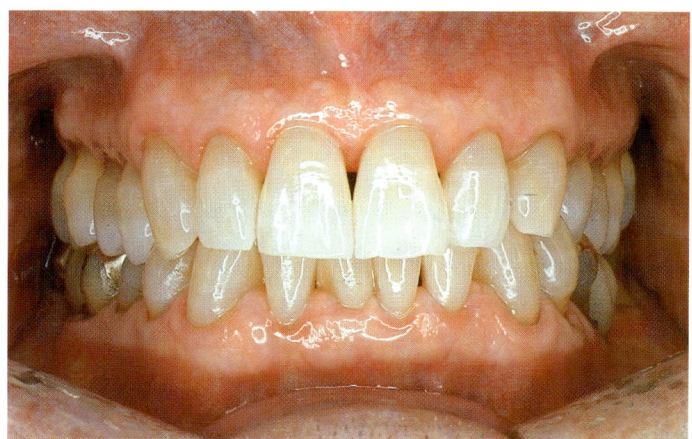

Fig 5-43c An 85-year-old man with nontraumatic natural occlusion showing large central incisors, shorter lateral incisors, and long canines. Note the attrition on the incisal edges of all of his anterior teeth.

Esthetics and Its Relationship to Function

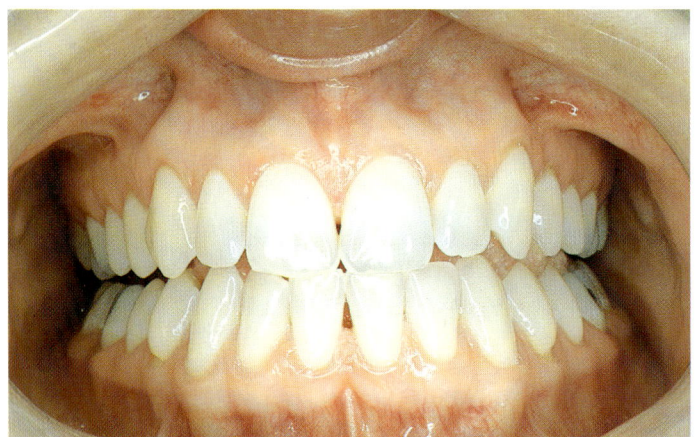

Fig 5-44a

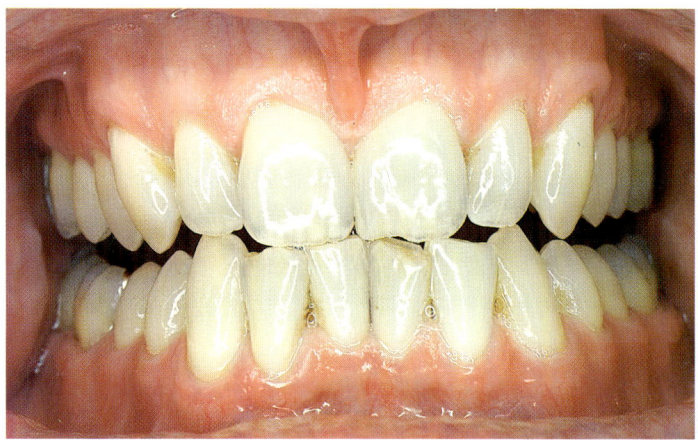

Fig 5-44b

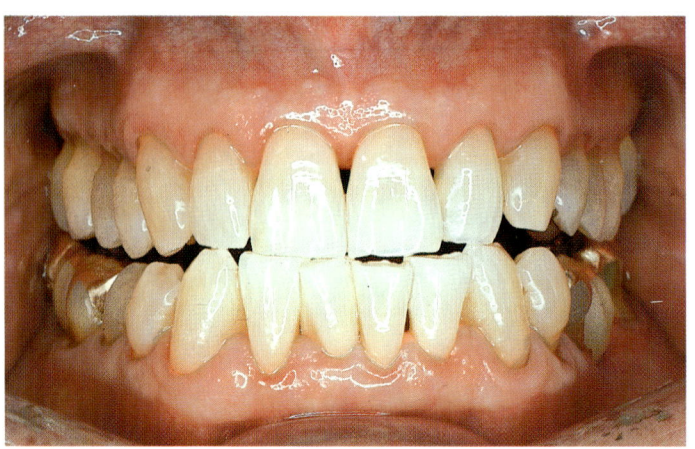

Fig 5-44c

Figs 5-44a to c · The same three patients as in Figs 5-43a to c, respectively, in an edge-to-edge incising position. Note that the incisal edge of the maxillary central incisors meets the incisal edges of the mandibular four incisors. The maxillary lateral incisors are higher on the incisal edges to make space for the cusp tips of the mandibular canines. There is a space of 2 to 3 mm between the posterior teeth cusps.

Physiology of occlusion

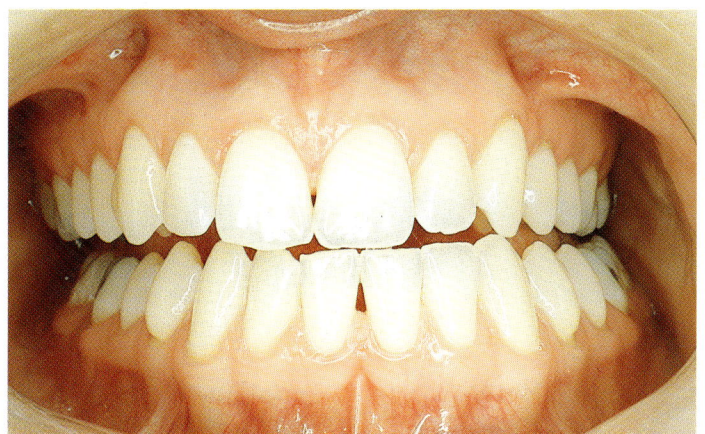

Fig 5-45a

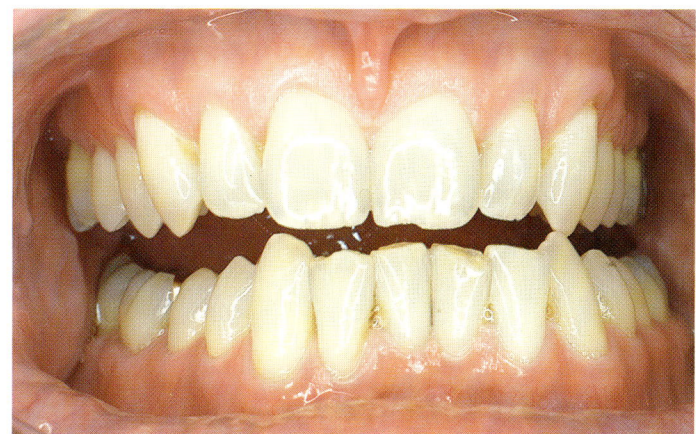

Fig 5-45b

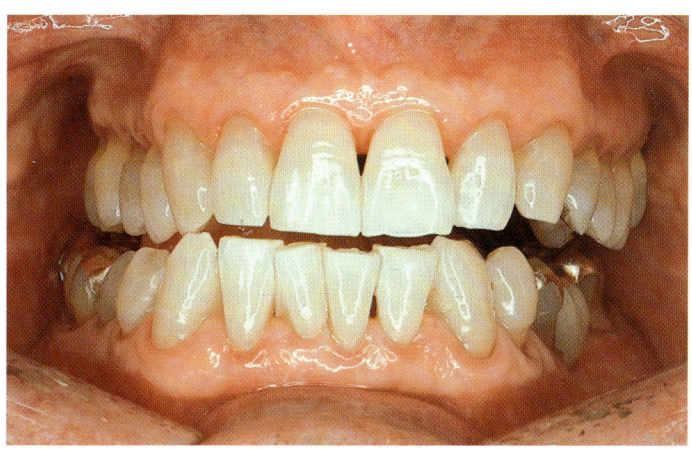

Fig 5-45c

Figs 5-45a to c The same three patients as in Figs 5-43a to c, respectively, in lateral jaw movement. Note that the canines are the only teeth in contact in this test position. Also note that the space between the posterior teeth chewing side (ipsilateral) ranges from about 1.5 to 2 mm. The nonchewing side (contralateral) space is greater, ranging from about 2 to 3 mm.

Esthetics and Its Relationship to Function

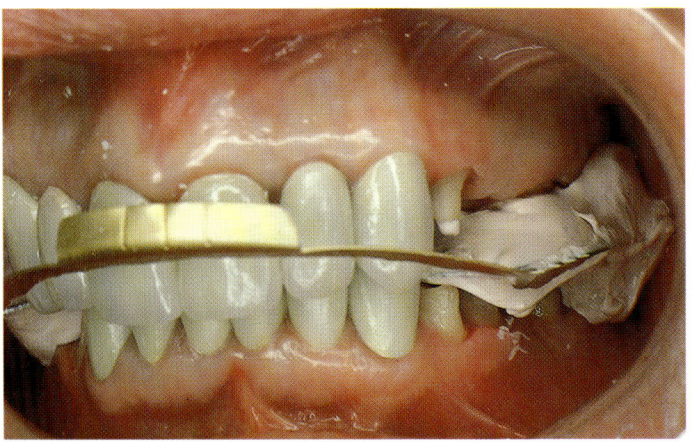

Fig 5-46 A closed bite CR record being made at the OVD established by anterior teeth. The posterior teeth have been prepared bilaterally for crowns and the anterior crowns are in even CR contact to act as an anterior stop that allows the condyles to move upward and forward to the CR position.

Condylar guidance

The transverse (hinge) axis is the only axis common to both condyles and the only one of clinical importance. In normal healthy joints the transverse (hinge) axis is constant to the condyles and thus to the mandibular teeth. A method for locating the transverse axis first suggested by Dr Robert Harlan was developed in 1924 by Dr B. B. McCollum and the Gnathological Society of California.[24] It still remains the basis for modern-day articulator design. Although condyles do not always exhibit as perfect a center of rotation as a spherical ball or a metal shaft, in normal joints the phenomenon is consistent enough to be of practical clinical value. The clinical value of accurately locating the hinge axis is related to the degree of jaw separation used in making open bite CR records, as well as the ability to change vertical dimension on the articulator and maintain accurate CR as the teeth are occluded. If the final vertical dimension

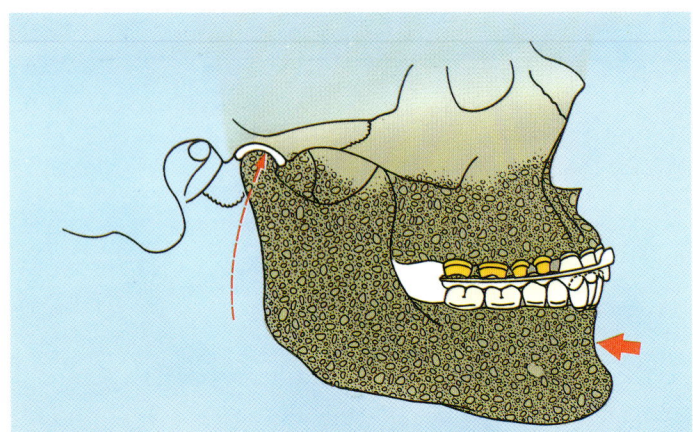

Fig 5-47a The mandible is retruded *(horizontal arrow)* with only anterior teeth in contact. The maxillary posterior teeth have been prepared bilaterally for crowns. The mandibular posterior teeth contact the soft bite registration material with no resistance while the condyles are positioned upward and forward in CR *(vertical arrow)* at the OVD established by the anterior teeth.

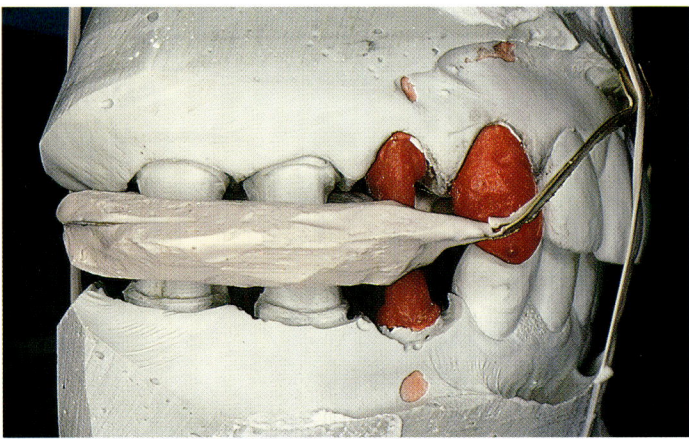

Fig 5-47b Mandibular cast mounted to maxillary cast on articulator with "closed bite" CR record at the OVD established by the anterior teeth.

Physiology of occlusion

of occlusion is established in the centric record, or with the anterior teeth together (closed bite CR record) as in the case of bilateral posterior tooth reduction, a precise location of the hinge axis is not mandatory (Fig 5-46 and Figs 5-47a and b). However, the accurate terminal hinge location and axis face-bow transfer of casts to the articulator is of vital importance during open-bite CR records since the occlusal vertical dimension will change when the CR record is removed (Fig 5-48 and Figs 5-49a and b). An open-bite CR record and a true hinge axis face bow mounting are always needed for remount occlusal adjustment procedures of artificial crowns in the laboratory.

Movements of the mandible can be described as simultaneous translations and rotations around vertical, sagittal, and transverse axes of the condyles (Fig 5-50).[25] The vertical and sagittal axes of the working side condyle are only of academic interest because they cannot be accurately located and because all movements of the

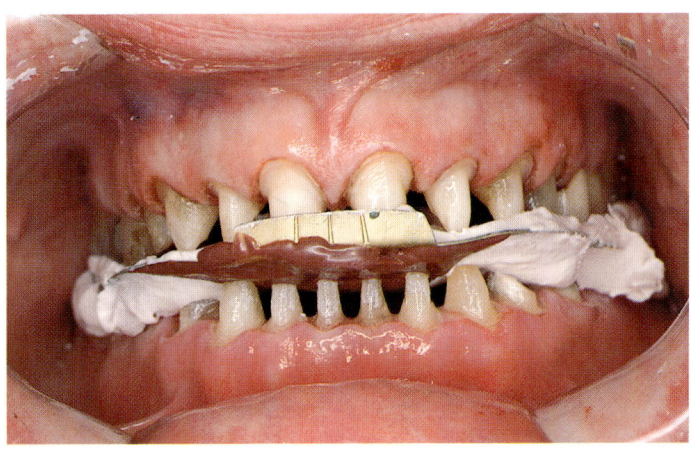

Fig 5-48 This "open bite" CR record has been taken at an increased OVD. Therefore, the casts should be mounted with a hinge axis facebow that will keep the casts in CR relation when the CR record is removed and the casts are closed together.

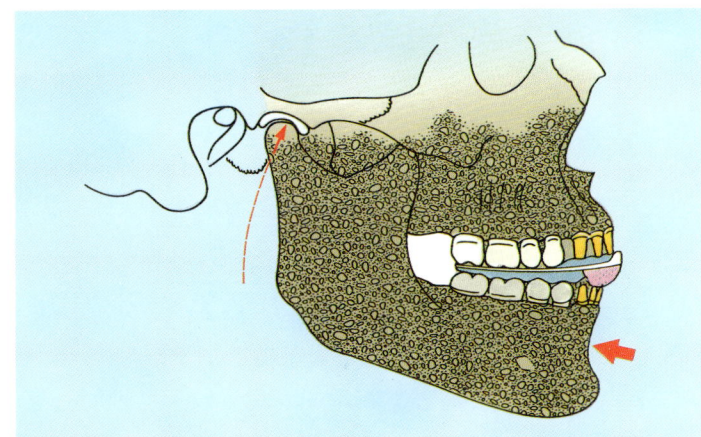

Fig 5-49a The maxillary and mandibular anterior teeth have been prepared for crowns. The bite registration material is first placed on the upper side of the bite tray to record the maxillary teeth position. Hot compound is added to the tray and water tempered in the mandibular incisor area. The mandible is *retruded* and elevated so that only the mandibular incisor preparations make contact with the soft compound to index the retruded position of the mandibular anterior teeth *(horizontal arrow)* and the compound is allowed to harden. Bite registration material is then placed on the lower side of the bite tray. In closing posterior teeth contact the soft bite registration material with no resistance, which allows the condyles to be positioned upward and forward in CR *(vertical arrow)*.

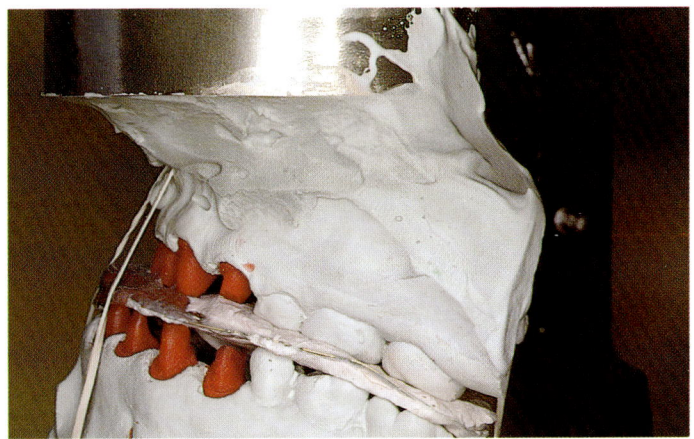

Fig 5-49b An "open bite" CR record being used to mount the mandibular cast to the previously axis-mounted maxillary cast. Premature posterior CR contacts must be removed if the OVD is reduced but the casts remain in centric relation because the maxillary cast was mounted with a true hinge bow. If the OVD is to be increased with the anterior crowns, posterior occlusal restorations (in at least one arch) will be necessary.

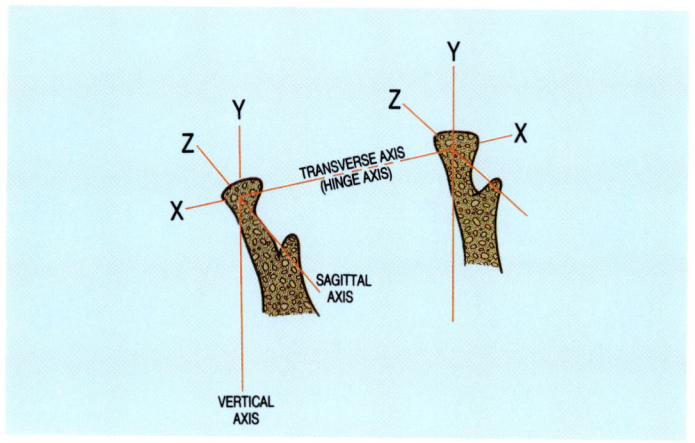

Fig 5-50 Movements of the mandible can be described as simultaneous translations and rotations around vertical, sagittal, and transverse (hinge) axes of the condyles.

condyles around these two axes can be reproduced by recording and reproducing the movements of any two points a fixed distance apart on the transverse (hinge) axis[26,27] (Figs 5-51 and 5-52). It has been shown that the effects of intercondylar distance in the functional range of lateral jaw movement have insignificant effects on posterior crown morphology.[28]

Condyle movements do not dictate natural tooth morphology. Along with anterior overbite and plane of occlusion, condylar movements only influence the path of approach of the mandibular to the maxillary teeth. Generally, the flatter the condylar paths, the greater the chance that the posterior teeth may come into contact in eccentric movements (Fig 5-53). The Bennett[29] shift phenomenon (loose joints) can also affect the path of approach of the posterior teeth (Fig 5-54). In the past emphasis has been placed by some dentists on recording and adjusting articulators to the exact Bennett paths so that "balanced occlusion" could be achieved.[24] Since D'Amico[20] presented the canine guided theory in 1958 the balanced occlusion concept was modified to include minimal canine disclusion for natural teeth.[30] Minimal canine guidance usually produces abnormally flat (low profile) posterior crown forms, which often results in

Physiology of occlusion

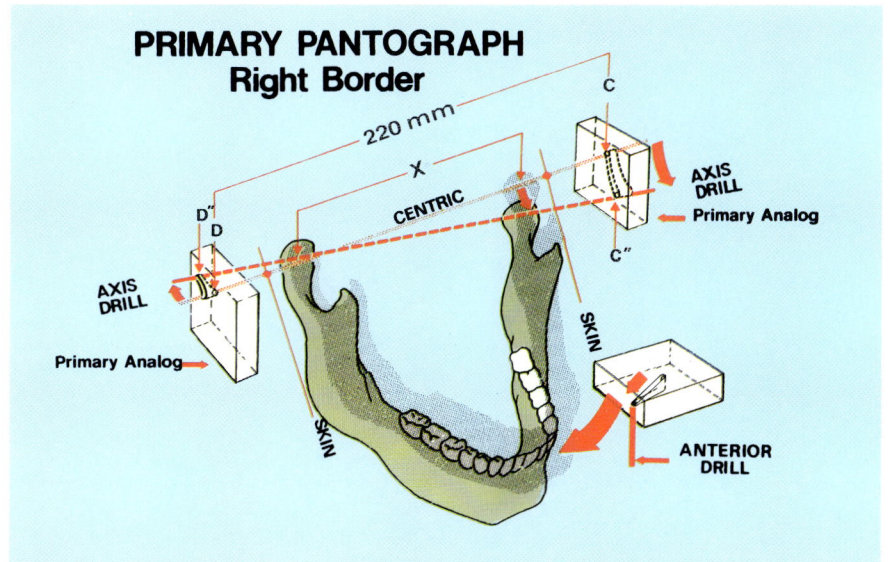

Fig 5-51 All movements of the mandible can be simulated by recording and reproducing the paths of any two points on the transverse axis a fixed distance apart because any movement around a vertical or sagittal axis will be reflected in the movement of the two fixed points on the transverse (hinge) axis.

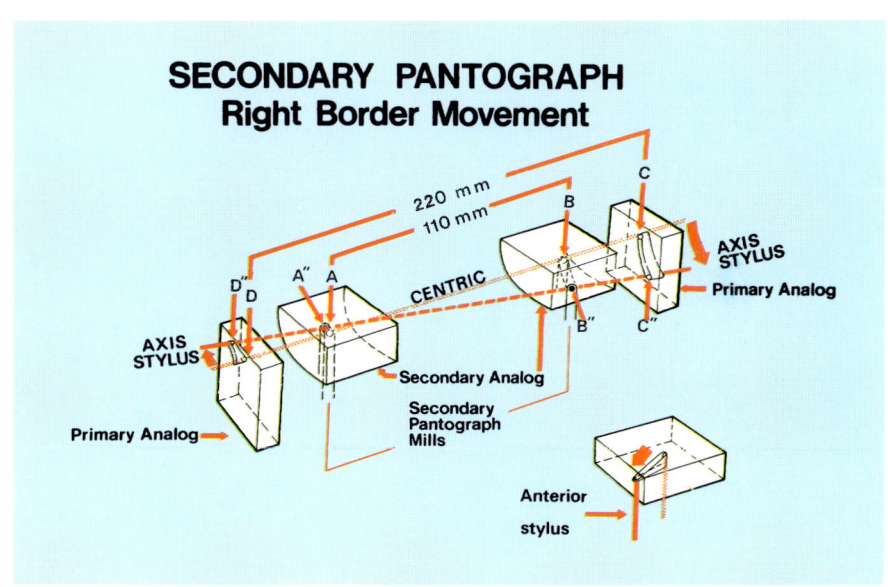

Fig 5-52 The paths of the original transverse axis recordings (motion analogs) can be used to generate other motion analogs at other locations on the hinge axis to produce a convenient-sized articulator for laboratory use.

163

Esthetics and Its Relationship to Function

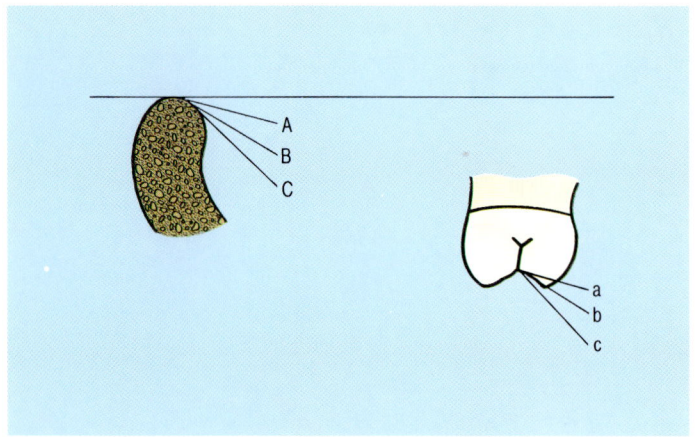

Fig 5-53   The more horizontal the protrusive condylar path, the greater the chance that the posterior teeth may come into contact in protrusive jaw movements. The other two factors in posterior tooth separation in protrusion are the overbite of the anterior teeth and the plane of occlusion.

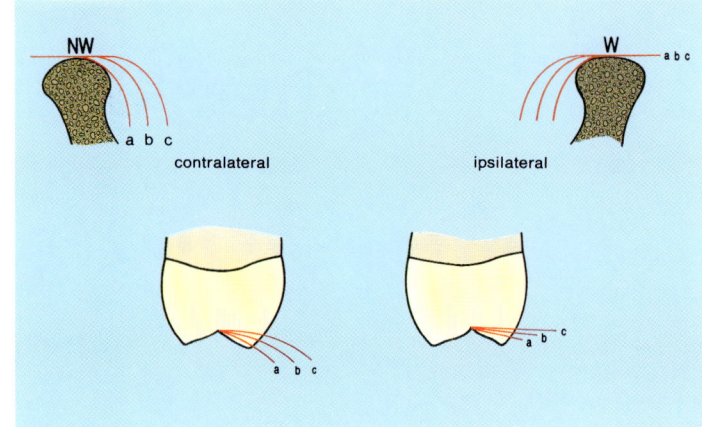

Fig 5-54   The greater the amount of Bennett movement (loose joints), the greater the chance of posterior eccentric contacts in protrusive and lateral jaw movements. With good canine overbite, the posterior teeth can usually be separated without reducing their genetic vertical profiles.

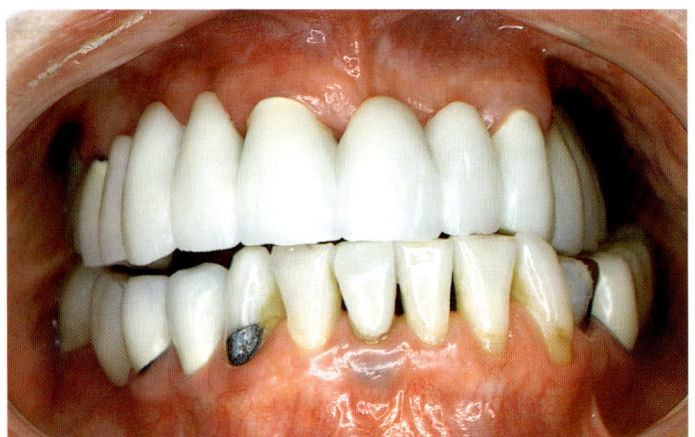

Fig 5-55a   Artificial crowns with minimum canine guidance in left lateral movement.

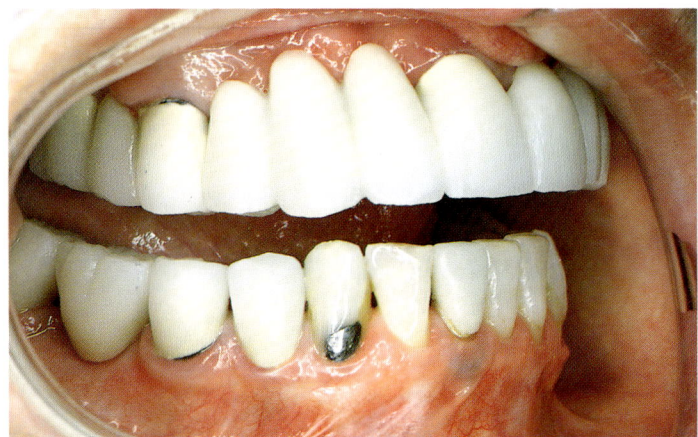

Fig 5-55b   Abnormally flat (unnatural) artificial crowns when minimal canine guidance was used.

Physiology of occlusion

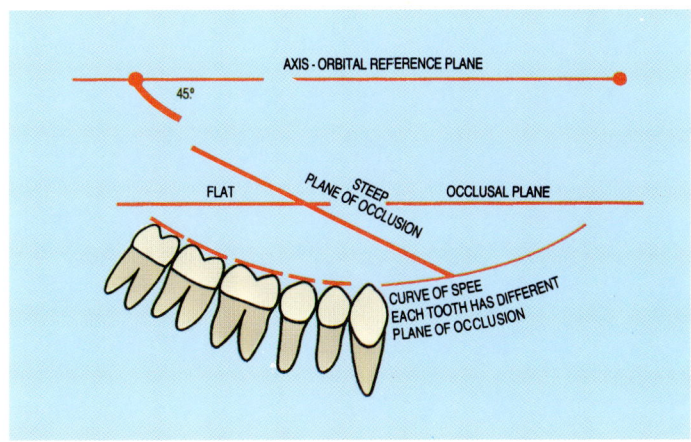

Fig 5-56 In flattening the occlusal plane to get better separation of the posterior teeth in eccentric jaw movements, one must also take into consideration the esthetics of the smile. By giving patients good anterior overbite, one is usually able to get good separation of posterior teeth in protrusive and lateral jaw movements and also allow the occlusal plane to be steeper for esthetics (see Figs 57a and b).

overload on the teeth and other components of the gnathic system (Figs 5-55a and b).

The closer the teeth are to the condyles (eg, second and third molars), the more the approaching pathways of these molars may be affected by Bennett movement and horizontal condylar paths. It has been found that giving patients naturally steep overbite of the canines (65° to 70°) greatly reduces the chances for posterior eccentric interferences even in the presence of flatter condylar paths and large amounts of Bennett movement. In no event should condyle movements be allowed to flatten the morphology of canines and premolars of artificial crowns when the occlusion is being treated. Occasionally, second and third molar buccolingual profiles may need to be flattened slightly to accommodate large amounts of Bennett movements. The mesiodistal profiles of molars, however, need not be reduced regardless of the amount of Bennett movement.

Occlusal plane

The plane of occlusion is important in function only when it is related to condylar paths and anterior overbite. The relation of these three factors (occlusal plane, anterior overbite, and condylar movements) controls the path and timing of the mandibular posterior teeth as they approach the maxillary posterior teeth. Generally, the steeper the plane of occlusion, the more difficult it is to prevent eccentric posterior tooth interferences because the plane of occlusion more closely equals the path of the condyles and therefore increases their occluding effect (Fig 5-56).

A curve of Spee and lateral curve of Wilson are usually minimal in good natural occlusions. In case of an accentuated curve of Spee, each tooth has a different plane of occlusion. The plane of occlusion of mesially inclined molars often approaches (or even exceeds) the descending path of the condyles, which explains why it is often difficult to avoid protrusive and lateral interferences of second and third molars that have tipped forward into a space created by an extracted tooth anterior to it.

A reverse plane of occlusion detracts from the es-

Esthetics and Its Relationship to Function

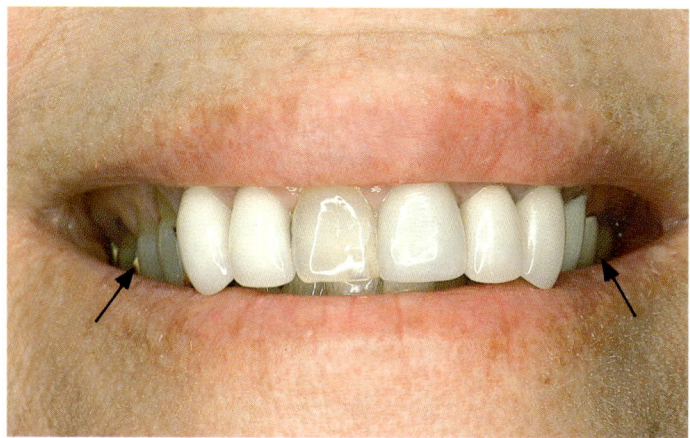

Fig 5-57a A 70-year-old woman with a severe reverse esthetic plane of occlusion caused by extruded maxillary molars (arrows).

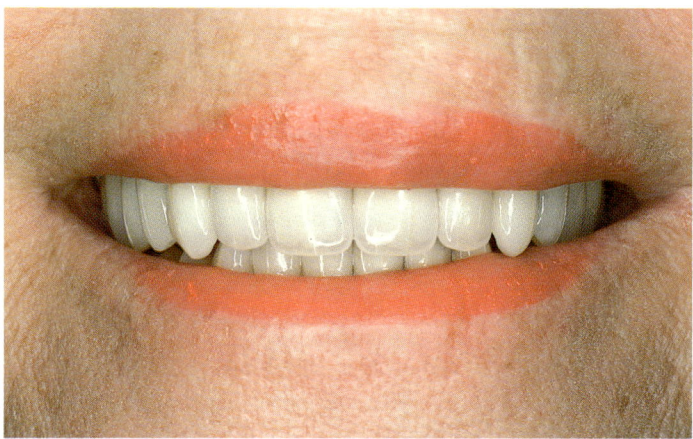

Fig 5-57b The esthetic results could have been better in the treatment if the posterior occlusal plane had been made steeper. The separation of the posterior teeth in protrusive and lateral movement was accomplished with good anterior overbite. The incisal edges of the maxillary central incisors could have been made longer for better esthetics.

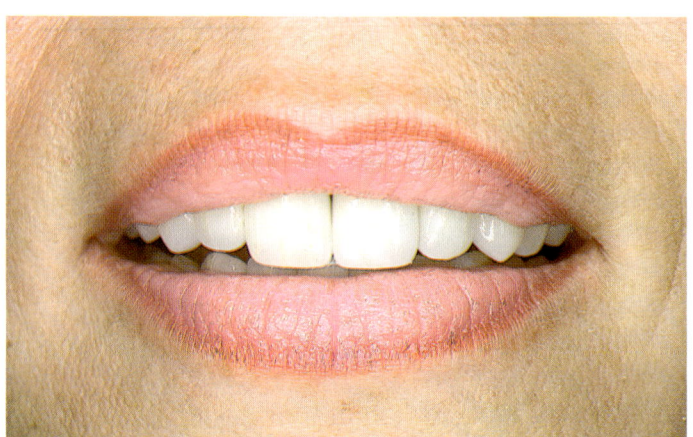

Fig 5-58 From an esthetic viewpoint, it is best when the posterior plane of occlusion generally follows the smile line of the lower lip, provided the smile line is symmetrical as shown in this patient with bioesthetic artificial crowns.

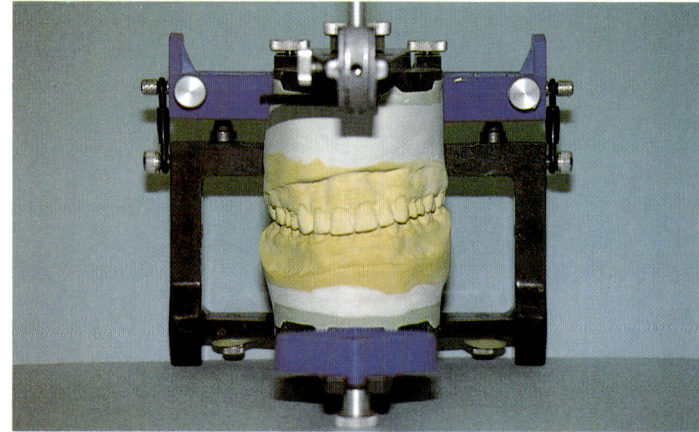

Fig 5-59 Face-bow mounted casts, although essential for good occlusion procedures, are esthetically misleading whenever they have a lateral tilt in the articulator. The dentist must communicate to the laboratory any difference between the esthetic occlusal plane and the anatomic occlusal plane. The esthetic plane should take priority. If good anterior overbite has been established, posterior tooth separation in jaw excursions will be accomplished even if the occlusal plane has to be modified for esthetic reasons.

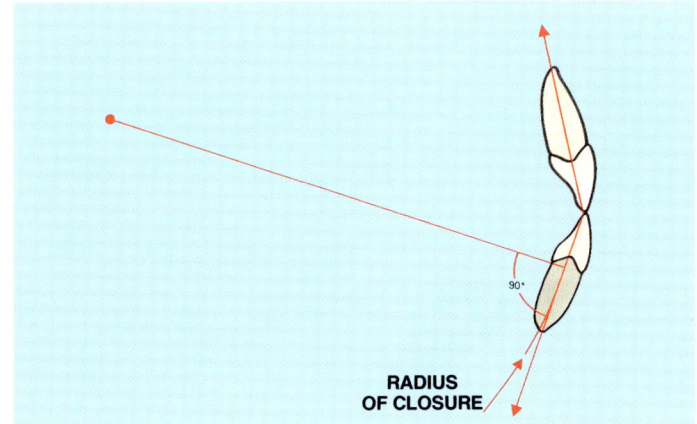

Fig 5-60 With naturally sharp incisors there is usually no more than 1 mm of retrusive shearing load, which is confined to the incisal edges of the teeth and loads both the maxillary and mandibular incisors in their long axes.

thetics of a smile. This problem is often faced in older patients in whom the maxillary teeth may have extruded over the years into edentulous areas of the mandibular arch (Figs 5-57a and b). A steep plane of occlusion can also cause a poor posterior esthetic smile line. From an esthetic viewpoint, it is best when the plane of occlusion generally follows the smile line of the lower lip, provided the smile line is symmetrical (Fig 5-58). The esthetic plane of occlusion is not always coincidental with the functional plane of occlusion. The esthetic plane is best when it is parallel to the horizon and the patient's head is perpendicular to horizontal. Anatomically (ear face-bow) and axis-mounted casts are sometimes misleading to technicians because the casts may be laterally tilted in the articulator (Fig 5-59). The dentist should communicate any discrepancy between the esthetic and anatomic plane of occlusion to the laboratory technician. Facial asymmetries should not be allowed to influence the esthetic plane of occlusion.

Mastication

Incising function

The simplest functional movement in mastication is opening the mouth to acquire the food. This movement takes place in the sagittal plane. It is primarily two-dimensional, with both condyles translating downward and forward on the eminentia (which protrudes the mandible). If food, such as bread, apples, and corn on the cob, is to be incised, the food is placed between the front teeth either by the hand or an eating utensil such as a fork. The mandible is elevated by the muscles so that the sharp incisal edges of the four mandibular incisors cut through the food to touch (or nearly touch) the incisal edge of the two maxillary central incisors. With naturally sharp unworn teeth there is usually no more than 1 mm of retrusive shearing load, which is confined to the incisal edges of the teeth. This function loads the maxillary incisors generally in their long axis (Fig 5-60). The mandibular incisors have a labial inclination that averages about 90° to the arc of closure around the hinge axis which loads them in their long axis (see Fig 5-60). Sometimes the incisors merely hold the food while the hand tears the food apart.

Esthetics and Its Relationship to Function

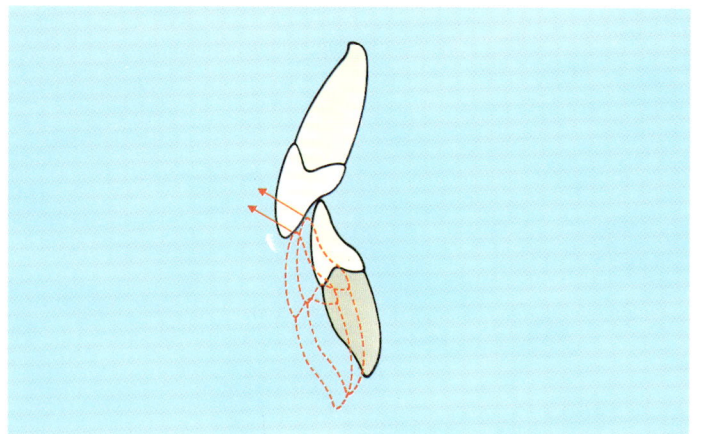

Fig 5-61   The labial inclination of the maxillary incisors appears unfavorable for lingual shearing forces. In an empty mouth test, however, the four mandibular incisors should maintain constant even contact with the lingual aspects of the maxillary incisors and no posterior teeth should interfere with the smooth, gliding movement back to CR occlusion.

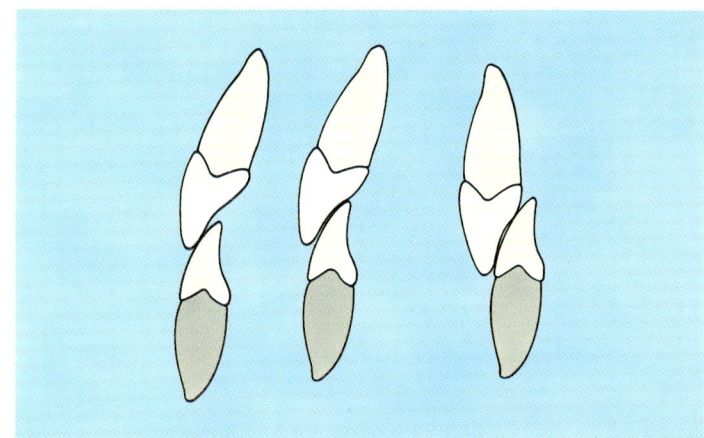

Fig 5-62   The labial surface of the mandibular incisors should not come in contact with the lingual surface of the maxillary incisors at any time.

It is probably a misconception that the incisal edges of the mandibular teeth should shear food against the lingual surfaces of the maxillary incisors. The irregular lingual surfaces (mesial, distal, and central ridges) of the maxillary incisors appear not to be designed for a shearing function. The labial inclination of the maxillary incisors also appears to be unfavorable for lingual shearing forces (Fig 5-61). The mesial, distal, and marginal central lingual ridge observed in natural incisors may deal more with trussing the relatively thin teeth as well as creating small IP contacts with the mandibular incisors. In an empty mouth test, however, the four mandibular incisors should maintain a constant even contact with the lingual aspects of the maxillary incisors, and no posterior teeth should interfere with the smooth, gliding movement back to CR occlusion (Fig 5-62). This even distribution of anterior lingual contacts probably helps to reduce bruxism and fremitus and to produce consistent horizontal overbite for speaking and rest positions. In addition, the maxillary anterior horizontal overbite provides freedom from incisor contacts in lateral mastication. The mesial incline of the mandibular first premolar often closely follows the distal incline of the maxillary canine as the jaw moves distally in an incisor guided motion, but this near-contact should never prevent the incisors from being the principal guiding factor. The *labial* surfaces of the mandibular incisors should not come in contact with the lingual surfaces of the maxillary incisors at any time in protrusive movements for at least two reasons:

1. Labial contacts on mandibular incisors may not allow for proper anterior posturing of the condyles in rest and speaking positions. This posterior confinement of the condyles may cause an adverse neuromuscular response leading to bruxism, craniofascial pain, or craniomandibular dysfunction.
2. Contacts on the labial surface of mandibular incisors overload the anterior teeth and may force the mandibular teeth lingually and the maxillary teeth labially.

The maxillary lateral incisors are shorter than the central incisors to make space for the cusp tips of the mandibular canines when the incisors are edge to edge

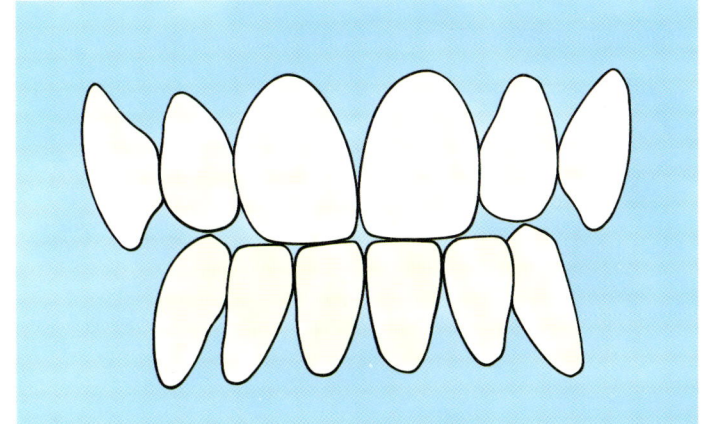

Figs 5-63 In the incisive position the maxillary lateral incisors are higher than the central incisors to provide space for the cusp tips of the mandibular canines in protrusion.

(Figs 5-63, 5-43b, 5-44b, 5-45b). This phenomenon is true in both men and women. This characteristic is also one of youthfulness and is usually perceived as a pleasant appearance in adults. In a good natural dentition, when the incisors are edge to edge in protrusion, there is usually about 2 mm of space between the cusp tips of the posterior teeth (see Figs 5-43b, 5-44b, 5-45b). This posterior space is controlled by the steepness of the condylar paths and the vertical overbite of the anterior teeth as they relate to the occlusal morphology of the posterior teeth and the horizontal plane of occlusion.

The protrusive paths of the condyles vary significantly from one patient to another and even between right and left sides in the same patient. In some patients the protrusive path nearly approaches horizontal, whereas in others it more nearly approaches vertical. The protrusive path of the condyles is the most significant movement to be simulated in an articulator. The recording and articulator setting for the path of the condyles in protrusion–retrusion is easily accomplished with an intraoral checkbite or simplified condyle movement recorder (Figs 5-64 to 5-67). Incisal guidance for bioesthetic occlusal function should be diagnosed and the treatment plan made on an individually adjusted articulator. If the diagnosis shows that the anterior teeth cannot be used in their natural state, restorative, orthodontic, and/or surgical means are indicated. Articulators do not have lips or smiles; therefore, some of the esthetics in this area remain a chairside procedure.

Incisal overbite affects canine length and guidance. For example, if canine restorations are given a natural vertical overbite to eliminate posterior lateral interferences and produce more vertical physiologic chewing patterns while the central incisors are allowed minimal vertical overbite (Figs 5-68 and 5-69), the patient's maxillary canines will rise up on the mesial side of the mandibular first premolars in protrusion and not allow the incisors to contact for proper incising function (Figs 5-70 and 5-71). Also, having a natural vertical overbite of the maxillary canines with a reduced overbite of the incisors may create a "vampire" look (Fig 5-72). If one shortens the canines for esthetics, the risk of producing

Esthetics and Its Relationship to Function

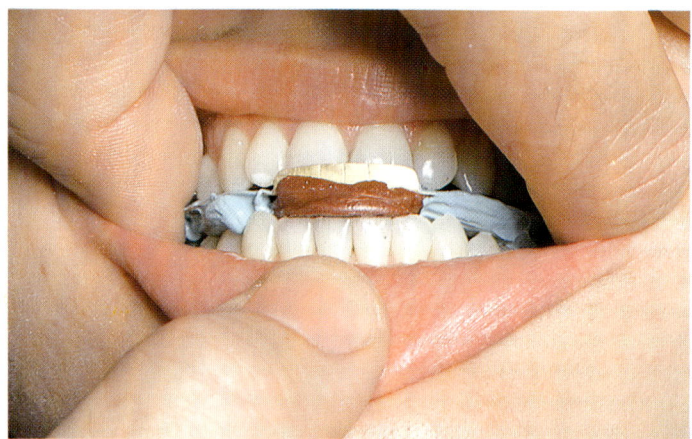

Fig 5-64 Recording the individual patient's protrusive path of the condyles is easily accomplished with the Panadent* intraoral checkbite.

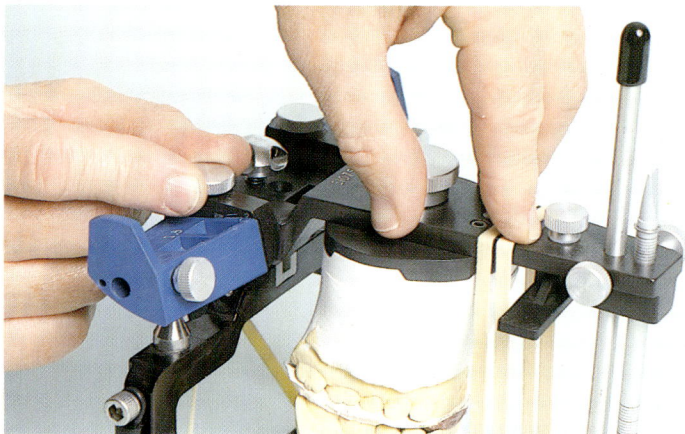

Fig 5-65 The Panadent articulator* motion analogs being adjusted to the protrusive path checkbite.

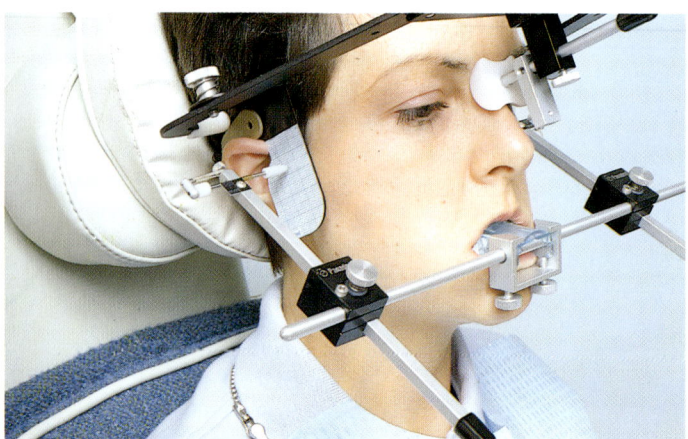

Fig 5-66 The Panadent Axi-Path Recorder* allows the complete protrusive path of the patient to be recorded graphically as well as the precise location of the hinge axis.

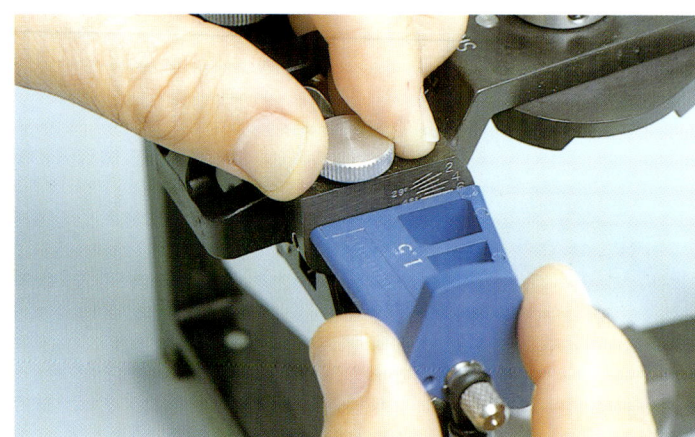

Fig 5-67 After the orbital axis reference line has been established on the protrusive graphs of the Panadent Axi-Path Recorder,* the angular adjustments of the Panadent articulator* are made.

* Panadent Corp, Grand Terrace, Calif.

Mastication

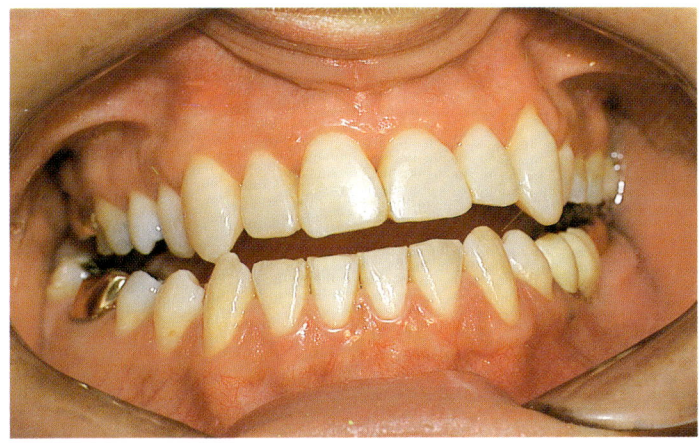

Fig 5-68 The worn-down canines of this patient have been restored to proper functional length with composite resin to prevent the posterior teeth from contacting in lateral jaw movement.

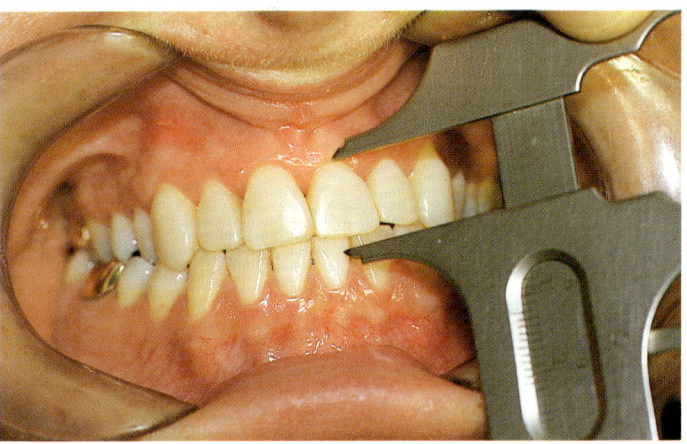

Fig 5-69 In protrusive movement the incisors would have to be lengthened concurrently, as indicated by the Boley gauge.

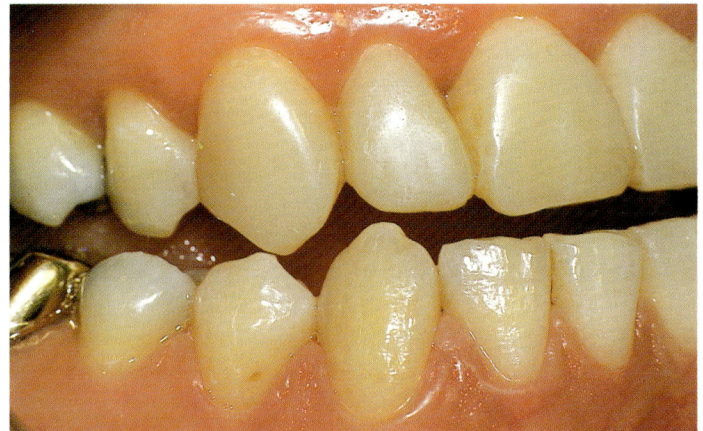

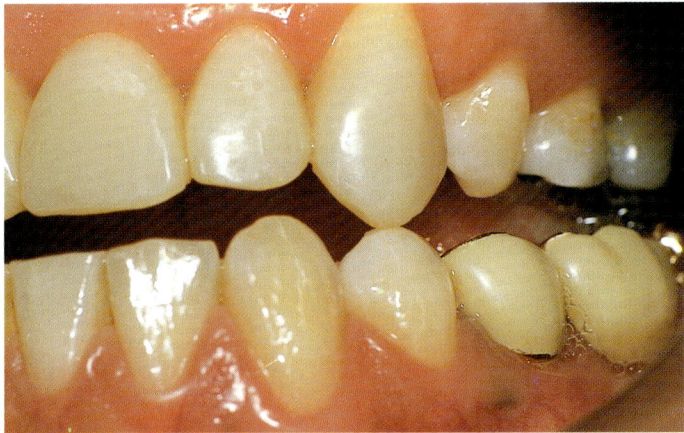

Figs 5-70 and 5-71 The incisors are prevented from contacting because the maxillary canines are touching the buccal cusp of the mandibular first premolars in protrusion.

171

Esthetics and Its Relationship to Function

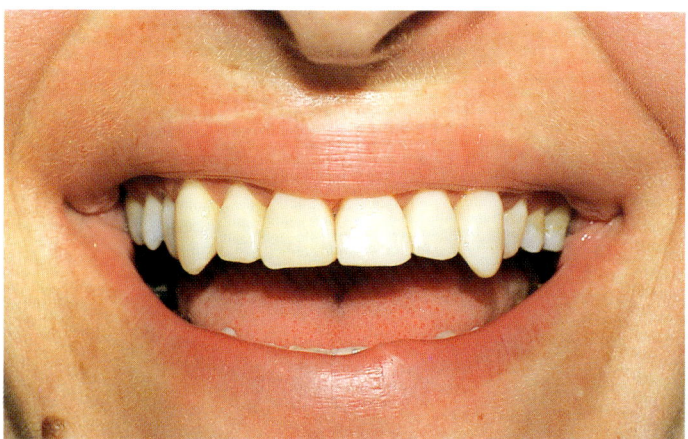

Fig 5-72 A "vampire" look is often created if only the canines are restored without restoring the incisors.

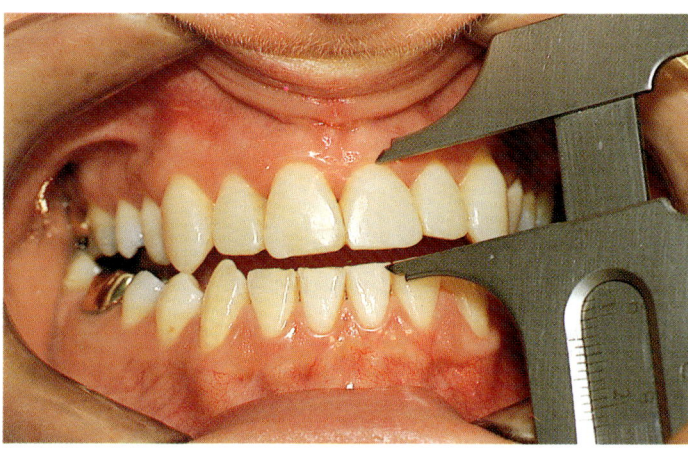

Fig 5-73 The Boley gauge shows that the incisors should be lengthened at least 2 mm in order to establish bioesthetics in addition to incisive function by separating the mandibular first premolars from contact with the maxillary canines.

"nonchewing side" (contralateral) interferences is increased. In these cases the lengths of the maxillary incisors must be increased to have proper esthetics and incising function (Fig 5-73).

Lateral chewing function

Opening phase
In preparation for lateral chewing function, the mouth is opened to accept the food and both condyles translate downward and forward in the sagittal plane. As the tongue places the bolus of food on the chewing side, the mandibular incisors move about 3 mm to that side. The chewing side (ipsilateral) condyle quickly shifts to a retruded lateral position while the nonchewing side (contralateral) condyle remains about 3 mm forward on the eminence and shifts medially the same amount that the chewing side condyle shifts laterally (Fig 5-74). The direction or path of the shift of both condyles is primarily a horizontal one at this point in the chewing cycle. This shifting phenomenon was observed in the working side condyle and first mentioned by Bennett in 1907.[29] It has subsequently been referred to as Bennett shift or side shift. The amount of lateral shifting (Bennett phenomenon) varies between people, ranging from zero to as much as 4 mm, depending on factors such as the looseness of the ligaments, boney configurations of the condyles and fossae, and the shape and condition of the discs. The average patient has a 1-mm Bennett shift in left lateral movement and a 1-mm Bennett shift in right lateral movement.[31] The amount of lateral shifting is also influenced neuromuscularly by the consistency of the food being chewed. Gibbs[32] reported that the tougher or harder the food, the greater the amount of shifting.[12] There is, however, a maximum that can be reached, which varies with each patient. There is often a difference in the amount of Bennett shift between right and left lateral chewing excursions in the same patient.

Early closing phase
With the mandibular incisors in a 3-mm lateral position (see Fig 5-74), the tongue places the bolus of food between the teeth on the chewing side. As the mandible begins its closure to full occlusion, the canines begin to proprioceptively guide the mandible more vertically in the coronal (frontal) plane. When the mandibular canine

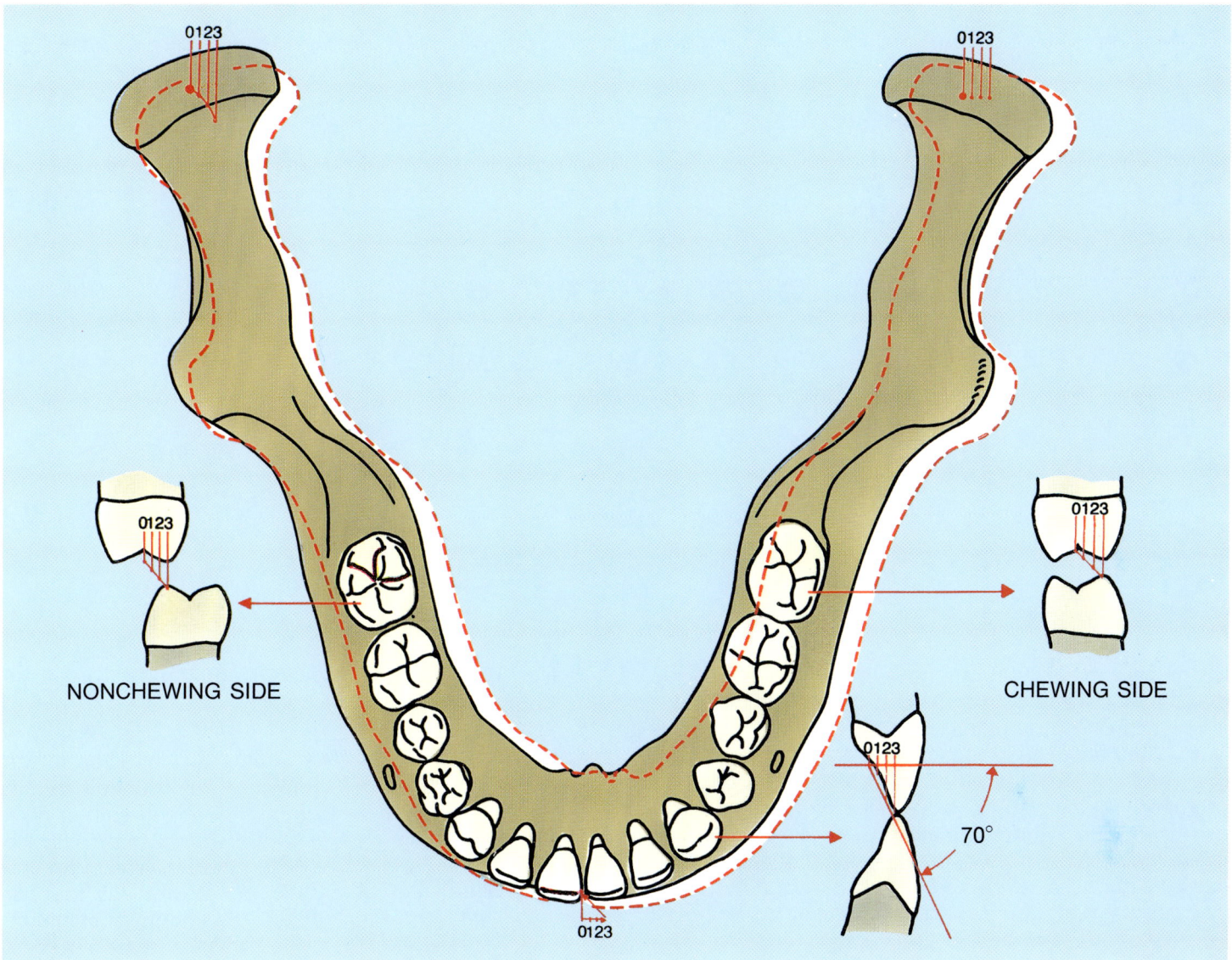

Fig 5-74 Approximate occluding path of molars during left side mastication as they relate to the guiding paths of the condyles and left canines. The condyles are shown in the horizontal plane while the second molars and left canines are shown in the frontal plane. Vertical arrows on condyles show that condyles move forward down the eminentia when the mouth is opened. The nonchewing side *(right)* condyle shifts medially *(horizontal arrow)* while the chewing side *(left)* condyle shifts laterally when Bennett movement is present.

Esthetics and Its Relationship to Function

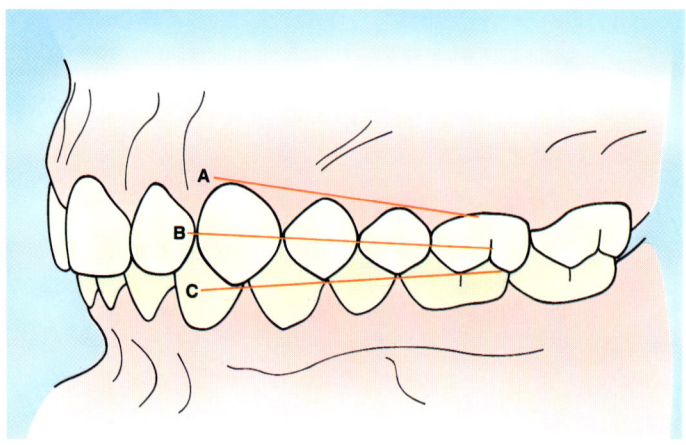

Fig 5-75 Line C shows the graduated group function position of the canine and buccal cusps of the first and second premolars ("second and third canines"), which aid the first canine in medial closure.

has moved medially about 1 mm from the cusp of the maxillary canine, the buccal cusp of the "second canine" (first premolar) begins to aid the "first canine." This is why the buccal cusp of the first premolar is prominent but slightly shorter than the canine (Fig 5-75). The natural morphology and position of the canine teeth produces about a 70° anterior closing path (from horizontal) in the coronal (frontal) plane as the mandible moves medially during a lateral chewing stroke (see Fig 5-74). In case the "first canine" should wear or be fractured or is out of position, the "second canine" (first premolar) becomes the surrogate and leads the teeth in medial guidance (Figs 5-76 and 5-77). This graduated chewing side group function appears to be more compatible with natural tooth morphology and the biomechanics of the human gnathic system than any other tooth arrangement. Lateral jaw movements should not be guided by incisor teeth for a number of reasons, including the following:

1. Incisors are not in a good position for lateral guidance because they nearly parallel the lateral movement of the mandible.
2. Possible overload and wear on anterior teeth because of their small size and fragility.
3. A tendency to force the condyles too far distally in lateral jaw movements.
4. Tendency for adverse neuromuscular response.

Also involved in the closing paths of the mandibular teeth are the ingrams in the brain which guide the mandible through learned reflexes. Although the chewing side (ipsilateral) condyle path is primarily horizontal in the function range of motion, the nonchewing side (contralateral) condyle moves in a curvilinear path simultaneously in the three planes of space: transverse (horizontal), sagittal (vertical), and coronal (frontal). There is often a significant component of the nonchewing side movement that takes place in the horizontal plane in patients who have larger amounts of Bennett movement (loose joints).

It is not known at this time what causes the looseness in the joints (Bennett movement).[25] It may be due to stretched ligaments, enlarged fossae, reduced condyle size, or a combination of factors. There is some evidence to indicate that horizontal occlusion may increase loose-

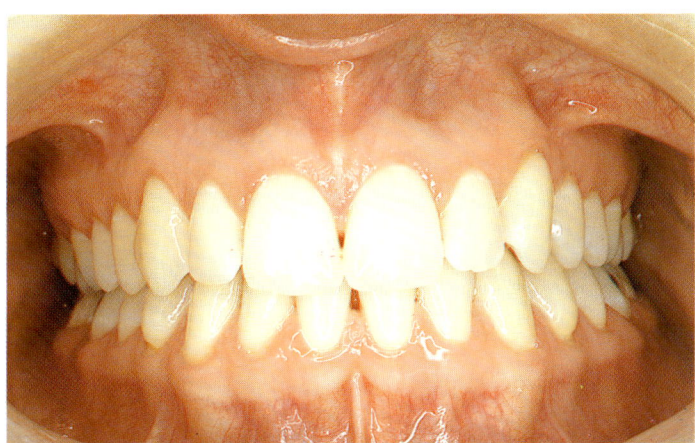

Fig 5-76 In full occlusion, the right side "first canine" of this patient is out of contact with the mandibular canine.

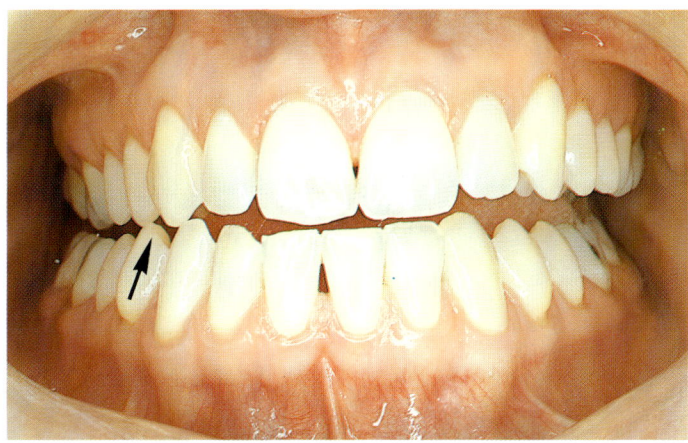

Fig 5-77 The "second canine" of the patient in Fig 5-76 acts as a surrogate to help guide the mandible in medial closure (arrow).

ness of the joints.[33] The curved Bennett path of the nonchewing side condyle varies greatly between patients.[34] It has been found that the greater the amount of Bennett shift, the greater is the radius of curvature of the nonchewing side Bennett path. It is the curved nonchewing side Bennett path that affects the approach of the cusps of the molars on that side significantly. The nonchewing side condylar Bennett path tends to bring the posterior teeth of that side of the mouth into premature medial contact during lateral function (see Fig 5-54). It is commonly agreed by authorities that lateral movement contacts of the nonchewing side teeth often lead to problems in the neuromuscular and TMJ mechanism and should be eliminated whenever a patient undergoes occlusal treatment.

Complex pantographs have been used to record the Bennett path of the condyles and transfer the movement to articulators. A simplified method for recording the Bennett movement of the condyles and simulating their curved paths in an articulator has been developed more recently (Figs 5-78a to d, Figs 5-79a to d). The adjusted articulator gives all of the needed jaw movement simulation for diagnosis and provides for maximum biocompatible artificial crowns. Because there is usually an attachment clutch over the occlusal surfaces of the teeth to hold the jaw movement recorder when Bennett movement is recorded and because the mandible is moved in the reverse direction of chewing (centric to eccentric), the neuromuscular system does not respond the same as when chewing occurs. When a jaw movement recorder is used, it is recommended that the operator artificially simulate a hard chew with hand pressure at the angle of the mandible where the pterygoid muscles attach in order to record the maximum Bennett movement (see Figs 5-78a to d, Figs 5-79a to d). Two to three times more Bennett movement can usually be achieved with operator inducement compared with allowing patients to move their own mandible in contact with the anterior discluder on the attachment clutch. The use of a paraocclusal clutch is not recommended when recording border movements to CR position because tooth contacts (when occlusal interferences exist) often prevent the condyles from reaching border paths (including CR).

When significant amounts of Bennett movement exist, the operator has two options: (1) flatten the posterior crown morphology and (2) steepen the "canine area"

Esthetics and Its Relationship to Function

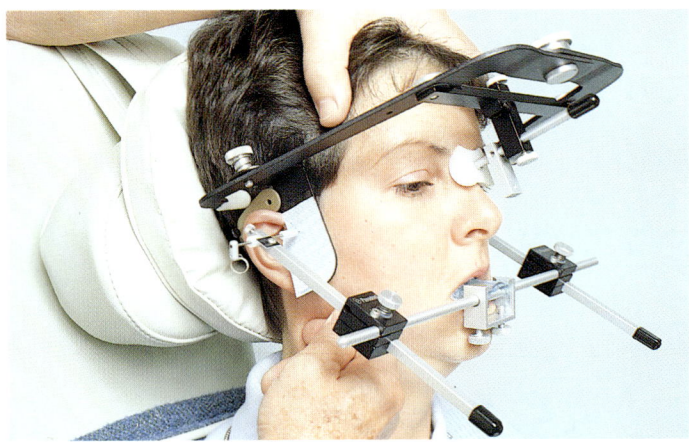

Fig 5-78a The Panadent Axi-Path Recorder is used to record the amount of Bennett movement.

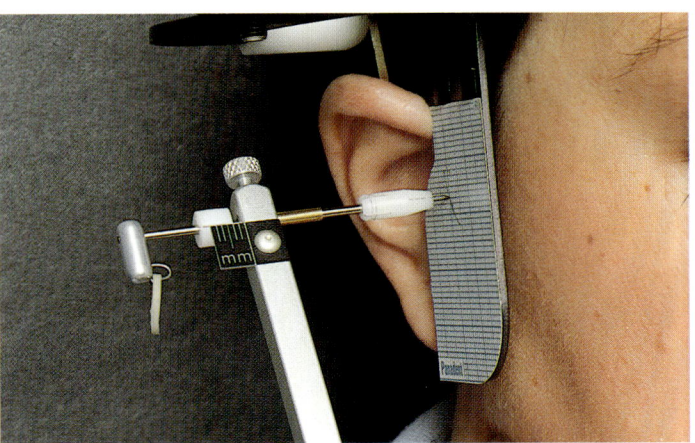

Fig 5-78b A close-up view of the recording arm shows the white ring registering the Bennett movement on the black millimeter scale.

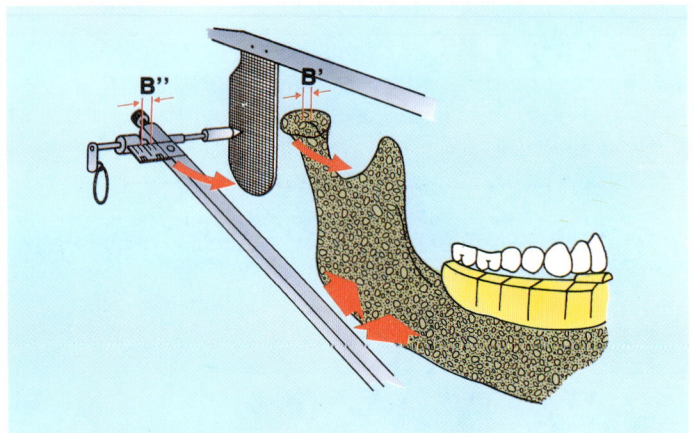

Fig 5-78c As the condyle is shifted medially on its characteristic Bennett path B', the movement is registered in the sagittal plane on the vertical graph and numerically in the horizontal plane B''.

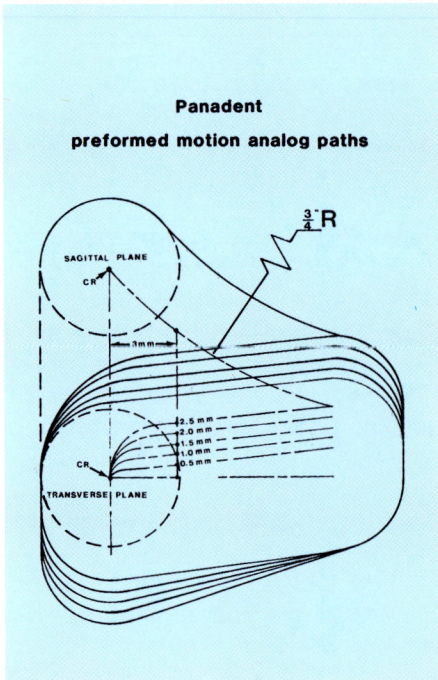

Fig 5-78d A schematic illustration of the Panadent preformed curved path motion analogs for the articulator guides.

176

Mastication

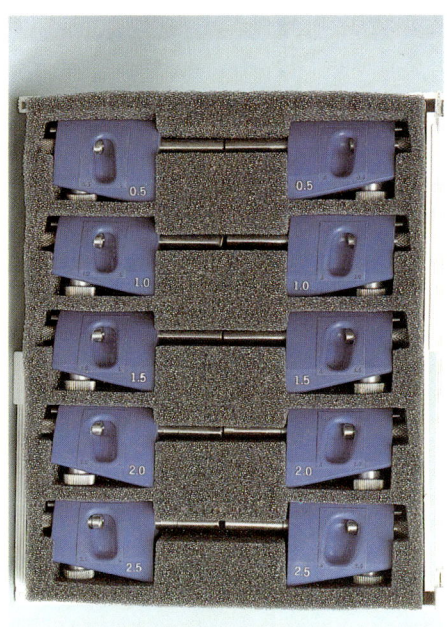

Fig 5-79a The Panadent preformed curved path condylar motion analogs are produced in five sizes: 0.5, 1.0, 1.5, 2.0 and 2.5 mm of three-plane curved path Bennett movement. They can be mixed to allow for differences between right and left side Bennett movement.

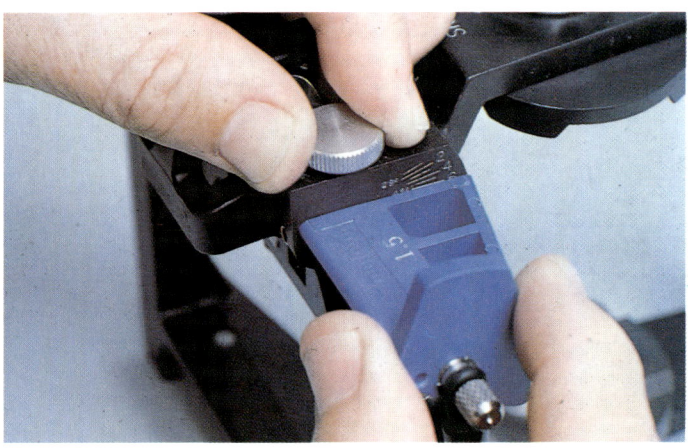

Fig 5-79b The analogs are rotatable to be adjusted to the patient's protrusive and lateral pathway.

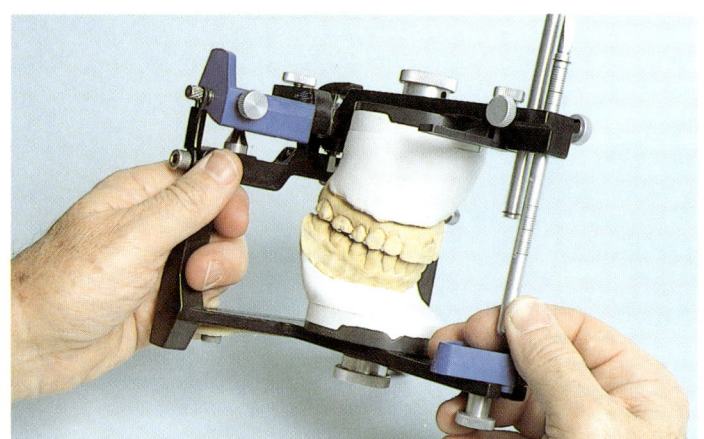

Fig 5-79c When using the Panadent motion analogs, the operator need only push on the incisal pin in lateral movements because of the unique resilient "Dyna-link" system and curved path motion analogs.

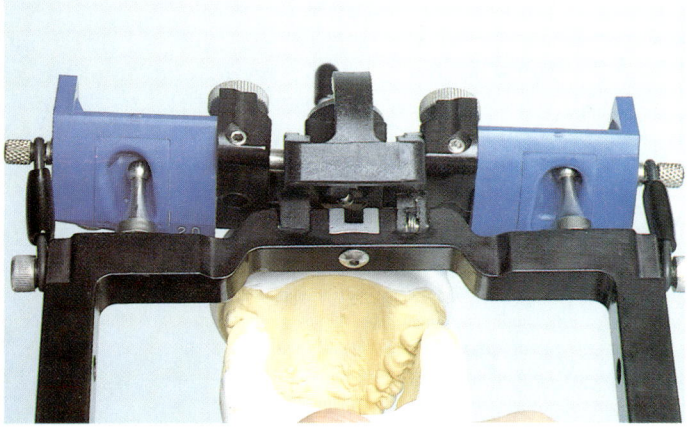

Fig 5-79d A rear view of the condylar elements shown in the functional range of lateral motion (3 mm). The right condylar element chewing side has shifted laterally while the left condylar element nonchewing side has moved downward, medial, and forward on the curved Bennett path of this patient.

Esthetics and Its Relationship to Function

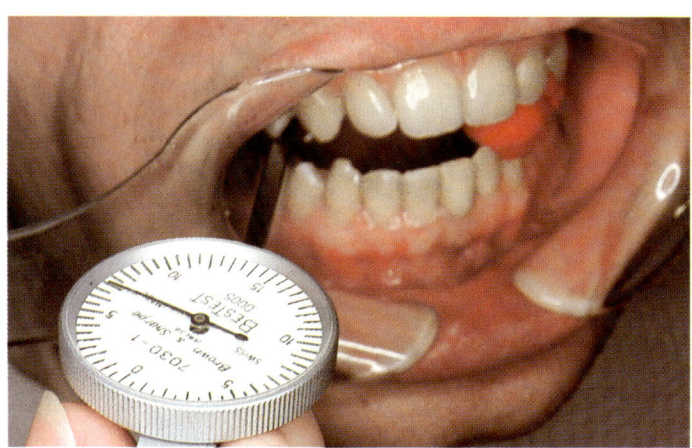

Fig 5-80 The functions of the posterior cusps.

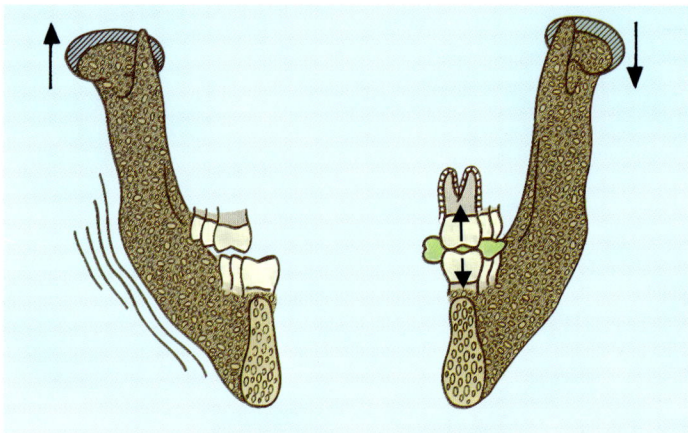

Fig 5-81 Because of biologic factors, such as flexions and compressions, teeth occlude differently in vivo than in vitro.

guidance. Every effort should be made to maximize the canine guidance to reduce the negative effects of Bennett movement to produce the best possible posterior crown morphology. Increasing canine guidance has a significant effect on posterior occlusion.[31]

Final closing phase

It is doubtful that total canine guidance exists in vivo. As the pressure of the food increases at the interface of the posterior teeth, it appears that the proprioceptive guidance transfers primarily from the canine to the posterior teeth. This is why it is important that there be compatible sharp posterior crown morphology to be in harmony with the naturally occurring steep canine guidance observed in good occlusions. Natural vertical guidance by the teeth does not negate or change the paths of the condyles but causes them to move along the Bennett (border) paths more rapidly to CR position before the major flexions and compressions of the gnathic system take place in the final phase of mastication (Fig 5-80).

Biomechanical factors take place in the last 1 to 2 mm of closure, such as: *(1)* flexion of the mandible, *(2)* compression of periodontal ligaments, *(3)* compression of TMJ discs, *(4)* movement at maxillary midline suture, and *(5)* distraction of working side condyle (Fig 5-81). Because of these factors, the teeth on the nonchewing side of the arch often touch first and also help guide the mandible proprioceptively into final closure (Figs 5-82a and b). In the final closing phase the teeth on the nonchewing side may also act as a mechanical stabilizing support to help the chewing side teeth penetrate tough food and make final occlusal contact (Fig 5-82c). In good occlusion with unworn posterior crown morphology these contacts take place near the intercuspal position of the teeth, thus directing the forces more vertically on the periodontium that conform to the natural biology of the gnathic system. The system is not a rigid but semirigid one. In mouths with flat teeth and poor canine guidance, the flexions and compressions are probably even greater because of greater chewing forces, resulting in the posterior teeth on the contralateral side coming into premature contacts on the inclines of the cusps *farther* away from IP (Fig 5-83). Avoidance patterns of these destructive posterior eccentric contacts often develop, causing excess wear on anterior teeth, and may eventually lead to bruxism, craniofacial pain, or craniomandibular disorders.

Mastication

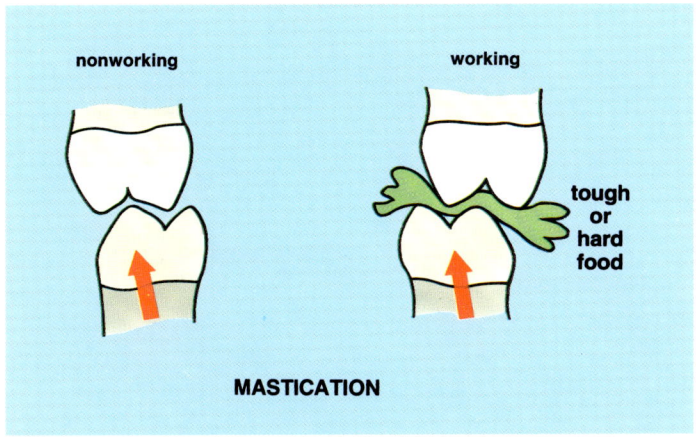

Fig 5-82a   In the early closing phase of mastication, the posterior teeth on both sides of the mouth are separated.

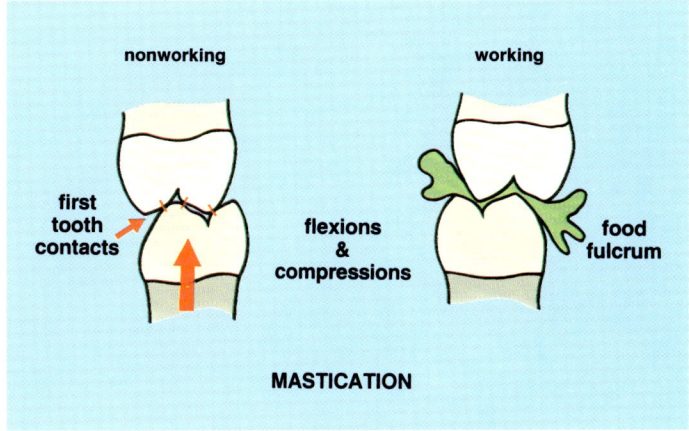

Fig 5-82b   In the final closing phase the consistency of tough or hard foods causes flexions and compression of the gnathic system, and the teeth on the nonchewing side often contact first. These contacts (if vertical) and near-CR of the condyles are noninjurious and compatible with the physiology of mastication.

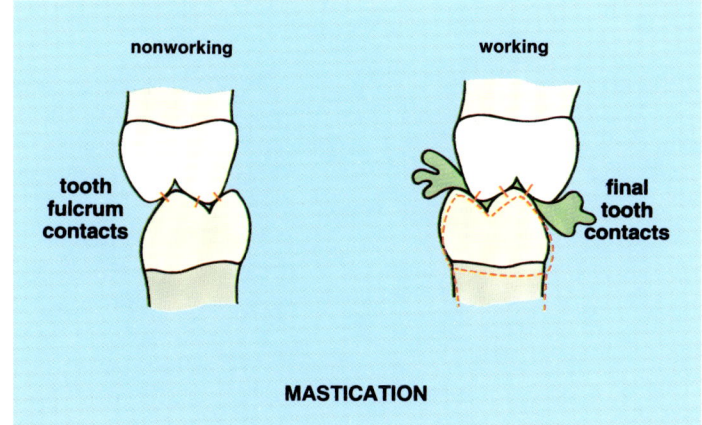

Fig 5-82c   In the final closing phase the occlusal contacts on the nonchewing side may act as stabilizing supports to help the cusps of the chewing side teeth make final contact through the bolus.

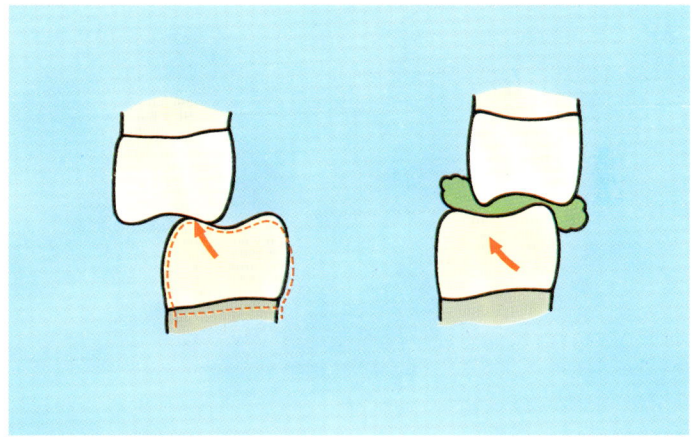

Fig 5-83   With flat teeth (horizontal occlusion) the biologic factors of flexion and compression still exist, but the nonchewing side contacts take place on the inclines farther away from CR. These types of occlusal contacts are nonphysiologic and are traumatic to the gnathic system.

Esthetics and Its Relationship to Function

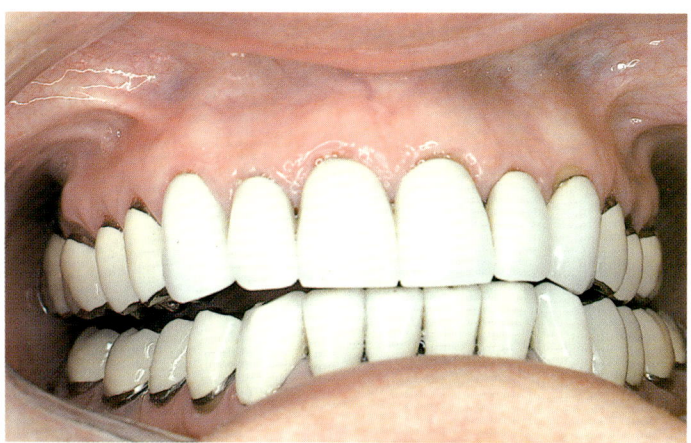

Fig 5-84a A nonbruxing patient (this patient was tested with biofeedback) who had undergone a full-mouth occlusal rehabilitation 6 years earlier. Note the excessive wear facets on the tips of the canines and incisal edges of the anterior teeth.

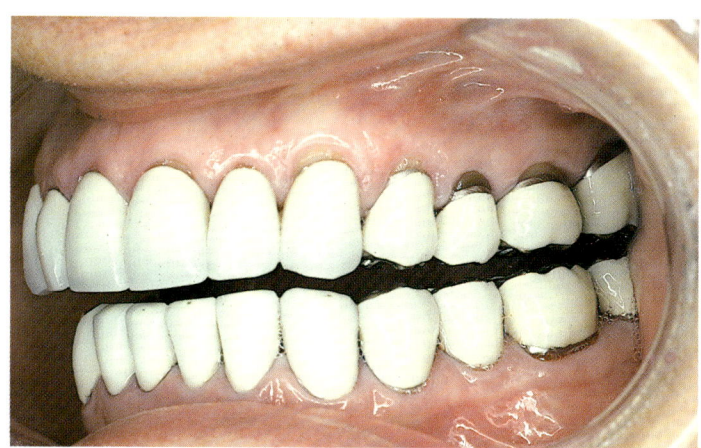

Figs 5-84b and c Left lateral views of the posterior crowns of the patient in Fig 5-84a reveal unnatural, low profile artificial crown forms that force the patient into horizontal chewing patterns, which no doubt are contributing to the early demise of the patient's crowns. Note also the excessive gingival recessions caused by overloading.

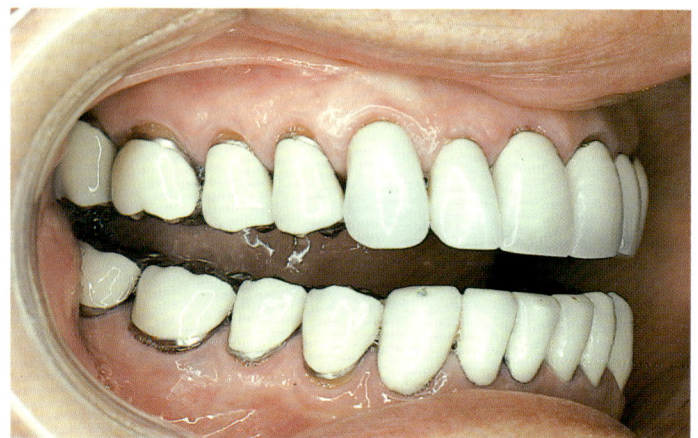

Fig 5-84c

Unworn, properly related posterior tooth forms are vital to guiding the mandible into more vertical physiologic closures. Sharp natural crown forms of the chewing side teeth guide the jaw closures in a more vertical mode. The sharp cusp points penetrate the tough foods whereas the sharp triangular and mesiodistal cusp ridges split, shear, and crush the food in a more vertical manner. The grooves and embrasures allow the food to extrude and reduce loading.

With good occluding unworn tooth morphology there are between 10 and 30 chewing strokes on a bolus of food before it is swallowed, depending on the consistency of the food. Normal physiologic lateral chewing strokes (65° to 70°) break down the large pieces of food into smaller ones while mixing them well with saliva so that swallowing is a comfortable, pleasurable, physiologic reflex. During mastication some chewing strokes may cause the mandible to cross the intercuspal position and briefly touch the canines together on the "non-chewing" side. These brief contacts, however, are relatively nondestructive to the teeth because the muscles are in the opening phase; therefore, little or no pressure is being applied.

Occlusal loading

The human body is subject to the physical laws of the universe, the laws of thermal dynamics and conservation of mass and energy.[35,36] The science of physics has long established the fact that there is less load, heat, friction, and molecular deformation created by sharp tools (teeth) compared with dull ones. In addition to poor functional occlusion, many of the patients that dentists are called upon to treat have compromises in their gnathic system such as (1) perforated or displaced TMJ discs, (2) bone loss caused by periodontal disease, (3) missing teeth, (4) resorbed ridges, (5) decayed teeth, (6) endodontic teeth (brittle), (7) worn teeth, (8) lost vertical dimension of occlusion, (9) skeletal disharmonies, (10) poor tooth alignment, and (11) poor arch forms. All of these mouths should have the load of mastication reduced as much as possible, and that this can be achieved better with sharp tools (teeth). Another argument in favor of sharp chewing tools (teeth) is for reducing chewing loads on high stress prosthodontic areas such as (1) longspan bridges, (2) solder joints, (3) bridge abutments, (4) clasps and attachments, (5) implants, (6) porcelain, and (7) removable prostheses.

It is well known that patients can masticate with either flat or sharp crowns. Patients learn (cortical) to chew with whatever natural or artificial tooth morphology they have in their mouths even though they overload and even destroy their teeth, joints, bone, and periodontium in the process. Probably the most insidious aspect of low profile (unnatural) posterior crowns is that patients chew with them and rarely complain. However, the more horizontal chewing patterns take their toll and subtly contribute to the demise of the dentition and other components of the gnathic system (Figs 5-84a to c). When doing individual crowns or segments of the mouth there may be a logical reason for keeping posterior crowns unnaturally flat to be compatible with existing worn teeth. However, there seems to be no logical rationale for aging (flattening) artificial crown morphology when the entire occlusion is being treated. In segmental dentistry if good anterior guidance is achieved by treating the anterior teeth first, subsequent posterior crowns can be made with more natural-like unworn forms; thus the entire occlusion can gradually be improved.

It is only logical that orthodontics and restorative dentistry should have the same goals for the final outcome of occlusal treatments. If we start with the premise that they should be one and the same, why should orthodontics use natural tooth morphology but fixed prosthodontics not use natural tooth morphology. Abnormal flattening of posterior artificial crown morphology may be caused by a lack of understanding of the importance of tooth morphology in occlusion or attempts to harmonize posterior crown morphology with poor anterior overbite. Crown and bridge technicians who do not understand the physiologic importance of restoring the original genetic crown morphology often make their posterior crowns too flat. Another reason for low profile posterior artificial crowns may be cause of the lack of interocclusal space to produce good tooth morphology. For these reasons, many dentists and technicians with outstanding skills are producing masterpieces of worn out artificial tooth anatomy.

Overloaded (flattened) occlusion may be evidenced by the following: (1) excessive wear on crowns, (2) broken prostheses, (3) lost vertical dimension of occlusion, (4) fractured teeth, (5) hypertrophic muscles, (6) exostoses, (7) TMJ overload, (8) tooth mobility, (9) tooth migration, (10) gingival recession, (11) periodontal over-

Esthetics and Its Relationship to Function

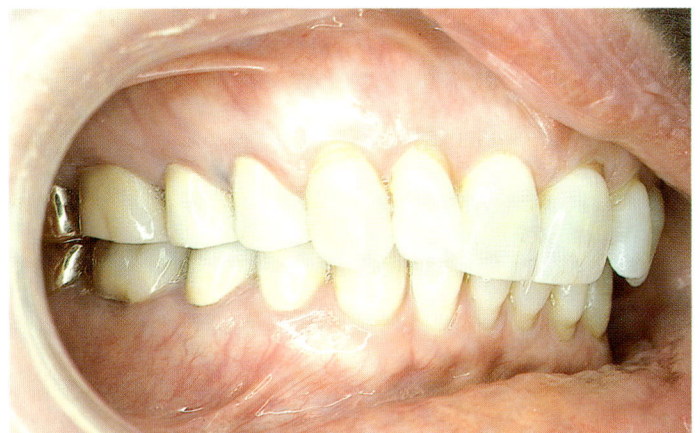

Fig 5-85a

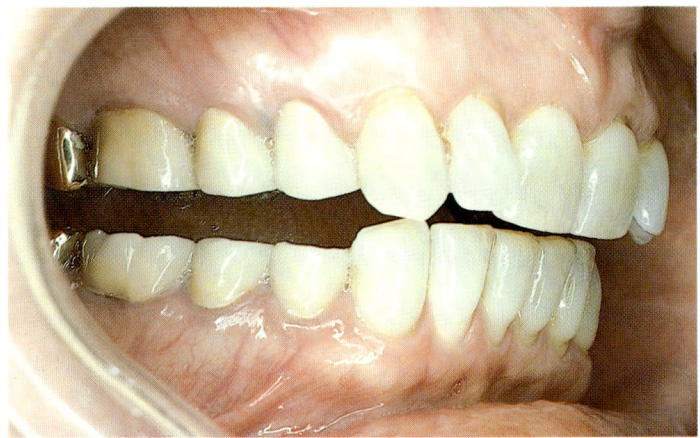

Fig 5-85b

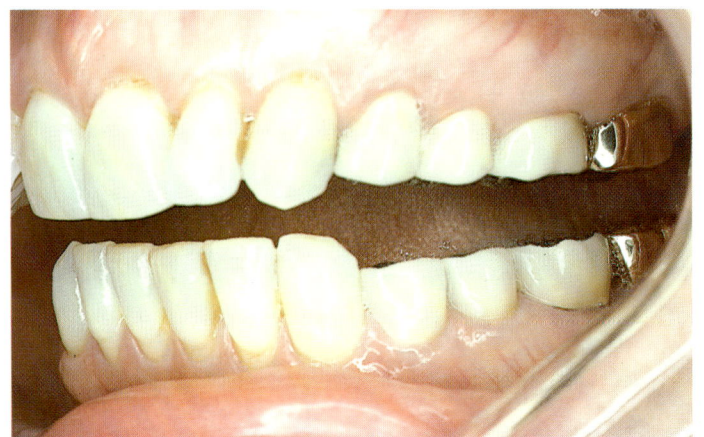

Fig 5-85c

Figs 5-85a to c   This Class II, division 2 patient had four quadrants of posterior crowns and the bite closed to obtain anterior guidance. However, because of lack of interocclusal space at the closed OVD, the posterior crowns were made cuspless. The incompatible guidance between the anterior and posterior teeth caused confusion to the patient's central nervous system because the anterior teeth mandated vertical chewing while the posterior teeth mandated horizontal chewing. A better diagnosis and treatment might have included orthodontics and/or orthognathic surgery to produce posterior occlusal space and obtain anterior guidance.

stress, *(12)* gingival clefting. Bruxism is often blamed for these conditions, when in many cases it is overloaded occlusion. Generally speaking, present-day fixed prosthodontics concepts do not include cusp forms (in the vertical profile) that simulate unworn natural teeth. Even with good anterior guidance, dentists who do not understand the importance of posterior tooth morphology can arrive at some very amorphic or bizarre posterior artificial crown anatomy (Figs 5-85a to c).

Since tooth anatomy is not specific to individuals, it seems logical that it is the responsibility of restorative dentists to give patients the best artificial tooth morphology possible as long as it does not inhibit condylar movements. The question is as follows: which is better? flat or steep occlusion? D'Amico[20] advocated steeper chewing patterns. Stallard and Stuart[30] stated that "chewing of modern foods for the most part is vertical..." Lee[22] advocated sharper (natural) posterior artificial crown morphology and steeper anterior guidance to produce more vertical chewing patterns. Gibbs[36] showed that patients with the best chewing patterns are steeper in the frontal plane. The best frontal plane chewing patterns are about 70° from horizontal.

The best way to learn tooth morphology is to understand its function and to observe teeth in their natural unworn, untreated states (Fig 5-86). Perhaps a biomechanically and physiologically "safe" guideline for posterior artificial crown forms (when good anterior guidance has been established) would be somewhere near the mean between the flattest and steepest observed in unworn natural teeth (see Figs 5-20 and 5-21).

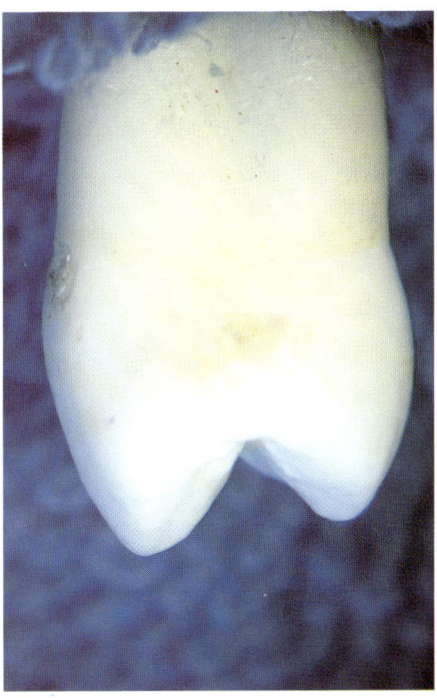

Fig 5-86 A typical natural unworn maxillary first premolar showing long sharp cusps. (Also see posterior natural tooth morphology in Figs 5-18, 5-20, and 5-21.)

Clinical aspects in bioesthetic function

Diagnosis

A proper diagnosis can only be made if one first understands bioesthetics, biomechanics, and the physiology of the gnathic system. The principal factors in long-range successful occlusal treatments for natural teeth or fixed prosthodontics include the following:

1. Stable comfortable most superior condyle position (CR).
2. CR = maximum intercuspal position (IP) of the teeth.
3. Adequate tooth support (periodontal).
4. Adequate number of stable teeth (or implants).
5. Good anterior overbite.
6. Good lateral guidance (65° to 70°).
7. Unworn posterior crown morphology (compatible with the good anterior guidance).
8. Absence of posterior eccentric tooth interferences in border, protrusive or intermediate movements of the condyles during function.
9. Good bioesthetics.

The safest sequence for treating a mouth to bioesthetic function is as follows: *(1)* good diagnosis and treatment planning, *(2)* patient education, *(3)* treating the periodontium, *(4)* stabilizing the craniomandibular relations in CR (occlusal splint), *(5)* restoring the anterior teeth to bioesthetic function, *(6)* restoring the posterior teeth to natural physiologic function, and *(7)* regular posttreatment maintenance.

A stable condyle position CR is best accomplished with a properly constructed, fitted, adjusted, and maintained anteriorly guided occlusal splint (Figs 5-87a to c). For best results the patient should wear the occlusal splint during eating and at all times (day and night)

Esthetics and Its Relationship to Function

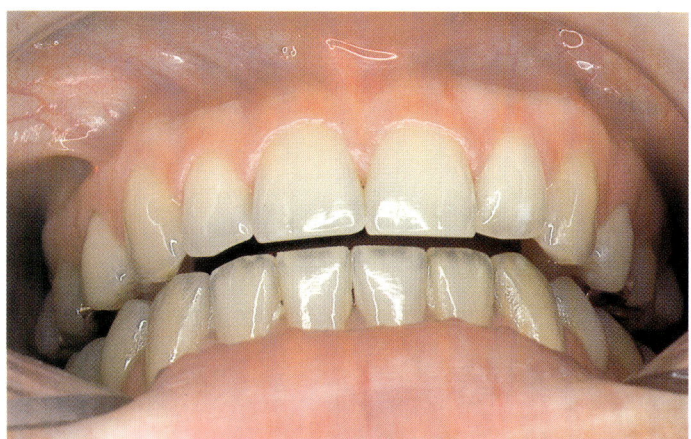

Fig 5-87a Open bite occlusal relation of a 24-year-old woman during bilateral manipulation to place the condyles in their most superior position CR before splint treatment.

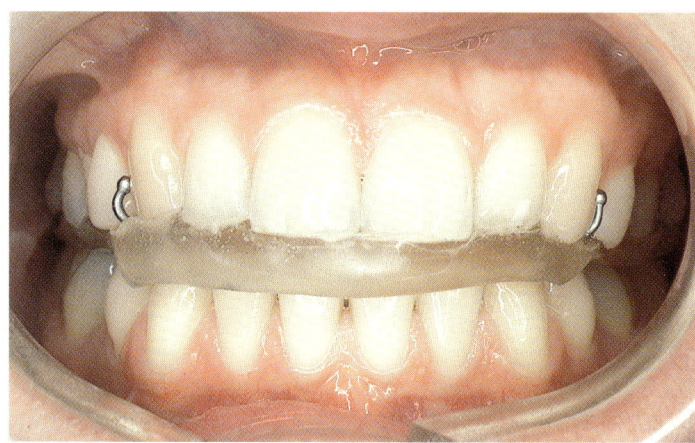

Fig 5-87b The patient in Fig 5-87a wore a properly constructed, fitted, and adjusted condyle CR repositioning splint for a few weeks to obtain joint stability and comfort.

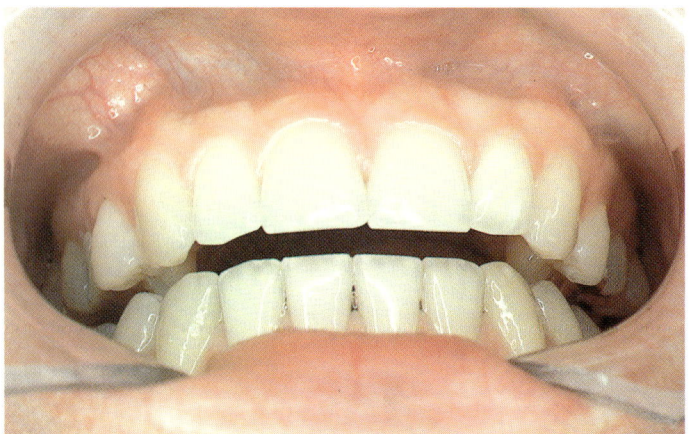

Fig 5-87c After condyle repositioning with the CR splint, the posterior teeth are striking earlier in CR hinge position because the condyles are higher in the fossae, which results in a more open bite relation of the anterior teeth. Final diagnosis and treatment should be made after the condyles are repositioned to their stable comfortable CR position.

Clinical aspects in bioesthetic function

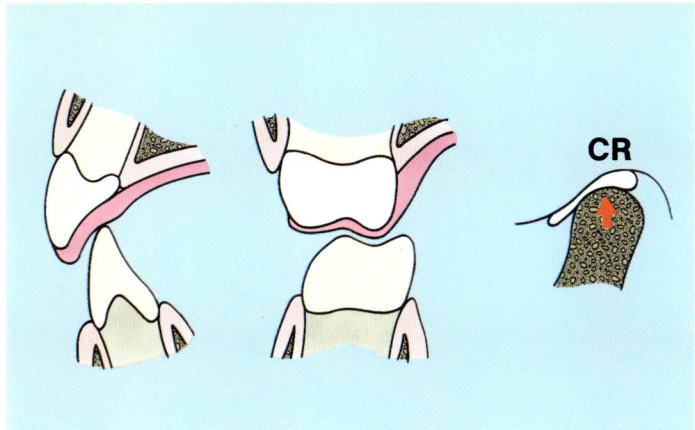

Fig 5-88a Phase I of condyle repositioning CR splint. The splint may be placed in the mouth without posterior occlusal contacts for a few days to allow for rapid seating of the condyles. Occlusal contacts should be made within 1 week by adding soft acrylic resin to prevent supereruption of mandibular posterior teeth.

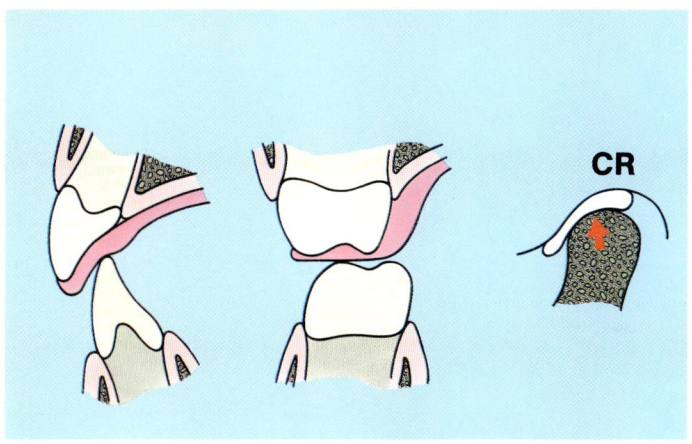

Fig 5-88b Phase II of condyle repositioning CR splint is accomplished by adding posterior occlusal contacts (soft resin). From this point the splint must have periodic posterior occlusal adjustments with bilateral manipulation to CR to allow the condyles to attain their highest position.

except for brushing and cleaning the teeth. The role of the splint is to remove all centric and eccentric occlusal interferences and allow the condyles to reach their most superior stable position (Figs 5-88a and b). The splint also gives assurance to the cerebral cortex that there will be no harmful posterior contacts; thus, the muscles are also treated. If a stable, comfortable CR position cannot be achieved on the occlusal splint, it is doubtful that definitive occlusal treatment will be successful. Patients with chronic craniofacial or TMJ pain should not receive extensive occlusal treatment until the craniomandibular relation has been stabilized and the pain has disappeared for a considerable period of time. Final diagnosis and the treatment planning should always be made with face bow mounted casts in CR following occlusal splint therapy. Posttreatment centrically related occlusal nighttime splints can also be of value for patients with nocturnal bruxism.

Probably the greatest challenge that dentists face in dealing with bioesthetic occlusion is to change poorly related anterior teeth to a safe biologic relationship that will help ensure the prospects for long-range successful treatment (Fig 5-89). The use of orthodontics, orthopedics, and orthognathic surgery should always be consid-

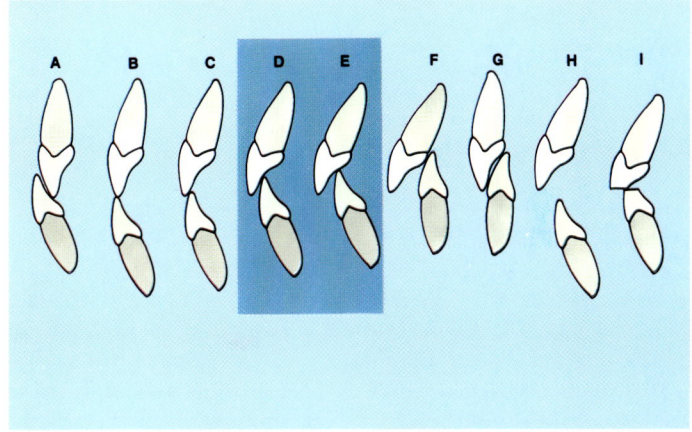

Fig 5-89 To obtain the highest degree of clinical success, dentists should use the best methods possible (ie, orthodontics, surgery, restorative dentistry) to change poorly related anterior teeth (A, B, C, F, G, H, and I) to physiologic relationship (D and E) that will help ensure long-range successful treatment.

Esthetics and Its Relationship to Function

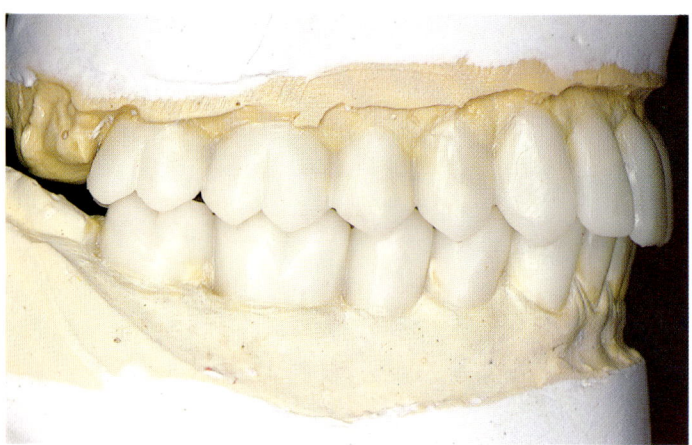 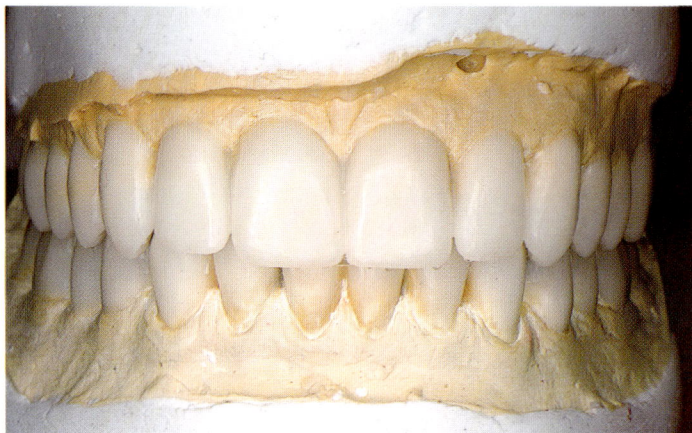

Figs 5-90a and b A diagnostic wax-up is one of the most valuable items in a restorative diagnosis and can be used effectively for patient education.

ered for treating cases in which the teeth are severely malpositioned. In any event, the anterior region of the mouth presents a double challenge because it deals not only with the vital anterior guidance system in occlusion but also the most predominant area of esthetics. Both objectives must be satisfied.

Fixed prosthodontics as a single treatment technique can solve many esthetic–occlusal problems. A diagnostic wax-up done with face bow centrically mounted casts on an individually adjusted articulator is one of the most valuable items in a bioesthetic rehabilitation (Figs 5-90a and b). The wax-up not only can be used for diagnosis, treatment planning, and patient education, but also to form plastic provisional crowns during treatment (Figs 5-91a to c). For patient education and consultation, psychologically it is best to use yellow stone casts with ivory colored wax or to take impressions of the diagnostic wax-up and pour white stone casts.

Operative dentistry

It is wrong to carve posterior restorations like glacier valleys. It is important when doing occlusal restorations with any material to keep the grooves naturally deep to reduce the load of mastication by allowing the pressure of the food to be reduced by extrusion and escape through the grooves. When single crown restorations are done, the cusps should be made as naturally steep and sharp as possible without causing interference with the existing occlusion. Even though resin occlusal restorations may be carved with good morphology, they lose it in a relatively short time under the abrasive action of food and toothbrushing. Porcelain inlays are good restorations (when indicated) as long as the occlusal anatomy is made deep like young natural teeth.

Clinical aspects in bioesthetic function

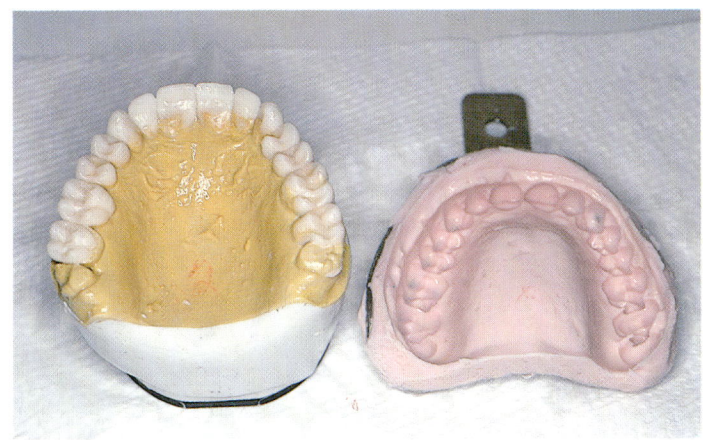

Fig 5-91a An alginate impression of the diagnostic waxup can be used to make provisional plastic crowns directly in the mouth. Self-curing resin is placed in the alginate impression of the waxup. The resin is lubricated and seated directly in the patient's mouth over the prepared teeth. After the plastic has hardened, it can be relined for better marginal fit.

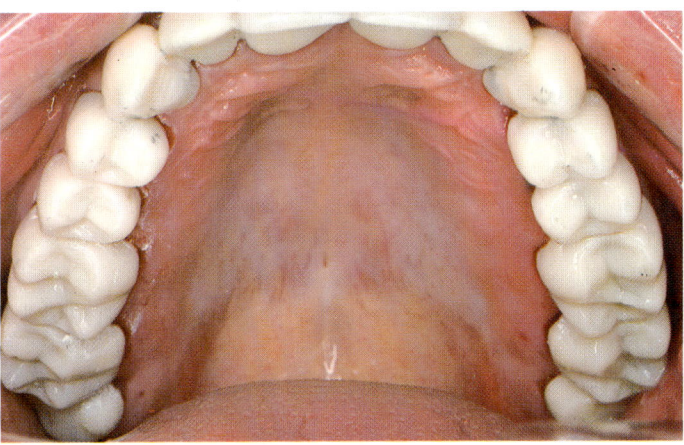

Fig 5-91b Plastic provisional crowns made from the impression of the wax-up cemented in the mouth give functional stability and esthetics until the final restorations can be placed.

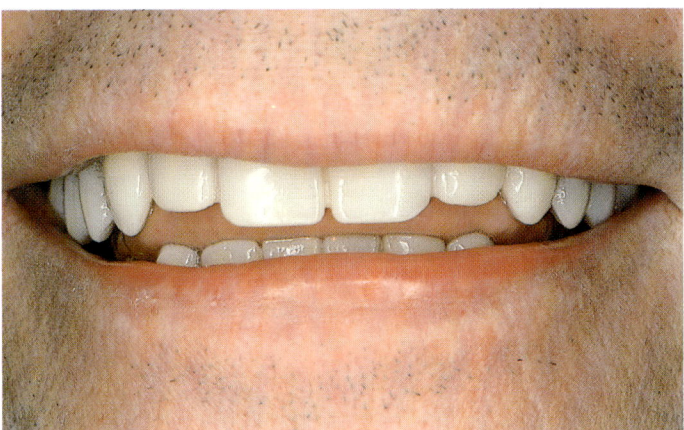

Fig 5-91c The provisional stage of treatment should receive utmost attention because it is the first time the patient gets a preview of what their appearance may be with the final crowns.

Esthetics and Its Relationship to Function

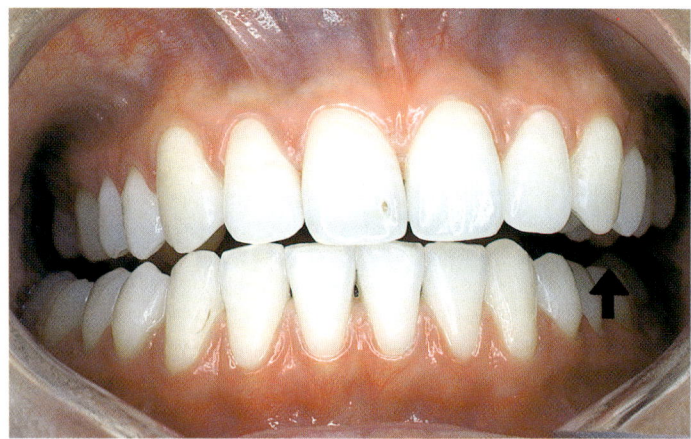

Fig 5-92a   Postorthodontic patient with wear on right canine causing contralateral (left side) interference.

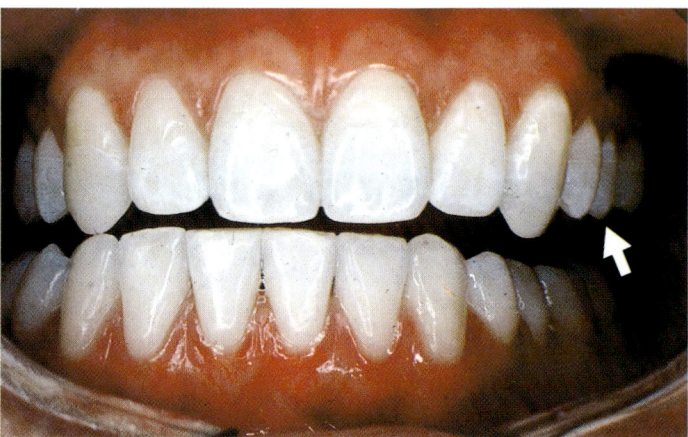

Fig 5-92b   Following coronaplastic to make IP–CR, composite resin was added to the maxillary right and left worn canines to eliminate the posterior lateral interferences rather than reduce (flatten) the molar morphology.

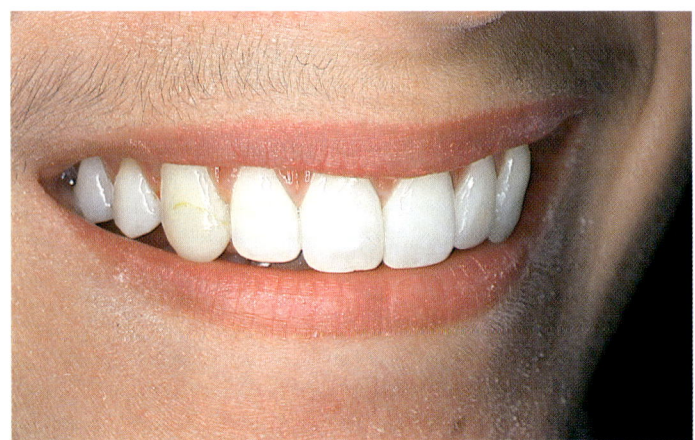

Fig 5-92c   The esthetic results are good and conservative, and normal physiology of occlusion is established.

Clinical aspects in bioesthetic function

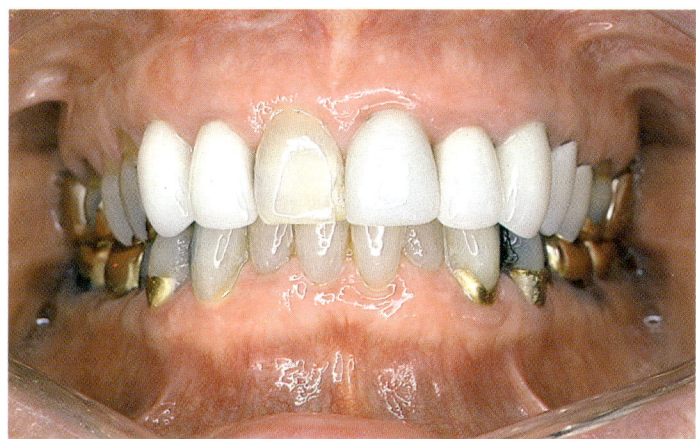

Fig 5-93a The much restored, overloaded, unesthetic dentition of a 70-year-old woman. Original smile of this patient can be seen in Fig 5-57a.

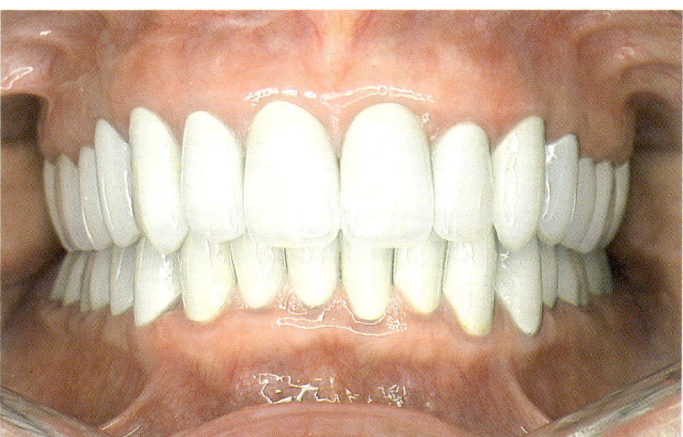

Fig 5-93b For mature patients with severely worn, decayed, or previously restored anterior teeth, the use of PFM or all-porcelain crowns are no doubt the materials of choice at the present time. The dentition of the patient in Fig 5-57a rejuvenated with bioesthetics and physiologic function. The changed smile of this patient can be seen in Fig 5-57b.

Anterior restorations

For young people in their teens and early 20s the use of composite resins on anterior teeth is probably the best available material because of its conservative nature to enamel (Figs 5-92a to c). If intercuspal position IP is equal to CR or made equal through coronaplasty (occlusal adjustments), the placement of bonded resins to worn anterior teeth usually lasts for long periods of time (several years). Porcelain veneers are esthetic and can be used to treat certain patients when the anterior functional relations are not too severe. For the mature patients with severely worn or decayed anterior teeth and/or existing restoration, the use of metal ceramic crowns or all-porcelain crowns is no doubt the material of choice at the present time (Figs 5-93a and b). All-porcelain crowns are esthetic but cannot be used for partial dentures. It is difficult to achieve harmonious esthetics if a combination or mixture of materials is used (eg, some crowns of the porcelain to metal type and other crowns of the all-porcelain type). Anterior restorative materials for artificial crowns should be matched in opposing teeth for best wear resistance and esthetics, eg, porcelain against porcelain instead of porcelain against enamel, resin, or gold.

Older patients should also have natural unworn crown morphology to meet the physiologic requirements to make and reduce functional loading on the gnathic system and help the patient look younger (Figs 5-94a and b). Darker shades and characterizations can be used to give the perception of maturity and make the teeth more believable. Contrary to most dentists' beliefs, it is the morphology and positions of teeth, more than shading, that has a greater effect on esthetics and believability.

Esthetics and Its Relationship to Function

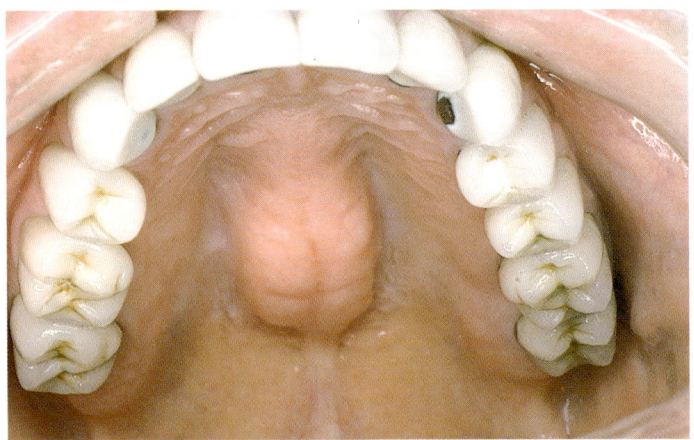

Figs 5-94a Older patients should have posterior unworn crown morphology to meet physiologic requirements and reduce functional loading, especially because many in this age group have compromised temporomandibular joints and supporting tissues of the teeth.

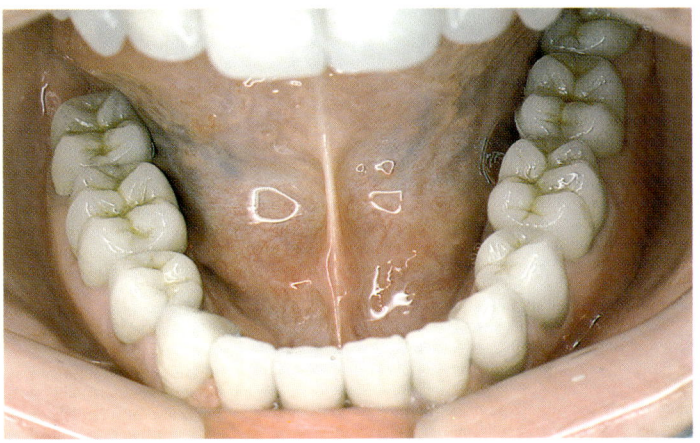

Fig 5-94b Occlusal surfaces of mandibular rejuvenated teeth of patient in Fig 5-93a.

Posterior restorations

When considering materials for restoring posterior teeth, it should be remembered that the hardest gold is too soft and the softest porcelain is too hard. At present we do not have the perfect biocompatible restorative material. The sharpest that the artificial crown morphology will probably ever be is the day the crown is cemented in the mouth. The normal contacts of opposing crowns in addition to abrasives in the food, air, water, and prophylaxis paste will gradually diminish the molecules of the restorative materials. Therefore, to ensure the best function and longevity of the restoration, one should start with the sharpest natural tooth form possible in harmony with the joint movements and teeth. Restorative materials for artificial posterior crowns should also be matched in opposing teeth for best abrasive resistances, ie, porcelain to porcelain, gold to gold.

Gold for occlusal surfaces of posterior teeth has been the standard of excellence in occlusal treatment for many decades. If yellow gold is used for posterior teeth, it should be hard (type 4). Full coverage yellow gold crowns can have facing of the newer microfilled light-cured type. These materials show better color stability than the older resins and plastics. However, they may change color with time. Adding a new veneer (if the facings darken with time) is easily performed in the mouth.

The use of ceramometal occlusal surfaces with porcelain facings poses problems both with esthetics and with obtaining crisp, clean tooth morphology. During the laboratory remount stage or when occlusal adjustments are made in the mouth, ceramic gold metalwork hardens, galls, and often becomes difficult to cut cleanly. If one polishes the roughened metal, occlusal contacts may be lost. Nonprecious metals are usually difficult to adjust occlusally due to their hardness. In the past most dentists and technicians have probably had more experience in the use of gold occlusal surfaces. Gold is not objectionable on molars or even bicuspids to some people (Figs 5-95a to d). There are patients, however, who do not want metal to show in their mouths. No doubt there will be an ever-increasing demand in the future for more esthetic occlusal restorations for both men and women. Regardless of how comfortable and functional a gold occlusal restoration may be, it is never as successful as it might have been to the esthetic-conscious patient.

A question often asked is whether good occlusion can

Clinical aspects in bioesthetic function

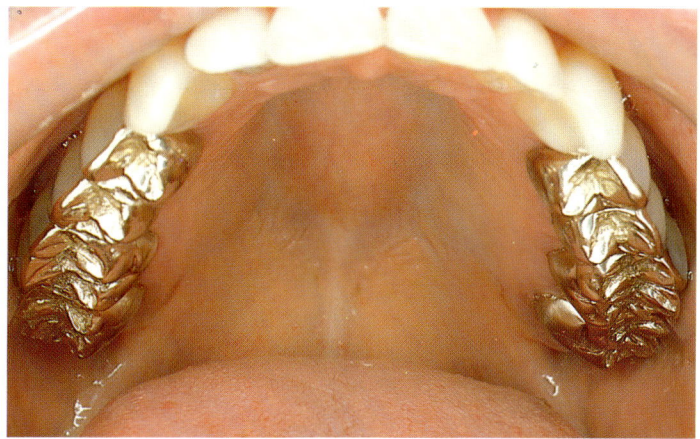

Fig 5-95a Occlusal view of maxillary gold onlays on a 27-year-old woman who requested that her posterior teeth be restored with onlays because her father had his mouth restored with gold onlays that were still in excellent functional condition after many years.

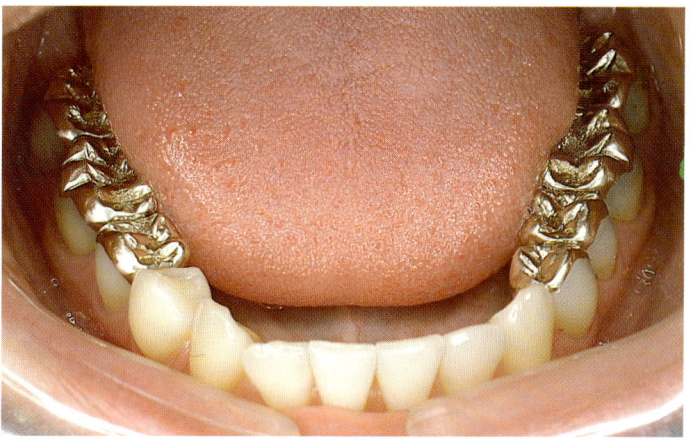

Fig 5-95b Occlusal view of mandibular gold onlays show the ultimate in artificial tooth morphology and function but are unacceptable esthetically to some patients.

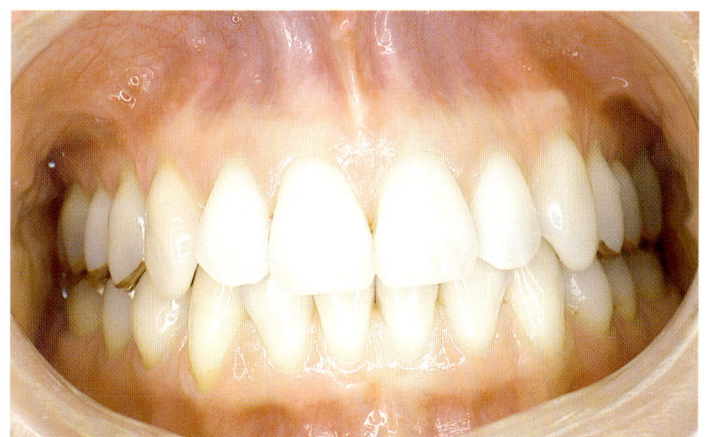

Fig 5-95c Results were achieved with minimum loss of tooth structure and optimum physiologic function. Worn maxillary canines were restored to proper function with acid-etched, light-cured resin on the canines.

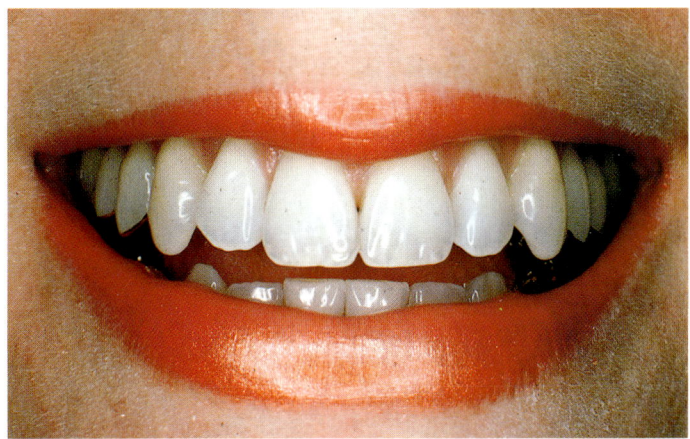

Fig 5-95d The beautiful bioesthetic smile will be protected for many years to come because the treatment included physiologic requirements.

Esthetics and Its Relationship to Function

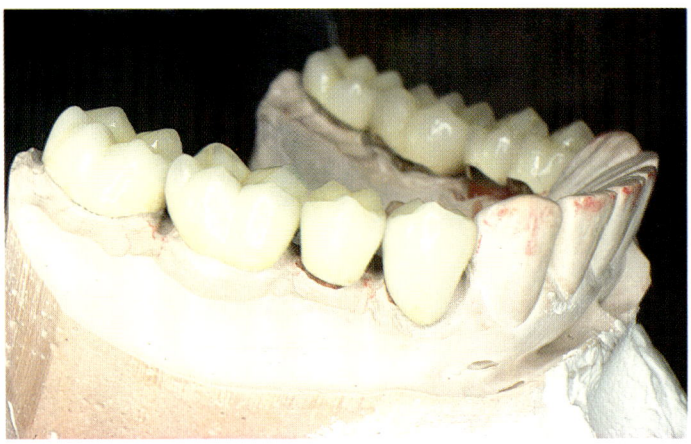

Fig 5-96a It is equally important when using porcelain posterior occlusal surfaces to rejuvenate them with unworn morphology to be compatible with the bioesthetics of the anterior teeth.

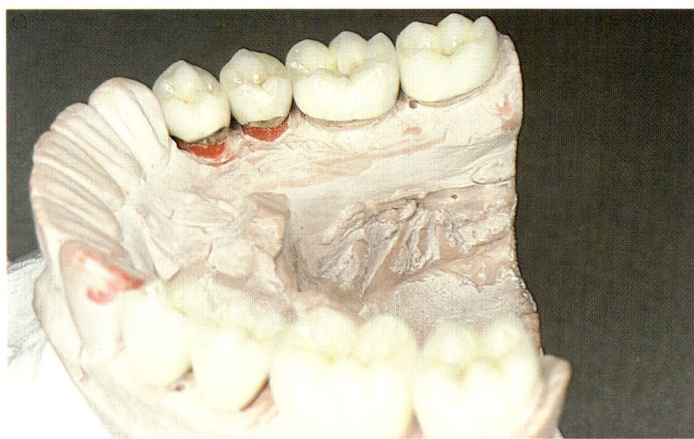

Fig 5-96b There is not only better physiologic function with good crown morphology but also less chance of fracturing because the chewing strokes are more vertical.

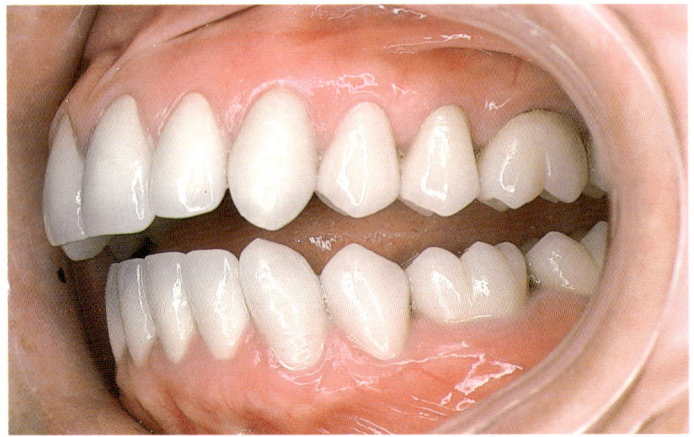

Fig 5-96c Lateral view of bioesthetic crowns in the mouth.

be achieved when porcelain is used on occlusal surfaces of posterior teeth. Some dentists believe that porcelain is too hard for occlusal surfaces and that it may be traumatic to the periodontium and teeth and encourage bruxism. The author has not experienced adverse effects on occlusion or negative tissue responses when verticalized bioesthetic occlusion has been used, provided of course, that other factors such as marginal fit and crown contours have not been violated. It is equally important when using porcelain to have sharp, rejuvenated posterior tooth morphology as it is with gold (Figs 5-96a and b). These beautifully sculpted crown forms not only produce the ultimate in esthetics but also can be made compatible with the patient's own characteristic jaw movements and the biologics of occlusion (Figs 5-97a to c). Surprisingly, sharp posterior porcelain tooth morphology reduces the chance of fracturing (when the total system is in harmony) because the loading is more vertical, whereas flat morphology enhances the chance of fracturing because of horizontal shearing forces.

Posterior occlusal technology is significantly different with porcelain than gold. Porcelain is probably less "forgiving" than gold. The dentist who uses porcelain posterior occlusal surfaces must understand the special

Clinical aspects in bioesthetic function

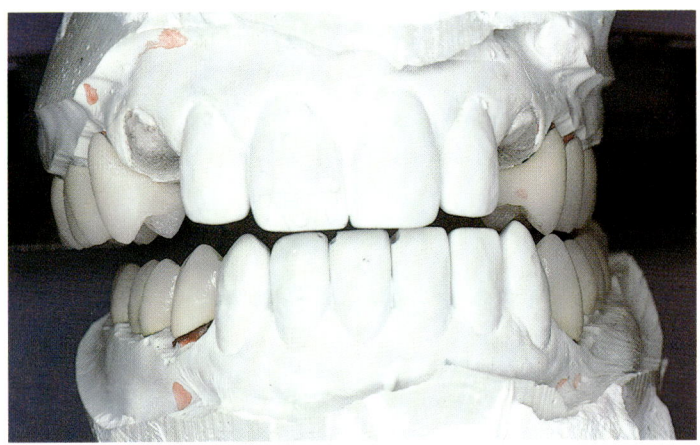

Fig 5-97a These beautifully sculpted crown forms not only produce the ultimate in esthetics, they can be made compatible with the patient's characteristic jaw movements on the individually adjusted analog articulator. The graduated "chewing" side group function is shown without the aid of the "first canine."

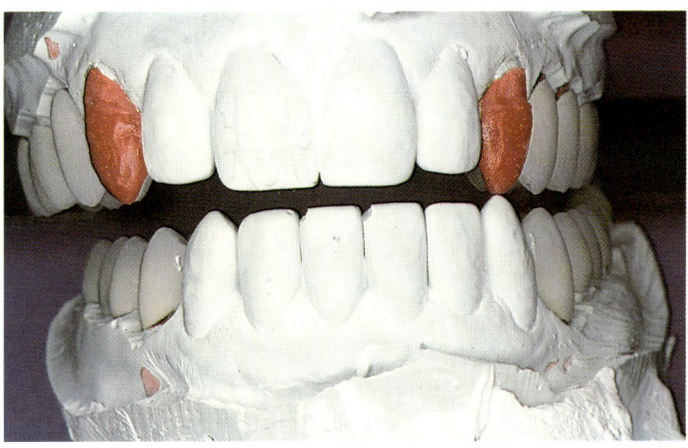

Fig 5-97b The canine in place causing more separation of the posterior teeth.

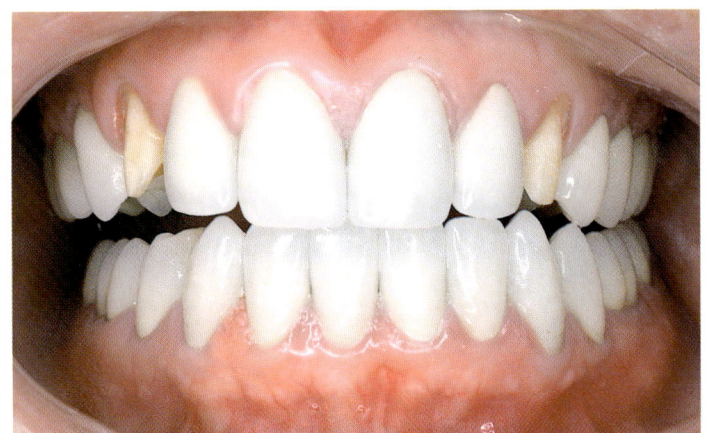

Fig 5-97c The same relation of the teeth in the mouth, without the canine.

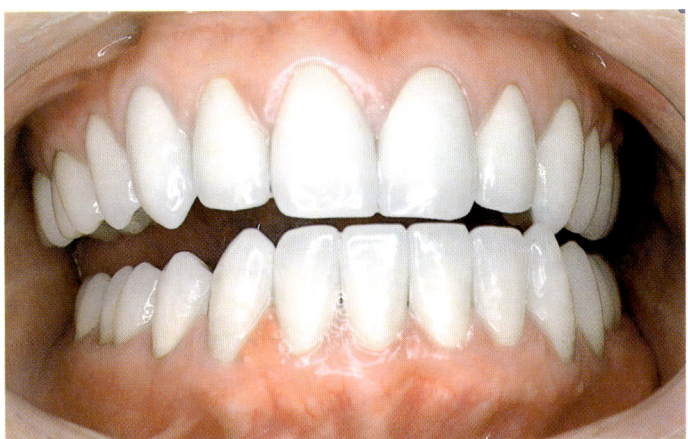

Fig 5-97d The increased separation of posterior teeth when the canine is in place.

Esthetics and Its Relationship to Function

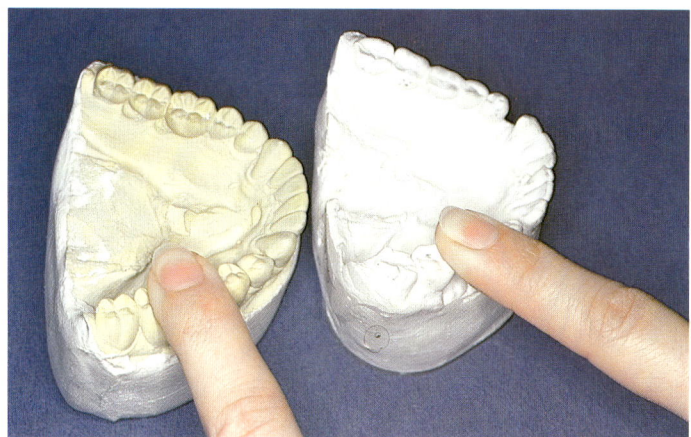

Fig 5-98 "Touch test" is performed by pressing with the fingers simultaneously on cast of cemented crowns and cast of unworn natural teeth to verify similarity of sharpness.

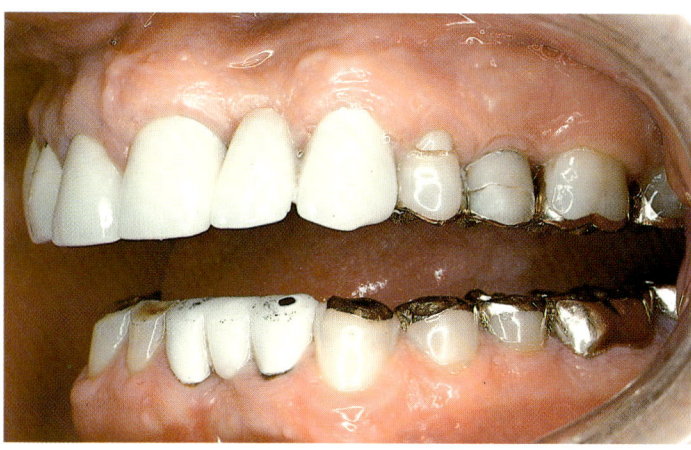

Fig 5-99 A nonbruxing patient shows the results of low profile posterior crowns, which increase functional wear on teeth.

problems associated with these materials and develop good communication with the technician, who is also required to develop new skills in bioesthetic occlusion. Multiple firing is almost mandatory when recreating lifelike (unworn) artificial tooth morphology concurrent with producing a stable, comfortable, physiological occlusion. Noble metals are preferable because they are more conducive to multiple firing.

A good test of the excellence of the final porcelain morphology is to make posttreatment stone casts of the crowns and compare them with casts of natural unworn teeth. The use of the touch test can also give a good indication of the efficiency of the tooth morphology for biologic occlusion (Fig 5-98). If the cusps of the artificial crowns do not feel sharp against one's finger like that of a young dentition, the crowns are probably too flat and may overload the porcelain.

Restoring the complete dentition

Nature intended tooth enamel to last a lifetime. However, many patients, including teenagers, have worn completely through the protective covering of enamel. Older patients often have worn into the pulp chambers of the teeth. Mandibular incisors often show the ravages of traumatic occlusion because of their small size and often-abused incisal edges. Traumatic occlusion often results in lost vertical dimension of occlusion.

Many patients' teeth are so severely worn that they appear to be Class III types. However, when placed at an OVD that will allow for normal unworn crown morphology, they are actually Class I or even Class II. The wear patterns usually start on the mesial cusp ridge of the maxillary canines and the distal cusp ridge of the mandibular canines (except in some severe open bite cases). Whenever a wear facet is seen on a canine, a contralateral posterior interference in lateral jaw movement can be demonstrated. The cause of the severe attrition is commonly believed by most dentists to be psychogenic bruxism. However, there is clinical evidence to indicate that the primary cause of wear on the anterior teeth of young people is caused by anterior contact

Clinical aspects in bioesthetic function

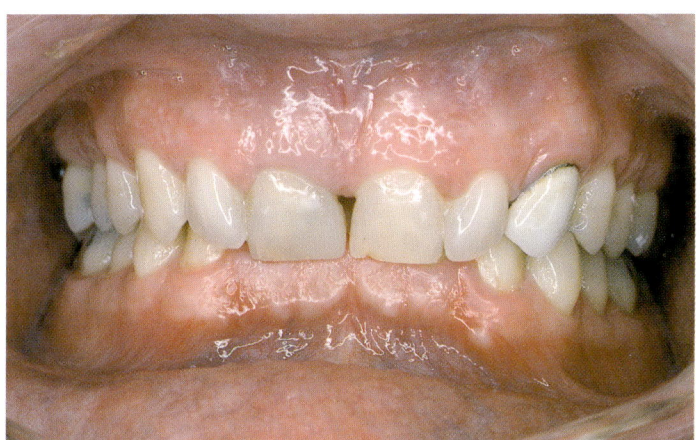

Fig 5-100a The anterior alveolar bone has migrated incisally in this Class II, division 2 patient.

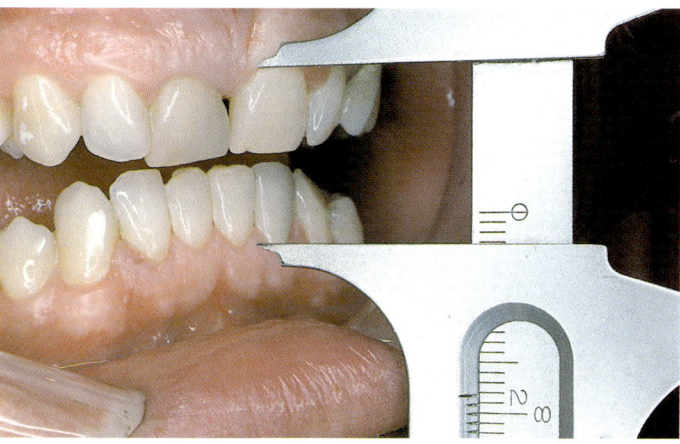

Fig 5-100b Because both the anterior and posterior teeth are relatively unworn and only the anterior alveolar bone has migrated incisally, the general rule of an average anterior upper to lower cementoenamel distance of 18 mm cannot be used without the chance of encroaching on the physiologic freeway space and rest positions. Orthodontics or surgery are needed to reposition the anterior teeth in order to gain the proper upper to lower cementoenamel distance.

guidance due to avoidance patterns of posterior interferences. By restricting their lateral chewing patterns (medial to border paths), these patients are able to avoid the traumatic posterior tooth interferences, but only at the expense of anterior tooth anatomy through contact guidance. It appears that the brain uses this continual light contact on the mesial cusp ridge of the maxillary canine against the distal cusp ridge of the mandibular canine to assure the cerebral cortex that the mandible will not inadvertently go into border paths and strike the contralateral posterior interferences. After the canines become worn down, posterior interferences can no longer be avoided, and the cortex restricts the chewing patterns more mesially using the lateral and central incisors as contact guides in an effort to assure the cortex that there will be no posterior occlusal interferences. During this sequence the patient is doing lateral chewing increasingly protrusively. Posselt[8] showed that whenever CO was not equal to CR, patients always chew in a restricted lateral fashion. Following the attrition of the anterior teeth, bruxism often develops, which destroys the occlusal morphology of the posterior teeth. Other major causes of wear on anterior teeth are iatrogenic due to flat restorations and low profile posterior artificial crowns or occlusal equilibrations which often cause patients to chew more horizontally (Fig 5-99).[22]

One of the most common challenges facing dentists is that of treating severely worn dentitions for both esthetics and function. With these worn down teeth it is virtually impossible to obtain enough tooth reduction to produce good tooth morphology and have adequate crown retention without increasing the existing OVD. Even if good canine guidance is established but the posterior crown morphology is too flat, the canines will be overloaded and develop wear facets because the patient is being forced into unphysiologic horizontal chewing patterns by the flat posterior crowns. A general rule for restoring lost OVD for most patients is to have the distance from maxillary to mandibular cementoenamel average about 18 mm. This allows for an average maxillary incisor (12 mm) and an average mandibular incisor (10 mm) with an average vertical overbite (4 mm) (see Fig 5-29). When treating Class II, division 2 patients where the anterior maxillary and/or mandibular alveolar processes have migrated incisally, one must be careful not to use the 18-mm average measurement between maxillary and mandibular cementoenamel junctions for establishing OVD (Figs 5-100a and b). In these severe

Esthetics and Its Relationship to Function

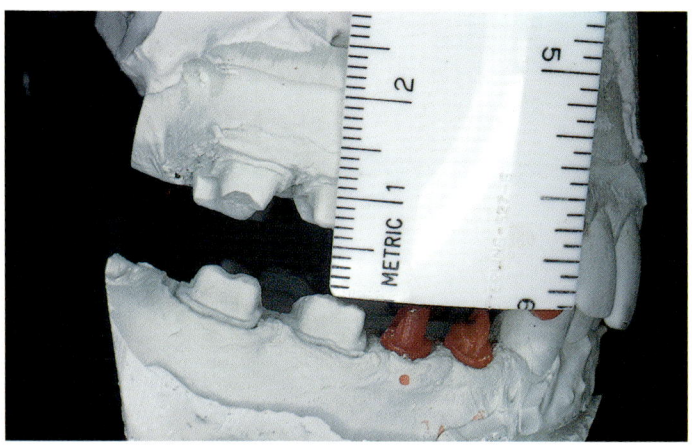

Fig 5-101a Mounted casts show interocclusal space of 6 mm.

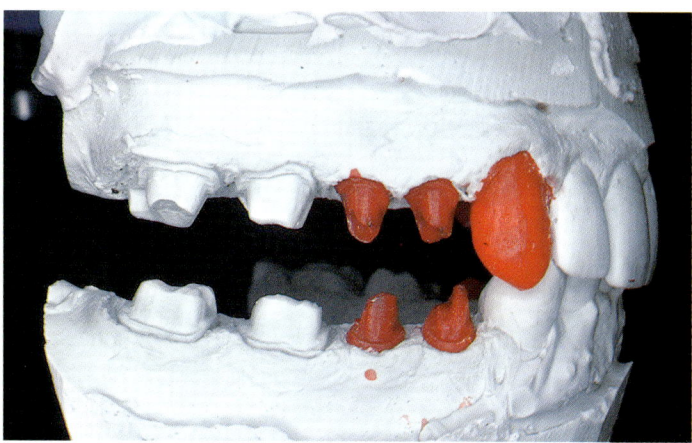

Fig 5-101b Laboratory technicians need approximately this much space for metal, opaques, and natural crown morphology, and to correct occlusal relationships.

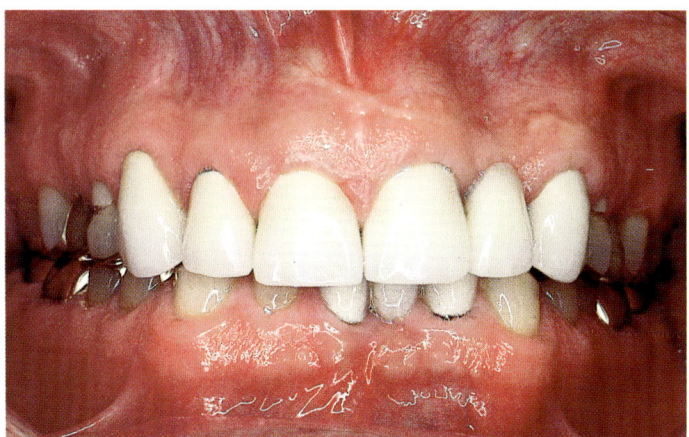

Fig 5-102a 55-year-old man in Fig 5-99 showing overclosed OVD.

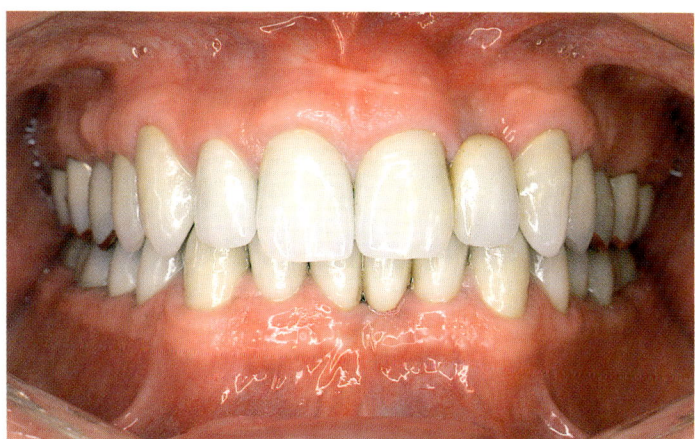

Fig 5-102b By increasing the distance from nasion to menton by 5 mm, normal crown morphology and bioesthetic function was restored.

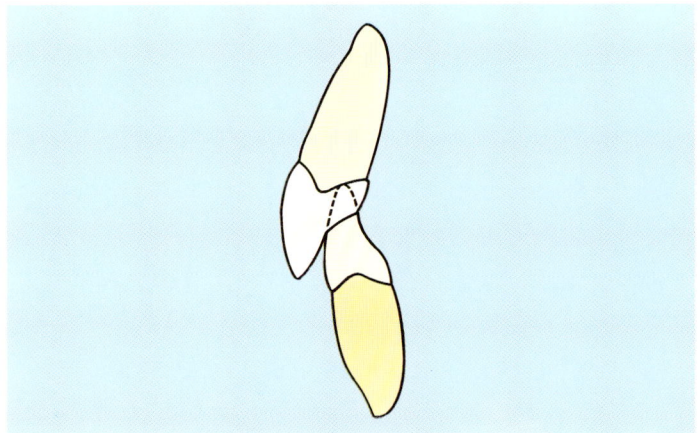

Fig 5-103 Much of the occlusal overload of function as well as parafunction results in attrition of the mandibular anterior incisal edges, which causes even more overload and lost OVD.

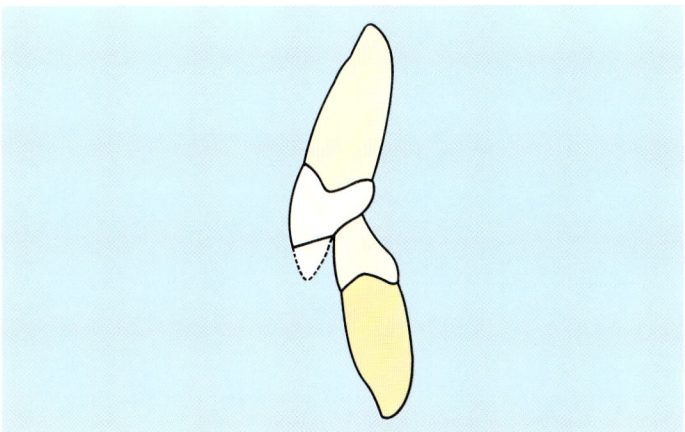

Fig 5-104 Wear on the incisal edges of maxillary teeth reduces anterior guidance.

skeletal deformities the use of orthodontics and/or orthognathic surgery should be considered to help establish the anterior cementoenamel distance for producing unworn anterior crown lengths and good physiologic overbite. When restoring severely worn anterior teeth, most of the regaining of lost OVD is accomplished by restoring the worn incisal lengths of the mandibular anterior teeth. The regaining of anterior guidance is primarily accomplished by restoring the incisal lengths of the maxillary anterior teeth.

The major complaint from crown-and-bridge technicians throughout the world is not enough interocclusal space to produce good crown morphology. The minimum posterior interocclusal space needed is about 2.5 mm for gold occlusal crowns and 3 mm for metal ceramic crowns. The interocclusal space should be about 6 mm when doing opposing arches (Figs 5-101a and b). Advantages of increasing OVD include the following: *(1)* space for better artificial crown morphology, *(2)* improved esthetics, *(3)* better facial profile, *(4)* improved lip lines, and *(5)* additional space to change the occlusal esthetic plane. Increasing OVD in patients with severe anterior attrition usually requires artificial crowns or other restorations on both the maxillary and mandibular anterior teeth (Figs 102a and b).

Much of the lost OVD is caused by wear on the mandibular anterior teeth. The worn incisal edges become less efficient and require more muscle force to function, thus increasing the wear on the teeth and load on supporting tissues (Fig 5-103). Wear on the incisal edges of maxillary teeth reduces the overbite for good anterior guidance (Fig 5-104). When the mandibular anterior teeth are severely worn, it is not uncommon to have lost 0.5 mm of crown width on each side of the six mandibular anterior teeth. The mandibular teeth usually tip lingually to close the interproximal spaces. The total lost dimension in the anterior curve of the arch is often as much as 6 mm (1 mm per tooth) (Figs 5-105a to c). Lingual tipping of the worn mandibular anterior teeth increases functional loading on the lower anterior teeth, muscles, and joints because the patient uses the labial surface of the mandibular incisors rather than the incisal edges. The increased incisal forces often encourage more lingual tilt of the mandibular incisors or even labial movement of the maxillary incisors (Fig 5-106).

Complicating factors due to this lingual tooth drift are

Esthetics and Its Relationship to Function

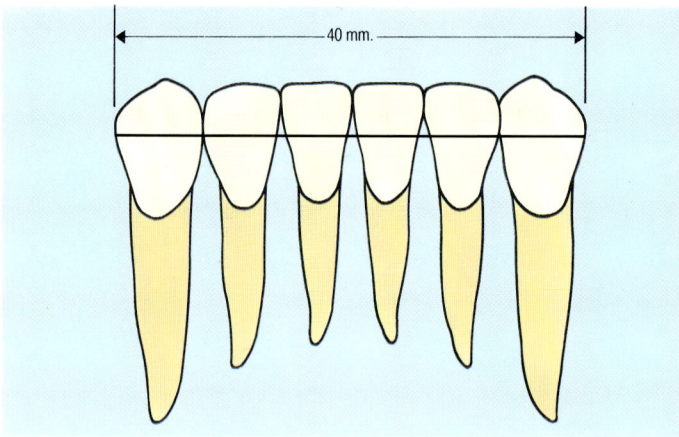

Fig 5-105a Horizontal line on teeth represents 50% reduction of clinical crown height, which is not uncommon in patients 50 years and older (especially men). The total anterior unworn occlusal arch length averages about 40 mm.

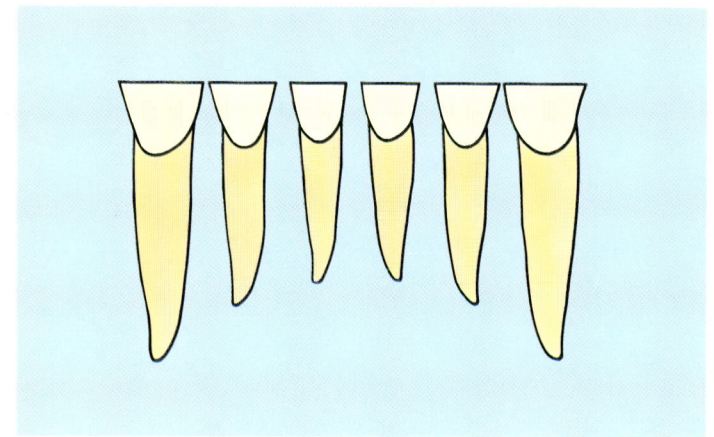

Fig 5-105b If the mandibular anterior teeth did not migrate lingually and are worn down from a 10-mm clinical crown length to 5 mm, there would be spaces at the interproximal contact areas of the anterior teeth. This space averages about 0.5 mm on each side of each of the six mandibular anterior teeth. The total space combined is about 6 mm.

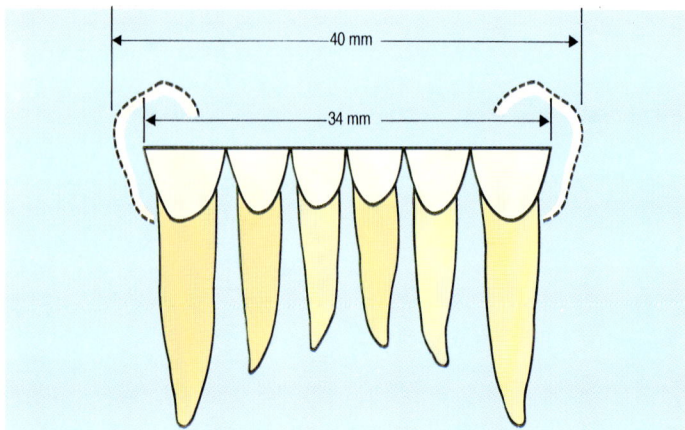

Fig 5-105c Usually the worn mandibular anterior teeth tilt lingually to close the spaces created by the wear. The original anterior occlusal arch length is reduced from 40 mm to about 34 mm. The lingual tilting causes the roots to get closer together, reduces space for interproximal gingival tissue, increases the Class II relationship, increases overload on the teeth and periodontium, and results in lost OVD and poor esthetics.

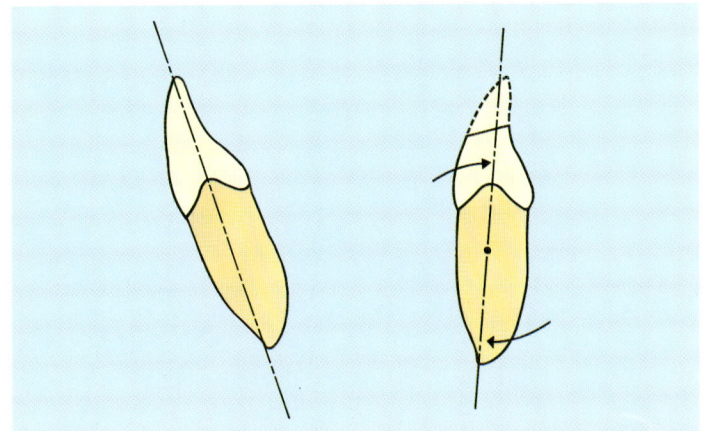 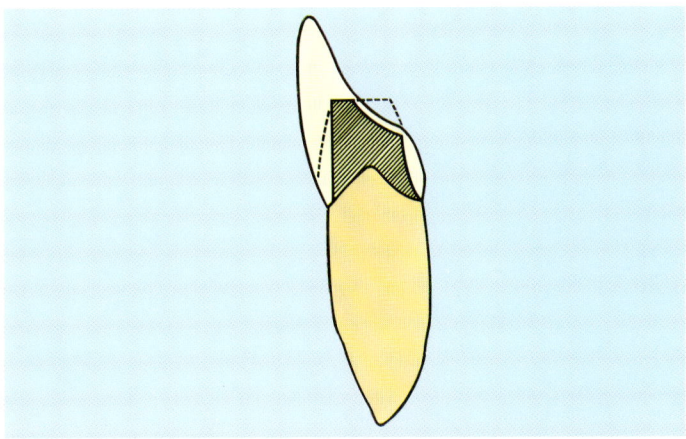

Fig 5-106 Increased incisal forces encourage more lingual tilt of the mandibular incisors.

Fig 5-107 Ideally, lingually tilted mandibular anterior teeth should be orthodontically repositioned before artificial crowns are placed. On patients who cannot be treated by prerestorative orthodontics, many times the worn mandibular anterior artificial crowns can be warped labially to establish anterior overbite and function within acceptable bioesthetics and physiologic range.

the following: (1) the roots move closer together and reduce the interdental papillae width; (2) the reduced interdental width makes gingival tooth preparation and tissue control for impressions difficult; (3) the final crown contours often overcrowd the interdental tissues and produce poor esthetics and unhealthy tissue. Even with none of these complicating factors, it is often difficult to reduce the mandibular anterior teeth enough to get space for metal, opaques, and porcelain. If the roots are not to be repositioned orthodontically, they should be prepared with heavy lingual reduction so that the porcelain can be warped anteriorly (Fig 5-107). In this way, a thicker labial buildup of porcelain usually gives better esthetic results. If the mandibular anterior porcelain crowns are warped too far labially (as in some Class II, division 1 patients), the crowns may become abnormally widened and occasionally create unfavorable esthetics. The incisal edges of the mandibular anterior teeth must be sharp to be efficient and to reduce incising loading. Even though the incising load is not ideally down the long axis of the mandibular incisors, this restorative compromise seems to work well clinically.

To reduce horizontal overbite to within the biological range (2 to 3 mm) and at the same time support the lips

Esthetics and Its Relationship to Function

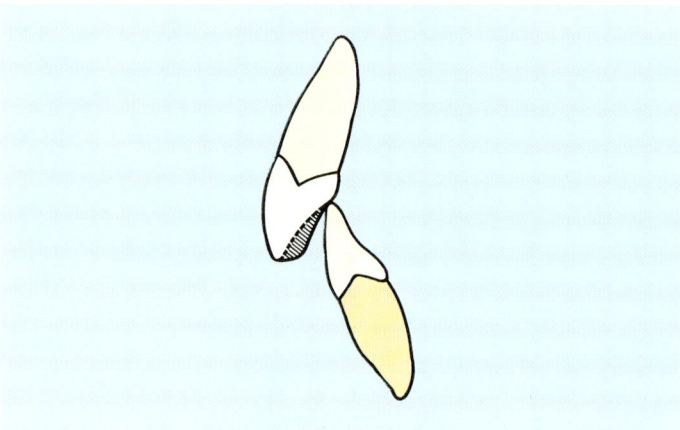

Fig 5-108 Another restorative method of simulating a physiologic bioesthetic maxillary anterior crown relationship for protruded maxillary teeth is to overcontour (thicken) the lingual incisal area of the crowns to produce a horizontal overjet for normal physiologic function.

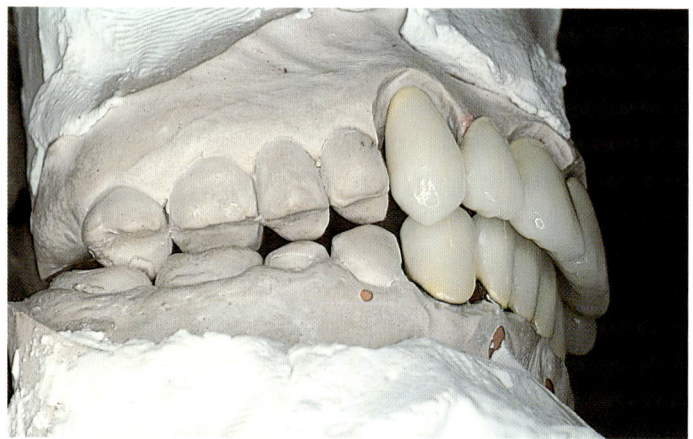

Fig 5-109a Thickened maxillary incisal edge reduces horizontal overbite for Class II patient.

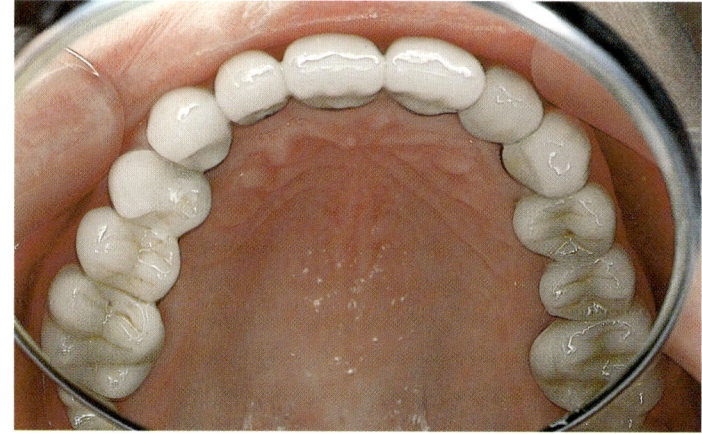

Fig 5-109b Crowns in mouth show thickened maxillary incisal edges to reduce horizontal overbite.

200

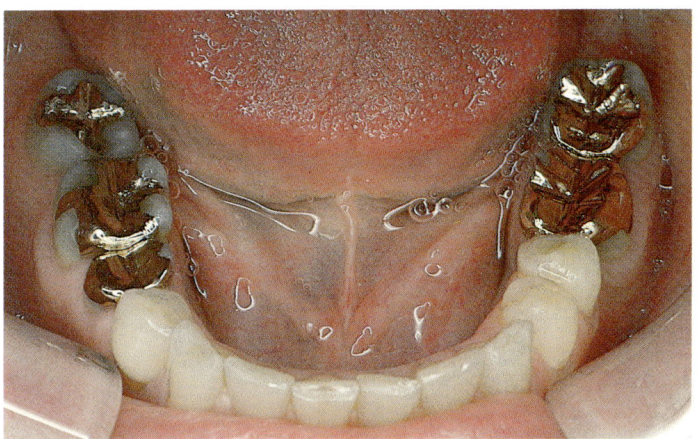

Fig 5-110a   Mandibular occlusal view before treatment.

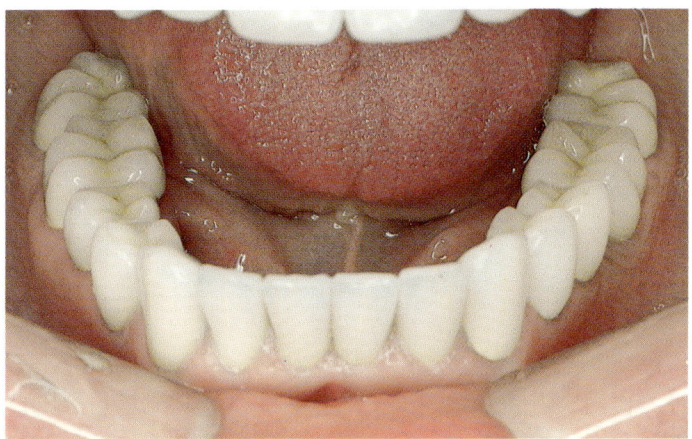

Fig 5-110b   Mandibular occlusal view after treatment.

(Class II, division 1), the incisal edges (labial–lingual) of maxillary anterior crowns can often be increased above normal thickness. This compromise can usually satisfy the esthetic demands and physiology of occlusion (Figs 5-108 and 5-109a and b). Closing anterior open bites by reducing posterior teeth occlusally (reducing OVD) to obtain anterior tooth relations can diminish the interocclusal space to the point that even with maximum posterior tooth reduction there may not be adequate space for producing unworn (natural) artificial crown morphology.

When doing occlusal rehabilitations with full crowns, it is better to flatten the entire occlusal surface of the preparation rather than follow normal rules for occlusal crown reduction. This flattening of the preparations allows more laboratory freedom for the cusps and fossae to be placed in better occlusal relations in the artificial crowns. In these cases the axial walls of the preparations should be made with minimal taper for maximum retention.

Figures 5-110 to 5-126 illustrate the use of bioesthetic occlusion to rejuvenate and rehabilitate the dentition of a 47-year-old woman presenting an overloaded unphysiologic and unesthetic mouth. The patient was advised that the final restorative results might be ideally better if she would have orthodontic treatment or orthognathic surgery because of a retrognathic mandible. However, the patient refused this suggestion and the mouth was treated only with crowns and fixed partial dentures.

Esthetics and Its Relationship to Function

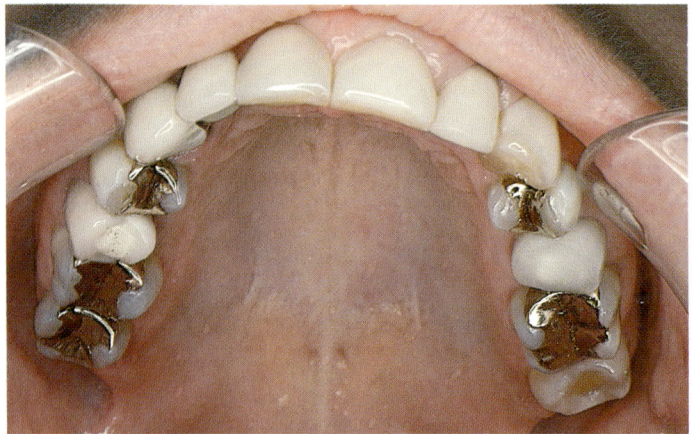

Fig 5-111a Maxillary occlusal view before treatment.

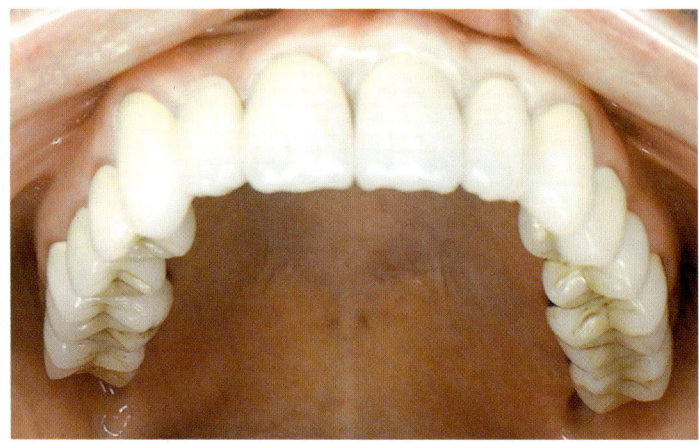

Fig 5-111b Maxillary occlusal view after treatment.

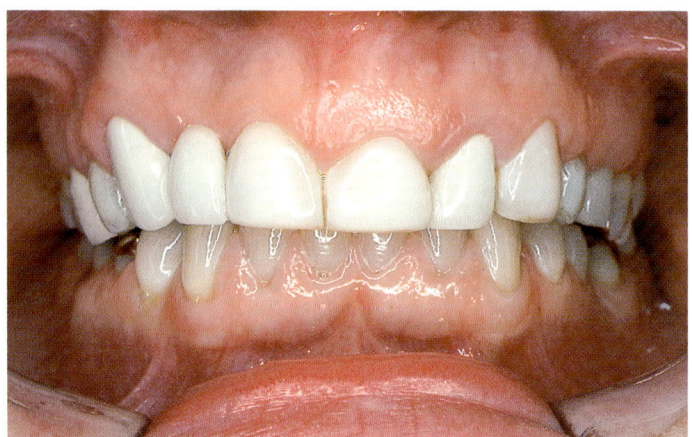

Fig 5-112a Centric occlusion before treatment.

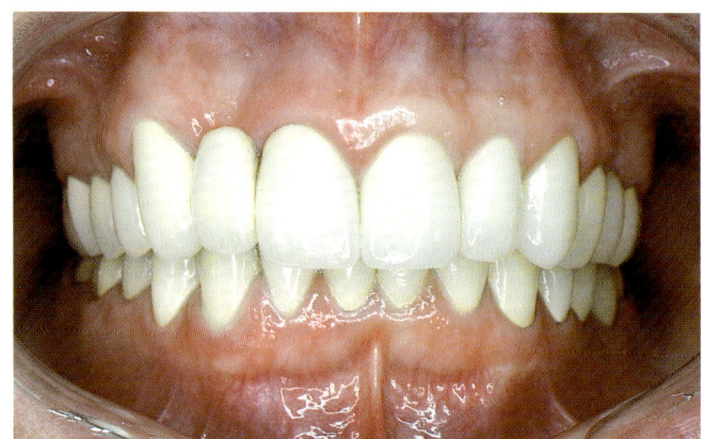

Fig 5-112b Centric related occlusion after treatment.

Clinical aspects in bioesthetic function

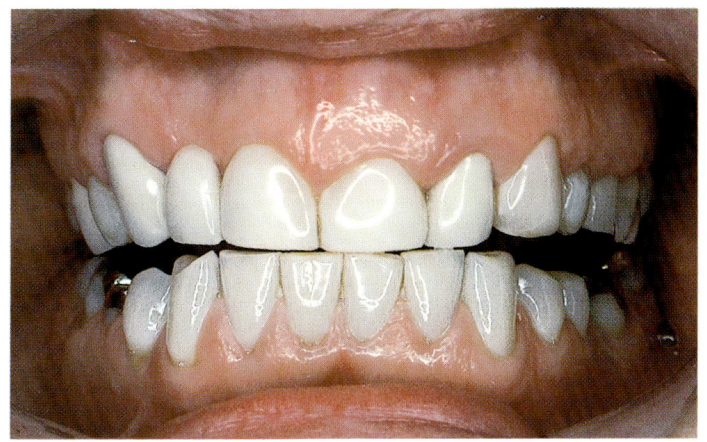

Fig 5-113a Incisive view before treatment.

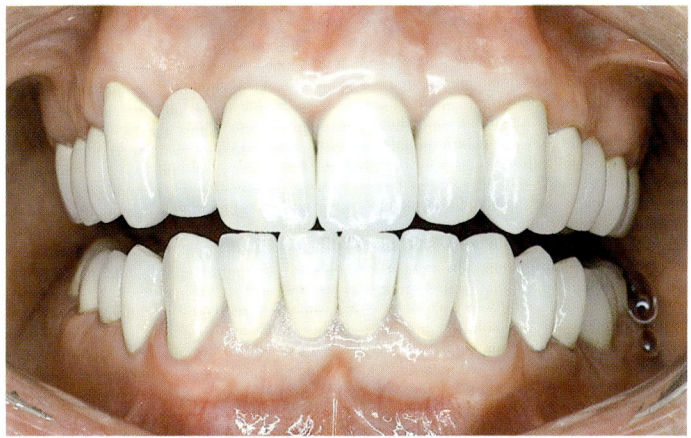

Fig 5-113b Incisive view after treatment.

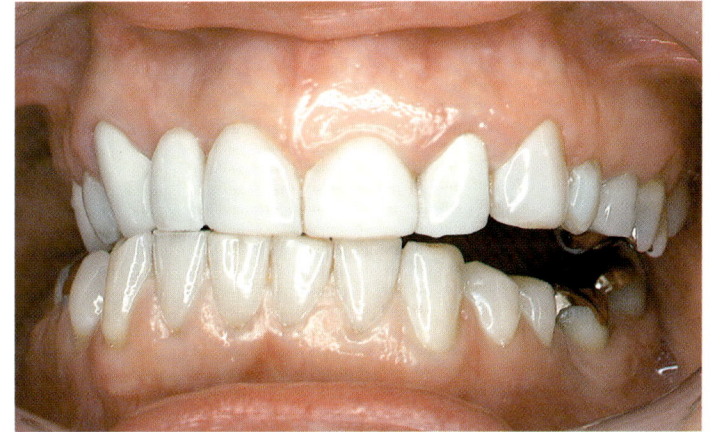

Fig 5-114a Right lateral occlusion before treatment.

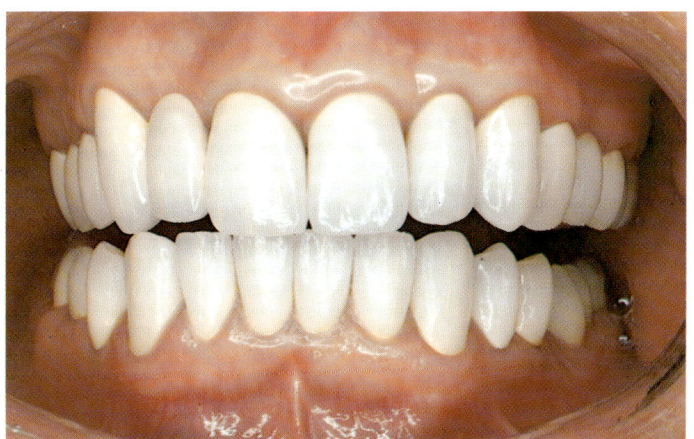

Fig 5-114b Right lateral occlusion after treatment.

Esthetics and Its Relationship to Function

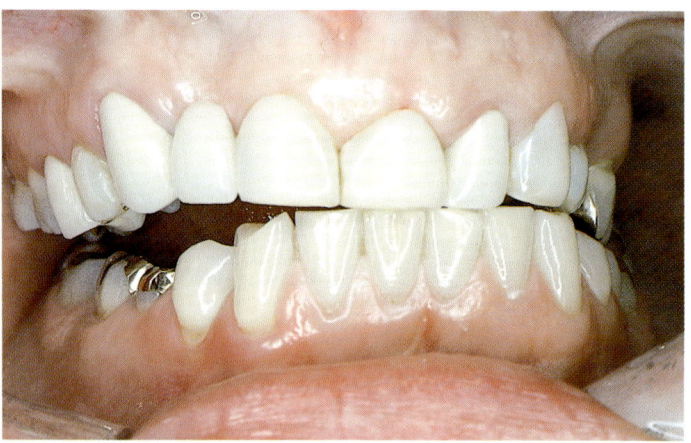

Fig 5-115a Left lateral occlusion before treatment.

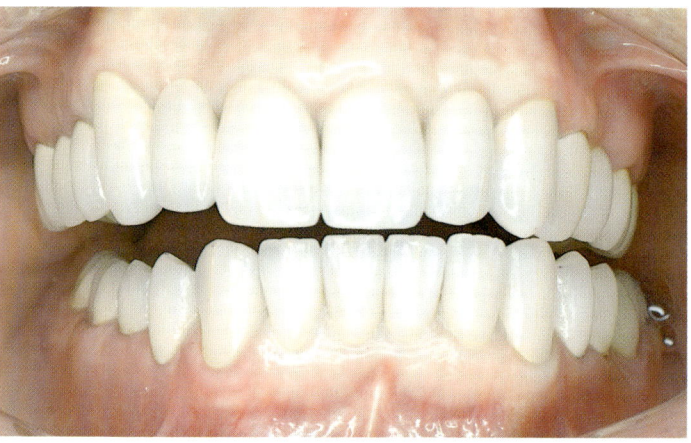

Fig 5-115b Left lateral occlusion after treatment. Note that the buccal cusp of the "second canine" first premolar is guiding the closure at this stage because of the severe retrognathic Class II mandibular relationship.

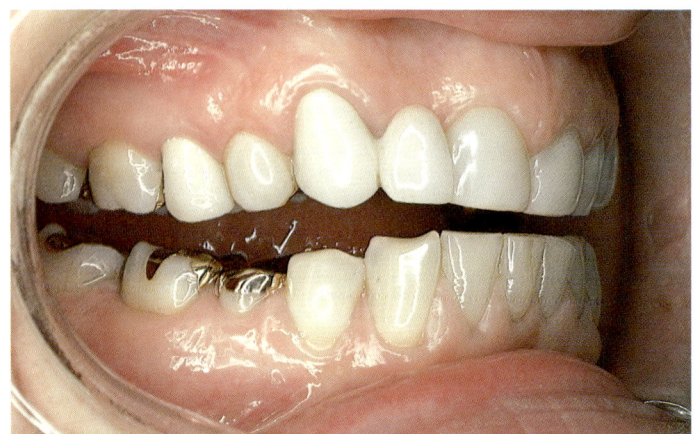

Fig 5-116a Right side view of worn cusps before treatment.

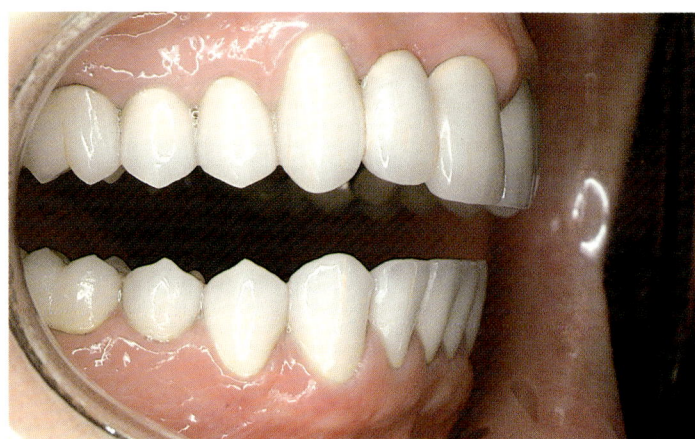

Fig 5-116b Right side view of rejuvenated cusps after treatment.

Clinical aspects in bioesthetic function

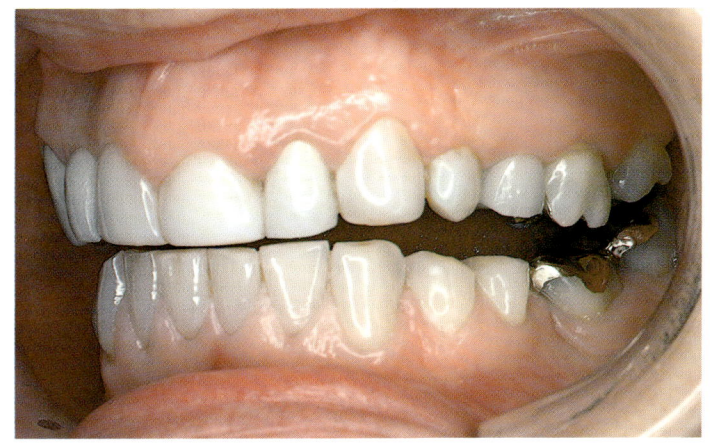

Fig 5-117a Left side view of worn cusps before treatment.

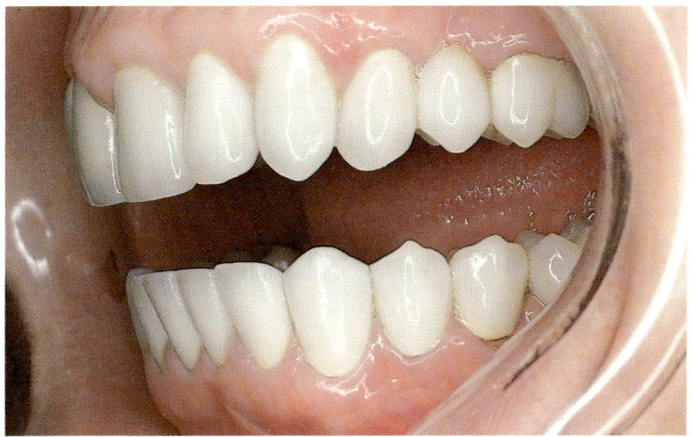

Fig 5-117b Left side view of rejuvenated cusps after treatment.

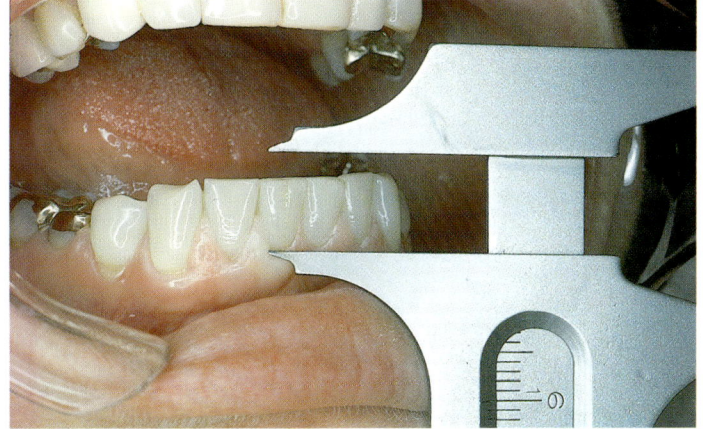

Fig 5-118a Boley gauge showing approximate amount of attrition on mandibular incisors before treatment.

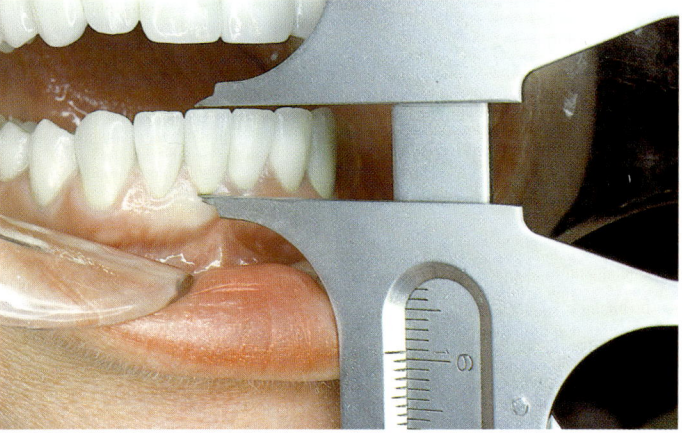

Fig 5-118b Boley gauge showing restored length of 9 mm to mandibular incisors after treatment.

205

Esthetics and Its Relationship to Function

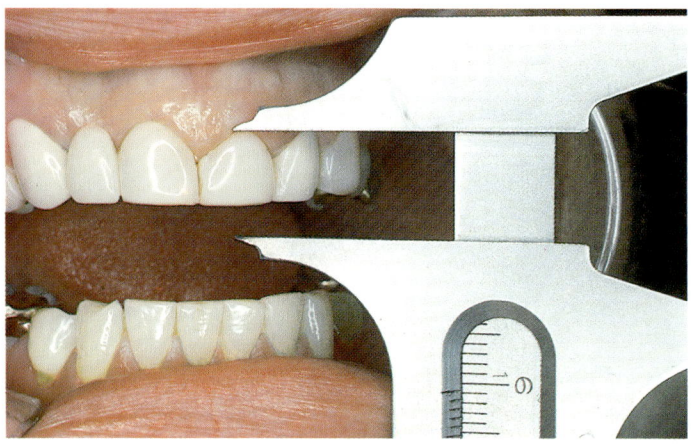

Fig 5-119a   Boley gauge showing approximate amount of attrition on maxillary incisors before treatment.

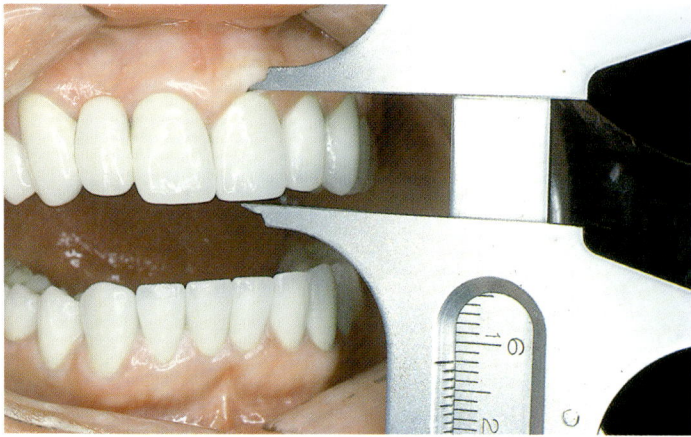

Fig 5-119b   Boley gauge showing 12 mm length of maxillary incisors after treatment.

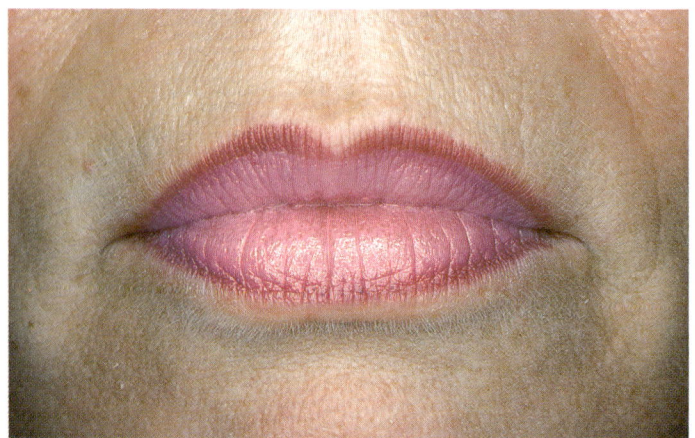

Fig 5-120   Posttreatment view shows relaxed sealed lips with teeth in full occlusion.

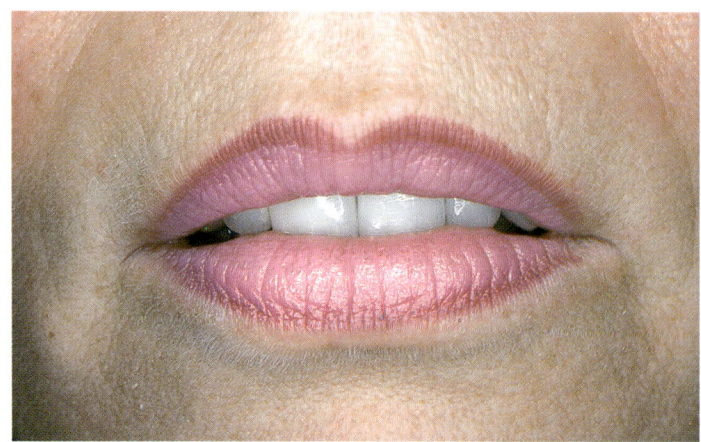

Fig 5-121   Posttreatment view shows lips separated with teeth in full occlusion.

Clinical aspects in bioesthetic function

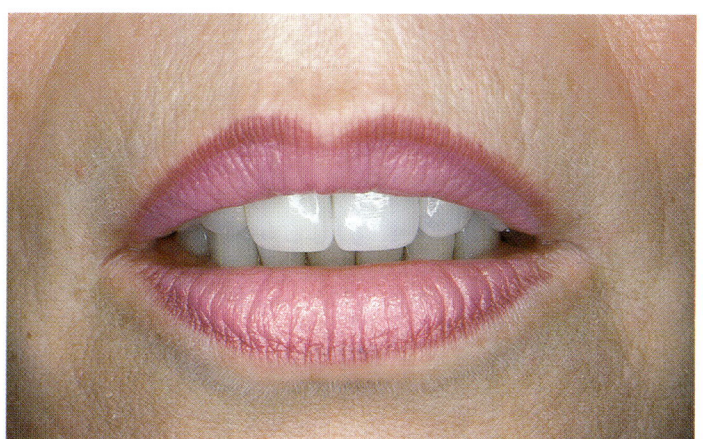

Fig 5-122 Posttreatment view shows lips separated to show mandibular teeth in full occlusion.

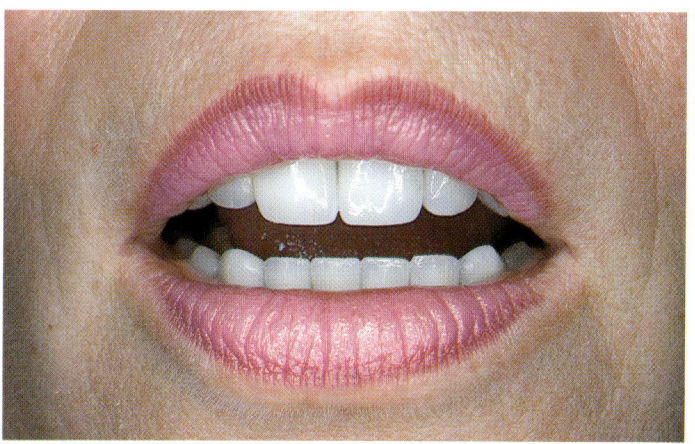

Fig 5-123 Posttreatment view shows lips separated and teeth separated to show incisal edges.

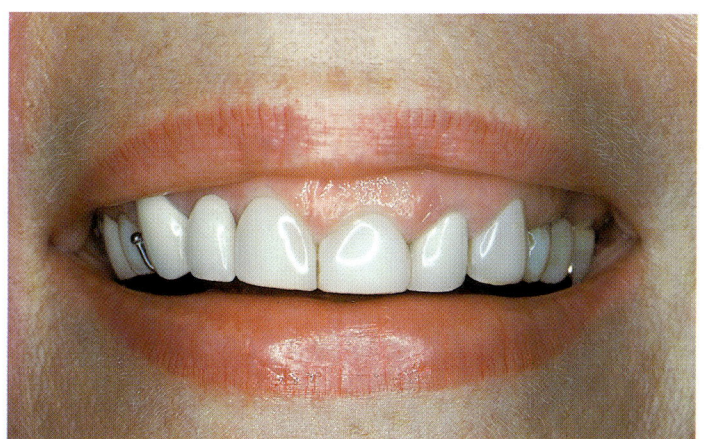

Fig 5-124 Pretreatment view shows straight incisal edges of maxillary teeth and asymmetrical gingival heights as well as lack of lip support.

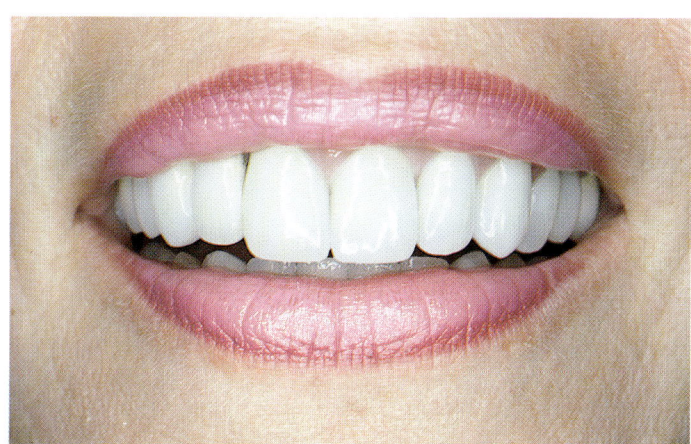

Fig 5-125 Posttreatment view shows bioesthetic incisal edges of both maxillary and mandibular crowns as well as restored symmetry to maxillary gingival heights.

207

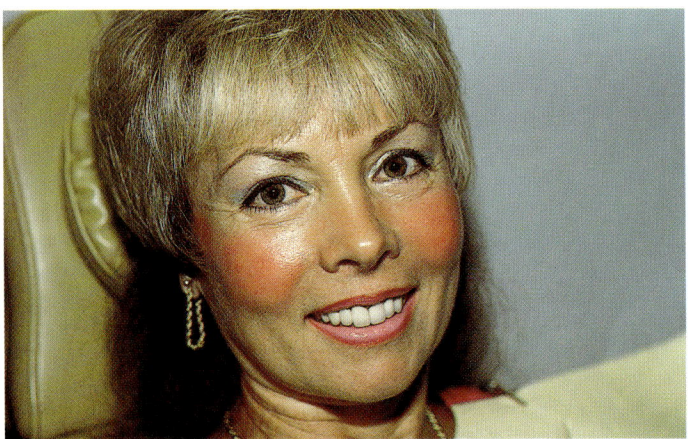

Fig 5-126 Smiling face of patient after treatment shows bioesthetic results.

Summary

Unworn (natural) crown morphology is essential for good esthetics and function. Patients with natural, long-lasting, nontraumatic occlusion show frontal chewing patterns of about 70° from the horizontal. These patients have good anterior crown lengths and overbite as well as unworn posterior crown morphology. All teeth affect occlusion; however, medial guidance in lateral function should be primarily from the "first canine" on the chewing side (ipsilateral) with the buccal cusps of the premolars following a graduated "canine area" guidance. Posterior tooth contacts should not be present on the nonchewing (contralateral) side of the mouth in lateral jaw movements. It is essential that posterior crown morphology be compatible with the anterior guidance. In good occlusion maximum intercuspation occurs when the mandible is retruded and the condyles are in their most superior anterior position. This condyle position not only reinforces the integrity of the disc during mastication and swallowing; it also allows for tooth contacts (IP) on the nonchewing side of the mouth to appear first because of flexions and compressions in the physiology of mastication.

Artificial crowns and other restorations should be made as nearly as possible like natural unworn crown forms. When the entire occlusion is to be restored, the restorations should simulate young tooth morphology (regardless of the patient's age) because natural tooth morphology is essential to the normal physiology of occlusion. Darker shades and external characterizations can be used to give the perception of maturity and aging to make them more believable.

To produce natural-like artificial crown morphology, it is often necessary to increase vertical dimension of occlusion from the worn-down level. With adequate interocclusal space it is possible to rejuvenate and rehabilitate worn out dentitions with porcelain occlusal surfaces that simulate natural unworn tooth morphology and meet the physiologic demands of function and the requirements for good esthetics.

Acknowledgments

I wish to thank Mick Illich, my private laboratory technician since 1978, for accepting this new challenge of bioesthetic occlusion and for his dedication to developing his skills during the past ten years to help make this concept a reality for many patients.

I also want to include my sincere appreciation to my word processor, Doris Stockman, for her patience with the numerous revisions of this manuscript.

And the most important, but least evident, contribution was that of my wife, Arlene, whose patience and confidence helped me find the time to organize and write my thoughts on this subject.

References

1. Linek HA. *Tooth Carving Manual.* New York, NY: Columbia Dentoform Corp; 1949.
2. Wheeler RC. *Dental Anatomy, Physiology and Occlusion.* 5th ed. Philadelphia, Pa: WB Saunders; 1984.
3. Fuller JL, Denehy GE. *Concise Dental Anatomy and Morphology.* 2nd ed. Chicago, Ill: Year Book Medical Publishers Inc; 1984.
4. Renner RP. *An Introduction to Dental Anatomy and Esthetics.* Chicago, Ill: Quintessence Publishing Co, Inc; 1985.
5. Stallard H, Stuart CE. *What Kind of Occlusion Should Recusped Teeth be Given?* Dental Clinics of North America. Philadelphia, Pa: WB Saunders; 1963.
6. Lucia VO. *Modern Gnathological Concepts.* 2nd ed. St. Louis, Mo: CV Mosby Co; 1987.
7. Kornfeld M. *Mouth Rehabilitation.* 2nd ed. St. Louis, Mo: CV Mosby Co; 1974.
8. Posselt HJ. *Physiology of Occlusion and Rehabilitation.* Philadelphia, Pa: FA Davis Co; 1962.
9. Shaw DM. Form and function in teeth and a rational unifying principle applied to interpretation. *Am J Orthodont.* 1924;10:703–718.
10. Lundeen HC. *Introduction to Occlusal Anatomy.* Gainesville, Fla: L & J Press; 1969–1984.
11. Dawson PE. *Evaluation, Diagnosis, and Treatment of Occlusal Problems.* 2nd ed. St. Louis, Mo: CV Mosby Co; 1989.
12. Lee R, Gregory G. Gaining vertical dimension for the deep bite restorative patient. *Dent Clin North Am* 1971;15:743–764.
13. Garnick JJ, Ramfjord SP. Rest position. *J Prosthet Dent.* 1962;12:895.
14. Ramfjord S, Ash M. *Occlusion.* 2nd ed. Philadelphia, Pa: WB Saunders; 1971.
15. Wickwire NA, Gibbs CH, Jacobson AP, Lundeen HC. Chewing patterns in normal children. *The Angle Orthodontist* Appleton, Wis: Vol 51, No 1, pp 48–60; 1981.
16. Graf H, Lander HA. Tooth contact patterns in mastication. *J Prosthet Dent.* 1963;13:1055–1066.
17. Scharer P, Stallard RE. The use of multiple radio transmitters in studies of tooth contact patterns. *Periodontics.* 1965;3:5–9.
18. Pameijer JHN, Glickman I, Roeber FW, Intraoral occlusal telemetry. Part II. Registration of tooth contacts in chewing and allowing. *J Prosthet Dent.* 1968;19:151–159.
19. Yeager JA. Mandibular path in the grinding phase of mastication: A review. *J Prosthet Dent.* 1978;39:569–573.
20. D'Amico A. The canine teeth. *J South Calif Dent Assoc.* 1958; 1,2,4,5,6,7:26.
21. Stuart C, Stallard H. Principles involved in restoring occlusion to natural teeth. *J Prosthet Dent.* 1960;10:304–313.
22. Lee RL. Anterior guidance. In Lundeen and Gibbs, eds. *Advances in Occlusion.* Boston, Ma: John Wright; 1982.
23. Kawamura Y. Neurophysiologic background of occlusion. *Periodontics.* 1967;5:175–183.
24. McCollum BB, Stuart CE. *A Research Report.* Scientific Press; South Pasadena, Calif; 1955.
25. De Pietro AJ. Concepts of occlusion: A system based on rotational centers of the mandible. *Dent Clin North Am.* 1963;607–620.
26. Lee RL. Jaw movements engraved in solid plastic for articulator controls, Part I: Recording apparatus. *J Prosthet Dent.* 1969; 22:209–324.
27. Lee RL. Jaw movements engraved in solid plastic for articulator controls, Part II: Transfer apparatus. *J Prosthet Dent.* 1969; 22:513–527.
28. Lee RL, Symposium on Teaching Aids, Equilibration Society Meeting, Chicago: Feb. 1980.
29. Bennett NG. A contribution to the study of the movements of the mandible. *Proc R Soc Med.* 1908;1:79–95.
30. Stuart CE, Stallard H. Principles involved in restoring occlusion to natural teeth. *J Prosthet Dent.* 1960;10:304–313.
31. Lundeen HC, Shryock EF, Gibbs CH. An evaluation of mandibular border movements: Their character and significance. *J Prosthet Dent.* 1978;40:442–452.
32. Gibbs CH, Lundeen HC, Mahan PE, Fujimoto J. Chewing movements in relation to border movements at the first molar. *J Prosthet Dent.* 1981;46:308–322.
33. Lundeen HC, Gibbs CH. *Advances in Occlusion.* Littleton, Ma: John Wright; 1982.
34. Lundeen CH, Wirth CG. Condylar movement patterns engraved in plastic blocks. *J Prosthet Dent.* 1973;30:866–875.
35. Caputo AA, Standlee JP. *Biomechanics in Clinical Dentistry.* Chicago: Quintessence Publishing Co, Inc; 1987.
36. McCoy G. On the longevity of teeth. *J Oral Impl.* 1983; Vol II: No 2.
37. Gibbs CH, Messerman T, Roswick JB, Derda HJ. Functional movements of the mandible. *J Prosthet Dent.* 1971;26:604–620.

Chapter 6

Facial Sculpture

Claude R. Rufenacht

Striated muscle: Physical and physiologic characteristics

The muscle fiber represents the basic unit of voluntary striated muscles.[1] Surrounded by an isolating connective tissue sheath, each muscle fiber may contract while the others remain inactivated. Bound together in bundles, supplied by nerves, lymph, and blood vessels, striated muscle fibers do not increase in number after birth; they only increase in diameter.

When a muscle fiber is stimulated, it contracts to its full extent; then, according to the strength of the demand, other fibers may contract. The muscle fiber is either fully contracted or fully relaxed.

In comparison with the muscle fiber, a muscle is always in a state of slight contraction. This apparent contradiction can be explained by the connection of the fibers with each other and the fact that the muscle fibers do not run the full length of the muscle. In a normal resting muscle certain fibers are fully contracted bringing a slight degree of tension to the entire muscle until they tire and are replaced by the contraction of other fibers. This process of maintaining a slight tension is called muscle tone.[2]

Muscle tone can also be defined as the passive resistance of muscles to stretch. In an increased passive resistance to stretch, muscles are said to be hypertonic, whereas in reference to a diminished passive resistance, they become hypotonic.

Reflex action

Muscle activity is the result of a reflex action in which impulses are transmitted to the brain by means of proprioceptive nerves where they are converted into stimuli that pass by way of motor fibers into the muscle where the response is an involuntary or automatic contraction.[3] For example, the tension exerted on the muscles of depression in the phenomenon of gravity stimulates the elevators and brings them into a state of slight contraction. In a similar fashion, the constant contraction of the elevators stimulates the depressors. This reflex action is called stretch reflex or myotatic reflex.[2,4] This explains the maintenance of the mandible in the rest position and the upright function of the head when no activity is present.

Muscle tonus is that part of muscle tone resulting from the myotatic reflex.[2] However, in a general sense, passive properties, such as the elasticity of the muscle and the surrounding tissues, and the myotatic reflexes, participate in the muscle tonus.

Muscle tonus and myotatic reflexes can be influenced and altered by inhibition or facilitation of the gamma or alpha motoneurons. As a result, a variety of factors, including psychologic, physical, emotional, and physiologic states, will affect muscle tonus.[5]

Muscular activity

The muscular contractions that are at the base of muscular activity are of the same nature and differ from myotatic reflex only by the number of fibers that are activated.

Muscular activity as the result of myotatic reflex re-

Change of muscle length	External muscle work	Function
Concentric = shortening = isotonic	positive	Acceleration
Eccentric = lengthening	negative	Deceleration
Isometric = same length	none	Fixation

Fig 6-1 Diagram of muscular activity. From Christensen.[7]

mains totally unconscious. When part of the impulses that are conveyed to the brain reach a level of consciousness, they are relayed to the voluntary motor area and are converted into voluntary or intentional motor stimuli that generate a voluntary contraction.

The physiologic principles of muscular[6] contraction may be summarized as follows:

1. When a single muscle fiber is activated, it contracts completely before a second fiber can contract.
2. Muscles are in a constant state of slight contraction (myotatic reflex).
3. The amount of strength produced by a muscle depends upon the number of fibers activated.
4. Muscles work in pairs. When a muscle contracts, the antagonist relaxes.

Movements occur through paired muscular activity and the individual muscle functions by being (1) a prime mover or initiator of the movement; (2) an antagonist, which relaxes when the mover contracts; (3) a fixator, in which a muscle establishes a stable basis for future complementary movement; and (4) a synergist, which may help the prime mover in its action.

The physiologic principles of muscular contraction and the movements exhibited during muscle function imply two types of muscle activity, dynamic and static[7,8] (Fig 6-1).

Dynamic muscle activities are divided into concentric contraction with shortening of the muscle fiber and production of positive work, and eccentric contraction with lengthening of the muscle fiber and production of negative work.[9] During positive work muscle tension overcomes external forces, whereas in negative work external forces overcome muscle tension.

Static muscle activity produces isometric contraction and takes place when variable levels of tension are exerted at a constant length of the fiber, such as maintaining weights immobile during the range of lifting movement.

Muscle motion mainly exhibits elements of dynamic and static activity. Pure static or dynamic contraction is difficult to find in nature.

Facial muscle characteristics

Facial muscles, highly integrated with one another, are characterized by a large variability in size and shape from one individual to another.

The absence of fascia and the integration of the fiber bundles explain the variety of combinations and the modulation of activity that takes place during facial expressions and express the characteristics of an individual, making him or her a distinct entity. The loss of these characteristics that may produce an important psychologic impact may become inevitable when facial movements requiring dental participation are affected by intraoral pathologies.

Subtle and highly individual facial expressions require the selected contraction of certain facial muscles, easily visualized by means of their delicate fibers or tendons attached to the skin and mucosa of the lip. They can show a variety of psychologic states[10,11] so that their meaning is clearly recognized and understood.[12]

The implication of movements of the lips, cheeks, and tongue during the movements of mastication and deglutition can be easily visualized, and a similar implication of coordinate movements of the mandible in the production of speech and facial expressions has been demonstrated. This suggests that unless strictly classified, none of the muscles involved in human oral and facial functions are totally independent[13] so that prosthodontists must recognize the importance of function in terms of restoration of movements of mastication, deglutition, speech, facial movements, and movements of expression.

The meticulous and progressive restoration of the dentogingival unit, tooth arrangement, vertical dimension, occlusion, and function is naturally integrated in daily practice.

If we accept the postulate that dental esthetics implies the restoration of the dentofacial environment, facial muscles that are part of its constitutive elements should receive attention proportionate to their esthetic and functional importance. Muscle retraining techniques that are aimed at putting back in action muscles or a group of muscles, which for any reason have lost their full range of activity and undergone atrophic changes, totally fulfill these requirements. Therefore, systematic recourse to these techniques, as a condition for a complete improvement of facial appearance, should be considered following any type of dental rehabilitation. However, one should keep in mind that improvement will only be obtained if the programmed aging process that throughout life erodes the integrity of the orofacial unit has not gone too far. This sequence of therapeutic techniques has to be respected before the patient can be referred to the specialist as a potential candidate for rhytidectomy. Conversely, some consideration of the facial implication of oral pathologies can be expected from plastic surgeons.

In integrating the muscle retraining techniques in the framework of the daily home care program, we ascribe to these techniques their true significance, which is the maintenance of a healthy dentofacial environment and a youthful appearance.

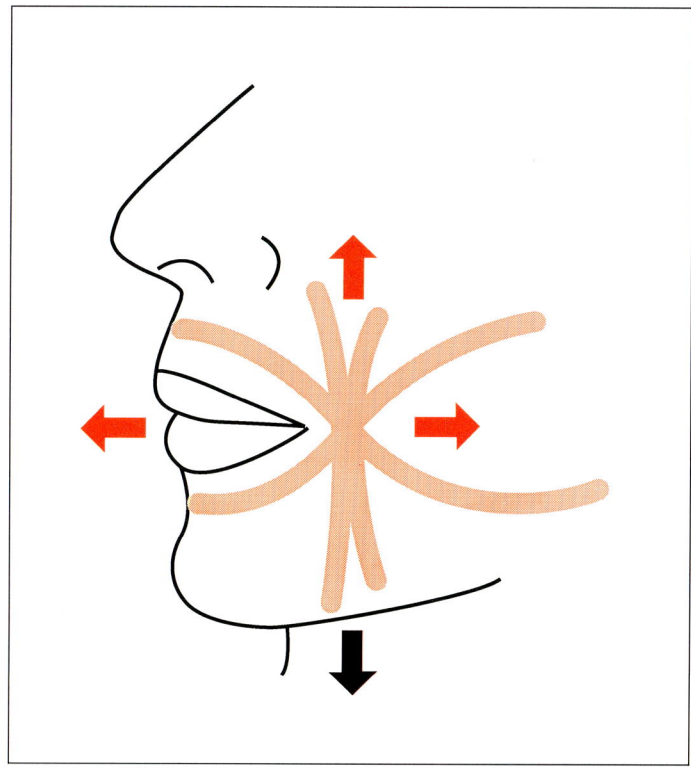

Fig 6-2 The modiolus, muscular knot in which mainly buccinator and orbicularis oris, caninus and triangularis oris, and zygomaticus interlace.

Perioral anatomy

According to Martone and Edwards,[14] the head and neck are divided into two distinct regions: fixed in the upper part of the face and movable in its lower part. Whereas the muscles of the upper part of the face exhibit limited facial movements, the movable lower bone region, depicted as an inverted pyramid extending from the sternum to the ears, houses the muscles that generate, in whole or in part, the functions of mastication, deglutition, speech, and a variety of facial expressions that involve oral participation. Knowledge of the muscles of the perioral structures that contribute to the movements of the lips and understanding of their range of action are prerequisites for the appropriate use of these techniques.

From a diagrammatic illustration, one can observe a bilateral convergence of a number of muscles toward the corner of the mouth where they form an interlacing knot called modiolus, approximately situated at the level of the first or second mandibular premolar (Fig 6-2). This thick, 3- to 4-mm-deep mass, which is extremely mobile and can be instantly and voluntarily moved or fixed by the synergic action of several of the facial muscles that interlace at this point of convergence,[15] has been recognized and described by prosthodontists.[16]

These muscles (Fig 6-3) in association with other facial muscles, are involved in the production of six types of movements that can be visualized in this area, comprising the participation of the muscles in Table 6-1.

Facial Sculpture

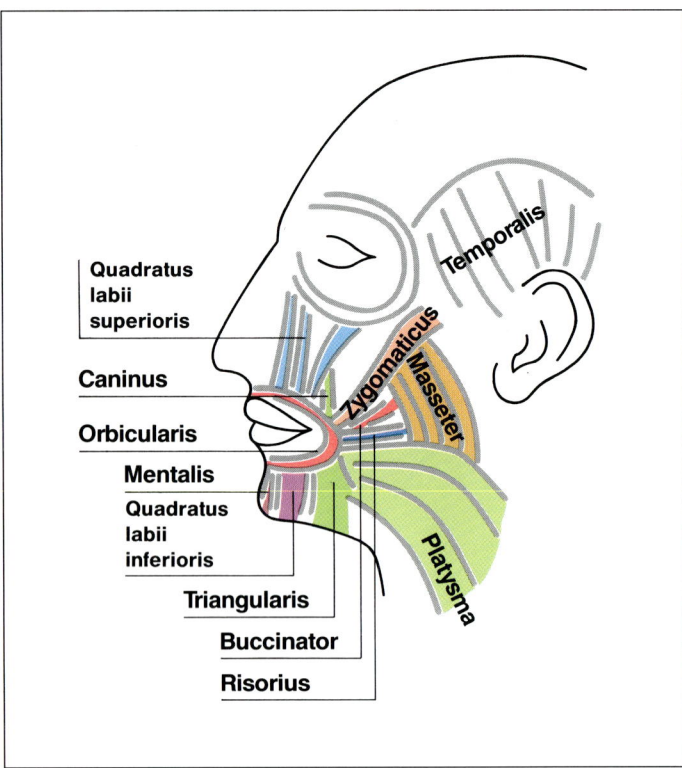

Fig 6-3   The muscles of facial expression.

Table 6-1   Movements and participating muscles

Elevation	Zygomaticus
	Quadratus labii superioris
	Caninus
Depression	Triangularis
	Quadratus labii inferioris
	Platysma
Retraction	Zygomaticus
	Risorius
	Triangularis
	Buccinator
	Platysma
Compression	Orbicularis, including labii superioris and inferioris
	Mentalis
Protrusion	Orbicularis oris (superficial fibers)
	Mentalis

This variety of facial movements always involves dental participation through the active contribution of the modiolus and the orbicularis oris.

Muscle retraining exercises

The maintenance of a firm face that is the privilege of youth becomes the symbol of physical health, vigor, and efficiency associated with that period of life, whereas older individuals usually exhibit sagging and wrinkles. The sagging of the face that cannot be totally explained through the phenomenon of gravity indicates that facial muscles are not used to their full capacity. Muscle conditioning, training, and strengthening through daily exercises will help to counterbalance the aging effect of gravity and disuse.[17]

It is amazing to state that during the progression of age most individuals totally lose control of a number of facial muscles that are not or are only slightly implicated in the development of usual facial expressions. One can understand that any specific exercise will be fruitless if an awareness of these muscles is not realized. Muscle awareness will be achieved through progressive training, enabling the control of facial movements that normally respond to a reflex action.

Smile exercise

As the production of a large variety and number of smiles is unconsciously experienced, the first basic exercise will consist of producing a voluntary smile that will bring into action the muscles involved in the movements of retraction and elevation of the oral structure that will rapidly be controlled. This exercise should be performed sitting or standing, with the help of a hand mirror, preferably slowly. It has been demonstrated that the faster the speed of the concentric contractions, the less the force produced by the muscle, and the force produced by the antagonist muscle is optimal at a high speed of eccentric contractions.[18,19] This exercise, like all the others, will produce concentric, eccentric, and isometric types of con-

Muscle retraining exercises

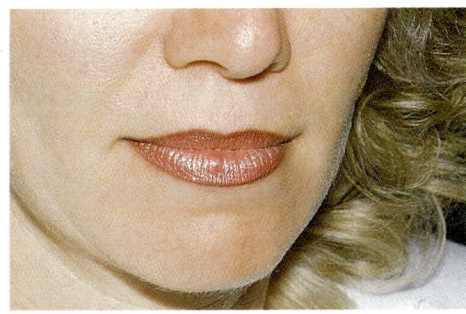

Fig 6-4 Have the face and lips in repose and the mind psychologically positive to slightly increase the contraction of the elevators.

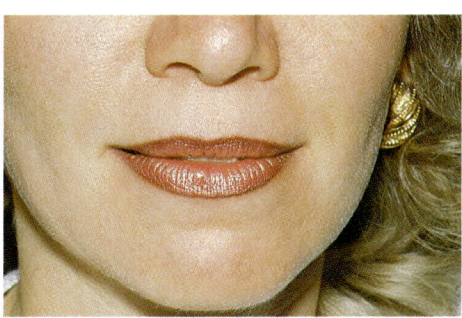

Fig 6-5 Begin to smile; stretch the corners of the mouth laterally keeping the lips in slight contact, and maintain this position for 10 seconds.

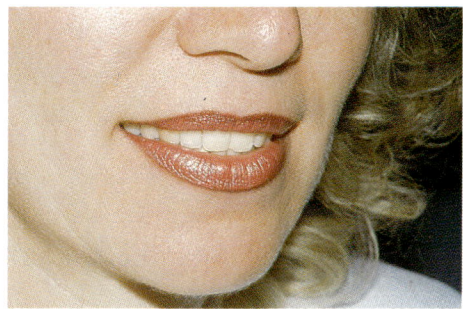

Fig 6-6 Expand the smile slightly laterally and upward to expose the edges of the teeth, control the parallelism of the corners of the mouth, and maintain this position for 10 seconds.

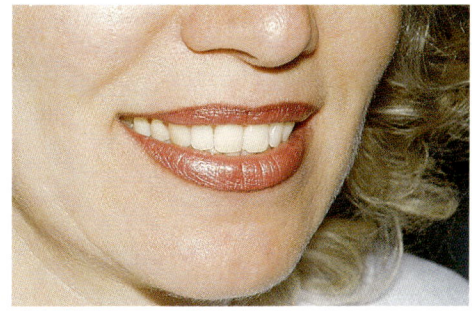

Fig 6-7 Increase the muscle tension, displaying a larger number and amount of teeth and exhibiting a lateral expansion of the cheeks, and observe that the relaxed lower part of the orbicularis oris follows the retraction and elevation of the corners of the mouth to cover the mandibular teeth. Keep this position for 10 seconds.

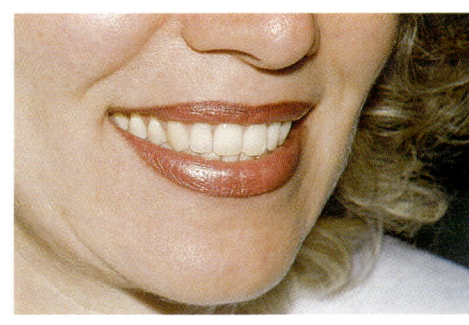

Fig 6-8 Give full tension to the muscles predominantly laterally, paying attention not to expose gingival tissue with the exception of the interdental papilla. Keep this position for 10 seconds.

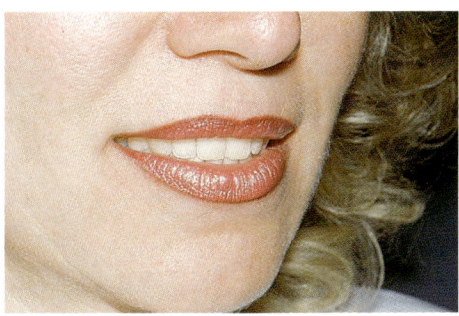

Fig 6-9 Slowly relax and maintain one half of the teeth visibility. Maintain this position for 10 seconds.

Figs 6-4 to 6-18 Smile exercise.

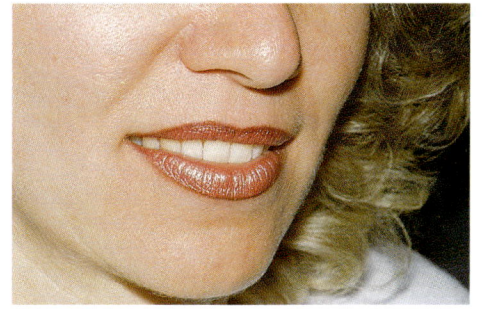

Fig 6-10 Continue relaxing, just keeping the edges of the maxillary anterior teeth visible, and maintain for 10 seconds.

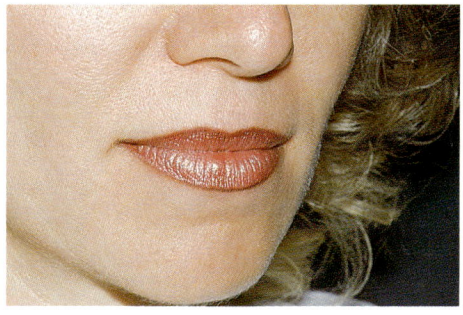

Fig 6-11 Go back to the initial position maintaining a slight tension of the elevators for 10 seconds. Relax.

Facial Sculpture

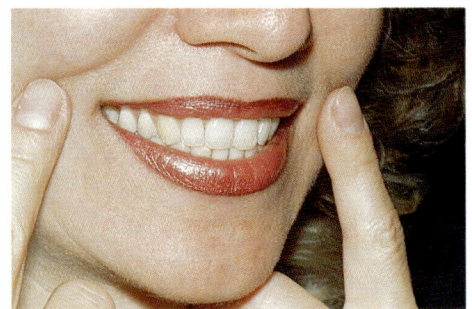

Fig 6-12 Form a full smile and maintain this smile with finger pressure at each corner.

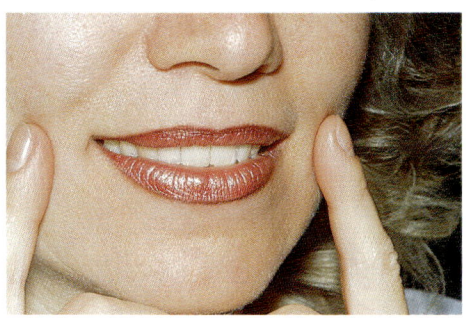

Fig 6-13 Close the smile halfway with a finger resisting the pull and hold pressure for 10 seconds.

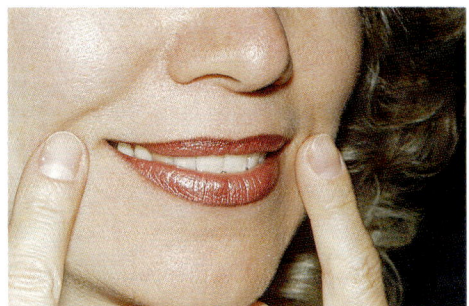

Fig 6-14 Try to close the smile completely with a finger resisting, having the lips trying to make contact in the middle part and maintain for 10 seconds. Relax.

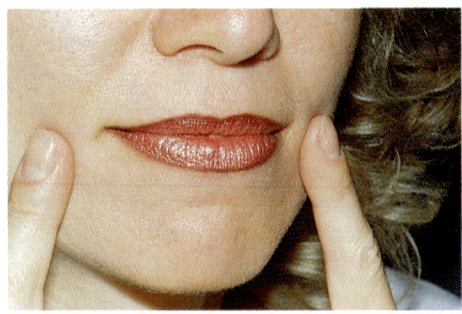

Fig 6-15 Reverse this exercise and place the fingers laterally at the corners of the mouth, slightly resisting muscle pull.

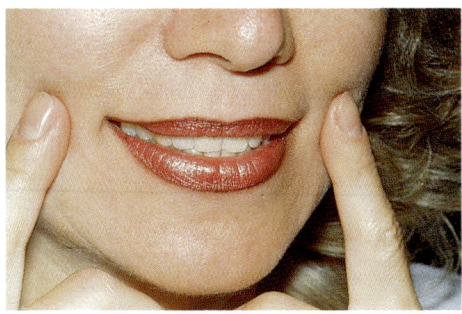

Fig 6-16 Maintain the pressure and try to expand the smile laterally and maintain for 10 seconds.

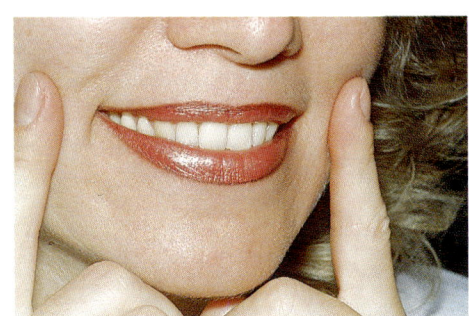

Fig 6-17 Expand the smile, reducing finger pressure.

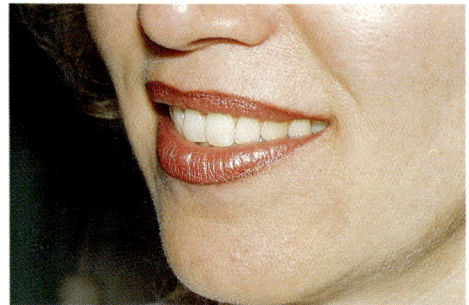

Fig 6-18 Relax and make a test.

traction. It has been advocated by Gibson[20] in his Smile Power Institute that within a few days, when practicing five times a day, complete control of the different levels of smile can be achieved (Figs 6-4 to 6-11).

One has to keep in mind that, following this training, these various degrees of smile will be automatically produced and play a key role in an individual's attractive power. The strengthening of the involved muscles that has naturally taken place during this exercise will be developed in using fingers as weights (Figs 6-12 to 6-18). The impact of this therapy varies according to the age of the patient and the type of pathology developed, but its control is a prerequisite to perform the other exercises with efficiency.

Face-lift exercise

The quadratus labii superioris, with its thin branches, caput angularis, caput orbitalis, and caput zygomaticum, is probably, together with the zygomaticus that has previously been trained in the smile exercise, the key muscle for maintaining a healthy and youthful facial appearance. The loss of its tonicity contributes with that of the zygomaticus to the sagging of the face, the effacement of lip contour, and the deepening of the nasolabial fold. The conditioning of this muscle will be achieved by means of two different exercises (Figs 6-19 to 6-26). The first one will be focused on its angularis branch that terminates at the wings of the nose for one part and on

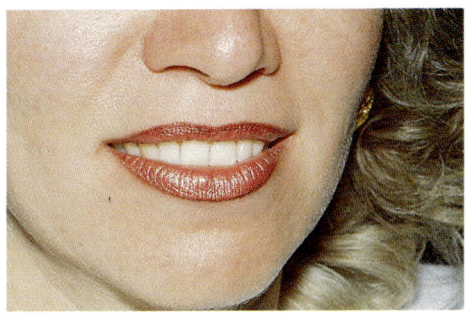

Fig 6-19 Have the mouth slightly open and flare the nostrils of the nose.

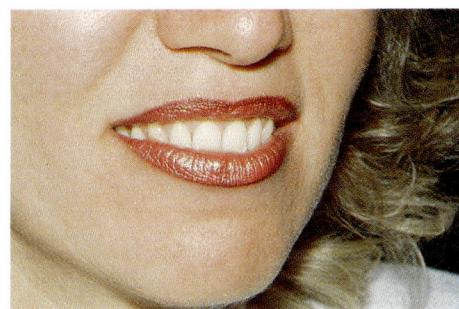

Fig 6-20 Wrinkle up the nose as far as possible and relax the upper lip.

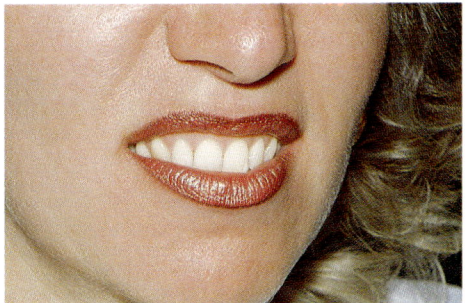

Fig 6-21 Slowly draw the upper lip upward as high as possible and maintain for 10 seconds.

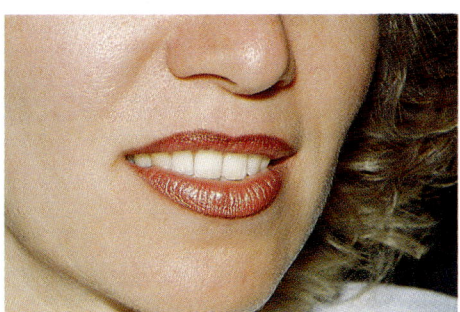

Fig 6-22 Concentrate on the upper lip and slowly bring it down. Relax.

Facial Sculpture

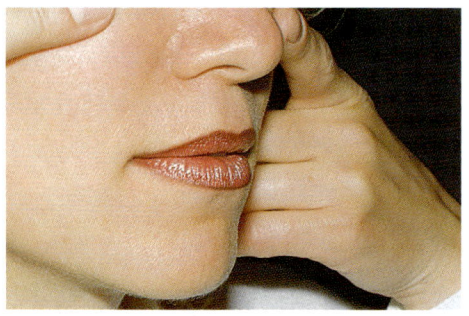

Fig 6-23 Have the mouth slightly open. Apply the middle, index, or annular fingers under the eye on the cheekbone and relax the upper lip.

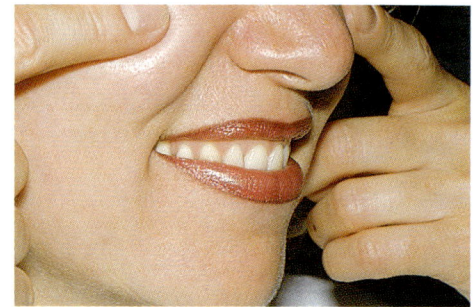

Fig 6-24 Curl the lip slowly up and maintain for 10 seconds.

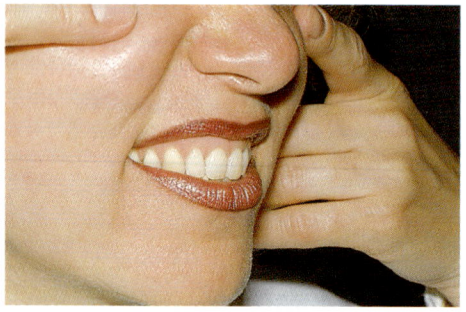

Fig 6-25 Curl up the lip as high as possible, maintaining the finger pressure, and keep this position for 10 seconds.

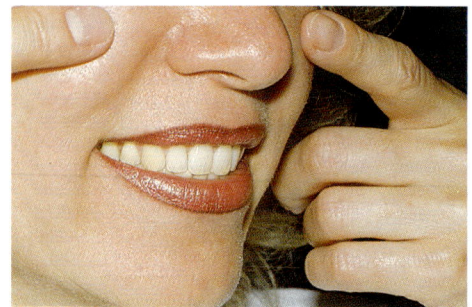

Fig 6-26 Return slowly to the initial position. Remove the fingers and relax.

the anterior part of the upper lip for the other. In developing the size of its fibers, the sunken area that runs along the base of the nose, which characterizes elderly people,[21] has a chance to be filled. The second will condition the orbitalis branch that terminates in the upper lip, where its fibers integrate with the orbicularis. It involves the participation of the caput zygomaticum and caninus and will contribute to the maintenance of the lip level and tooth visibility. These two exercises have to be performed following the smile exercises, thus strengthening the infraorbital musculature. The results become visible in varying degrees after a period of 3 to 5 months, greatly depending upon the diligence of their daily application.

Chewing exercise

It was felt that the systematic introduction of the verticalization of occlusion in practice would make necessary the training of a vertical chewing pathway. However, with or without this exercise the large majority of patients adapted in a relatively short period of time until it became a simple reflex movement (Figs 6-21 to 6-29). At the same time, this functional exercise may also strengthen the jaw and refine its contours. It is advisable, however, to provide patients with a biteguard to carry out this exercise when they show a reduced periodontal support.

Muscle retraining exercises

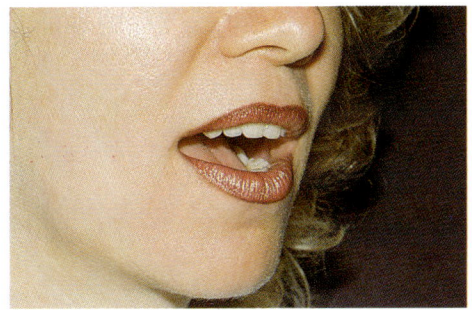

Fig 6-27 Have the patient open and close slowly two or three times.

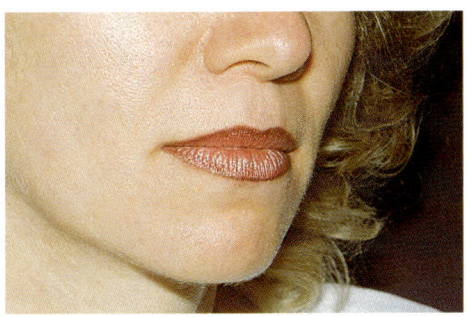

Fig 6-28 Close in centric without any special pressure.

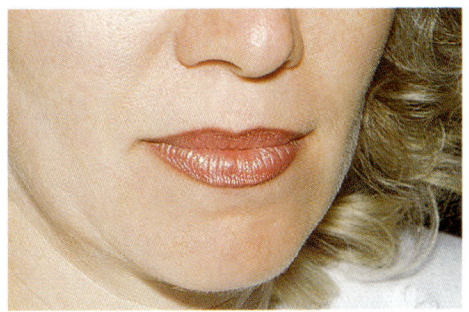

Fig 6-29 Bite hard and maintain the pressure for 5 seconds. Relax.

Lip exercise

Many years ago the orbicularis oris was the focus of so much of our attention that it totally obscured the esthetic importance of other muscles. Increasingly, we realized that an adequate placement of the six or eight anterior teeth in the horizontal, vertical, and frontal planes was the condition necessary to restore the original contour and lip design to permit the natural functional activity of the orbicularis during mastication, deglutition, speech, and facial expressions. However, under the pressure of female patients disturbed by the vertical wrinkles that mark not only the margin but so often the body of the lip, we had to recommend and demonstrate an exercise specific to the orbicularis and complementary to the face-lift exercise (Figs 6-30 to 6-32).

It should be noted that its impact, although rather encouraging with respect to the vertical lines of the lip body, remains poor concerning the wrinkles that surround its margin. However, this exercise, probably by increasing the blood flow, contributes to give a more natural and live color to the fleshy portion of the lip.

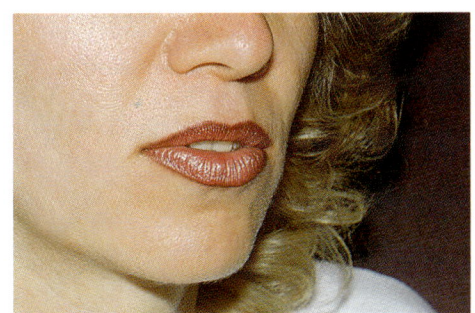

Fig 6-30 Have the mouth slightly open, with the upper and lower lips relaxed.

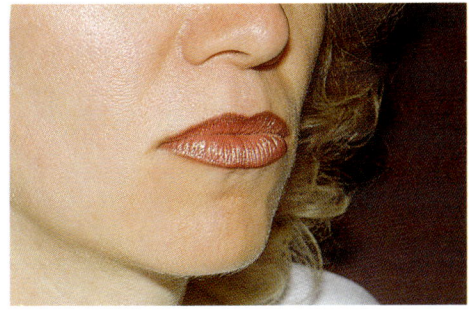

Fig 6-31 Bring the lower lip forward to contact the upper lip.

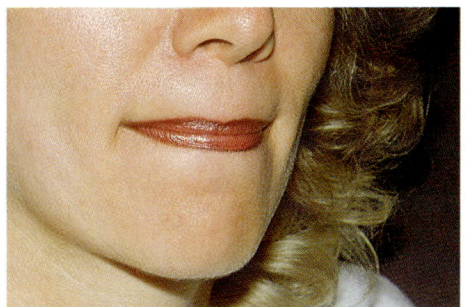

Fig 6-32 Turn the upper and lower lip inward and exert pressure. Relax.

Facial Sculpture

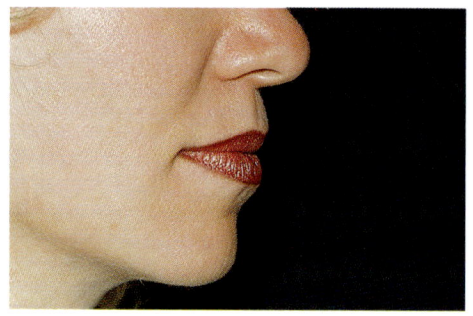

Fig 6-33 Keep teeth and lip slightly closed.

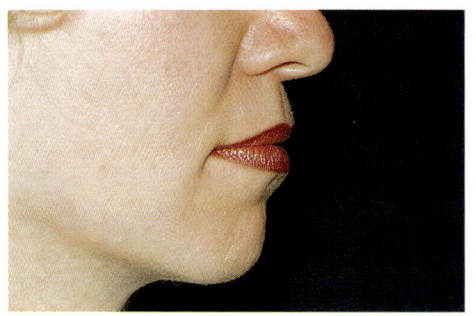

Fig 6-34 Separate the teeth as much as possible without separating the lips.

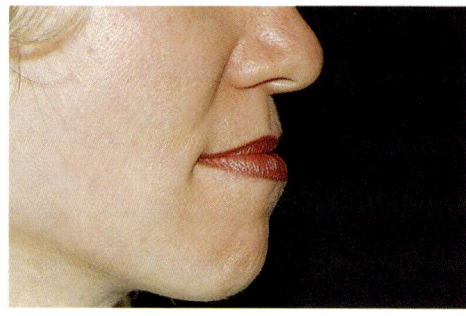

Fig 6-35 Bring the mandible slowly and continuously forward.

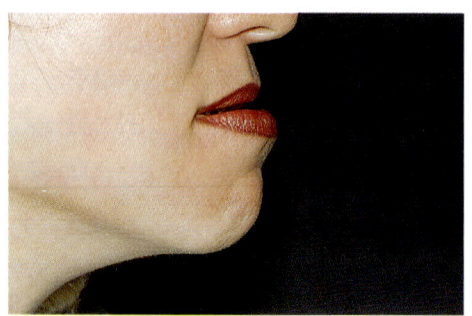

Fig 6-36 Stretch the lower lip in an upward direction, and maintain for 5 seconds in this position.

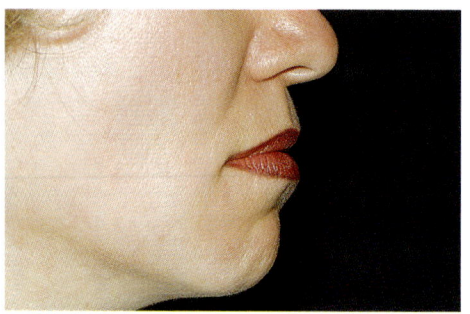

Fig 6-37 Come back slowly to the initial position, bringing back lip and mandible.

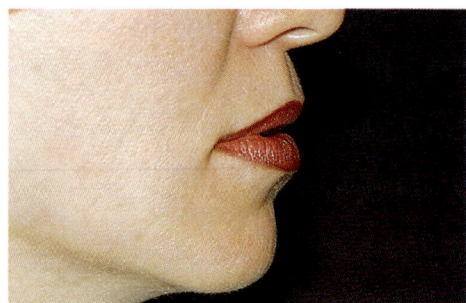

Fig 6-38 Relax and breathe.

Strengthening the mandibular shape

To maintain facial harmony it is advisable not only to focus attention on the muscles exerting a lifting motion but also to strengthen and condition the muscles and skin of the mandibular area (Figs 6-33 to 6-38).

This movement, which involves temporalis, external pterygoid, digastric, mentalis, platysma, and the lower part of the orbicularis oris, will fight a double chin and prevent aging grooves in the lower part of the face.

These exercises have been selected to cover most of the activity of the facial muscles and to maintain a harmonious facial composition. After the first month following rehabilitation, during which the recall system maintains the motivation, one should not expect patients to consume as much time in the home care program. Most of the time it will be restricted to oral hygiene and smile and face-lift exercises that are sufficient as long as the action exerted on muscles during the initial phase of treatment has been positive.

Muscle retraining techniques form a natural part of the range of activities of a dental office and conform to the philosophy that the profession does not restrict its interest and competence to the dentogingival unit but extends them to the orofacial environment.

References

1. Schneider E. *Physiology of Muscular Activity*. Philadelphia, Pa: WB Saunders; 1939.
2. Ramfjord SP, Ash M. *Occlusion*. Philadelphia, Pa: WB Saunders; 1966.
3. Hammond PH, Merton PA, Sutton GG. Nervous graduation of muscular contraction. *Br Med Bull*. 1956;12:214.
4. Szentagothai J. Anatomical consideration of monosynoptic reflex arc. *J Neurophysiol*. 1948;11:445.
5. Sherrington CS. *The Integrative Action of the Nervous System*. New York, NY: Charles Scribner's Sons; 1906.
6. Rogers AP. A restatement of the myofunctional concept in orthodontics. *Am Assoc Orthod*. 1950.
7. Christensen LV. Physiology and pathophysiology of skeletal muscle contractions. Part I. *J Oral Rehabil*. 1986;13:451–461.
8. Christensen LV. Physiology and pathophysiology of skeletal muscle contractions, Part II. *J Oral Rehabil*. 1986;13:463–477.
9. Asmussen E. Positive and negative work. *Acta Physiol Scand*. 1952;28:364.
10. Matthews PBC. Muscle spindles and their motor control. *Physiol Rev*. 1964;44:219.
11. Livingstone RB. Some brain stem mechanisms relating to psychosomatic functions. *Psychosom Med*. 1955;17:347.
12. Martone AL. Anatomy of facial expression and its prosthodontic significance. *J Prosthet Dent*. 1962;12:1020–1042.
13. Brodie A. Anatomy and physiology of head and neck musculature. *Am J Orthod*. 1950;11:831.
14. Martone AL, Edwards LF. Anatomy of the mouth and related structures. *J Prosthet Dent*. 1966;12:4–27.
15. Lightoller GS. Facial muscles: The modiolus and muscles surrounding the Rima Oris with some remarks about the Panniculus Adiposus. *J Anat*. 1926;60:1–85.
16. Glossary of prosthodontic terms. *J Prosthet Dent*. 1977;38:70–109.
17. Howald H. Training induced morphological and functional changes in skeletal muscles. *Int J Sports Med*. 1982;3:1.
18. Abbott BC, Bigland B, Ritchie JM. The physiological cost of negative work. *J Physiol*. 1952;117:370.
19. Bigland B, Lippold OCJ. The relation between force, velocity and integrated electrical activity in human muscle. *J Physiol*. 1954;123:214.
20. Gibson RM. *The Miracle of Smile Power*. Smile Power Institute; 1977.
21. Johnson T. Age related differences in isometric and dynamic strength and endurance. *Phys Ther*. 1982;62:985.

Part III
Esthetic Restoration of the Smile

Chapter 7

Esthetic Management of the Dentogingival Unit

Claude R. Rufenacht

The preservation of a healthy periodontal attachment is a prerequisite for successful restorative procedures. It has been demonstrated that margin placement, fit of restoration, restorative material, emergence profile, and tooth contour are factors that may contribute to the disturbance of this state of health.[1-5] Even the best clinician must face postinsertion gingival inflammation as a consequence of an overlooked evaluation of the clinical situation or as a result of faulty clinical procedures.

Sound knowledge of the normal anatomy of the dentogingival unit should be present if the clinician wants to avoid violating the conditions necessary for maintaining health or jeopardizing the physiologic and esthetic result of any restorative procedure.

The dentogingival unit

The dentogingival unit is composed of two parts: (1) the connective fibrous tissue attachment, and (2) the epithelial attachment or junctional epithelium.[6,7]

In a study that involved 325 measurements taken from clinically normal specimens, it has been established[8] that there is some form of proportional dimensional relationship among the crest of the alveolar bone, the connective tissue attachment, and the junctional epithelium, as well as a repetitive consistency in these proportions.

It has been shown (Fig 7-1) that the sulcus depth averages 0.69 mm, the junctional epithelium averages 0.97 mm, and the connective fibrous tissue attachment averages 1.07 mm. Of these three tissue components the supracrestal connective fibrous attachment seems to exhibit the least variability. The combined dimension of the connective tissue attachment and the junctional epithe-

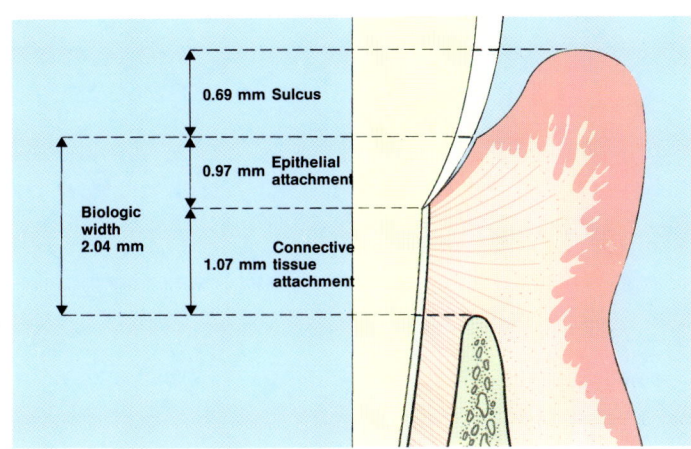

Fig 7-1 This diagrammatic representation has been progressively developed by the studies of a number of authors. It describes the dimensions and relations of the different elements of the dentogingival unit. It should be impressed and visualized whenever clinical practice reaches the gingival level.

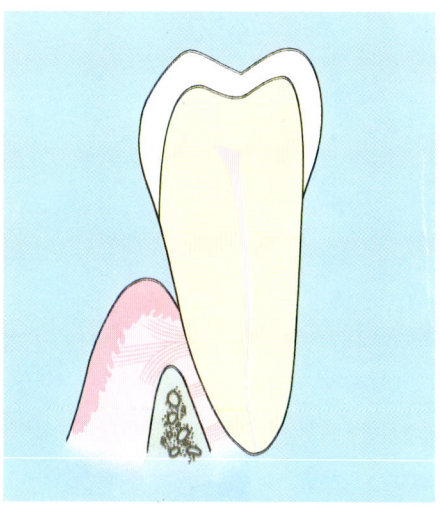

Fig 7-2 Passive eruption describes the apical shift of the gingival attachment along the root surface.

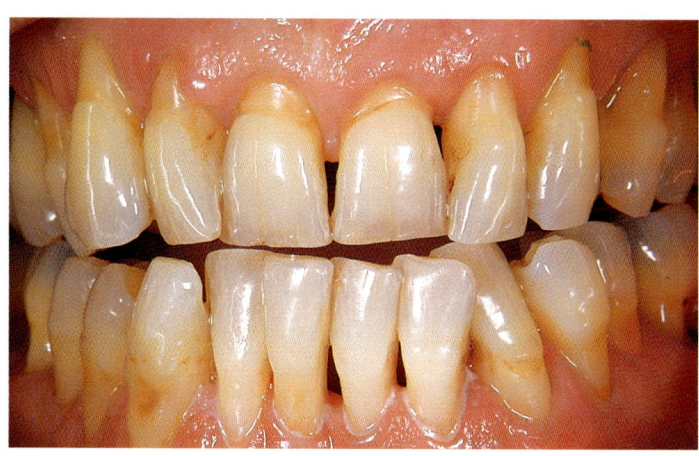

Fig 7-3 Clinical view of a passive eruption that is held by many as the result of successive chronic or acute inflammatory processes.

lium reaches 2.04 mm and is referred to as the biologic width. The biologic width appears to exist in any periodontium, and the importance of not violating this physiologic dimension was suggested by Ochsenbein and Ross[9] and stressed by other authors.[1,10-12] When margin placement impinges into the biologic width, inflammation and bleeding cannot be avoided; as a result, a loss of attachment with apical migration of the junctional epithelium and periodontal pocket formation occurs.

Passive eruption

The location of the bottom of the gingival attachment at the cementoenamel junction (CEJ) is considered by many a transitional stage. As age progresses the epithelium is apt to proliferate in an apical direction. In so doing it establishes a firm union with the cemental surface. The apical shift of the dentogingival junction is termed passive eruption (Figs 7-2 and 7-3). This concept of passive eruption as a physiologic process seems to derive mainly from microscopic examination of human teeth at different ages, in which the bottom of the sulcus is visualized at different levels below the CEJ. It may be that passive eruption or the apical shift of the gingivoepithelial junction is not a physiologic process. This could be explained by considering the fact that nearly all civilized adults have had a history of acute or chronic tissue inflammation, with a concomitant destruction of the connective fibrous attachment. The clinical picture is then characterized by the recession of the gingival margin or the retention of the original level and a deepening of the pocket.

Delayed passive eruption

Many adults exhibit short anatomic crowns with gingival tissue located occlusally or incisally. As opposed to passive eruption, this clinical situation is referred to as delayed passive eruption in which the junctional epithelium did not migrate apically and remains along the convexity of the anatomic crown, giving the impression of a transitional stage in the phase of a normal tooth eruption. Lip, tongue, and muscle interferences have been suggested among the reasons that prevent teeth from ex-

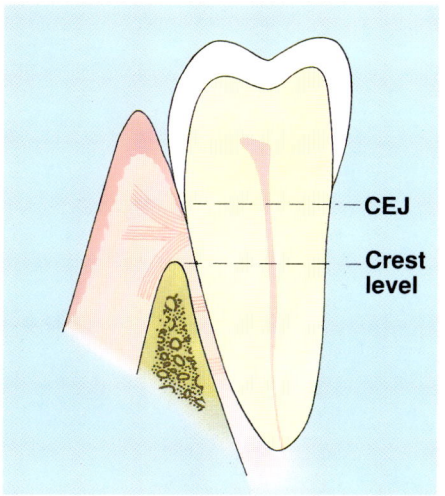

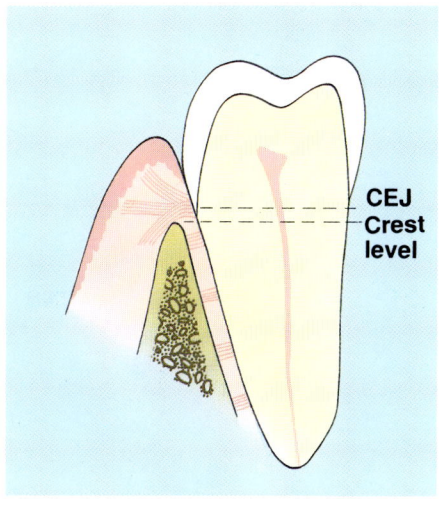

Fig 7-4 Differential diagnosis of delayed tooth eruption. An excessive amount of gingiva covering in the occlusal direction of the anatomic crown can be noted. The mucogingival junction is apical to the alveolar crest. (From Coslet et al.[14])

Fig 7-5 Differential diagnosis of delayed tooth eruption. The alveolar crest is situated at the level of the cementoenamel junction and the mucogingival junction apical to the alveolar crest. (From Coslet et al.[14])

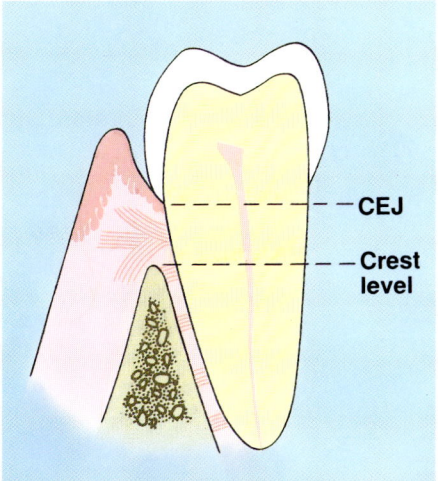

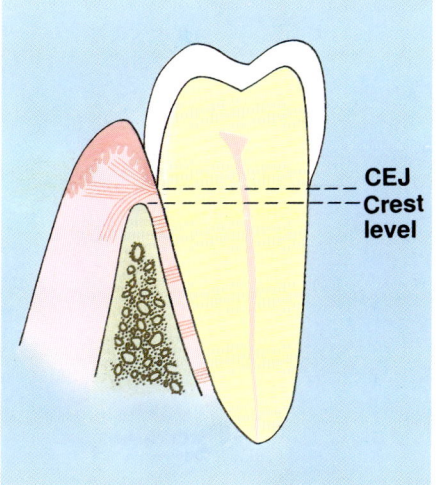

Fig 7-6 Differential diagnosis of delayed tooth eruption. The mucogingival junction is situated at a level coronal to the alveolar crest, and the anatomic relationships existing between the other elements appear normal. (From Coslet et al.[14]).

Fig 7-7 Differential diagnosis of delayed tooth eruption. The position of cementoenamel junction relative to the alveolar crest does not allow the normal insertion of the connective tissue attachment. The mucogingival junction is located coronal or at the level of the alveolar crest. (From Coslet et al.[14])

Esthetic Management of the Dentogingival Unit

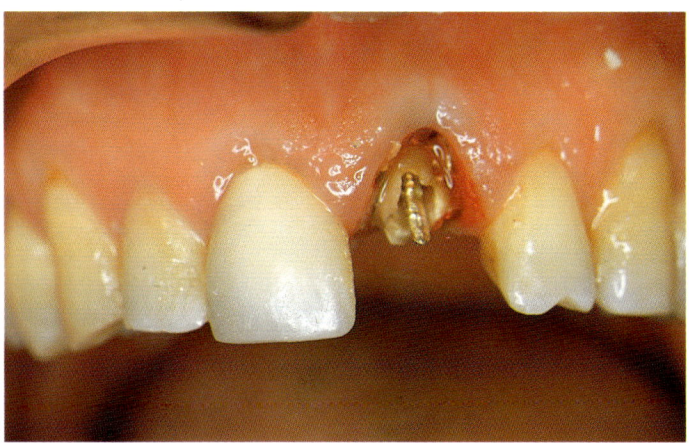

Fig 7-8 Subgingival root fracture. This clinical situation presents, on the buccal level, similarities to that described in Fig 7-5, and suggests treatment possibilities.

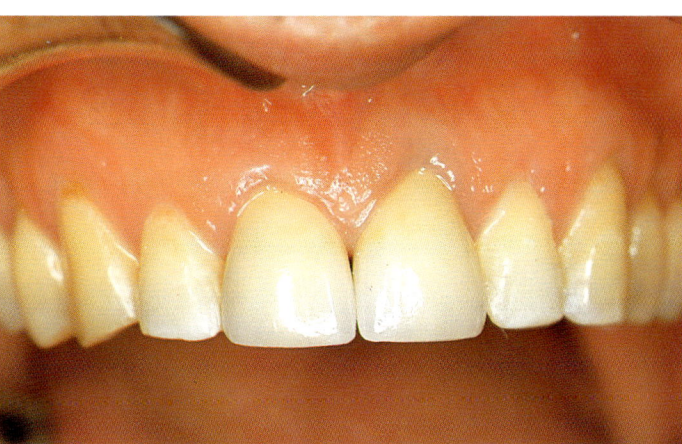

Fig 7-9 Clinical situation following minimal tooth lengthening by means of forced eruption with fiber resection. This procedure made possible margin placement without violating the biological width.

hibiting a normal and total eruption. In a healthy state, the gingival margin is generally located on the enamel and the junctional epithelium from the base of the sulcus to the CEJ, and the gingival fiber apparatus takes place between the osseous crest and the CEJ.[13] The mucogingival junction is considered in a normal location when positioned either coronal or apical to the crest of the bone. A more precise classification, based on histologic findings of clinical situations in the adult exhibiting deviations from this normality, has been proposed.[14]

With reference to the norm, an excessive amount of gingival tissue or an inadequate position of the osseous crest related to the CEJ can be stated. These types of situations that have been also named altered passive eruption can be evaluated according to the following factors:

1. Location of the mucogingival junction.
2. Location of the gingival margin.
3. Location of the CEJ.
4. Location of the osseous crest.

This approach will enable the clinician to evaluate the situation and to adopt the appropriate method of treatment, limited to gingival and mucogingival procedures or extended to osseous surgical procedures (Figs 7-4 to 7-7).

Clinical situations

The complexity of the necessary clinical and technical steps to routinely construct restorations without damaging the healthy periodontium should give credit to those who advise supragingival margin placement of restoration.[15,16–18] However, daily practice does not allow for routine supragingival margin placement, which is judged esthetically unacceptable in the anterior area[19] or inadequate in the posterior area when dealing with reduced crown height where emphasis should be put on mechanical retentions. Intrasulcular margin placement must be accepted as inevitable. In modern dentistry appropriate management of these factors with respect to the environment has been widely described. Healthy gingival tissue surrounding dental elements or dental restoration is part of structural beauty, and a protocol of treatment to maintain this state will be proposed in chapter 10. Unfortunately, proper intrasulcular margin placement is often impossible because of the deep location of caries and previous overzealous tooth preparations.

The same impossibility can be stated regarding clinical situations exhibiting high located horizontal root fractures or endodontic perforation (Figs 7-8 and 7-9).

Tooth maintenance does not leave any alternative for treatment other than lengthening the dental element to expose sufficient sound tooth structure coronally to the junctional epithelium for proper placement of the margin of the restoration.

To summarize, the foreseen impossibility of establishing or maintaining a normal biologic width and the absence of a sufficient sound tooth structure are the key elements that will lead to the decision for lengthening procedures.

Tooth lengthening

Tooth lengthening procedures can be classified in two categories: forced orthodontic eruption and surgical. These methods must be appraised in relation to the final objective of the treatment. In case of a contraindication with respect to the two procedures, a strategic extraction must be envisaged because it always represents a reliable alternative in dentistry.

Forced orthodontic eruption

Forced orthodontic eruption is a dependable and elegant alternative to periodontal surgery for lengthening tooth structure. This procedure is not limited and may also offer effective treatment potentialities of certain types of localized infrabony pockets.[20-23]

Rationale of treatment

When an orthodontic force is applied axially to erupt a tooth,[22] it stretches the gingival and periodontal fibers bringing tension in the bone and generating a coronal shift of the alveolar crest and the gingiva relative to the adjacent teeth as though alveolar bone attached to the teeth via periodontal fibers accompanied the tooth in its movement[20,23-25] (Figs 7-10 to 7-12). As a consequence, a reverse bone architecture is created around the erupted root, which is then surgically leveled to restore the physiologic anatomy without sacrificing bone and gingival attachment on the adjacent teeth.

The tension existing on the periodontal fibers seems to induce the deposition of bone to fill the tooth socket. This deposition of bone is a compensatory mechanism, aimed at returning the periodontal membrane to its original width. It has been documented that such bone deposition is a constant following a tension stimulus.[26-28] In addition, a considerable increase of cementum on the side of the tension has been observed on the root surface[29] with a predominant deposition in the area of the apex.

The histologic observation of the extrusion phenomenon revealed that the alveolar housing follows the tooth occlusally and is later followed by bone deposition at the alveolar crest.[30] This confirms a histologic study done 40 years earlier, which stated that the alveolar housing follows the tooth occlusally as long as a uniform light force is used that enables the maintenance of periodontal fibers and an osteoid deposition. On the contrary, when a strong force is used, some fibers do tear, and osteoid forms only where fibers remain uninjured. Some have stressed the fact that there could exist an inverse relationship between the speed of the eruption and the period of time during which the alveolar housing can catch up with the progression.[31]

The above statements suggested to some clinicians, in selected cases in which only tooth eruption without changes of crestal bone level was desired, to rapidly extrude the tooth and separate surgically the connective tissue attachment from the original osseous level before the bone has a chance to follow the course of the tooth.

In severing alveolar crystal fibers during the extrusion, the tension transmitted to the alveolar bone is eliminated and with it the stimulus necessary for bone deposition. This has been called "the rapid extrusion with fiber resection"[32] (Figs 7-13 to 7-15).

From forced eruption to rapid extrusion with fiber resection, the clinician is provided with a wide range of tooth lengthening procedures that can be modified depending upon radiologic and clinical situations.

These procedures, which are easy to perform and predictable in their results, should be carried out, keeping in mind two important restrictions.

Esthetic Management of the Dentogingival Unit

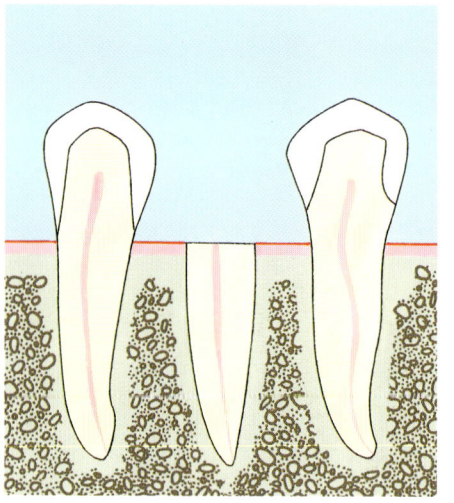
Fig 7-10

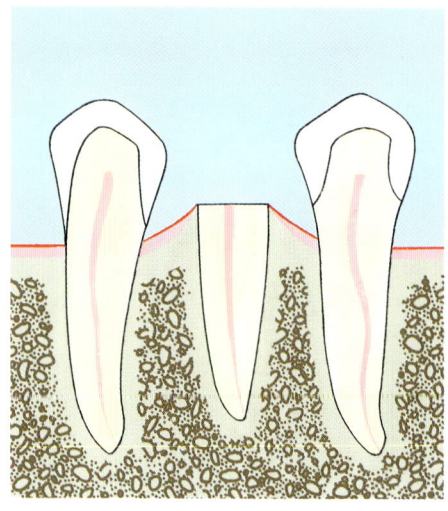
Fig 7-11

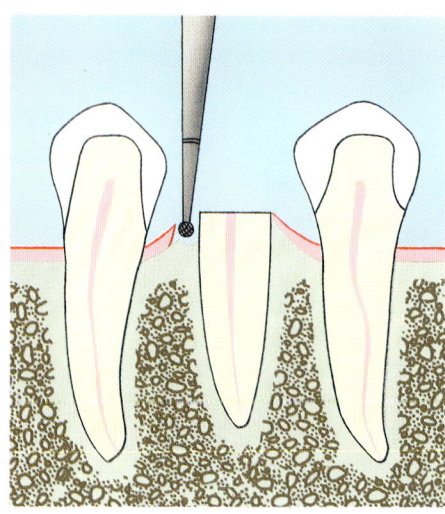
Fig 7-12

Figs 7-10 to 7-12 Whenever an orthodontic force is applied to erupt a tooth the movement draws the surrounding structures (Fig 7-11) but maintains with them identical anatomic relationships (Figs 7-10 and 7-11). A subsequent surgical procedure is necessary to restore crest level (Fig 7-12).

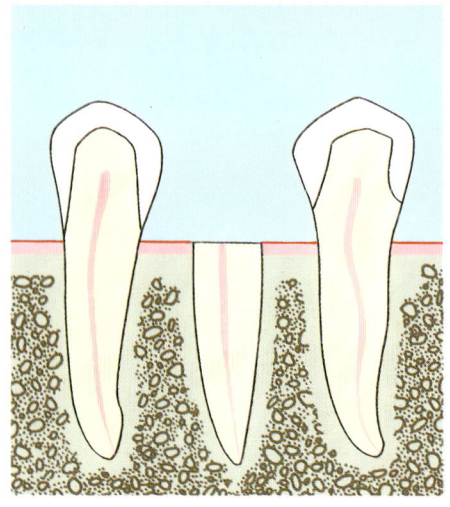
Fig 7-13

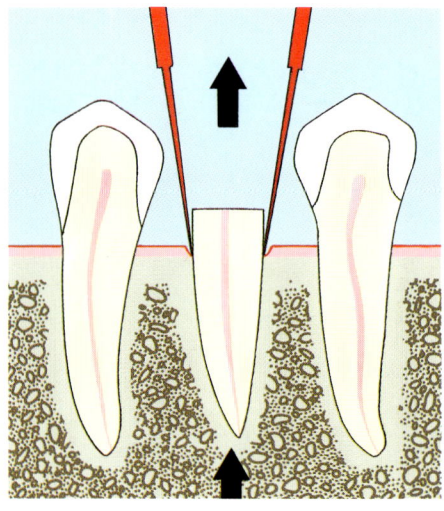
Fig 7-14

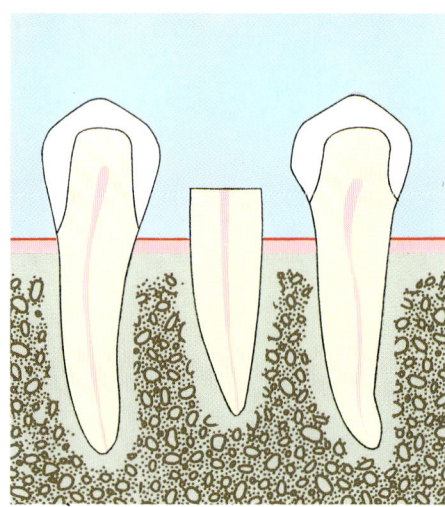
Fig 7-15

Figs 7-13 to 7-15 The maintenance of the bone at its original level (Fig 7-13) is possible when a surgical separation of the connective tissue attachment from the underlining tissue (Fig 7-14) takes place during the orthodontic movement (Fig 7-15).

1. Developing a healthy attachment along with the tooth eruption is doubtful in the presence of inflammation, and this could cause a deepening of osseous defects.[33] Initial periodontal therapy including plaque control, root planing, and curettage should be done prior to the eruption.[34]

2. In any normal orthodontic movement, some periodontal fibers are stretched while others are compressed against the wall of the socket. In so doing, an excessive force may produce undermining resorption away from the socket wall. The resulting potential damage seems to be resolved by dispersal over a large area of neighboring bone. This safety mechanism is not present in the eruption process, because in the absence of occlusal bone, resorption does not occur. As a consequence, the rapidity combined with the force exerted during the extrusion may produce pulpal necrosis and/or root resorption.

It can be recommended prior to any restorative procedure to treat endodontically teeth that have undergone forced eruption and that presented some degree of root denudation or deep caries prior to this eruption. It appears that the pulps carefully memorize successive traumas and choose to exhibit them during the postinsertion period. This is always a traumatic experience for the practitioner.

Surgical approach

Lengthening the clinical crown by removing the marginal supporting structures is the solution that is generally recommended and first envisaged. However, the variety of clinical conditions existing in this type of situation will require the use of specific periodontal surgical procedures. It is therefore indicated that once the diagnosis is established and the surgical procedure selected, to evaluate the results of the therapy should be according to the following factors:

1. *Esthetic:* in the anterior area surgery may result in esthetic deformities.
2. *Remaining root implantation:* surgery should not compromise tooth stability.
3. *Furcation involvement:* surgery should not expose root furcation and introduce new potential pathologic factors.

It should be emphasized that, whatever the approach selected, the finalization of the treatment is the formation of a normal sulcular or junctional epithelium at any level of the root, ie, the restoration of a healthy and biologic gingival attachment. Considering the biologic width and the requirement to maintain it unviolated, a sound tooth structure of a minimum of 3 to 4 mm must be present from the osseous crest level to provide adequate placement and seal of the restoration. It should also be kept in mind that the rise and fall of normal osseous topography along the CEJ of the tooth must be respected and that osseous removal should invariably be extended to adjacent elements, not only for esthetic reasons but also to blend in with this new topography and to provide future tissue stability.

This modality of treatment requires the removal of buccal and lingual bone to restore the scalloped type of anatomy when dealing with the elimination of interdental craters to prevent further recessions or pocket formation.[35] Therefore, the indications for this type of treatment appear limited to areas without esthetic importance, areas where preexisting periodontal problems can be involved in the surgical procedure, and areas where teeth are adjacent to edentulous areas.

Surgical versus orthodontical tooth lengthening

From a strictly clinical point of view, each of these different modalities of treatment is aimed at exposing sufficient tooth structure to maintain the biologic integrity of the dentogingival unit that is going to be restored. Probably because it is a standard field of activity of the dental team, surgical procedure is first considered whenever tooth lengthening is required.

However, when esthetics come into consideration and even if a one session procedure may appeal to both the dentist and the patient, many factors should be evaluated in the therapeutic choice of tooth lengthening. These will depend upon the overall configuration of the mouth, clinical and radiologic findings, and the patient's motivation and availability (Figs 7-16 to 7-19).

In the case in which an orthodontic treatment is considered, the patient must be informed about the potential discomfort produced by brackets, wires, the frequency of checks, and the difficult predictability of the treatment duration that usually does not exceed 8 weeks. Although out-of-town orthodontic patients are generally a source

Esthetic Management of the Dentogingival Unit

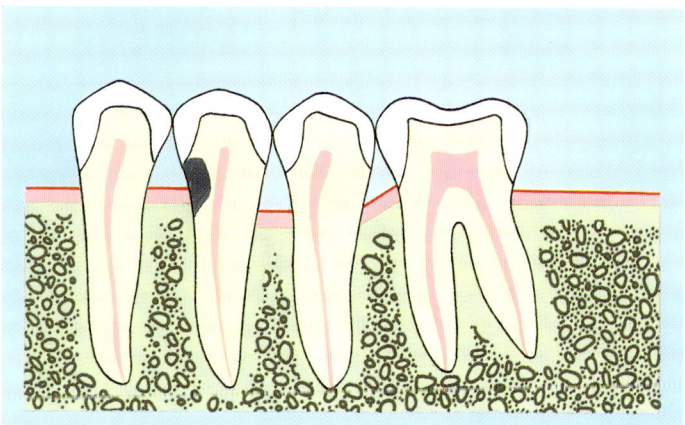

Fig 7-16 Hypothetical initial clinical situation showing a carious lesion located below the crest level and periodontal pocket on an adjacent tooth. Modalities of treatment are left to the judgment of the operator.

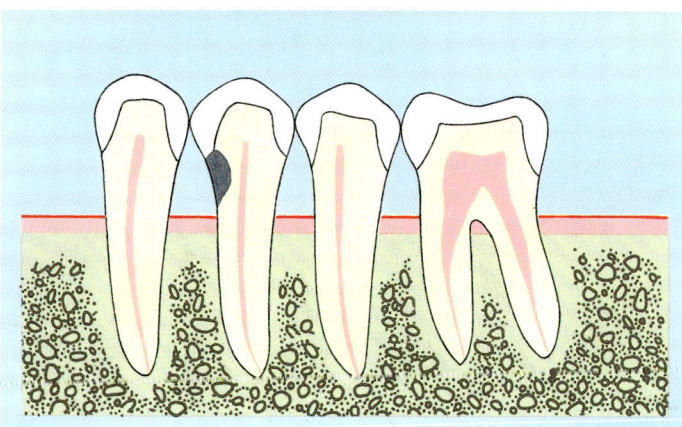

Fig 7-17 The usually selected one-stage surgical procedure has to be carefully evaluated depending upon the particularities of the oral cavity, basically the presence of furcation. Esthetics must be considered whenever performed in the anterior area.

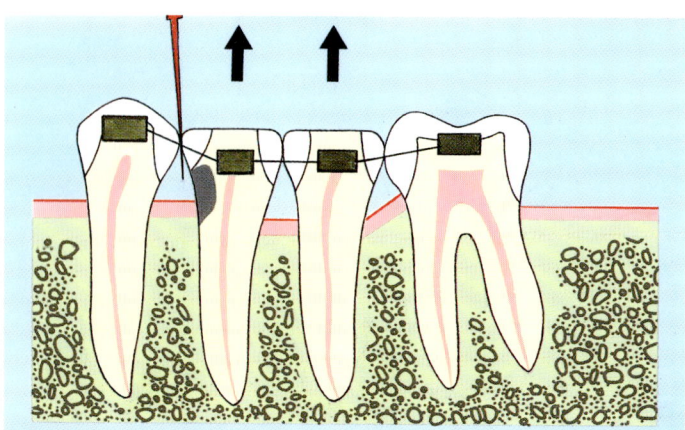

Fig 7-18 Depending upon the situation, orthodontic eruption offers to the clinician a selected approach: from forced eruption to forced eruption with fiber resection.

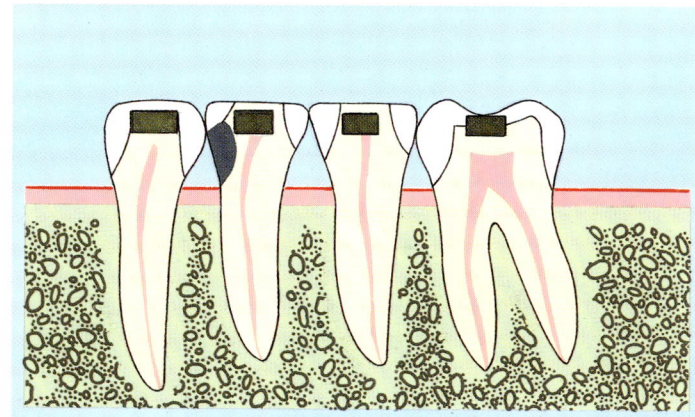

Fig 7-19 In this event, one must deal with a multiappointment procedure requiring the patient's cooperation for hygiene maintenance. The elegance of the procedure enabling the treatment of infrabony pockets is most appealing.

Tooth lengthening

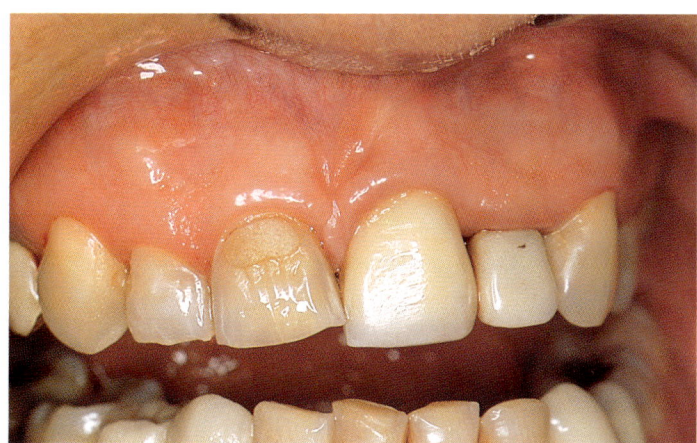

Fig 7-20 The maxillary anterior segment shows an altered or delayed eruption of both lateral incisors, minor malposition of a central incisor, and in general poor restorative dentistry and puffy gingival tissue.

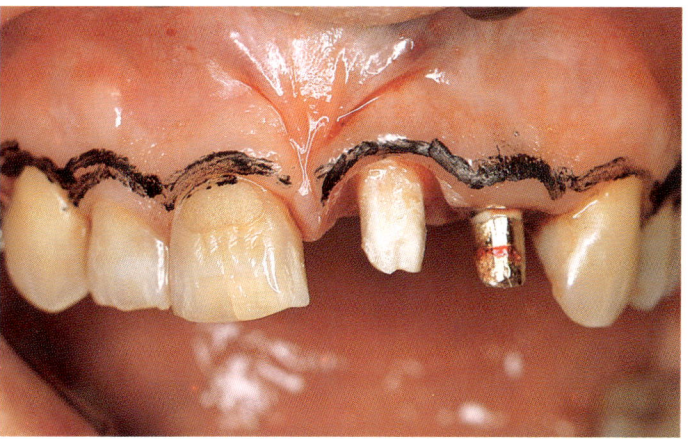

Fig 7-21 The left central incisor presents a shallow infrabony pocket. All these factors contributed to an unesthetic result that was planned to be improved by means of a one-stage resective surgical procedure and the future insertion of restorations.

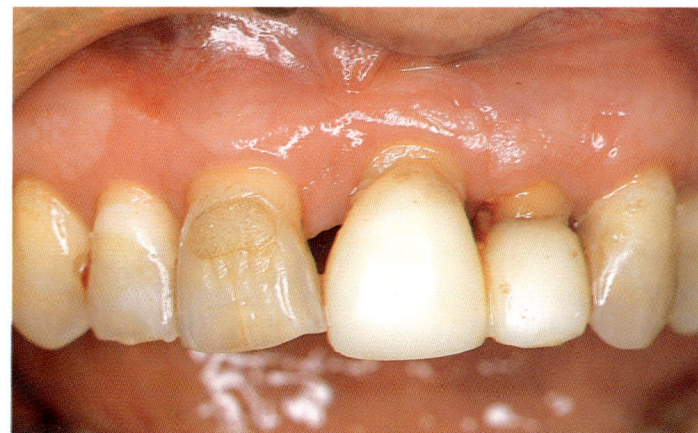

Fig 7-22 The depth of the pocket affecting the maxillary left central incisor was underevaluated and the surgical procedure could not be completed, culminating in this unexpected situation. A decision was made to move the central incisor orthodontically to restore normal gingival and osseous relationships.

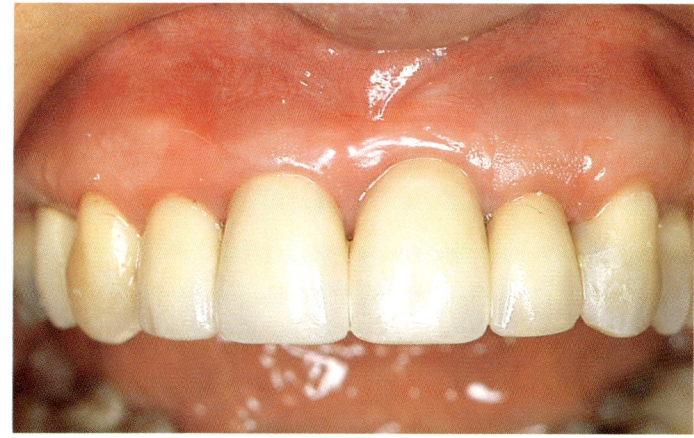

Fig 7-23 A fixed anterior acrylic resin fixed partial denture of four elements with a pontic hiding a rubber band for erupting the central incisor was inserted. The marginal level of the pontic was trimmed out to allow for tooth movement. Unfortunately, the patient was not seen for 6 months and the amount of tooth eruption could not be verified. Tissue swelling increased.

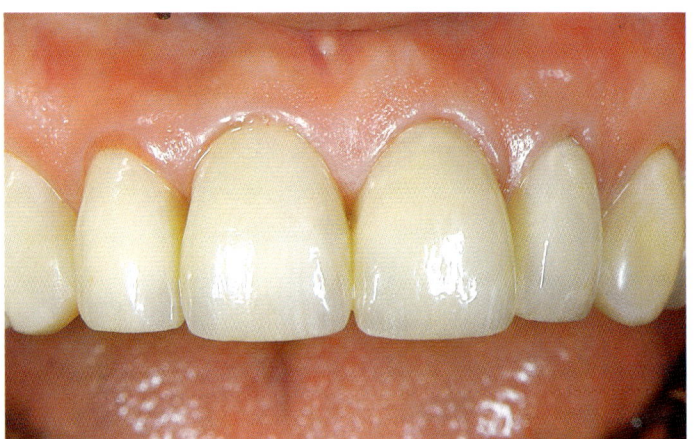

Fig 7-24 The development of nonanatomic osseous design made necessary the recontouring of the osseous support. At the same time, tissue thickness was refined and a frenectomy performed. Four anterior crowns and two veneer facets (canines) were finally inserted. These last therapeutic measures and improvement in the patient's dental hygiene contributed to the restoration of tissue health.

of problems, orthodontics in general, and for adult patients in particular, is not an experience that is a glorious period in life unless imagination and the clinical situation open the possibility of insertion of an adequate device for eruption within the acrylic resin frame of a provisional fixed partial denture.

Considering the elements of clinical evaluation, posterior teeth exhibiting greater osseous support, greater root surface, flatter interdental form, and fewer esthetic requirements are more amenable to osseous surgery than to orthodontic eruption. However, particular attention should be paid not to open furcation during the resective procedures. The same attention must be paid to carefully evaluate molar root proximity if orthodontic eruption is carried out.

The anterior area is the adequate location for orthodontic eruption to prevent esthetic deformities evidenced by large embrasures consecutive to surgical procedures. Single anterior teeth, the position of which disturbs the structural beauty of the rise and fall of gingival tissue, are elements of choice for orthodontic eruption. More frequently, in the presence of fracture or root caries affecting the anterior dental elements, rapid extension with fiber resection represents the ideal indication to expose sufficient tooth structure and to maintain a healthy dentogingival unit (Figs 7-20 to 7-24).

References

1. Björn AC, Björn H, Erkovic B. Marginal fit of restorations and its relation to periodontal bone level, Part II: Crowns. *Odontol Rev.* 1970;21:337.
2. Leon AR. The periodontium and restorative procedures. *J Oral Rehabil.* 1977;4:105.
3. Ingraham R et al. *Der Goldguss.* Berlin: Quintessenz; 1968.
4. Ramfjord S. Periodontal aspects of restorative dentistry. *J Oral Rehabil.* 1974;1:107.
5. Silness J. Periodontal conditions in patients treated with dental bridges. The influence of full and partial crowns on plaque accumulation, development of gingivitis and pocket formation. *J Periodont Res.* 1970;5:219.
6. Sicher H. Changing concepts of the supporting dental structures. *Oral Surg.* 1959;12:31–35.
7. Schroeder HE, Listgarten RA. Fine structures of the developing epithelial attachment in human teeth. *Monographs in Developmental Biology.* Basel: S Karger; 1971:2.
8. Garguilo AW, Wentz FM, Orban B. Dimensions of the dento-gingival junction in humans. *J Periodontol.* 1961;32:261–267.
9. Ochsenbein C, Ross SE. A reevaluation of osseous surgery. *Dent Clin North Am.* 1969;13:87–102.
10. Björn AC, Björn H. Crkovic B. Marginal fit of restorations and its relation to periodontal bone level, Part I: Metal fillings. *Odontol Rev.* 1969;20:311.
11. Maynard JG Jr, Wilson RD. Physiologic dimensions of the periodontium significant to the restorative dentist. *J Periodontol.* 1979;50:170.
12. Ingber JS, Rose LF, Coslet JG. The biologic width concept in periodontics and restorative dentistry. *Alpha Omegan.* 1977;70:62.
13. Löe H, Ainamo J. Anatomical characteristics of the gingivae: A clinical and microscopic study of free and attached gingivae. *J Periodontol.* 1966;37:5–13.
14. Coslet JG, Vanarsdall RC, Weinsgold A. Diagnosis and classification of delayed eruption of the dento-gingival junction in the adult. *Alpha Omegan.* 1977.
15. Silness J. Periodontal conditions in patients treated with dental bridges: The relationship between the location of the crown margin and the periodontal condition. *J Periodont Res.* 1970;5:225.
16. Goldstein R. *Esthetics in Dentistry.* Philadelphia, Pa: JB Lippincott; 1976:338.
17. Newcomb GM. The relationship between the location of sublingual crown margins and gingival inflammation. *J Periodontol.* 1979;45:151.
18. Waerhaug J. Tissue reactions around artificial crowns. *J Periodontol.* 1983;54:172.
19. Kay HB. Esthetic considerations in the definite periodontal prosthetic management of the maxillary anterior segment. *Int J Periodont Rest Dent.* 1982;3:45.
20. Ingber J. Forced eruption, Part I: Methods of treating isolated one and two walls infrabony osseous defects: Rationale and case report. *J Periodontol.* 1974;45:199–206.
21. Langer B, Wagenberg BD. Methods of altering crestal levels: Clinical case report. *J Periodontol.* 1975;520–532.
22. Potasknick SR, Rosenberg ER. Forced eruption: Principles in periodontics and restorative dentistry. *J Prosthet Dent.* 1982;48:141–148.
23. Stein N, Becher A. Forced eruption: Biological and clinical considerations. *J Oral Rehabil.* 1980;7:395.
24. Ingber J. Forced eruption, Part II: Method of treating nonrestorable teeth: Periodontal and restorative considerations. *J Periodontol.* 1974;47:203.
25. Palomo F, Kopczyk R. Rationale and methods for tooth lengthening. *J Am Dent Assoc.* 1978;96:257–260.
26. Reitan K. Effects of force magnitude and direction of tooth movement on different alveolar bone types. *Angle Orthod.* 1964;34:244.
27. Reitan K. Clinical and histological observations on tooth movement during and after orthodontic treatment. *Am J Orthod.* 1967;55:721.
28. Reitan K. Biomechanical principles and reactions. In Graber TM (ed). *Current Orthodontic Concepts and Techniques.* Philadelphia, Pa: WB Saunders; 1969;1:56.
29. Polson A et al. Periodontal response after tooth movement into infrabony defects. *J Periodontol.* 1984;55:201.
30. Simon JH, Lythgoe et al. Extrusion of endodontically treated teeth. *J Am Dent Assoc.* 1978;97:17.
31. Oppenheim A. Artificial elongation of the teeth. *Am J Orthod Oral Surg.* 1940;26:931.
32. Pontoriero R, Celenza F Jr, Ricci G, Carnevale G. Rapid extrusion with fiber resection: A combined orthodontic–periodontic treatment modality. *Int J Periodont Rest Dent.* 1987;5:31–43.
33. Amsterdam M. *Graduate Seminar Series.* Philadelphia, Pa: University of Pennsylvania, School of Dental Medicine; 1969–1972.
34. Batenhorst KF, Bowen GM, Williams JE. Tissue changes resulting from facial tipping and extrusion of incisors in monkeys. *J Periodontol.* 1974;45:660.
35. Ochsenbein C, Ross SE. A re-evaluation of osseous surgery. *Dent Clin North Am.* 1969;13:87–102.

Chapter 8

Gingival Recessions

Giano Ricci

Introduction

A frequent occurrence in periodontal and nonperiodontal cases is the presence of localized gingival recession, which may jeopardize the patient's esthetics.

Definition

A gingival recession may be defined as the exposition of the radicular surface of the tooth due to the destruction of the marginal gingiva and of the epithelial attachment that will be reestablished at a more apical position. The recession may appear as a cleft of the gingival margin or may consist of the partial or complete loss of the gingiva on the radicular aspect of the tooth (Figs 8-1 and 8-2). A fenestration can be defined as the situation in which the buccal plate of bone is partially missing and part of the root is exposed but the marginal bone is intact (Fig 8-3). When the marginal bone is also missing, a dehiscence is present (Fig 8-4). In this case the root is just covered with soft tissue; therefore, it can be easy to have a recession in that area if plaque alone or plaque associated with trauma is present in the area.

Symptomatology

The symptomatology of the gingival recession may consist of dentinal hypersensitivity, marginal inflammation, root decay, pulpal pathology, and psychologic and esthetic problems, especially if the recession is present in the anterior region in a patient with a high smile line.

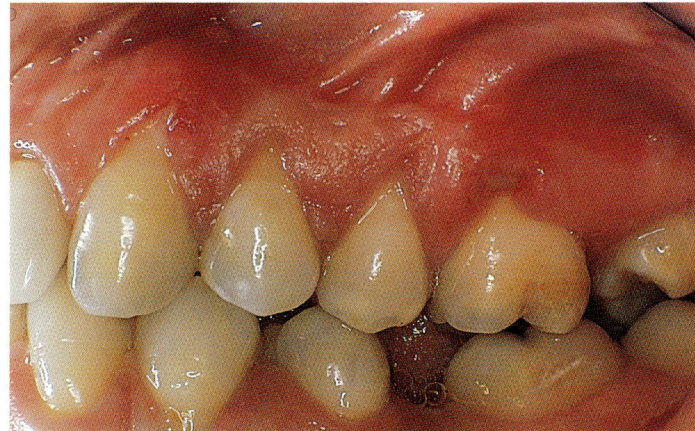

Fig 8-1 Deep and narrow localized gingival recession (clefts).

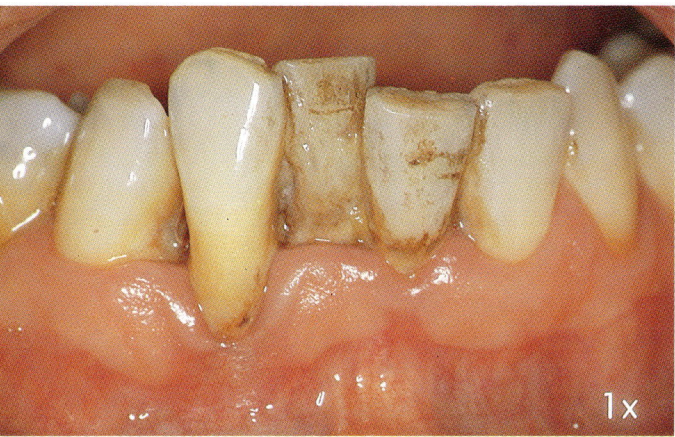

Fig 8-2 Large and shallow localized gingival recession in a case of advanced periodontitis.

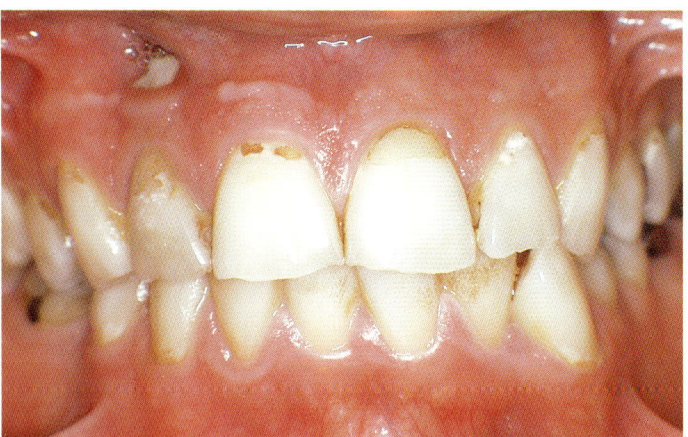

Fig 8-3　Fenestration.

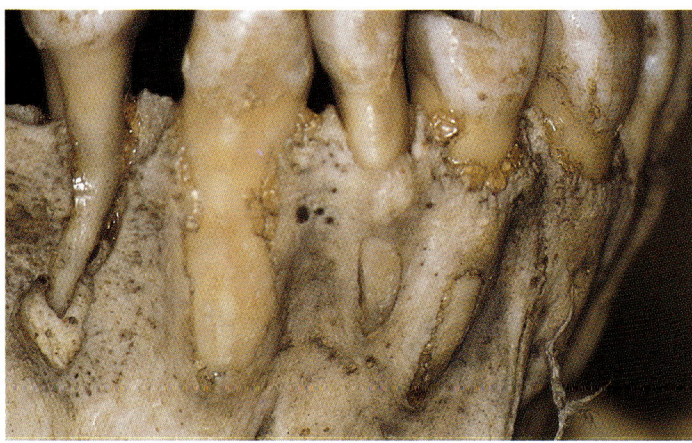

Fig 8-4　Dehiscences and fenestrations in a skull.

Etiology

The etiology of gingival recessions consists of determinant factors and cofactors (Table 8-1).

Table 8-1　Etiology of gingival recessions

Determinant factors	Cofactors
Bacterial plaque	Tooth malposition
Trauma from toothbrushing	Unfavorable anatomy
Iatrogenic factors	Occlusal trauma
Habits	Ortho movements

The most important of determinant factors is the bacterial plaque. O'Leary et al[1] found a direct correlation between the increase of plaque index and the increase of gingival recessions. Trauma from toothbrushing is another factor and it is frequently associated with erosion of the root's surface. This is the major etiologic factor in the establishment of gingival recessions in young patients who, in an effort to perform good oral hygiene, damage the gingival tissue by using an improper technique or a wrong toothbrush. The horizontal use of the toothbrush is one of the major causes of recessions on canines and premolars.[2] These lesions are frequently observed on the opposite side of the hand that the patient normally uses (left side for a right-handed person). Also, iatrogenic factors, such as amalgam or prosthetic overhangs, clasps, and orthodontic appliances that impinge on the soft tissue, can determine gingival recessions for mechanical aggression or because they facilitate the accumulation of plaque.

Procedures for impression taking, such as the improper use of a retraction cord and electrosurgery on a thin gingival tissue, can cause gingival recessions. The trauma induced by habits, such as toying with the soft tissues with fingernails or foreign objects, is also a cause. Tooth malposition, such as buccally displaced teeth or rotated teeth because of the altered tooth–bone relationship, may act as a cofactor in the onset of gingival recessions, as well as anatomic situations, such as high frenum insertions and a shallow buccal fold that will produce tension on the marginal gingiva. In the past gingival recessions have also been associated with trauma from occlusion,[3] but more recently this concept has been refuted.[4]

Pathogenesis

The pathogenesis of the recessions in most instances can be related to the presence of a localized inflam-

Historical rationale and treatment techniques

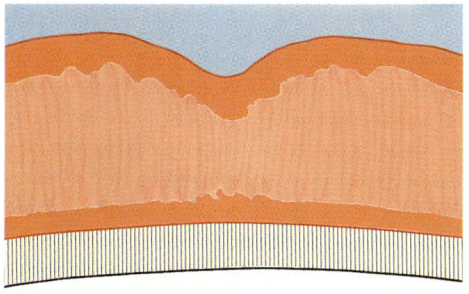 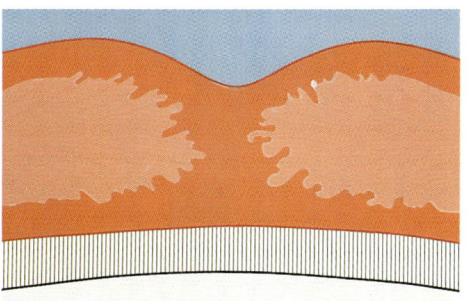 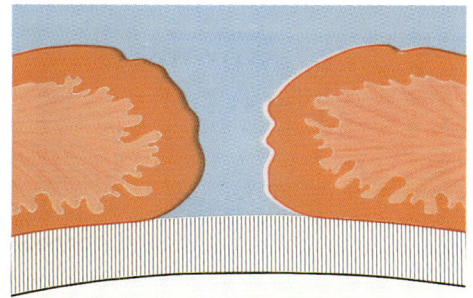

Figs 8-5a to c   Schematic representation of the pathogenesis of a gingival recession. The sulcular epithelium proliferates through the connective tissue and joins the oral epithelium. The epithelium undergoes necrosis and a recession is formed.

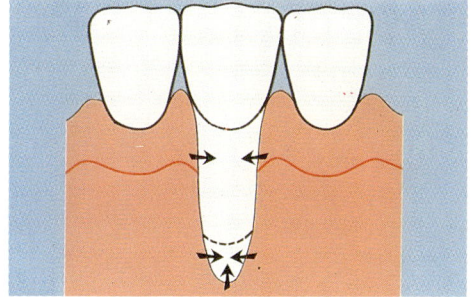 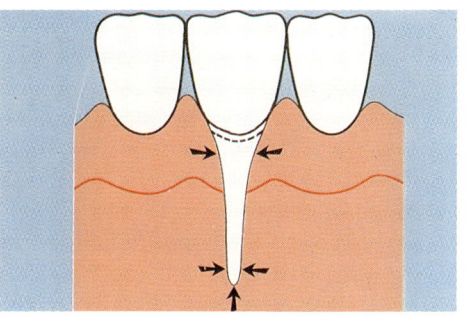 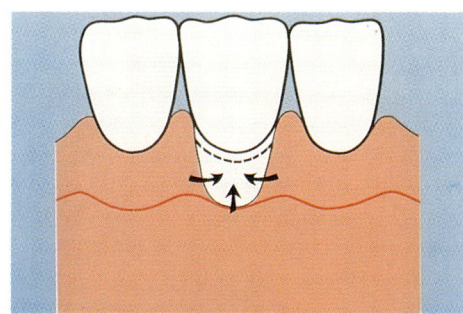

Fig 8-6a   Wide and deep recession.   Fig 8-6b   Narrow and deep recession.   Fig 8-6c   Wide and shallow recession.

Fig 8-6d   Narrow and shallow recession.

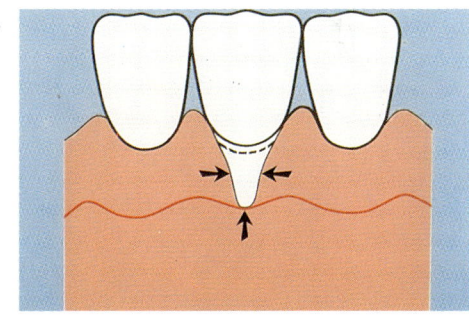

Figs 8-6a to d   Classification of gingival recessions according to Sullivan and Atkins. Arrows indicate the source of vascular proliferation for the establishment of vascular bridging to ensure taking of a graft.

mation that destroys the epithelium and the connective tissue. The epithelium tends to migrate through the connective tissue and, when the two epithelium layers meet, the recession occurs (Figs 8-5a to c). In the case of recession from brushing or from other habits, this recession takes place because of the trauma itself and no inflammation is present.

Historical rationale and treatment techniques

The predictability of the root coverage is much higher with the use of pedicles than with free grafts, especially in the presence of wide and deep defects according to the classification made by Sullivan and Atkins[5] (Figs 8-6a to d).

Gingival Recessions

Figs 8-7a to d   Split-thickness laterally positioned flap.

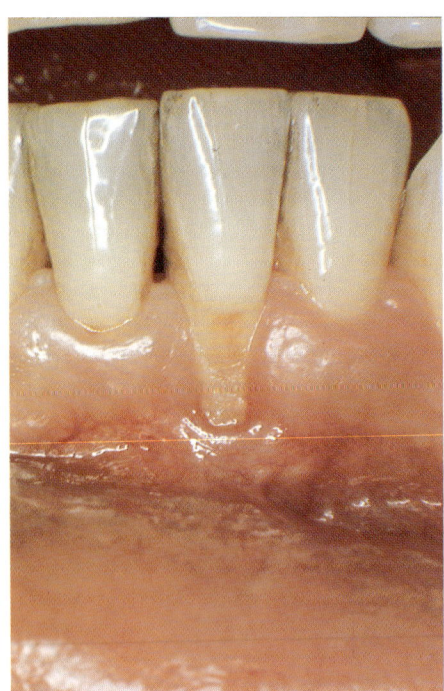

Fig 8-7a   Case of advanced periodontitis before treatment.

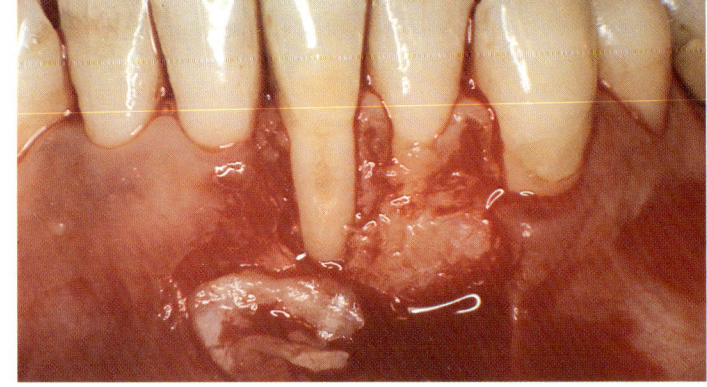

Fig 8-7b   Recipient site preparation. Note donor site covered by periosteum.

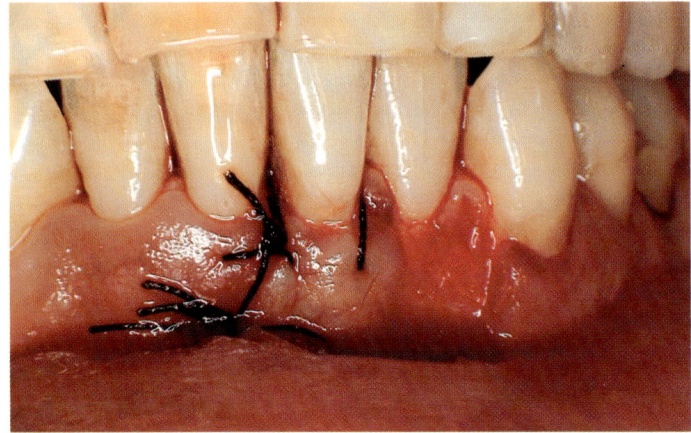

Fig 8-7c   Split-thickness flap sutured on the area of gingival recession.

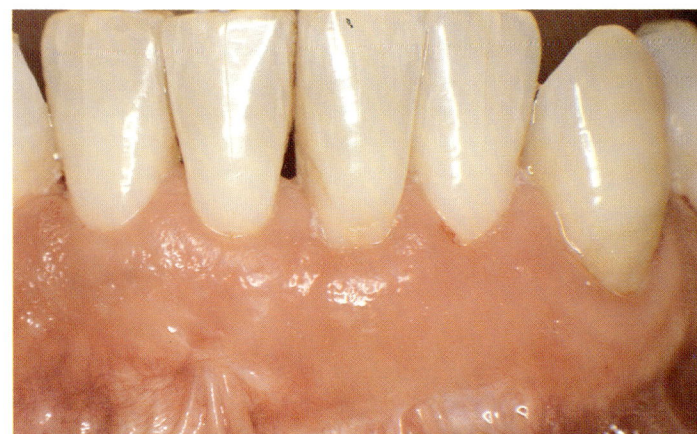

Fig 8-7d   Healing after 2 years.

More recently new techniques have been developed to take advantage of both procedures using a free connective tissue autograft, over which a pedicle is placed,[6,7] or by placing a connective tissue autograft in a mucosal pouch to provide better nourishment to the graft.[8] Root coverage may also be enhanced through a creeping attachment, a phenomenon by which the gingiva tends to migrate coronally through the years as long as the roots are plaque-free. After a year the average migration of attachment can be 0.46 to 0.89 mm.[9] This phenomenon is frequent with the use of free grafts but can also be noticed with pedicle grafts. Occasionally, a recession on the donor site of the pedicle can be noticed. For this reason Guinard and Caffesse[10] have proposed the use of a free graft to protect the donor site with good results. The same results can be obtained by using dura mater.[11]

To enhance the healing potential of a pedicle over the root, Goldman and Smukler[12] proposed the transfer of a full-thickness flap with stimulated periosteum. The procedure consists of irritating and therefore stimulating the cellular proliferation at the donor site with a needle 20 days before transferring a full-thickness pedicle graft over the denuded root. The results of this technique have yet to be proven.

Therapeutic possibilities

The type of therapy of gingival recessions depends on the quality and quantity of gingiva that is present near the area of recession. If there is an adequate zone of attached gingiva that can be used, it is possible to perform a surgical procedure that will consist of the following:

1. Laterally positioned flap (partial-thickness, full-thickness, and mixed-thickness).
2. Double papilla flap.
3. Coronally positioned flap.

When an adequate zone of attached gingiva is not present in the surrounding area, it is then possible to use the following:

1. Free gingival graft.
2. Free gingival graft and coronally positioned flap.
3. Free connective tissue graft (envelope technique).
4. Free connective tissue graft and pedicle (subpedicle connective tissue graft).

Laterally positioned flap

The first surgical approach to the therapy of isolated gingival recession has been proposed by Groupe and Warren.[13] The technique (Figs 8-7a to d) consists of the following steps:

1. Preparation of the exposed root with scaling, root planing, use of chemicals, and flattening of the root curvature.
2. Incision and removal of a thin band of marginal gingiva around the recession, exposure, and preparation of a firm periosteal bed to allow perfect adaptation between the pedicle and the recipient site.
3. Exposure and stimulation of periodontal ligament.

Gingival Recessions

Figs 8-8a to f Full-thickness laterally positioned flap. Protection of donor site with microfibrillar collagen.

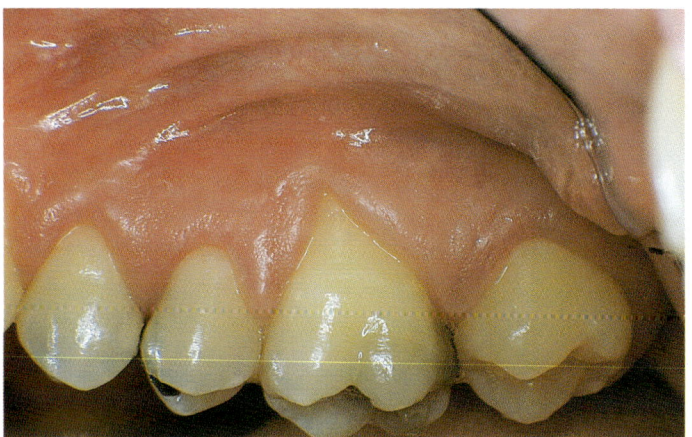

Fig 8-8a Initial lesion.

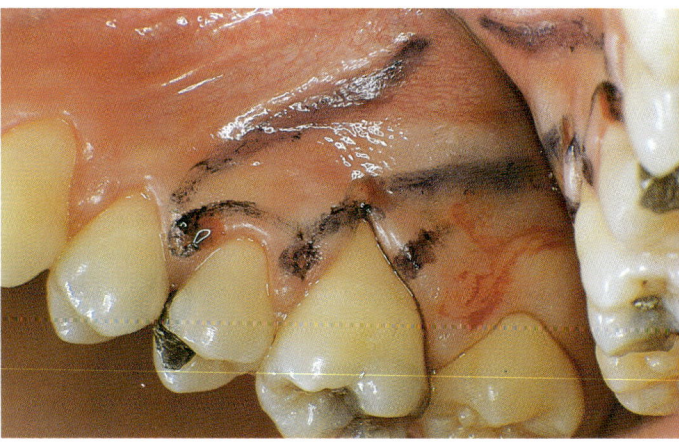

Fig 8-8b Outline of flap design.

4. Full-thickness flap including the marginal gingiva with vertical incisions oriented toward the base of the defect raised from the donor site. The base of the pedicle must correspond to the recipient site. If tension is present on the pedicle, a horizontal incision can be added to the vertical incisions (cut back).
5. Full-thickness flap is sutured in the most coronal position on the recipient site.
6. Protection of the donor site with a split-thickness flap, a free gingival graft, dura mater, or microfibrillar collagen (Figs 8-8a to f).

Therapeutic possibilities

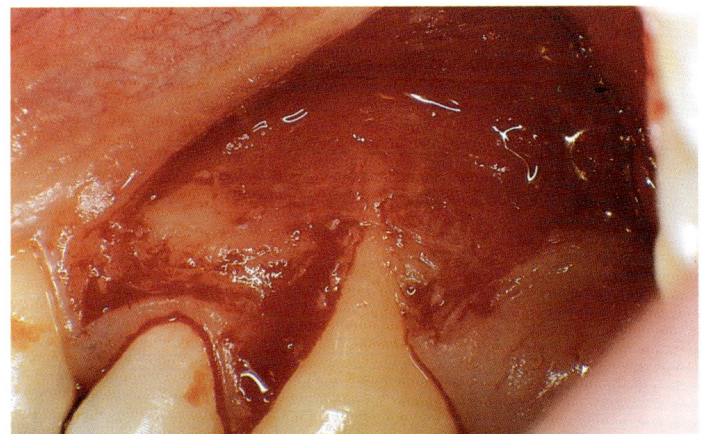

Fig 8-8c Recipient site prepared (note exposed bone on donor site).

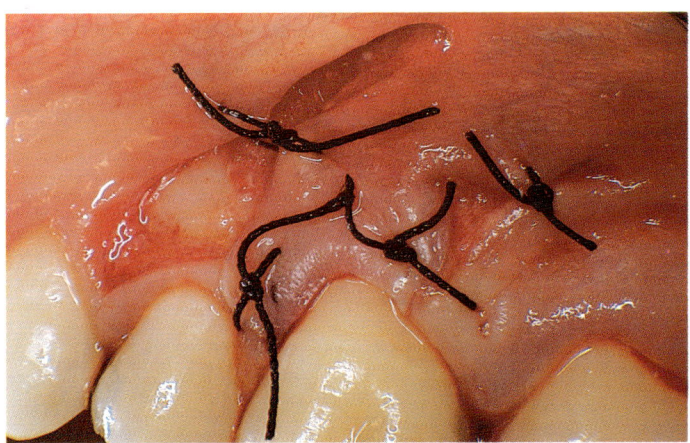

Fig 8-8d Flap sutured.

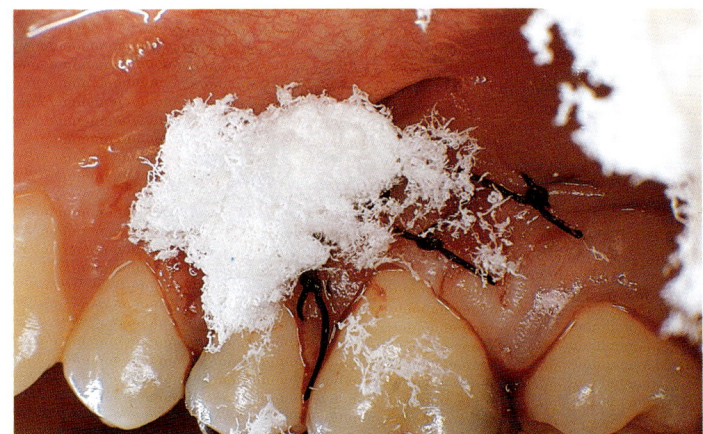

Fig 8-8e Donor site protected with microfibrillar collagen.

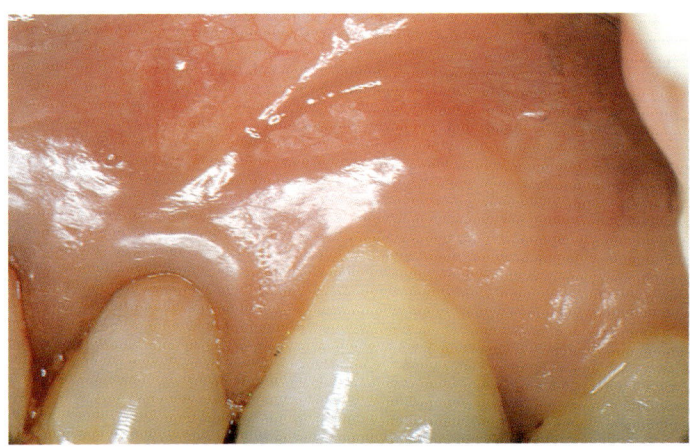

Fig 8-8f Healing after 5 years.

Figs 8-9a to f Split-thickness laterally positioned flap and root preparation with citric acid.

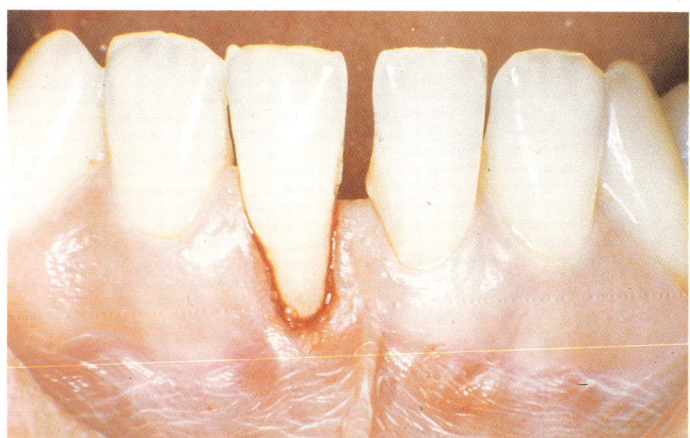

Fig 8-9a Initial lesion after curettage.

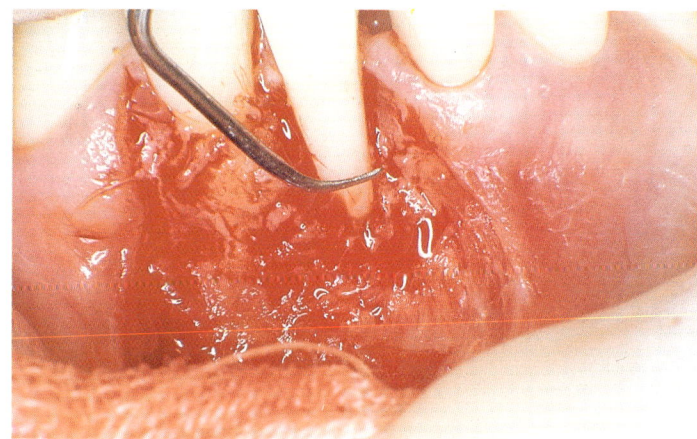

Fig 8-9b Root preparation with a curette.

This last step was later added to the original procedure proposed by Groupe and Warren.[13]

Root preparation at the recipient site is a critical step in improving the rate of success of root coverage. To obtain maximum root coverage, Aleo et al[14] proposed the use of phenol to remove all the toxins that may be present from the root surface. Register and Burdick[15] suggested the use of citric acid to be applied to the root surface to expose collagen fibers from cementum or dentin, which should then anastomose with the collagen fibers of the flap (Figs 8-9a to f). Tetracycline application has been proposed for the same reason, whereas fibronectin applied to the root should also enhance the possibility of root coverage by facilitating the attachment of

Therapeutic possibilities

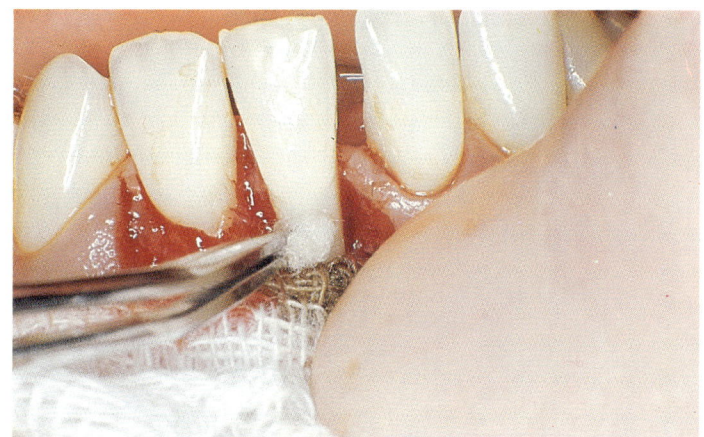

Fig 8-9c   Root preparation with citric acid.

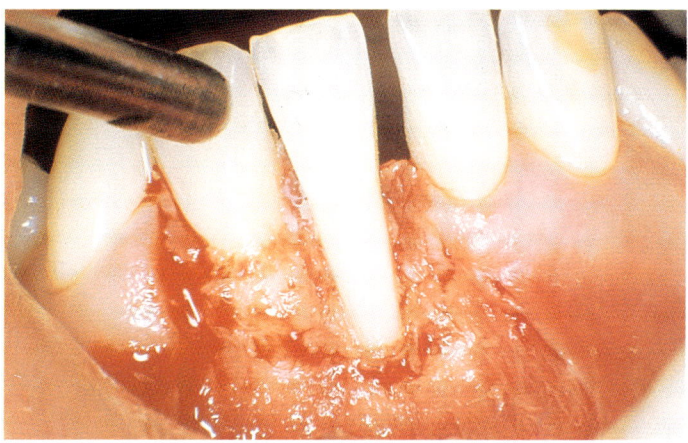

Fig 8-9d   Preparation of donor and recipient site completed.

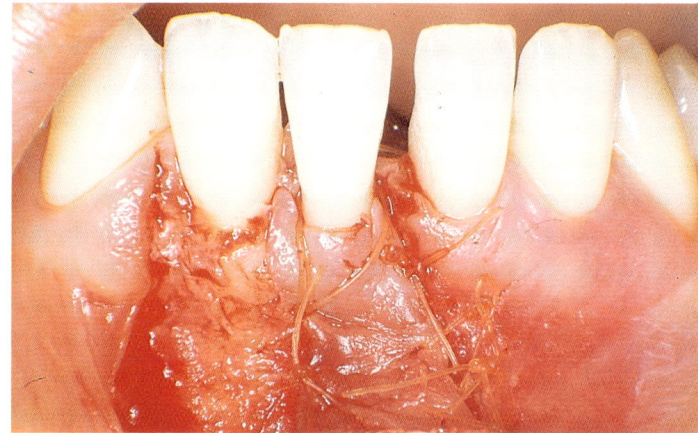

Fig 8-9e   Flap sutured.

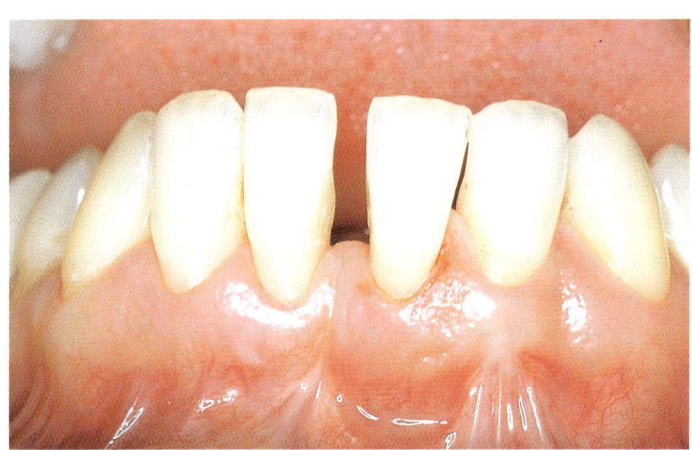

Fig 8-9f   Healing after 5 years.

Figs 8-10a to e   Split-thickness laterally positioned flap and protection of donor site with dura mater.

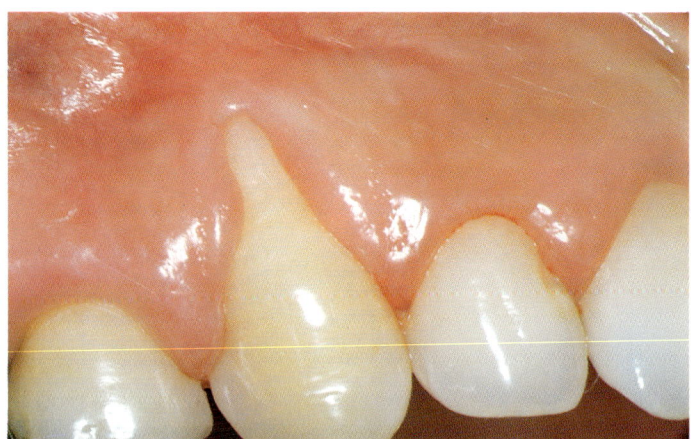

Fig 8-10a   Initial lesion.

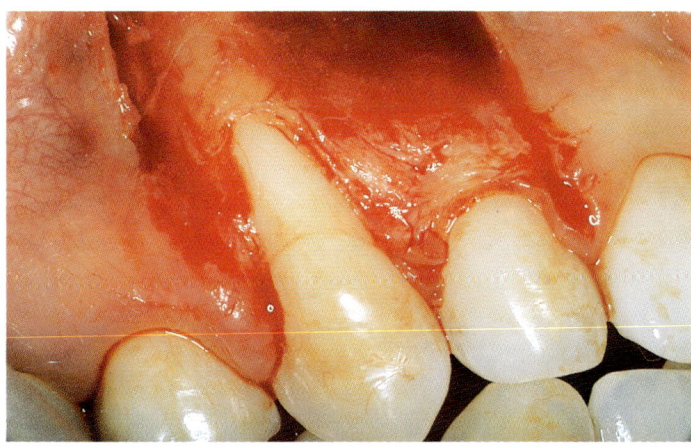

Fig 8-10b   Split-thickness flap is raised from adjacent area.

fibroblast to the root. The morphology of the root surface plays an important role in the final result. Because it is known that the potential for repair depends for the most part on the periodontal ligament cells of the recipient site and because it is also known that they can migrate for about 2 mm in a mesiodistal or an apicocoronal direction, the area that can be covered with a pedicle cannot exceed an area of 4 mm^2.

The original technique suggested by Groupe and Warren[13] was to utilize a full-thickness flap and to take the marginal gingiva from the donor site. This could cause gingival recession on the area. To avoid this problem, Staffileno[16] proposed the utilization of a split-thickness flap leaving the periosteum to cover the donor site, but it has been shown that the healing following the use of a split-thickness flap is more difficult and of different quality when compared with the healing obtained with a full-thickness flap.[17]

With the same objective, Ruben et al[18] proposed the use of a mixed-thickness flap where a full-thickness flap is moved over the defect, a partial-thickness flap covers the donor site, and the area from which the split-thickness flap is taken is covered by the periosteum.

To prevent recession, a submarginal flap rather than a marginal one from the donor site can be used. Espinel and Caffesse[19] proposed instead the use of a free graft to protect the donor site and they showed that no gingival recession occurs on the donor site. The same favorable results can be obtained with the use of dura (Figs 8-10a to e).

As a consequence of all the modifications introduced to the original technique proposed by Groupe and Warren,[13] today the use of a laterally positioned flap to cover a denuded root is considered a predictable surgical procedure with no undesirable consequences on the donor site.

Therapeutic possibilities

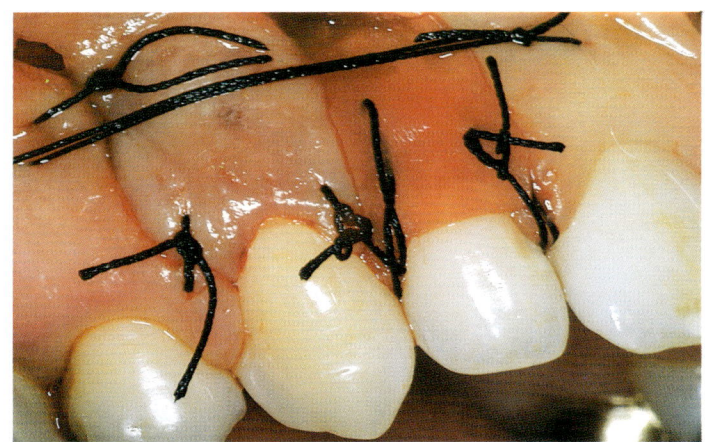

Fig 8-10c Flap sutured over recession and protection of donor site with dura.

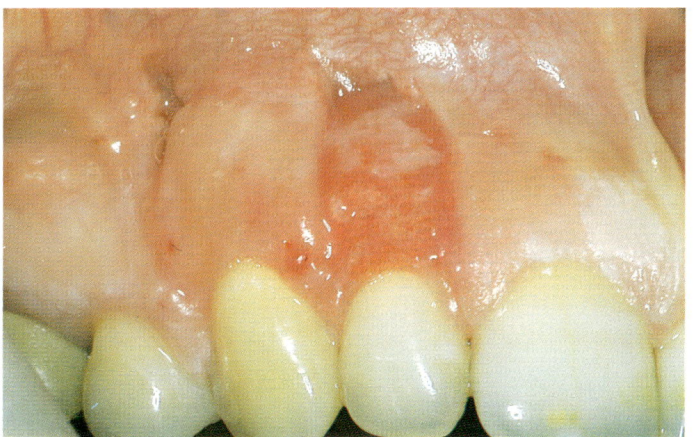

Fig 8-10d Healing after 10 days.

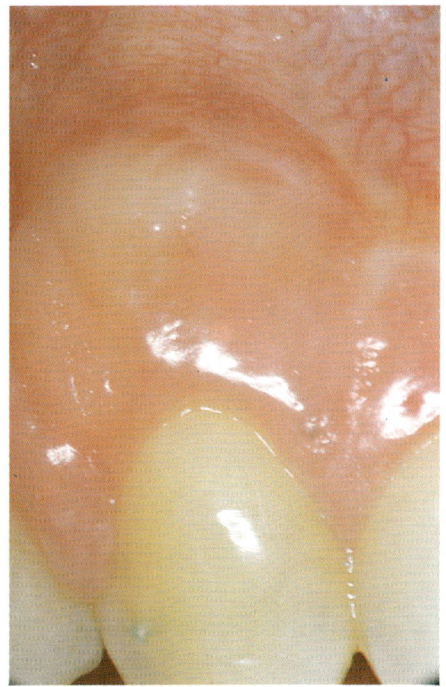

Fig 8-10e Result after 1 year.

Figs 8-11a to d   Double papilla flap.

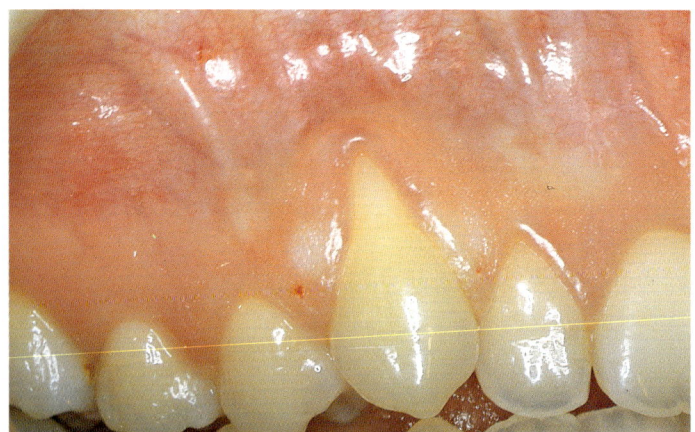

Fig 8-11a   The defect at the time of surgery.

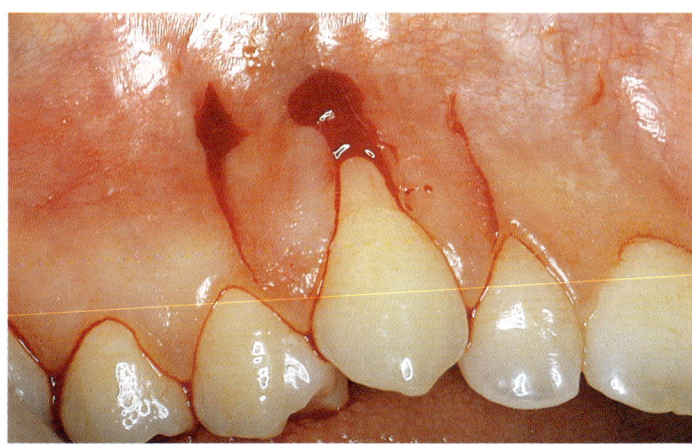

Fig 8-11b   Flap design. The two adjacent papillae are undermined and ready to be transferred.

Double papilla flap

The double papilla flap procedure was proposed in 1968 by Cohen and Ross[20] to increase the zone of attached gingiva or to obtain root coverage. This type of surgical approach requires the presence of interdental papillae of adequate dimension adjacent to the root that needs to be treated. The advantage of this procedure results in minimal, if any, exposure of the radicular surface on the donor site favoring the wound healing process and causing minimum damage. The disadvantage consists of difficulties in the surgical manipulation, especially at the time of suturing, because of the limited dimension of the two papillae. This, in turn, may lead to an inadequate thickness of the connective tissue just in the area of maximum convexity of the root during the healing process, therefore causing a recurrence of the lesion. For this reason, the double papilla flap procedure to cover exposed roots should be performed by an expert clinician who has selected the case carefully (Figs 8-11a to d).

Therapeutic possibilities

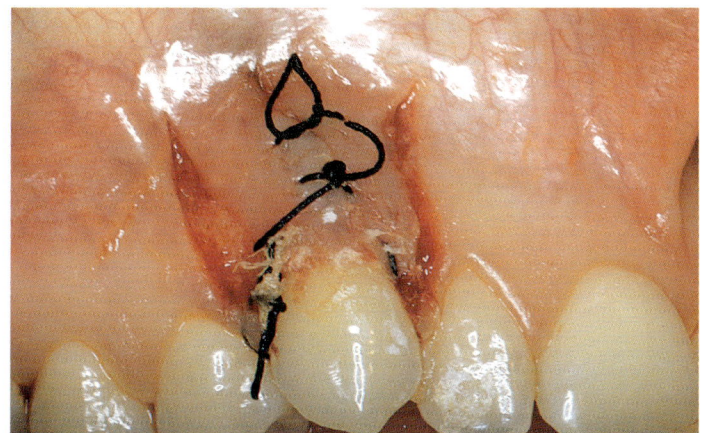

Fig 8-11c Flap adapted and sutured on recipient site. Note that cyanoacrylate has also been used coronally to better stabilize the flap.

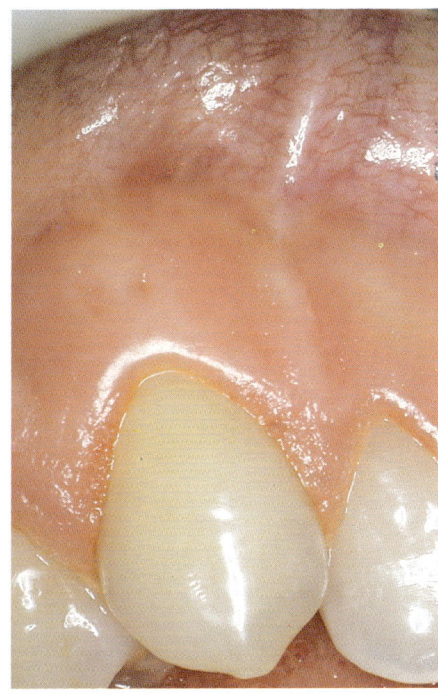

Fig 8-11d Healing after 6 months.

Figs 8-12a to f   Coronally positioned flap.

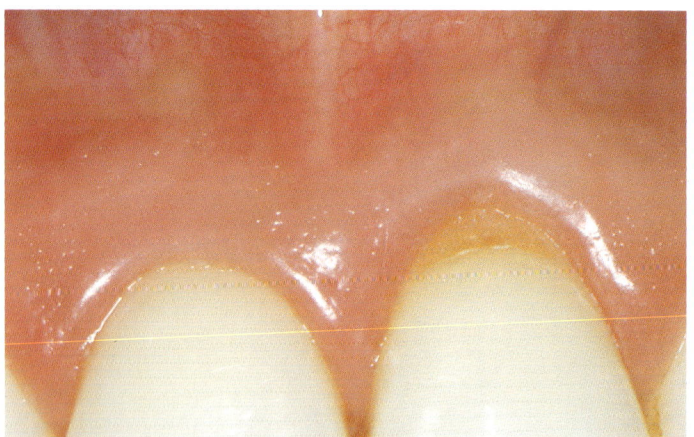

Fig 8-12a   Initial defect. Note the uneven level of gingiva causing big esthetic problems to a young patient with a high smile line.

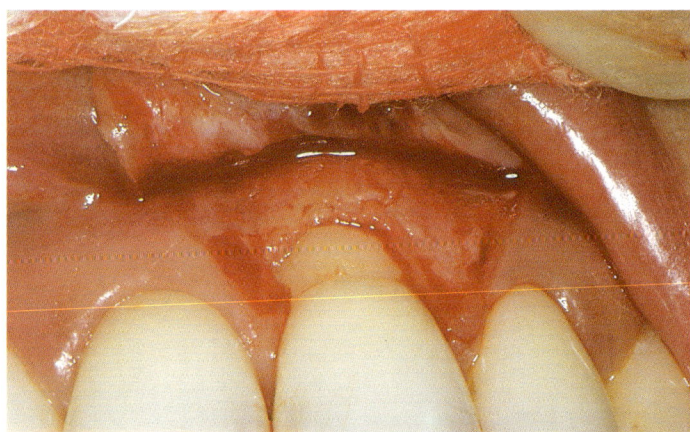

Fig 8-12b   A full-thickness flap is raised.

Coronally positioned flap

Norsberg in 1926 was the first to suggest the use of coronally positioned flaps to solve esthetic problems in the anterior region. Kalmi et al[21] in 1949 and Nordenram and Landt[22] in 1969 introduced modifications to the original method, but the predictability of results was questionable because of inadequate blood supply for large flaps. Harvey[23] and Restrepo[24] suggested the use of the coronally positioned flap for the treatment of isolated recessions. The flap is a full-thickness flap that is moved coronally and sutured in this position (Figs 8-12a to f).

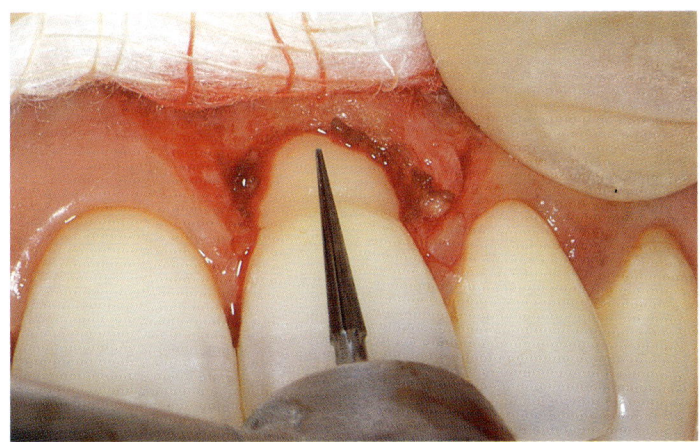

Fig 8-12c The cementoenamel junction is flattened with a carbide bur to facilitate flap adaptation.

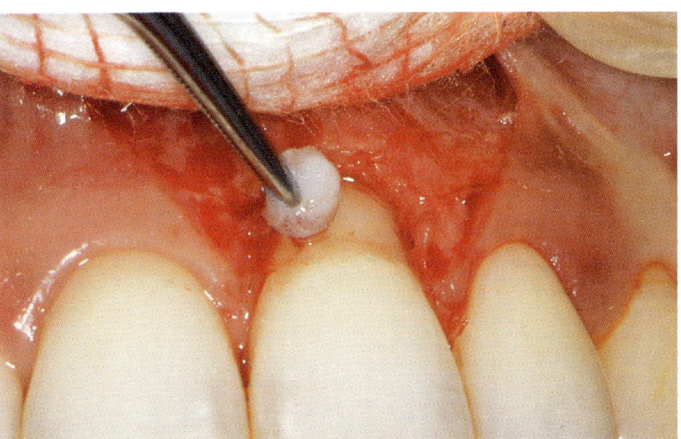

Fig 8-12d Root conditioning with citric acid.

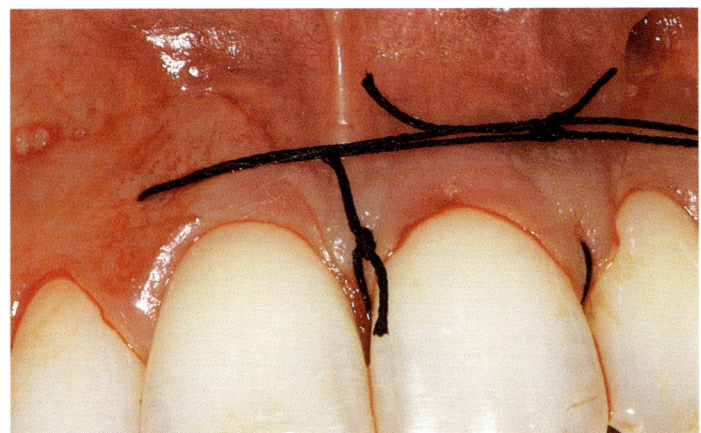

Fig 8-12e Flap sutured. The horizontal suture keeps the flap in close approximation with root surface.

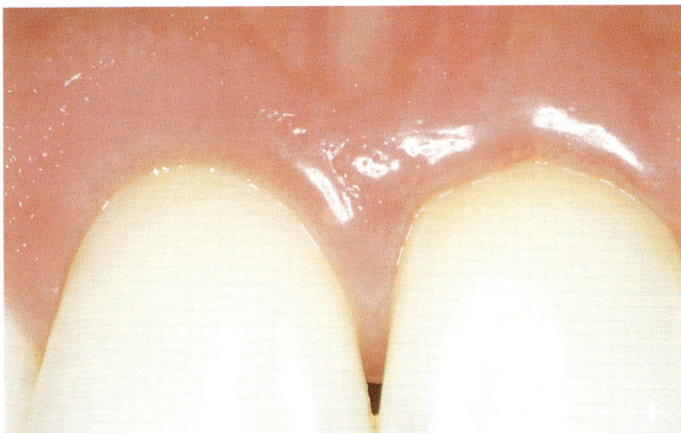

Fig 8-12f The result after 3 months. The gingival margins are now even.

Gingival Recessions

Figs 8-13a to c Free gingival graft.

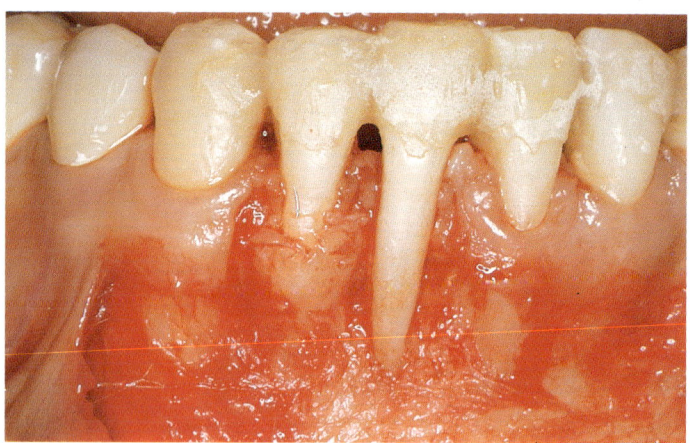

Fig 8-13a Gingival recession in a postorthodontic case. Teeth have been splinted temporarily.

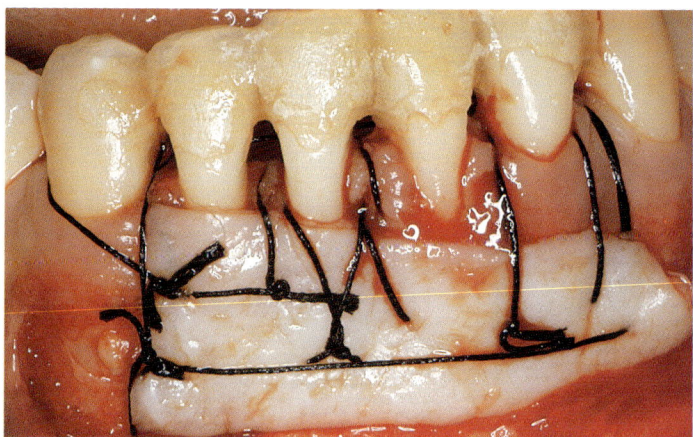

Fig 8-13b Free graft placed on denuded root.

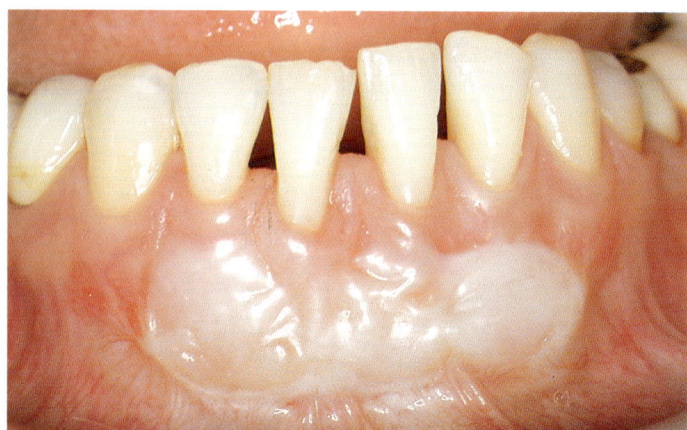

Fig 8-13c Healing with almost complete root coverage after 5 years. Temporary splint has been removed.

Figs 8-14a and b "Bridging" phenomenon.

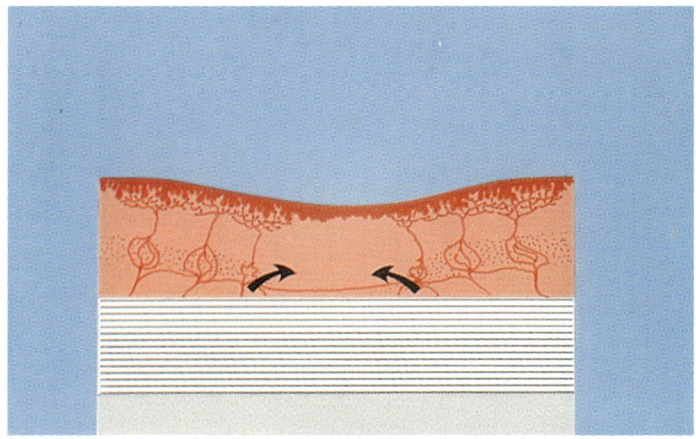

Fig 8-14a The area with no vascularization is small; therefore, the free gingival graft can survive.

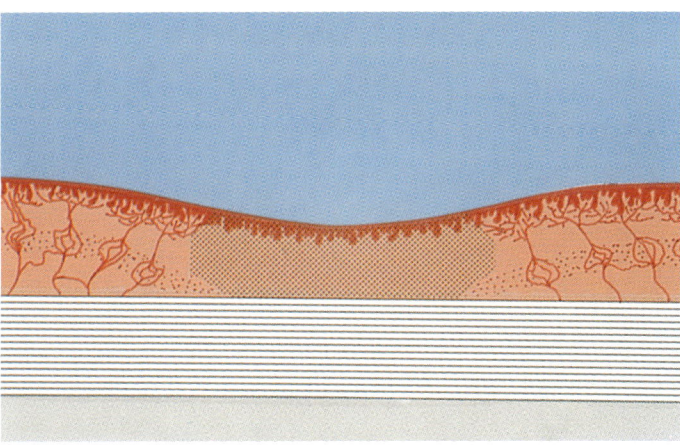

Fig 8-14b If the area of no vascularization is larger, the free graft will undergo necrosis in the central part (dotted area).

Free gingival graft

In 1966 Nabers[25] proposed the use of free gingival grafts in the treatment of gingival recessions. Sullivan and Atkins[5] described the possibility of obtaining root coverage by using this technique (Figs 8-13a to c). According to their classification, the best results could be obtained in cases in which narrow defects were present because collateral circulation could be easily provided. In such cases positive results have been reported by several investigators.[26-32] When areas of wide and deep recession are present, the rate of success in root coverage decreases dramatically because the survival of the graft depends on the "bridging" phenomenon. This consists of the formation of vascular bridges from the vascular portion of the recipient site. The wider the recession, the less likely is the formation of a new vascular network over the denuded root (Figs 8-14a and b). Following completion of healing, a coronal migration of the free gingival margin can occur as a result of the creeping attachment mechanism.

Creeping attachment occurs more frequently in the presence of narrow recession, high interproximal bone levels, and absence of tooth malpositioning and good plaque control.[33]

Miller and Cimasoni[34] and Holbrook and Ochsenbein[35] showed that by using different surgical modifications and additions to the traditional technique, such as extensive root planing to reduce root convexity, the use of a graft 1.5 to 2.0 mm thick, and different types of suturing techniques, predictably favorable results can be obtained even in the presence of wide and deep recessions.

Figs 8-15a to f   Free graft and coronally positioned flap.

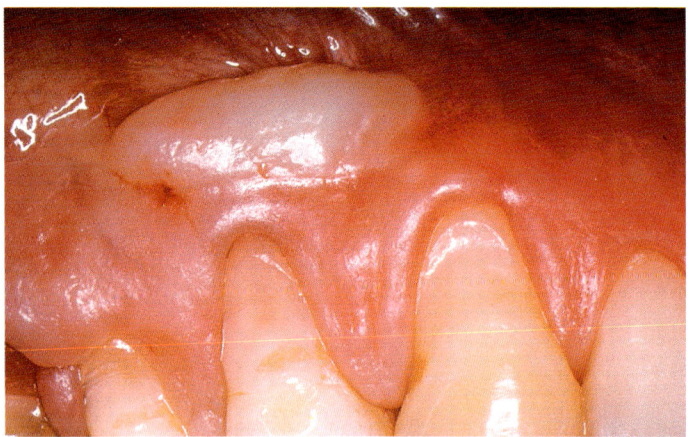

Fig 8-15a   Surgical site before the coronally positioned flap. A free graft had been previously performed to increase the amount of attached gingiva.

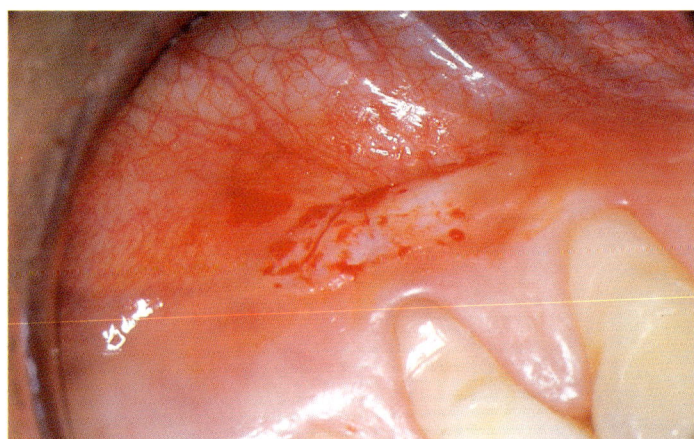

Fig 8-15b   A plasty of the area is first performed.

Free graft and coronally positioned flap

In cases in which there is not an adequate zone of attached gingiva to be moved coronally, Harvey,[23] Bernimoulin,[36] and Caffesse and Guinard[37,38] proposed a two-stage procedure in which an increase of the zone of attached gingiva is first obtained through a free gingival graft and, at a later time, the newly formed tissue is moved to a more coronal position (Figs 8-15a to f).

Free connective tissue graft (the envelope technique)

This technique, recently proposed by Raetzke,[8] consists of a bilaminar procedure by which a connective tissue graft is placed over the exposed root inside an envelope, previously created by undermining with a partial-thickness incision the tissues surrounding the defect. The wound healing mechanism of this surgical procedure is based on maximal blood supply to the graft from the surrounding tissues and a decreased tendency for graft shrinkage.

Advantages

The advantages of this method consist of minimal surgical trauma at recipient site, minor surface wound at donor site, and good esthetic appearance because the graft matches the surrounding tissues well.

Indications

The indications are the treatment of localized areas of recession with or without sufficient keratinized and attached gingiva or areas of recession next to crown margins in cases in which the prosthesis is considered adequate (Figs 8-16 and 8-17).

Therapeutic possibilities

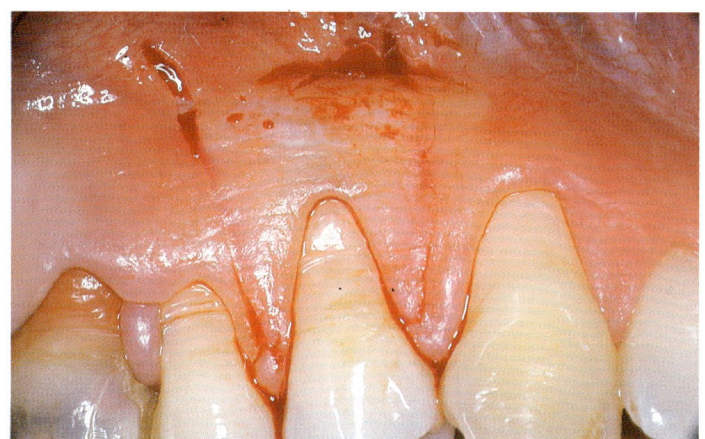

Fig 8-15c Vertical incisions are made without jeopardizing the adjacent areas.

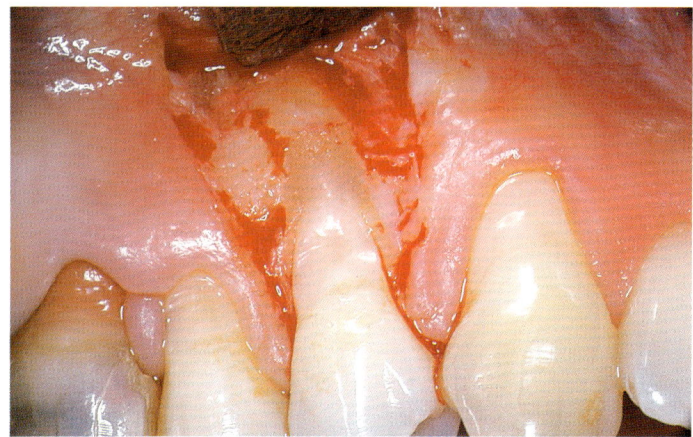

Fig 8-15d A full-thickness flap is raised.

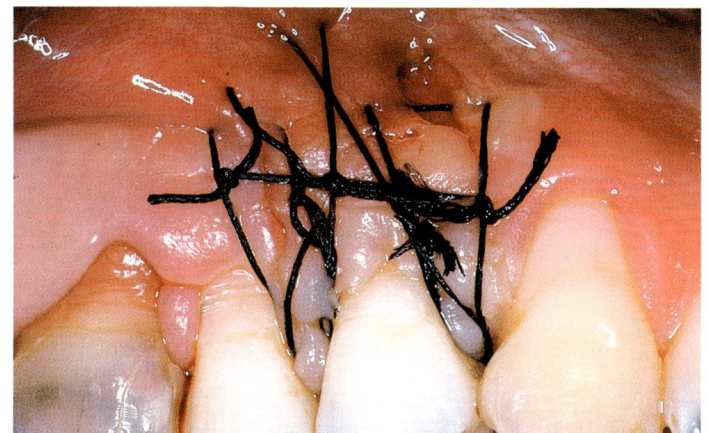

Fig 8-15e Different types of sutures maintain the flap in close approximation to root surface.

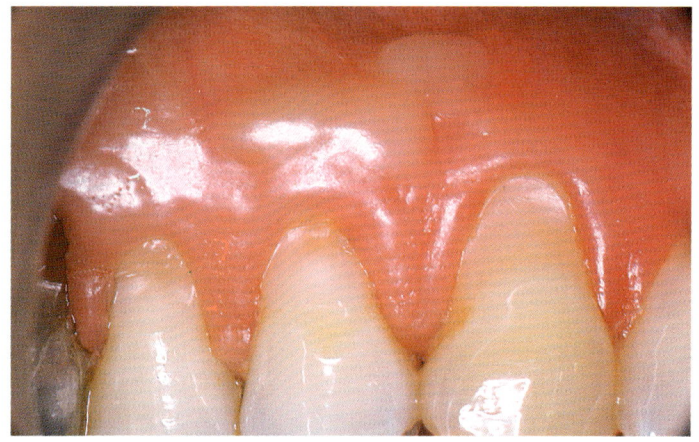

Fig 8-15f The result after 1 year.

Gingival Recessions

Figs 8-16a to j The envelope technique.

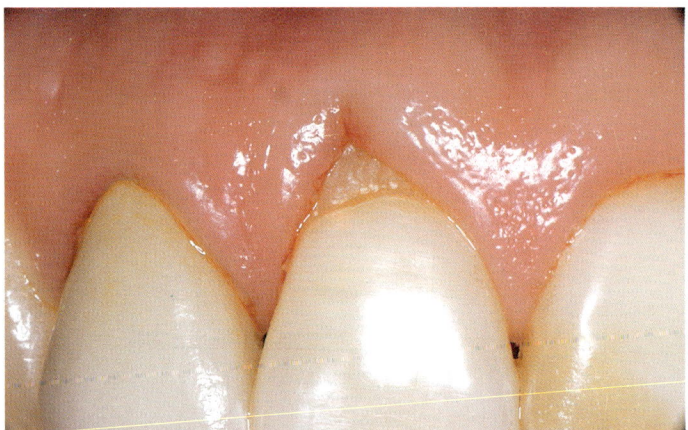

Fig 8-16a Localized gingival recession. Note the uneven gingival margins.

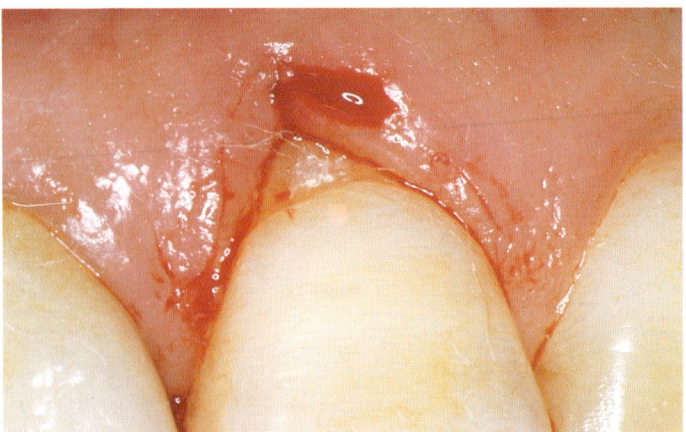

Fig 8-16b Incision of marginal tissue of recipient site.

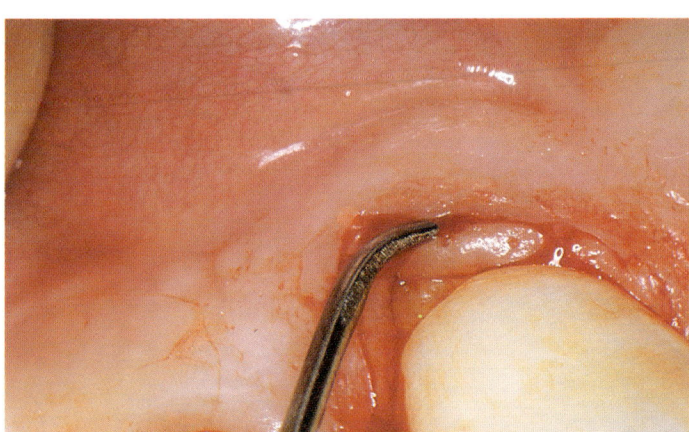

Fig 8-16c Collar of marginal tissue is excised.

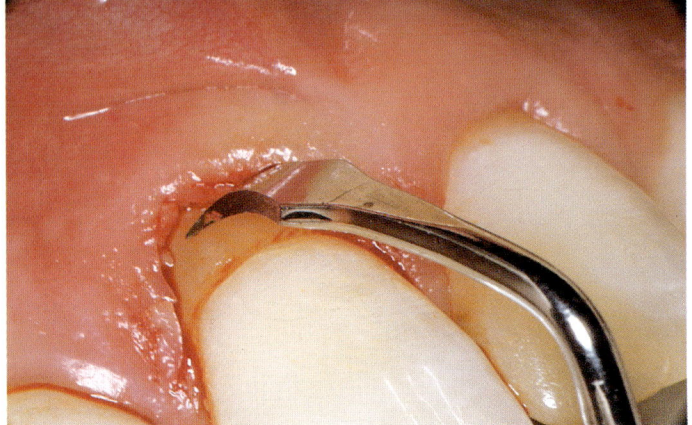

Fig 8-16d Root is debrided and planed.

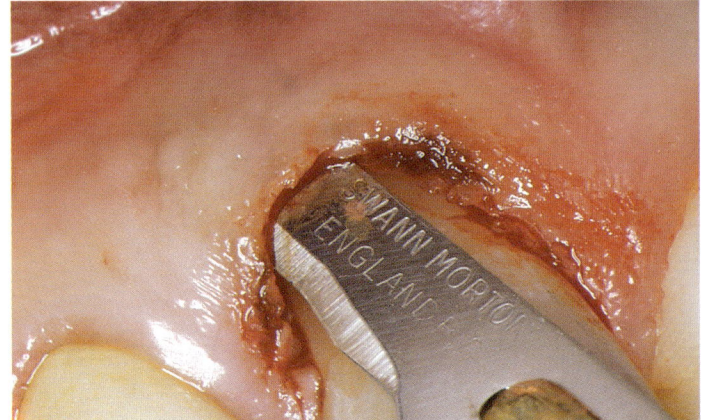

Fig 8-16e Undermining partial-thickness incision to create the "envelope."

Therapeutic possibilities

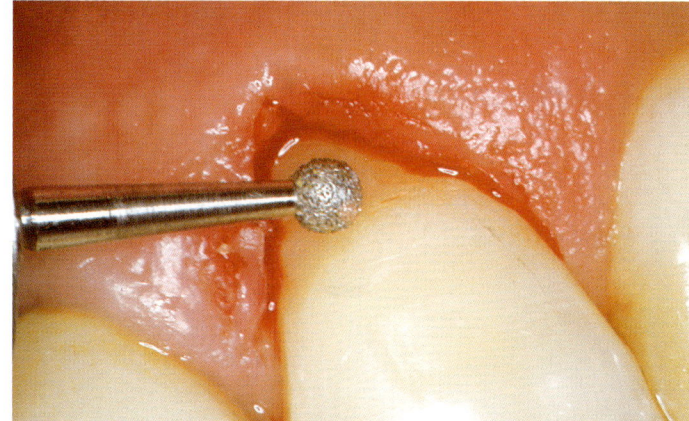

Fig 8-16f The cementoenamel junction is flattened to facilitate flap adaptation.

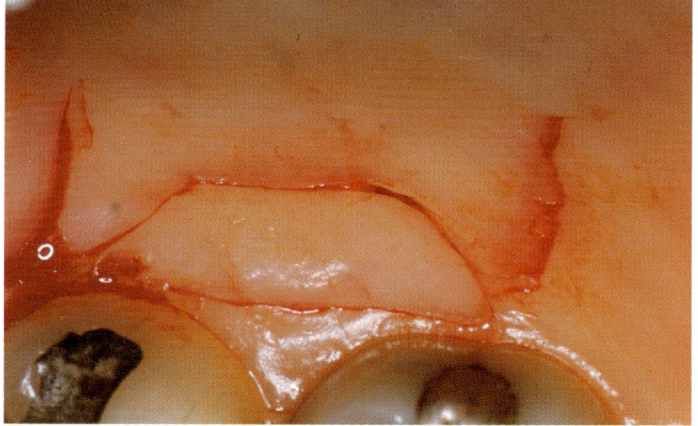

Fig 8-16g Connective tissue wedge is removed from the palatal side.

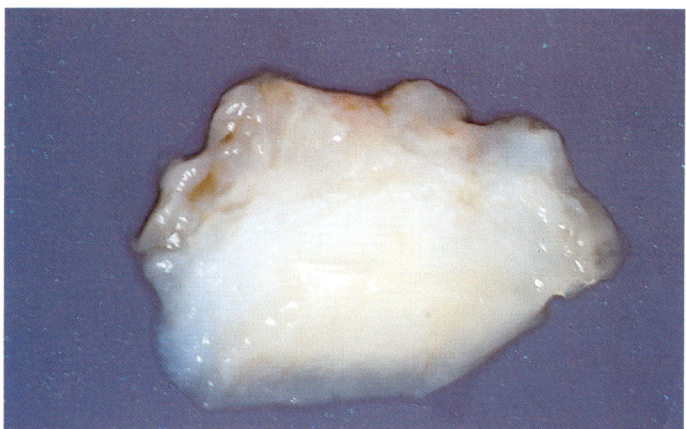

Fig 8-16h Graft before suturing. Note that epithelium has been left on the marginal part.

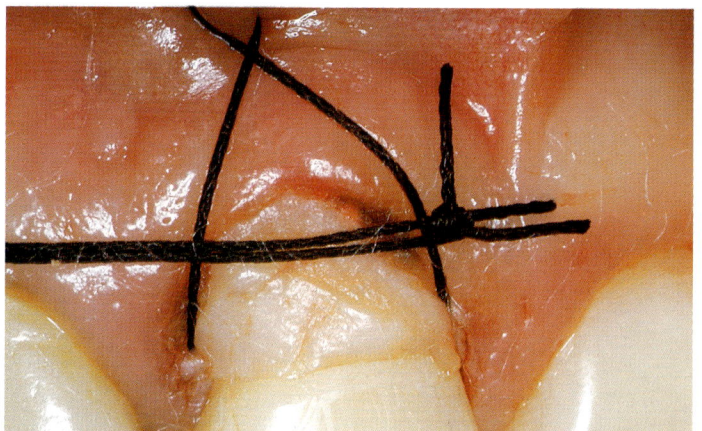

Fig 8-16i Graft sutured to get close approximation with root surface.

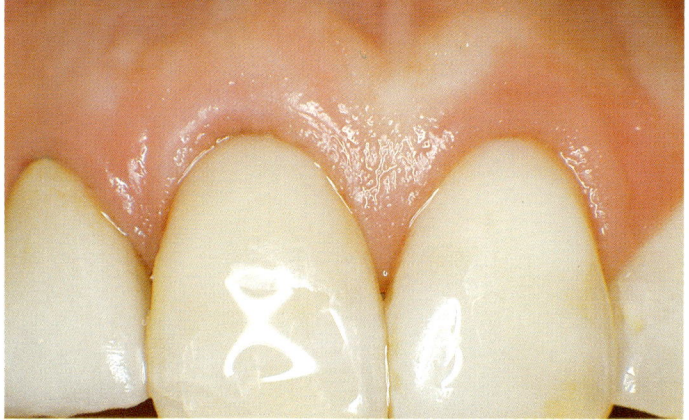

Fig 8-16j Final result after reshaping of crown on cervical area.

Gingival Recessions

Figs 8-17a to d   The envelope technique. Courtesy of Dr Bianchessi.

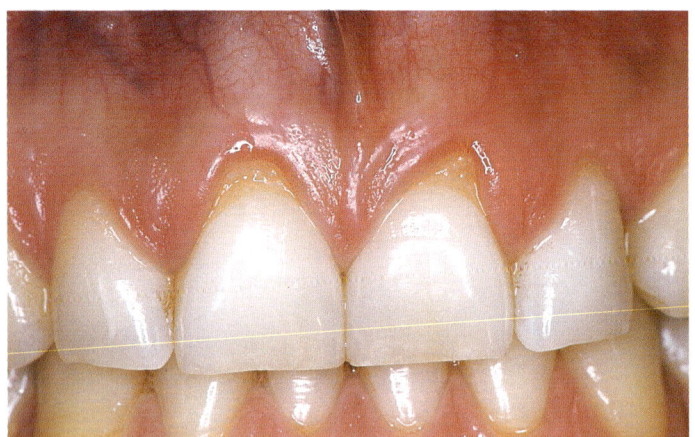

Fig 8-17a   Localized recessions causing esthetic problems in a patient with a high smile line.

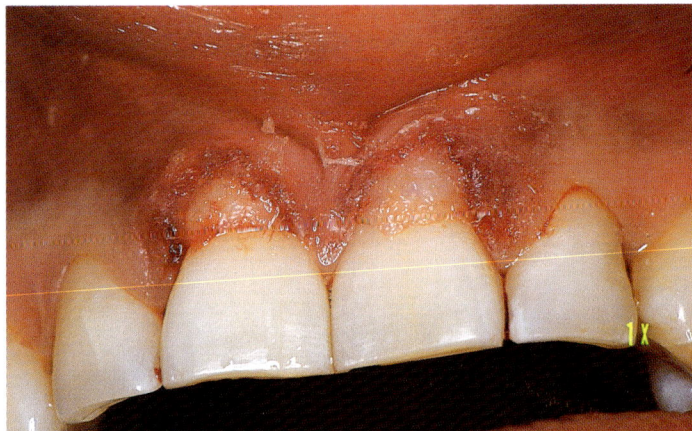

Fig 8-17b   Graft adapted and kept on recipient site with cyanoacrylate.

Therapeutic possibilities

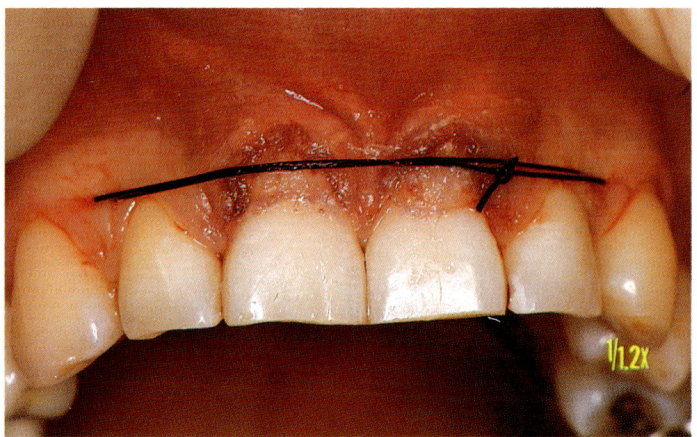

Fig 8-17c Graft sutured.

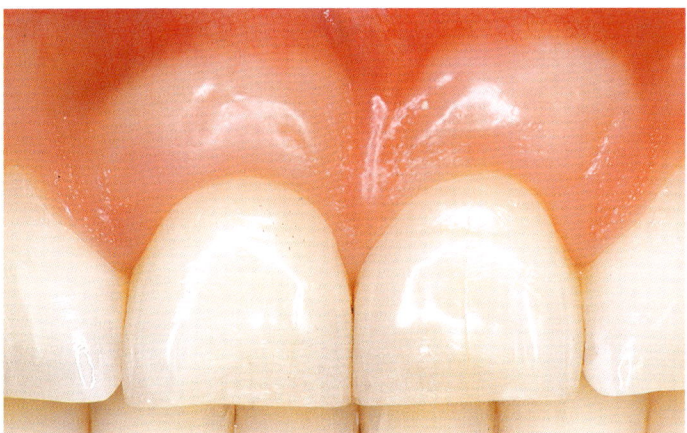

Fig 8-17d Final result after 5 months.

Subpedicle connective tissue graft

This mucogingival grafting procedure has been recently developed and proposed by Langer[6] and Nelson[7] to cover denuded root surfaces. The subpedicle connective tissue graft is a bilaminar graft that is composed of a free connective tissue graft and an overlying pedicle graft. This technique allows survival of that section of the free graft that covers the denuded root surface by supplying an adequate plasmatic circulation from capillaries of the pedicle. The subpedicle connective tissue graft is a delicate operation that requires careful attention. The connective tissue graft should be 1.5 to 2.0 mm thick, the interdental papilla should be retained in the pedicle graft, the pedicle should be positioned over the area of maximal convexity of the root to be covered, and adequate follow-up care should be performed (Figs 8-18a to f).

Advantages

This method has the advantage of being a single-stage procedure that allows covering of the denuded root surface in a predictable way when there is inadequate keratinized gingiva for a pedicle and when the prognosis is poor for root coverage with a free gingival graft.

Indications

This probably provides the best kind of mucogingival grafts in cases of advanced gingival recession in which there is thin gingiva and thin radicular bone on the adjacent teeth.

Gingival Recessions

Figs 8-18a to f The subpedicle connective tissue graft.

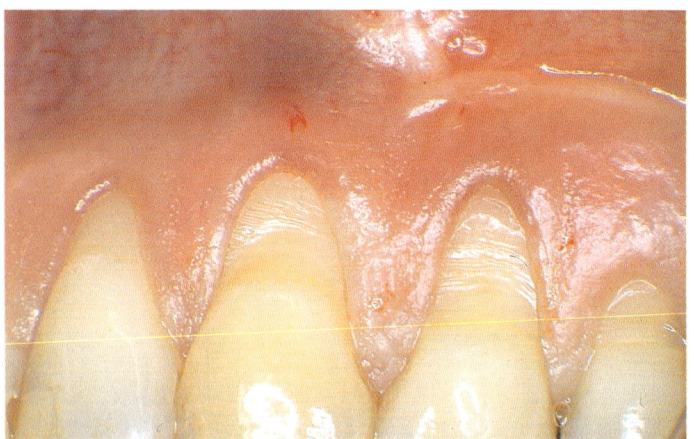

Fig 8-18a Gingival recessions in the anterior region with sensitivity and esthetic problems in a young woman.

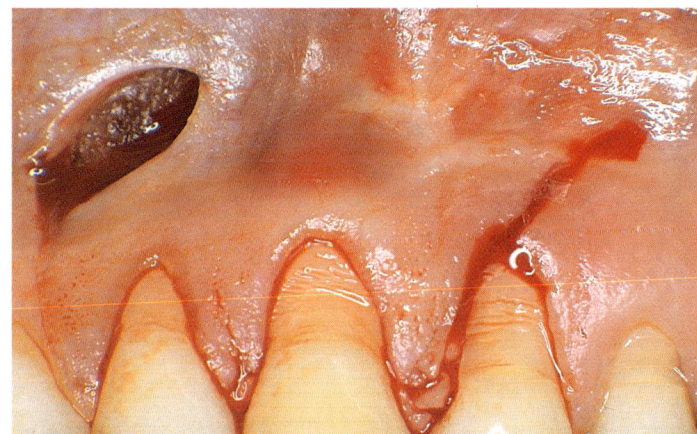

Fig 8-18b Flap incision.

Conclusion

In summary, today the clinician has several therapeutic possibilities and different surgical techniques available. It is through the selection of the appropriate technique, along with proper evaluation of the potential for repair of the surgical site, that the clinician can accomplish optimal results in the treatment of gingival recessions and enhance the structural beauty of the dentogingival unit.

Therapeutic possibilities

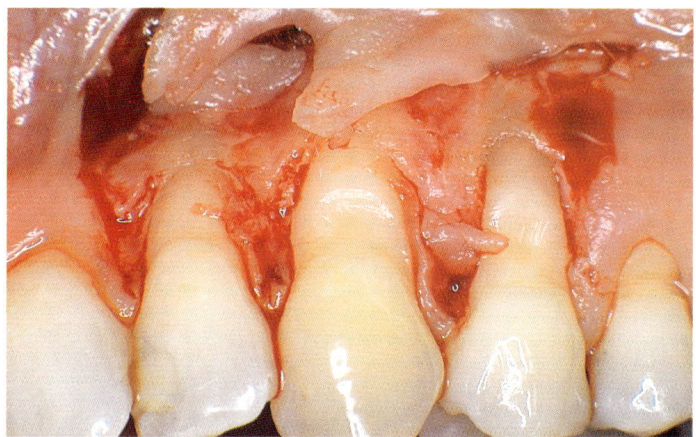

Fig 8-18c Pedicle graft reflected, showing the extent of recessions.

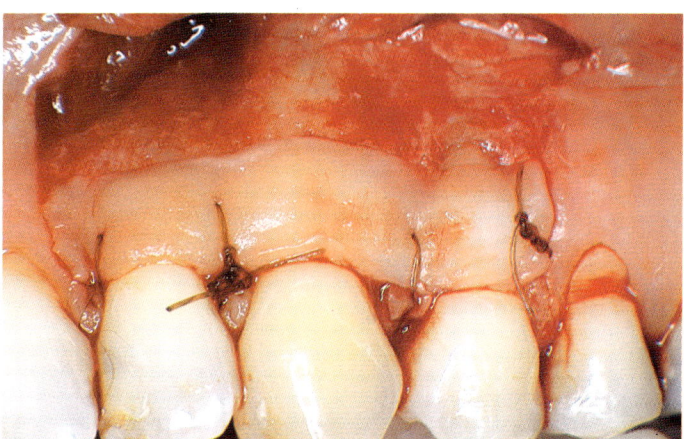

Fig 8-18d Free gingival connective tissue graft sutured.

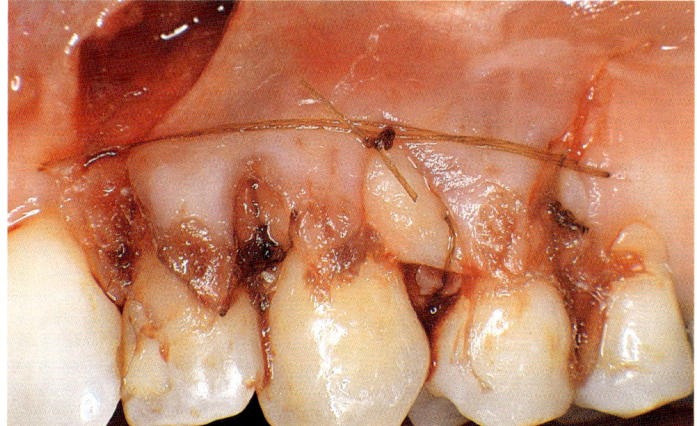

Fig 8-18e The pedicle graft sutured over free connective tissue graft. To enhance marginal stability to the pedicle graft, cyanoacrylate has been used.

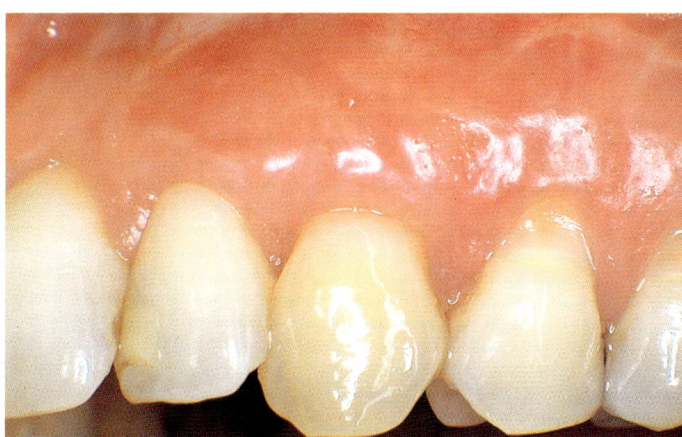

Fig 8-18f The final result 9 months later.

References

1. O'Leary TJ, Drake RB, Crump PP, Allen MF. The incidence of recession in young males: A further study. *J Periodontol.* 1971;42:264.
2. Schluger S, Youdelis RA, Page RC. *Periodontal Disease.* Philadelphia, Pa: Lea & Febiger; 1977.
3. Stillman PR. Early clinical evidences of disease in the gingiva and pericementum. *J Dent Res.* 1921;3:25.
4. Lindhe J, Svanberger G. Influence of trauma from occlusion on progression of experimental periodontitis in the beagle dog. *J Clin Periodontol.* 1974;1:3.
5. Sullivan HC, Atkins JH. The role of free gingival grafts in periodontal therapy. *Dent Clin North Am.* 1969.
6. Langer B. Subepithelial connective tissue graft technique for root coverage. *J Periodontol.* 1985;56:715.
7. Nelson SW. The subpedicle connective tissue graft. *J Periodontol.* 1987;58:95.
8. Raetzke PB. Covering localized areas of root exposure employing the envelope technique. *J Periodontol.* 1985;56:397.
9. Bell A, Valluzzo TA, Garnick JJ, Pennel BM. The presence of "creeping attachment" in human gingiva. *J Periodontol.* 1978;49:513.
10. Guinard EA, Caffesse RG. Treatment of localized gingival recession, Part I: Lateral sliding flap. *J Periodontol.* 1978;49:351.
11. Sterrantino SF, Carnevale G, Ricci G. Biometrical studies using dura mater on the donor site of lateral sliding flaps. *Int J Periodont Rest Dent.* 1987;3:43.
12. Goldman HM, Smukler H. Controlled surgical stimulation of periosteum. *J Periodontol.* 1978;49:518.
13. Groupe HE, Warren RF. Repair of gingival defects by a sliding flap operation. *J Periodontol.* 1956;27:92.
14. Aleo JJ, De Renzis FA, Farber PA, Varbocoeur AP. The presence and biologic activity of cementum-bound endotoxin. *J Periodontol.* 1974;45:672.
15. Register AA, Burdick FA. Accelerated reattachment with cementogenesis to dentin demineralized in situ. *J Periodontol.* 1976;47:497.
16. Staffileno H. Management of gingival recession and root exposure problems associated with periodontal disease. *Dent Clin North Am.* 1964.
17. Pfeifer JS, Heller R. Histologic evaluation of full and partial thickness lateral reposition flaps: A pilot study. *J Periodontol.* 1971;42:331.
18. Ruben M, Goldman HM, Janson W. In Sthal SS, ed. *Periodontal Surgery: Biological Basis and Technique.* Springfield, Ill: Charles C Thomas, Publisher; 1976.
19. Espinel MC, Caffesse RG. Comparison of the results obtained with the laterally positioned pedicle sliding flap revised technique and the lateral sliding flap with a free gingival graft technique in the treatment of localized gingival recessions. *Int J Periodont Rest Dent.* 1981;6:31.
20. Cohen DW, Ross SE. The double papillae repositioned flap in periodontal therapy. *J Periodontol.* 1968;39:65.
21. Kalmi J, Moscor M, Goranov Z. The solution of the aesthetic problem in the treatment of periodontal disease of anterior teeth: Gingivoplastic operation. *Paradentologie.* 1949;3:53.
22. Nordenram A, Landt H. Evaluation of a surgical technique in the periodontal treatment of maxillary anterior teeth. *Acta Odontol Scand.* 1969;27:283.
23. Harvey PM. Management of advanced periodontitis: Preliminary report of a method of surgical reconstruction. *N Z Dent J.* 1965;61:180.
24. Restrepo OJ. Coronally repositioned flap: Report of four cases. *J Periodontol.* 1973;44:564.
25. Nabers JM. Extension of the vestibular fornix utilizing a gingival graft. *Periodontics.* 1966;4:77.
26. Sugarman EF. A clinical and histological study of the attachment of grafted tissue to bone and teeth. *J Periodontol.* 1969;40:381.
27. Hawley CE. Staffileno H. Clinical evaluation of free gingival grafts in periodontal surgery. *J Periodontol.* 1970;41:105.
28. Corn H. Mucogingival surgery and associate problems. In Goldman H, Cohen DW, eds. *Periodontal Therapy.* St. Louis, Mo: CV Mosby Co; 1973:713–741.
29. Vandersall DC. Management of gingival recession and a surgical dehiscence with a soft tissue autograft: 4-year observation. *J Periodontol.* 1974;45:274.
30. Ward VJ. A clinical assessment of the use of the free gingival graft for correcting localized recession associated with frenal pull. *J Periodontol.* 1974;45:78.
31. Livingstone HL. Total coverage of multiple and adjacent denuded root surfaces with a free gingival autograft: A case report. *J Periodontol.* 1975;46:209.
32. Douglas GL. Mucogingival repairs in periodontal surgery. *Dent Clin North Am.* 1976;20:107.
33. Matter J, Cimasoni G. Creeping attachment after free gingival grafts. *J Periodontol.* 1976;47:574.
34. Miller PD. Root coverage using a free soft tissue autograft following citric acid application, Part I: Technique. *Int J Periodont Rest Dent.* 1982;1:65.
35. Holbrook T, Ochsenbein C. Complete coverage of the denuded root surface with a one-stage gingival graft. *Int J Periodont Rest Dent.* 1983;3:9.
36. Bernimoulin JP. Deckung gingivaler Rezessionen mit koronaler Verschiebungsplastik. *Dtsch Zahnaerztl Z.* 1973;28:1222.
37. Caffesse RG, Guinard EA. Treatment of localized gingival recessions, Part II: Coronally repositioned flap with a free gingival graft. *J Periodontol.* 1978;49:357.
38. Caffesse RG, Guinard EA. Treatment of localized gingival recessions, Part IV: Results after 3 years. *J Periodontol.* 1980;51:167.

Chapter 9

Ridge-Pontic Relationship

Claude R. Rufenacht

In areas where missing teeth have to be replaced with fixed prosthodontics, the clinician has to face the task not only of fabricating pontics that fulfill the requirements in form, function, and esthetics of a normal tooth but also of maintaining the health of the adjacent periodontium. These requirements are usually conflicting.

The relationship of the pontic to the underlying ridge is more than complex because of the various deformities that this ridge may exhibit. The ultimate physical and anatomic form of the pontic's recipient site results directly from the periodontal and dental state prior to the extraction and the maneuvers exerted during this procedure. Periapical and periodontal pathology, trauma, and the healing potentialities of the body are important factors in determining the future design of the pontic recipient site.

If we assume that the edentulous ridge may retain the general shape and mass of bone that existed prior to the extraction of the tooth, we will be confronted with an adequate or normal ridge. Even classified as normal, the ridge may not be normal in many respects. The eminences that existed in the bone over the root in a prominent arch position usually disappear as bone remodels during healing. The interdental papilla and the scalloped form of the marginal gingiva no longer exist and the smooth tissue surface of the edentulous ridge does not mimic the preexisting "orange peel" appearance of the gingiva.

In fixed prosthodontics a correctly placed pontic tooth rests on the top of a smooth tissue, lacks root prominence and marginal and interdental papillae, and does not fool a critical or simply discerning eye.

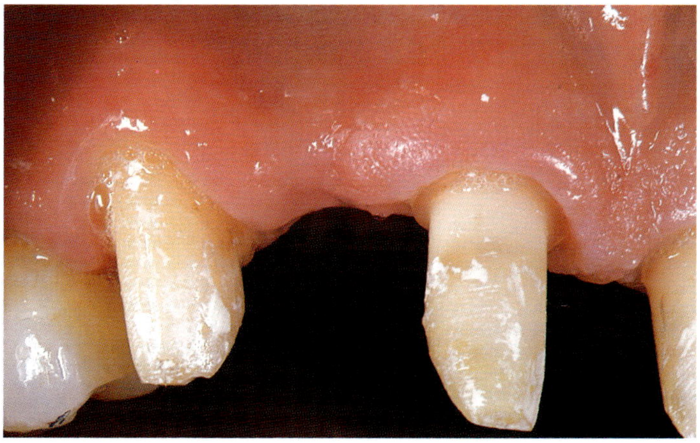

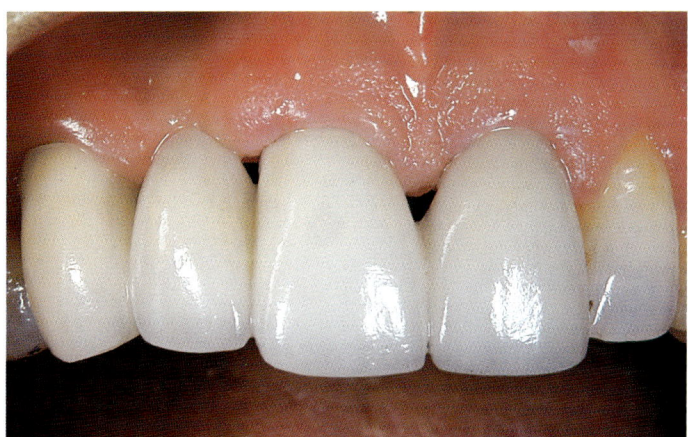

Fig 9-1 An edentulous area barely maintains the mass of bone that existed prior to the extraction.

Fig 9-2 The pontic rests on a tissue from which prominences and the usual particularities marking gingival tooth relationships have disappeared. From this point a "gingivabrasion" would improve tissue color blending.

If one wishes to restore the tooth and tissue contour that existed prior to extraction, it will be impossible, even if the edentulous area is considered normal (Figs 9-1 and 9-2). Consequently, one must compromise with these restrictions and modify the environment in adopting modalities of treatment that will help to restore the previous situation.

Prevention of ridge collapse

Ridge collapse consecutive to extraction may be considered inevitable. The attempt to maintain the edentulous alveolar ridge is an old concept that was applied in the last century.[1] The retention of endodontically treated roots[2,3] was recommended together with the submerging of vital roots.

Implants that act as fillers after extractions provide mechanical support, prevent the collapse of both labial and lingual plates of bone, and delay or diminish bone loss.[4-9]

Once the tooth is extracted, the soft granulation tissue, properly removed with curettes, synthetic graft material (hydroxyapatite, HA) in granules is introduced in the socket with a sterile amalgam carrier. Excess of hemorrhage is carefully sponged from the extraction site opening and the socket is filled to a level approximating the free gingival margin. If the graft material is a solid HA root, it should be placed 2 to 3 mm below the marginal crest of bone, and attention must be paid to carefully rounding its occlusal surface. At this moment the superficial part of the socket should be sealed by means of three procedures:

1. A gelatine or collagen material is applied, compressed on the area and maintained with surgical dressing.
2. Freeze-dried cadaver skin is placed over the graft and sutured. Sutures and the cadaver skin are removed 10 days postoperatively. The results of this approach seem to be stable.
3. A free gingival graft or partial-thickness flap prepared from the palatal side of the socket is placed over the implant material to assure initial healing.

Maximal preservation of the alveolar requires immediate placement of HA implants after tooth extraction. Both animal and clinical studies have proved HA to be safe and capable of retarding postextraction bone resorption.[10] Control sockets after 1 year are significantly smaller than the roots or particle-filled sockets. Based on a 31-month follow-up study, it has been demonstrated that with HA implants twice as much alveolar bone was maintained than in the unimplanted control sites.[11,12]

Predictability of the procedure is best assured when implant material is placed into a socket provided with adequate bone support. When we respect this basic clinical principle and assure the seal of the socket over the implant, no evidence of rejective phenomenon, such as inflammation, ulceration, fistula and pain, has been stated. However, a loss of the cortical plate following extraction or periodontal disease constitutes a contraindication.

Indeed, the difficulty of preventing the possible migration of HA particles into the alveolar mucosa is coupled with the risk of tear that, affecting the thin remaining alveolar gingiva, may compromise the healing process. When facing this type of situation, the socket is best left for normal healing in the knowledge that a surgical corrective procedure can be easily carried out later.

Morphology of the ridge

The correction of an edentulous ridge has to be performed prior to the construction of the fixed prosthesis and is aimed at making the ridge accept the pontic rather than making the pontic fit and adapt into the edentulous area. The modification of an undesirable contour and the creation of the adequate space are the most frequent problems that have to be treated.

Two types of situations have to be faced: *(1)* a reduced available space, and *(2)* an increased available space with the subsequent problem created by the location of the mucogingival junction and the width of the attached gingiva.

Morphology of the ridge

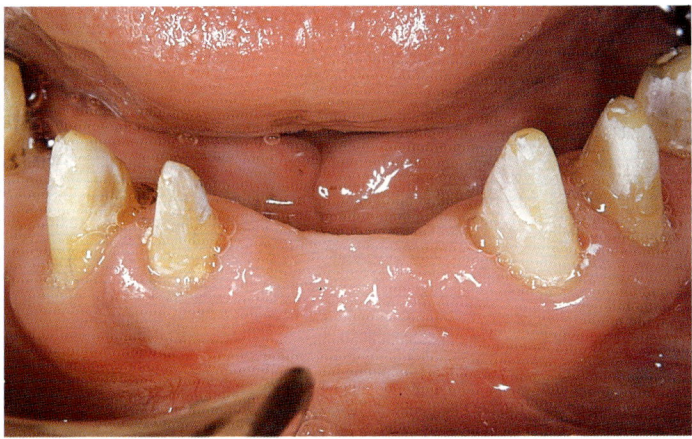

Fig 9-3 The surgical coaptation of buccal and oral flaps most often leads to the necessity of restoring the edentulous area with an adequate width of attached gingiva.

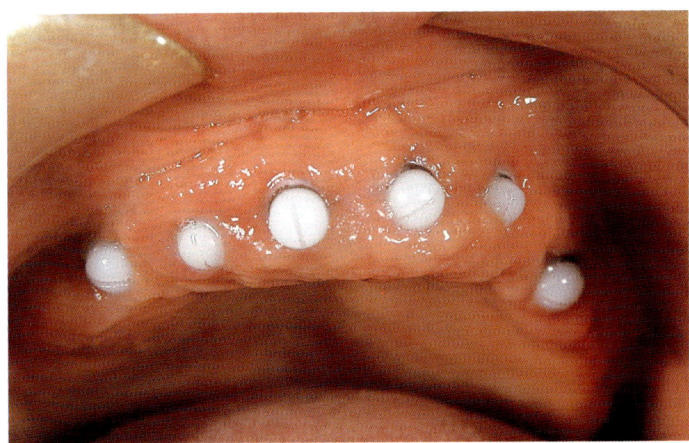

Fig 9-4 This edentulous maxillary has received six endosseous implants (IMZ) in an area going from the right to the left second premolar.

Width of the attached gingiva and location of the mucogingival junction in the edentulous ridge

The amount of attached gingiva, the location of the mucogingival junction in edentulous areas, and the presence of frenula should be carefully evaluated. Should they interfere with the placement of the apicobuccal margin of the pontic, proper management of this problem should be undertaken. In chapter 4 we gave the description of the usual and natural width and position of the attached gingiva. In this respect the edentulous area should be approached, considered, and treated the same way as dentulous areas because they have to fulfill the same requirements. Usually, this factor is either ignored or neglected by practitioners. Furthermore, one has to consider that conflicts in therapeutic modalities and goals inevitably exist between specialists and more precisely between the extractionist and the prosthodontist.

The coaption and suturing of buccal and lingual flaps to control hemorrhage and add to the patient's postoperative comfort leave such an edentulous area covered with a reduced amount of gingiva that correct pontic placement is only possible if a subsequent mucogingival procedure is carried out (Fig 9-3).

Correction of a reduced available pontic space

The correction of reduced available pontic space, which requires the reduction of the thickness of connective tissue overlying the bone or the reduction of the osseous support, is a procedure that can be performed within the range of activity of a general practice.

These minor surgical corrective procedures permit the creation of an adequate vertical space for the pontic element and of an edentulous ridge that is similar in width and height to the adjacent ridge and, assuming that the mucogingival junction is in continuity with that of the adjacent teeth, we find ourselves in the presence of what we called a normal edentulous ridge.

Ridge-Pontic Relationship

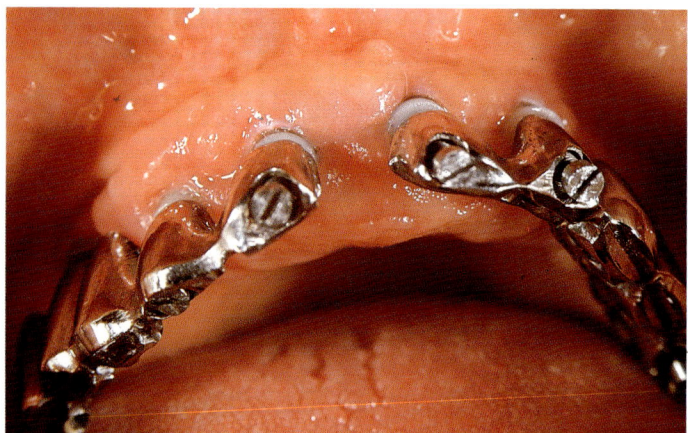

Fig 9-5 A primary suprastructure is connected to each implant by means of a long screw.

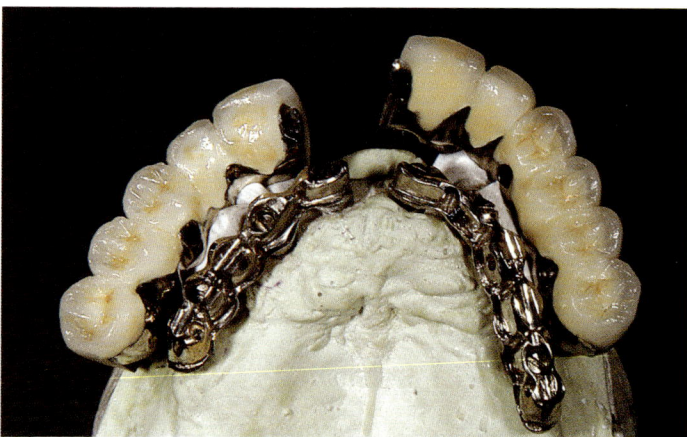

Fig 9-6 A precise insertion over this primary suprastructure of two ceramometallic fixed partial dentures interlocked by a precision attachment has been realized. Maintenance on the primary suprastructure is ensured by means of four microscrews.

Correction of an increased available space

Prosthodontic approach

From clinical and scientific observation it can be stated that the residual ridge that forms after the extraction of teeth is usually characterized by a loss of substance compared with the dentulous ridge. The rate of loss can vary in different sites within the same individual, is dependent upon biologic, anatomic, and mechanical factors, and may result in a deformed or collapsed type of ridge.

It was long believed that these deformities could only be compensated by prosthodontic means. Consequently, the shape of the pontic was modified and oversized to fit in the concavity of the residual ridge and its base modeled to be a precise mirror image of the tissue surface it contacted. This created a situation that was unacceptable esthetically and biologically because we assume that access for oral hygiene should be at all times respected. Most patients feel frustrated by the situation created by the elongated and nonanatomic pontic element and express justified complaints.

In an attempt to create some kind of harmony and give a visual perception of continuity with the remaining dentition, a pink gingival color, such as acrylic or porcelain flange, has been designed at the cervical end of the pontic to simulate normal tooth length. Unfortunately, this approach never responds fully to the esthetic expectations because of the difficulties of matching the gingival color and texture.

Another concept used in large defects has been to build up a false removable gingival flange, which can be adapted and locked in the interdental areas. Techniques have been described using rigid or soft acrylic resins. The addition of this flange aids in making the prosthesis look more lifelike by filling the dark triangle between elongated teeth, giving the illusion of papilla and marginal gingiva. At the same time, phonetics and air flow can be improved. This removable flange is indicated in all situations in which surgical procedures for one reason or another have failed or have not been used.

It seems that, with the increased use and success of osseointegrated implants, the poor esthetic appearance of emergence connecting devices, and the amount of vertical ridge collapse that most of these cases exhibit, this type of device will have to be improved (Figs 9-4 to

Correction of an increased available space

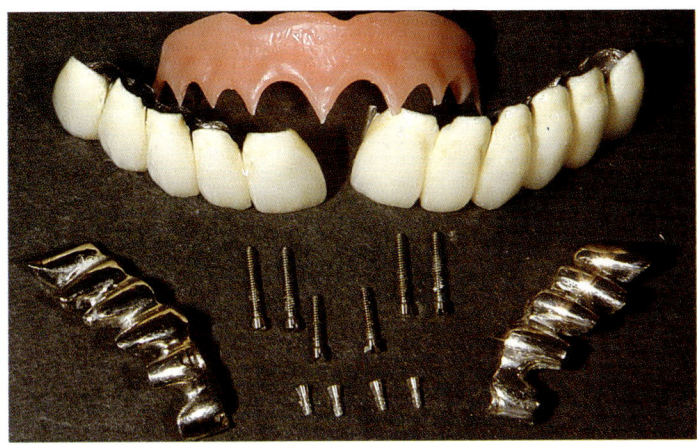

Fig 9-7 An overview of the elements of the puzzle that require an average of 20 minutes either for insertion or desinsertion.

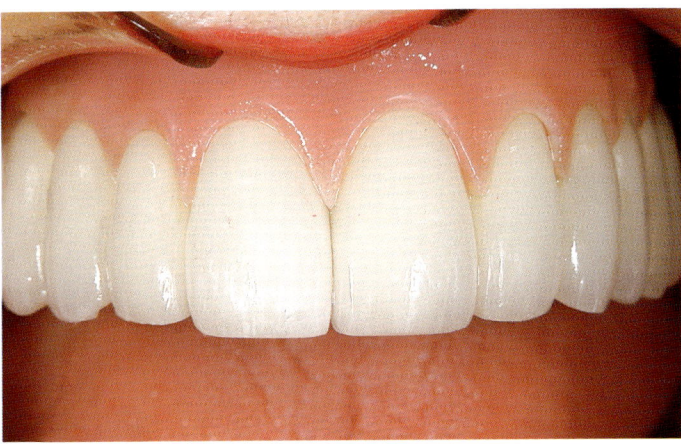

Fig 9-8 Patient desire and insistence to receive a fixed restoration could not be totally satisfied because a removable gingival flange locked in the interdental spaces had to be proposed to hide the anesthetic metallic emergence of the implants as well as tooth length reaching 18 mm.

9-9). However, one should be realistic enough to admit that, at the present time, the majority of edentulous patients requiring implants are technically, functionally, economically, and esthetically better provided for with a removable denture base than with fixed prosthodontics when osseous ridge collapse has proceeded too far. This statement, based only on observation, should not prevent the implantologist, whose attention has been focused on the biologic success of the procedure, from providing systems with emergence devices that mimic dental roots in color and approximate diameter.

One should see that the correction of an increased pontic space in height and width by means of a fixed or removable prosthesis will be progressively abandoned in favor of surgical procedures, the developments of which present a challenge for our profession. Esthetic goals require providing the patient with a prosthesis that restores function and natural appearance.

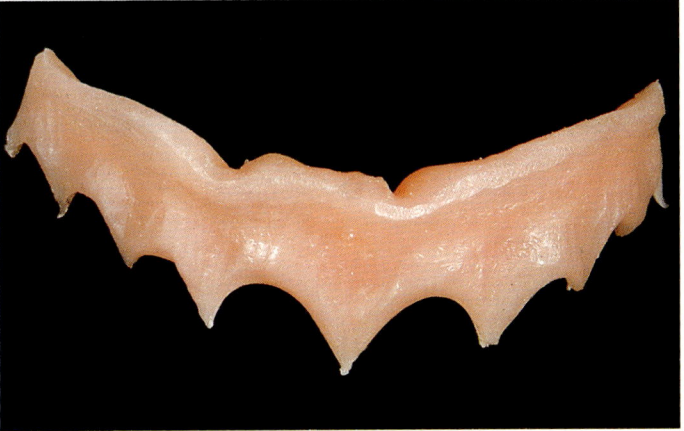

Fig 9-9 Gingival acrylic resin movable flange, or when old concepts come to help updated technology.

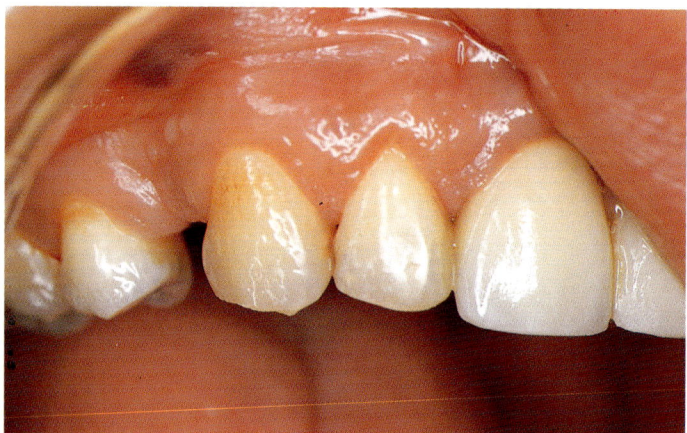

Fig 9-10 Postextraction horizontal or buccolingual bone loss.

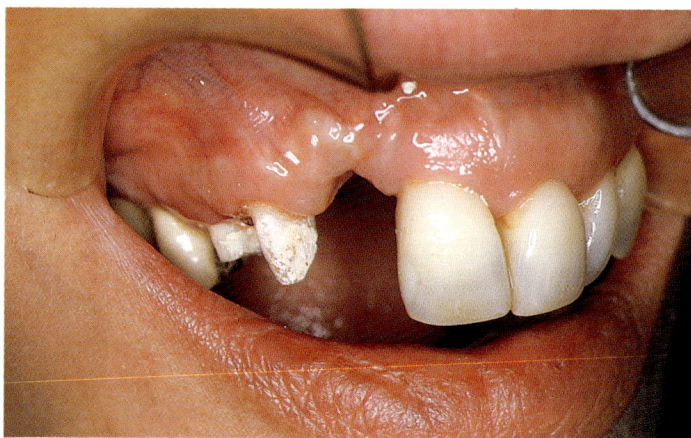

Fig 9-11 Postextraction vertical or coronoapical bone loss.

Surgical approach

The topographic observation of a residual ridge that has to be restored to its normal dimension through surgical procedures can be classified in three categories[13]:

1. Horizontal buccolingual loss of tissue with normal apicocoronal dimension (Fig 9-10).
2. Vertical apicocoronal loss of tissue with normal horizontal dimension (Fig 9-11).
3. A combination of buccolingual and apicocoronal defects resulting from the loss of tissue in height and width.

In addition, another classification was proposed in which the ridge deformities are classified by assessing the depth of the defect in relation to the adjacent ridge[14]: mild, less than 3 mm; moderate, from 3 to 6 mm; and severe, greater than 6 mm.

The second classification probably constitutes the best warning of possible complications and multiplication of the procedures necessary to achieve the desired result. This can ease the dentist–patient relationship in the sense that subsequent surgical procedures will be considered as foreseen and not the result of the failure of the first one.

Protocol for ridge augmentation

The basic requirements for success in the reconstruction of the collapsed ridge depend upon the following factors:

1. Understanding of the various types of defects.
2. Evaluation of the quantity and quality of soft tissue in the edentulous area to allow elevation of a flap and avoid perforation.
3. Evaluation of the blood supply in the area.
4. Absence of periodontal pockets on the adjacent teeth.
5. Preservation of the marginal papillae of the adjacent teeth.
6. Proper evaluation of the quantity and quality of grafting material from the donor site or choice of the implant material.
7. Evaluation of the number of surgical procedures necessary to achieve an optimal result.

Graft material and donor site

Autogenous subepithelial connective tissue graft

The sources of the dense connective tissue autograft may be one of the several areas of the patient's oral cavity. The most readily available sources of donor tissue are found in the lateral aspect of the palate and in the tuberosity region. Any edentulous posterior area presenting an adequate thickness of tissue may be used as well as gingivectomy tissue. The best area in the palate is located on the ridge near the teeth, posterior to the most distal ruga, away from the opening of the anterior palatinal foramen. The length of the horizontal incision is dependent upon the concavity to be filled.

Sequence

A split-thickness flap is dissected, elevated, and separated from the underlying bone[15] to be used as donor material. The epithelialized superficial flap is placed over the denuded bone and coapted to the gingiva. The procedure can only be executed by hand dissection and is far from easy. As an alternative, one can proceed to the initial deepithelialization of the donor site with a rotary coarse diamond instrument and the elevation of the donor material with a hand scalpel or motor mucotom. The palatal area that is used as a preferential donor site for epithelial connective tissue graft most often does not provide subepithelial connective tissue grafts of a sufficient thickness. On the tuberosity region, the graft may be removed as part of a maxillary periodontal procedure or as an individual procedure. Several methods have been described to reduce the tuberosity and retromolar tabs. Whenever possible, the selection of the retromolar area should be favored because it aids in normalizing the sulcus depth and the accessibility to oral hygiene and provides, depending on the technique used, epithelial or subepithelial tissue graft of sufficient thickness for reconstructive goals.[16,17] Postoperative discomfort is minimized when graft material is dissected from the retromolar area.

Implant material

The availability of autogenous subepithelial tissue may sometimes be limited to the anatomic specificities of the oral cavity or the amount of tissue needed for the reconstruction of the ridge. Autogenous bone graft material taken from the iliac crest and rib have been utilized for the past three decades in edentulous ridge augmentation, but this procedure encountered the problem of the progressive loss of bone in the grafted areas.[18,19] Various technical modifications have decreased the amount of bone resorption, but no really satisfactory results have been obtained, whatever the technique used. As a result, this material was never taken into consideration in partially edentulous ridge reconstruction.[20,21] This problem stimulated research for a synthetic inorganic product available to support repair, both for periodontal defects and for ridge augmentation. To perform successful ridge augmentation, any biomaterial should satisfy the following criteria[22]:

1. Easily carved and molded.
2. Biocompatible and stable.
3. Firmly bond with bone and soft tissue.
4. Soft tissue healing after implant exposure.
5. Resistant to infection.
6. Acceptance for subsequent vestibuloplasty when necessary.
7. No adverse effect on adjacent bone.

Existing information has shown calcium phosphate ceramics to be safe and effective for clinical applications.[23–25] They differ from previous hard tissue implant materials by their basic biocompatibility, which includes a lack of toxicity and inflammatory response.[26–28] Calcium phosphate ceramics present the ability to become apparently bonded to bone by natural bond cementary mechanisms,[21] but the nature of this bonding is still under investigation. The material is well tolerated by soft tissue[25–27] and no really significant difference in the inflammatory response from different shapes of particles has been evidenced.[21,29,30] Phosphate ceramics do not induce bone formation in soft tissue and therefore are not osteogenic, but they can be considered osteoconductive because they provide a physical matrix suitable for deposition of new bone.[31] Investigators and clinicians have limited their attention to the performance of nonresorbable, high-density HA and porous HA and a potentially bioresorbable form of beta-tricalcium phosphate (TCP). The investigations on TCP with reference to animal and clinical studies concluded that the material provides a biocompatible matrix but has a tendency to resorb in an unpredictable fashion. Whereas some particles resorb, others remain as biologic foreign bodies or "fillers." No mention is made of the use of this material in ridge augmentation, and investigations have been limited to the repair of periodontal defects.[32]

Hydroxyapatite

HA is a dense calcium phosphate ceramic material possessing considerable compressive strength and consequently limited mechanical properties. To minimize the problem of brittleness that was observed in HA tooth implants, dense calcium phosphate ceramic particles were produced. The reparative matrix of bone invasion surrounding the particles provided strength to the implant. Particles are available in different forms: irregular and multifaceted, smooth and rounded. Although highly biocompatible, HA undergoes some degradation in the tissue. The degradation rate depends on variations in the formation of ceramic, crystallographic structures and the rate of cooling and porosity. Several types of HA can be observed:

1. Solid, dense HA with almost no void spaces, extremely stable in the tissues and undergoing no resorption;
2. Porous HA whose porosity may be of two types:
    a. microporosity with pores of about 1 to 5 μm in diameter left in the material as a consequence of an incomplete fusion during the sintering process. Micropore HA has too small pores for tissue penetration and slowly degrades.
    b. macroporosity, including synthetic HA with pores between 100 to 300 μm in diameter, intentionally introduced in the material to allow ingrowth of bone and connective tissue and porous coralline HA (interpore) derived from the calcium carbonate skeleton of a reef-building coral that is converted into calcium phosphate with this unique interconnecting pore surface. Coralline HA has an average pore diameter of 200 μm and about 60% of void surface.

Porous versus dense implant material

Macroporous HA presents the disadvantage of a decrease in strength proportionally to the increase in porosity. However, pores of 150 to 200 μm have been shown to be optimal for the ingrowth of mineralized bone so that mechanical properties can be modulated in the preparation of the synthetic form.

The coralline porous form of HA offers the advantage of being easily carved and has pores that can provide a firm fixation of the implant through tissue ingrowth that will increase its compressive strength as shown by laboratory studies.[33] Unfortunately, if bone ingrowth into the porous surface of the implant has been observed,[34] it has also been observed to be slow and incomplete in comparison with the bone invasion around dense HA particles, and undesirable bone remodeling has been noted. The reason may be in the notorious particularities of osseous tissues that remodel according to their own biomechanical dictates, apparently best achieved around dense HA particles rather than through unnatural pore pathways.

Improved techniques for localized ridge augmentation

Roll technique

The basic concept of this procedure consists of the creation of a deepithelialized tissue pedicle over and palatal to the residual crest. The pedicle used as donor is rolled in upon itself and placed in a labially prepared pouch[34,35] (Figs 9-12 to 9-17). Free bleeding shows evidence of epithelial removal, and an adequate thickness of connective tissue eases the desinsertion of the flap that is designed to preserve the marginal gingiva of the adjacent teeth. The palatal donor site will slowly granulate in and fill.

A preventive mucogingival-free graft can be inserted at this moment if secondary surgical treatment is considered or simply to improve the palatal design of the crest. In both cases the area is dressed and allowed to heal for 10 days. Thin palatal tissues are a contraindication for this type of procedure and for most of the others because they do not allow for sufficient blood supply and therefore compromise the success of the

Improved techniques for localized ridge augmentation

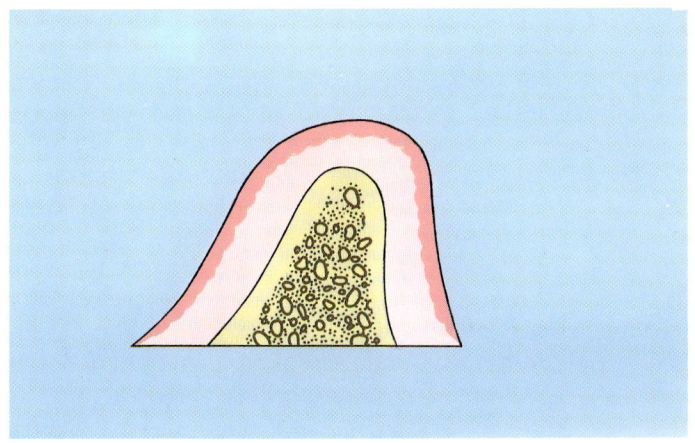

Fig 9-12 Diagrammatic representation of the initial situation. Usually the thickness of the epithelium averages 0.5 mm.

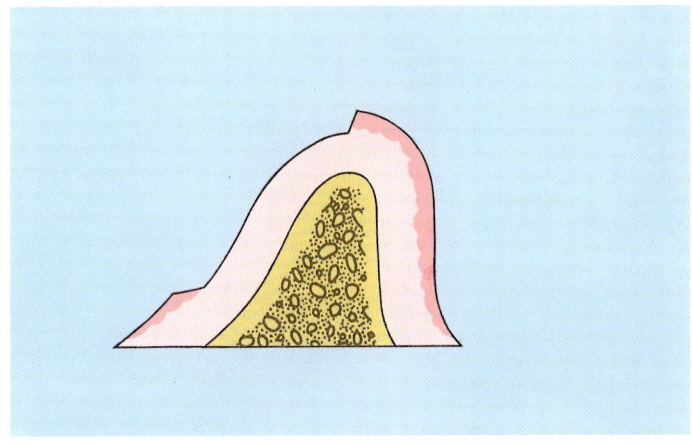

Fig 9-13 The epithelium is removed by firm dissection or with the use of rotary diamond instruments.

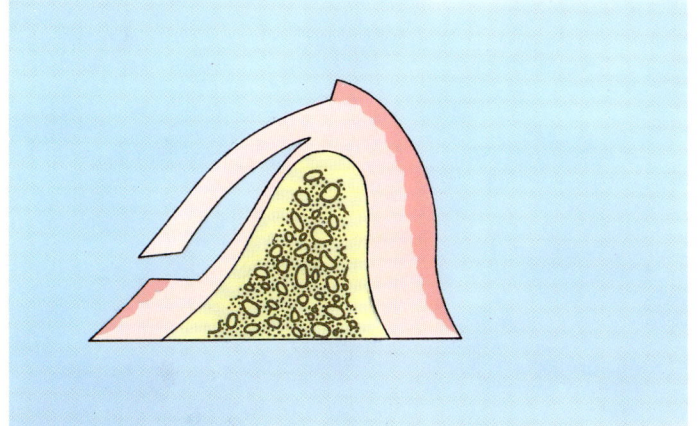

Fig 9-14 The pedicle is designed from the palate toward the buccal angle of the crest.

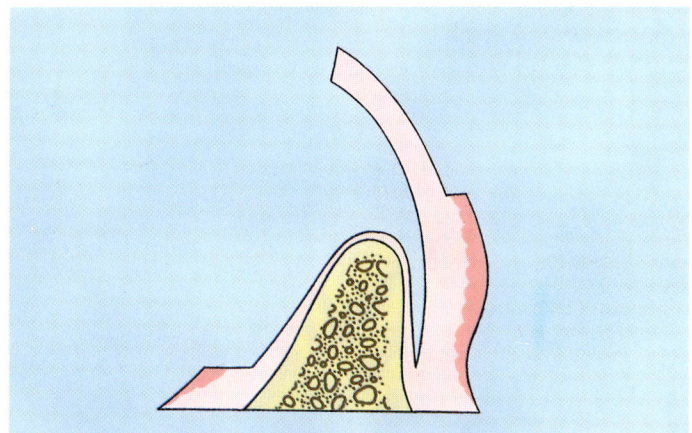

Fig 9-15 The flap is elevated and the incision is extended in a apical direction.

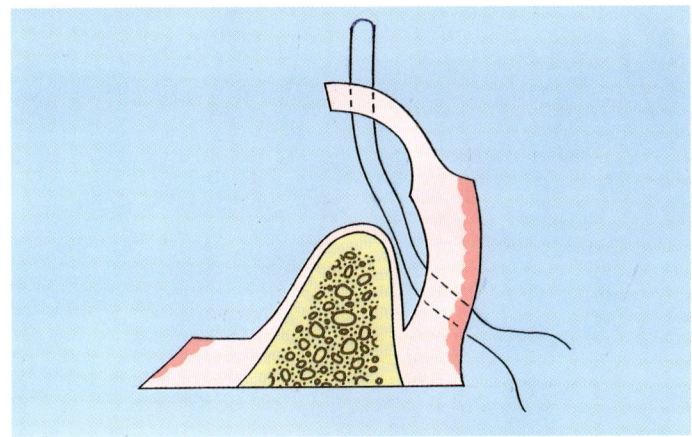

Fig 9-16 The elevation of the flap permits the insertion of suture material around its free end and at the same time at the base of the buccal incision.

271

Ridge-Pontic Relationship

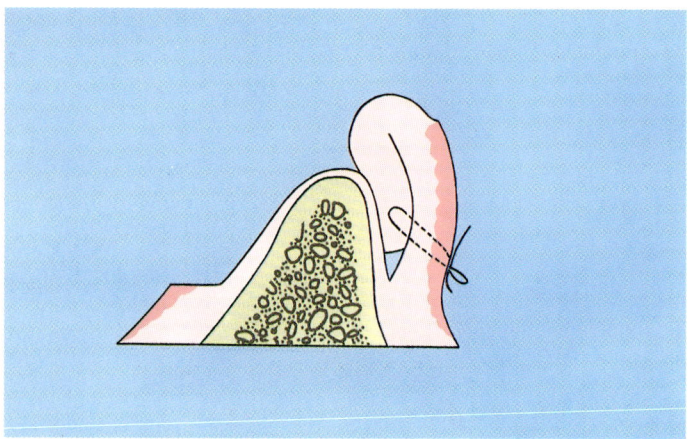

Fig 9-17 This permits it to be rolled, by gentle guided pull, invertedly into the buccal insertion where it is firmly sutured. (Suggested by L. Abrams.)

procedures. The use of this technique is indicated to correct mild or moderate horizontal defects. Depending upon the thickness of the flap and the buccal extension of the recipient site, little improvement of a vertical bone loss can be obtained with this approach.

Clinical experience has demonstrated the importance of tissue thickness in the donor site to allow sufficient blood supply and ease the elevation of the flap and in the recipient site when implant material has to be used. The roll technique is then indicated to increase tissue thickness in a first-stage procedure, preventing future tissue laceration with the introduction of implant material and healing phase of a second stage procedure (Figs 9-18 and 9-19).

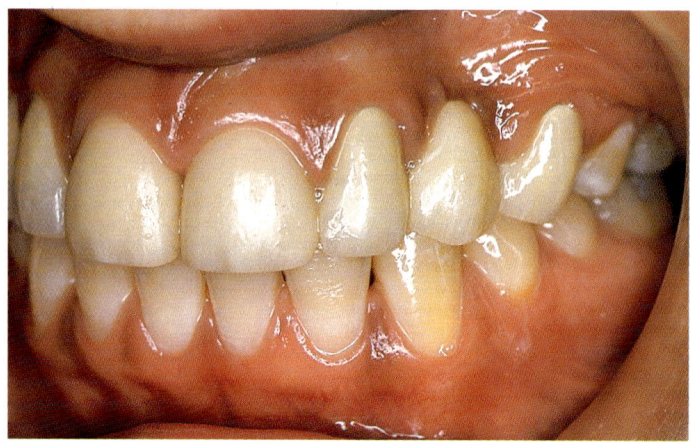

Fig 9-18 Clinical situation of horizontal defect created by a traumatic extraction. The extreme thinness of the gingival tissue on the recipient site required previous correction in a first-stage surgical procedure (roll technique).

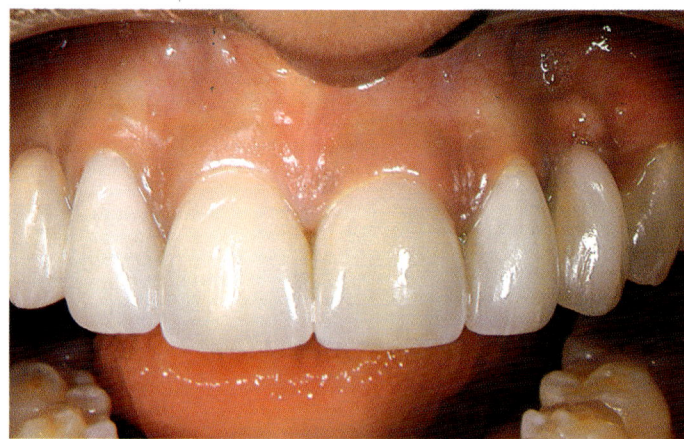

Fig 9-19 A second-stage surgical procedure permitted the insertion of an implant material to fill the horizontal defect and create a rootlike prominence over the pontic.

Improved techniques for localized ridge augmentation

Flap procedure

This is the most used and useful procedure for correcting both horizontal and moderate vertical deformities. The design of the flap should be carried out depending on the location and extension of the defect and relating to the specificity of the reconstructive donor material because the flap procedure requires the subsequent adaptation of an autogenous subepithelial connective tissue graft or the placement of an HA implant material (Figs 9-20 to 9-23).

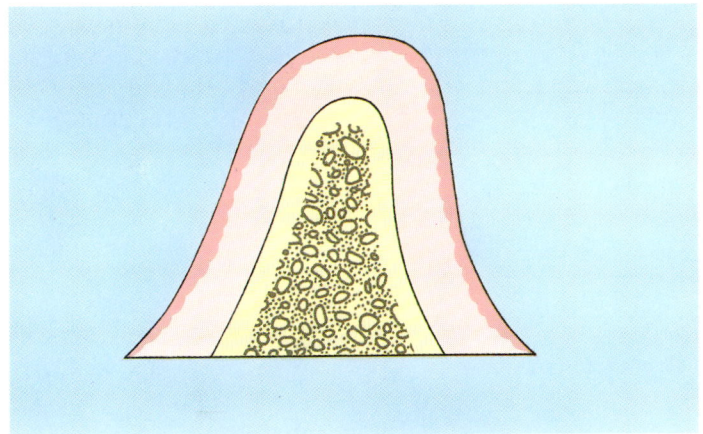

Fig 9-20 The elevation of a split-thickness flap requires an adequate tissue thickness.

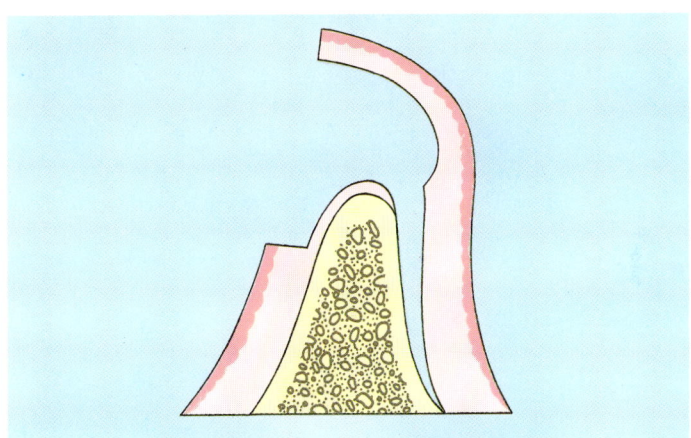

Fig 9-21 The procedure is carried out from the palatal side by sharp dissection until it reaches the defect on the crest or on its buccal side. From this point a full-thickness flap is elevated.

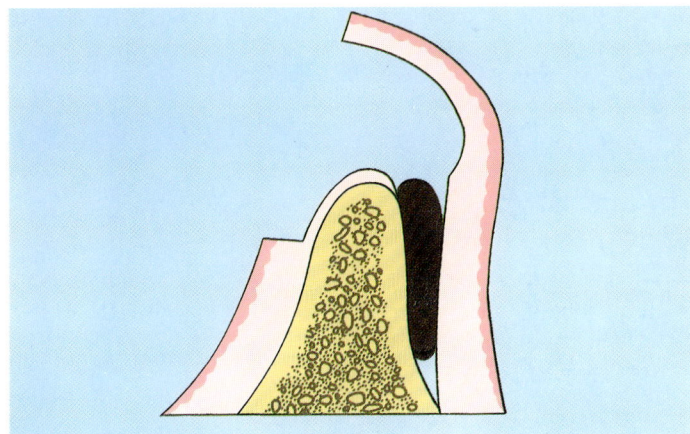

Fig 9-22 When adequate tissue thickness does exist, buccal vertical incisions are limited to the opening of a pouch, created to receive implant material or a subepithelial tissue graft.

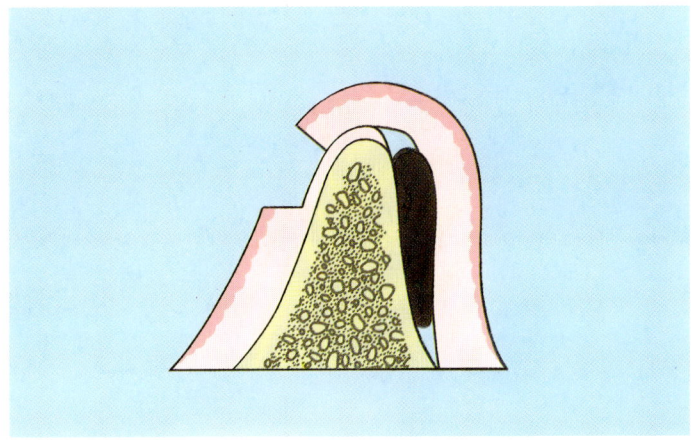

Fig 9-23 The pedicle is then reflected back and secured at all margins. Because of its displacement, a small area is left to granulate and fill in at the palatal side.

Ridge-Pontic Relationship

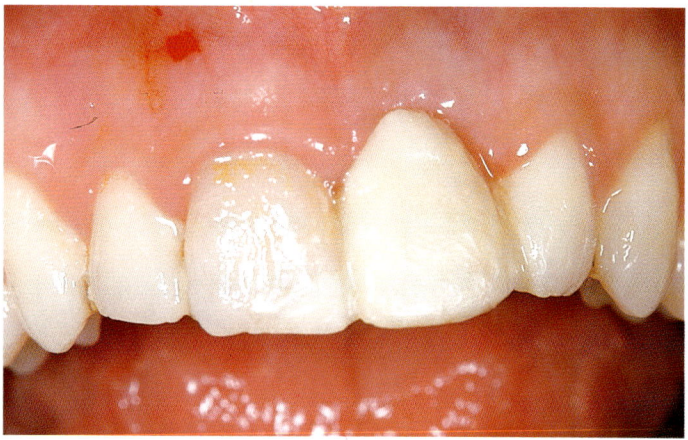

Fig 9-24 Combination of vertical and horizontal defect of accidental origin corrected by means of a one-stage flap procedure using coralline HA.

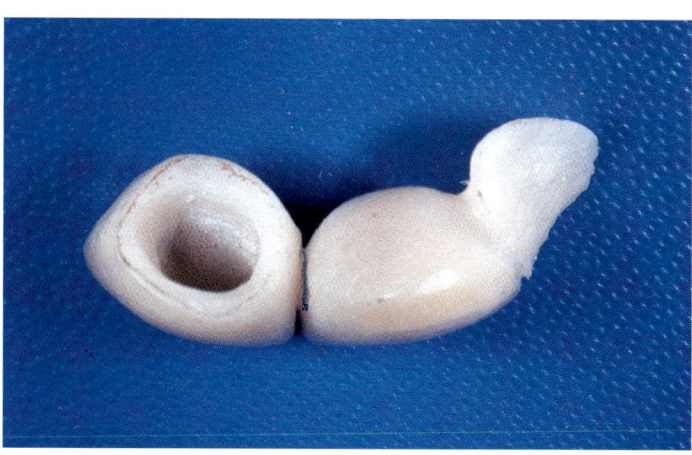

Fig 9-25 Free metal porcelain fixed partial denture with extension on the palatal side of the left lateral incisor.

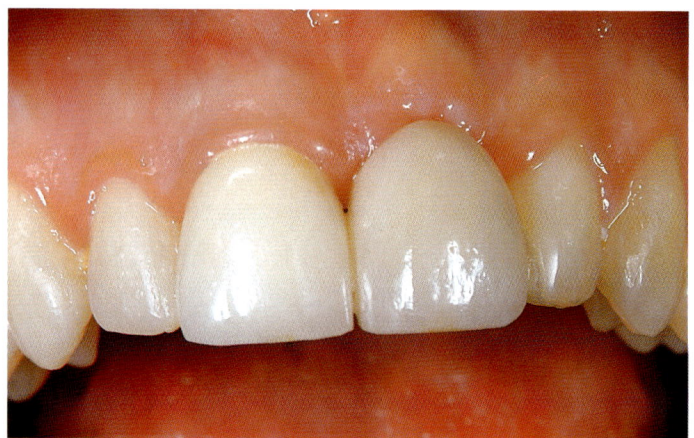

Fig 9-26 The overextension of the root prominence in the apical direction results from a slide of the coralline apatite that was left unsecured in this area.

Recipient site for connective subepithelial tissue

A split-thickness flap is elevated proximal to the adjacent teeth. Periosteum and connective tissue are allowed to remain over the alveolar ridge, which will become a source of blood supply and nourish the autogenous connective tissue graft. The flap is sutured over the donor tissue to maintain it in the desired position and dressed for 10 days. The augmentation only becomes stable 2 months after the graft procedure.[15,35–37]

Recipient site for HA implant

The design of the flap must necessarily be extended to the palatal site according to the location and importance of the defect. An adequate thickness of tissue is the basic condition for the success of the procedure. It should be noted that the use of coralline HA, which is easy to mold to the appropriate shape, opens interesting possibilities and results. At the difference in crest augmentation in edentulous areas, where future pressure from denture base should be exerted, no pressure is exerted in the edentulous pontic area; consequently, crush or resorption of the material does not happen. The elevation of a flap is a common practice in all disciplines of dentistry, and there should be no reluctance to select this treatment technique.

The HA implant material offers the advantage over the subepithelial connective tissue graft of being stable, requiring one surgical site, and providing an unlimited amount of material. However, the use of HA should be limited to large edentulous areas because the future coaptation of the flap margins to the surrounding tissue over the implant material can hardly be assured when dealing with restricted mesiodistal edentulous areas. The procedure is then best achieved with a deepithelialized connective tissue graft. Attention must be paid that no pressure is exerted during the initial stage of healing.[38–40] Both horizontal and moderate vertical defects respond favorably to this approach (Figs 9-24 to 9-26). Vertical defects treated in using Interfore 200 present encouraging results, whereas HA particles are more difficult to handle, interfering with the pedicle margin during suturing and lacerating the gingival cover.

Pouch procedure

This procedure is used to correct situations in which the deformity is horizontal and the mucogingival junction in line with that of the adjacent teeth. Basically there are three different procedures that have been designed depending upon the direction of the entry incision and the subsequent dissection: *(1)* coronoapical (Fig 9-27), *(2)* apicocoronal (Fig 9-28), and *(3)* lateral (Fig 9-29).

Sequence

A subepithelial pouch is created by split dissection of the tissue overlying the ridge extending slightly beyond the deformity. The concave shape of the deformity allows for an easy elevation of the buccal tissue and permits the insertion into the pouch of a free autogenous subepithelial graft (Fig 9-30) or implant material that is accordingly molded to create the desired ridge contour. The opening incision is carefully sutured and dressed whenever possible. This technique is indicated when the elevation of a flap may become impossible due to the thinness of the tissue, compromising the results of the procedure. Provided an adequate zone of attached gin-

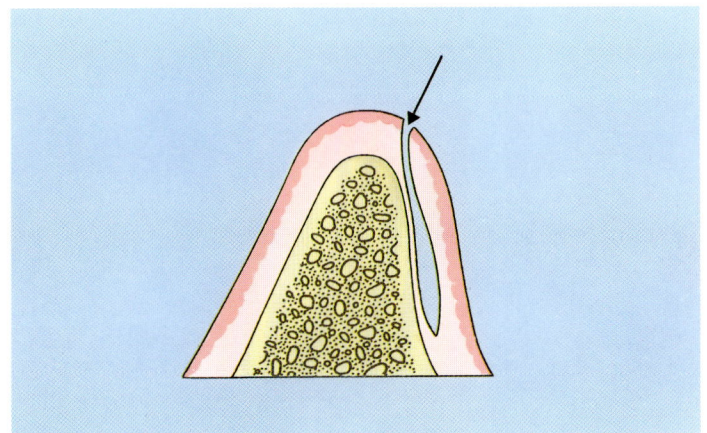

Fig 9-27 Diagrammatic representation of a pouch prepared by an occlusal opening, the most commonly used approach.

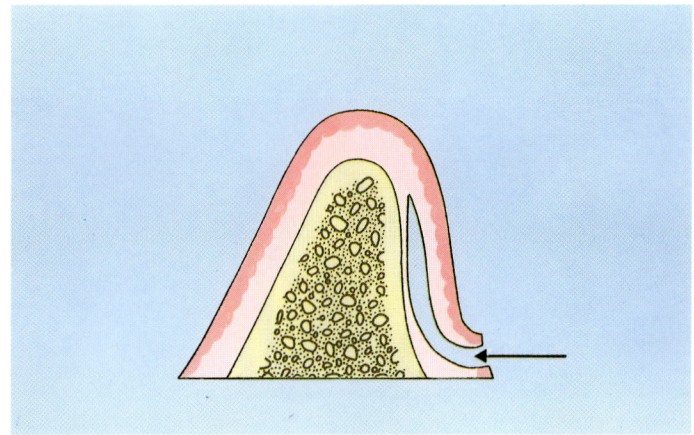

Fig 9-28 The apical opening of a pouch is an interesting approach, but it is limited to cases in which specific anatomic conditions permit its preparation.

Ridge-Pontic Relationship

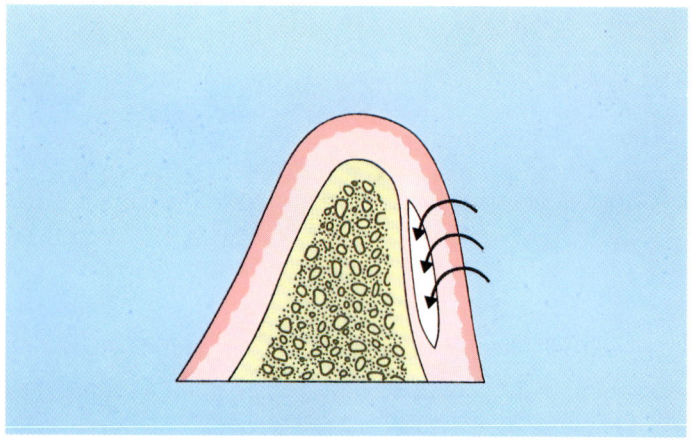

Fig 9-29 The lateral opening of a pouch permits the easy insertion of subepithelial grafts.

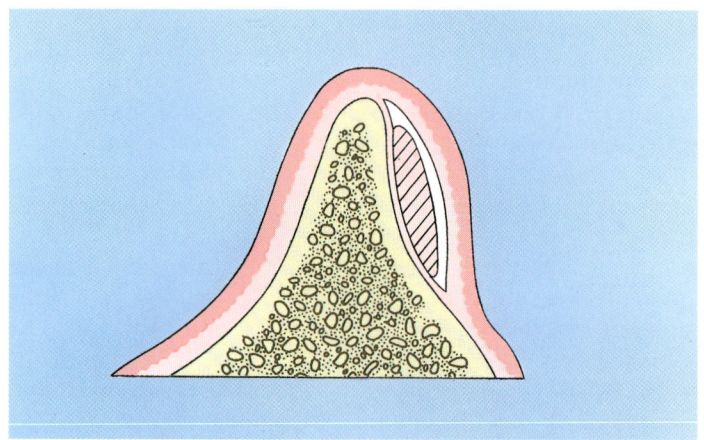

Fig 9-30 Draft of the positioning of a subepithelial graft in a coronoapical pouch. The graft must be secured with sutures.

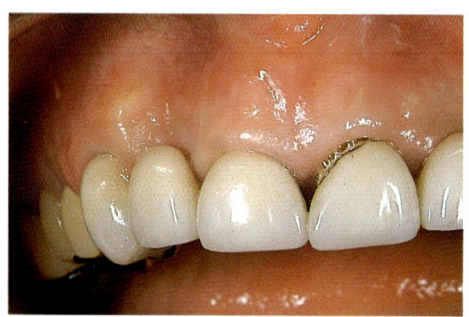

Fig 9-31 Important buccal horizontal osseous defect extending to the alveolar mucosa.

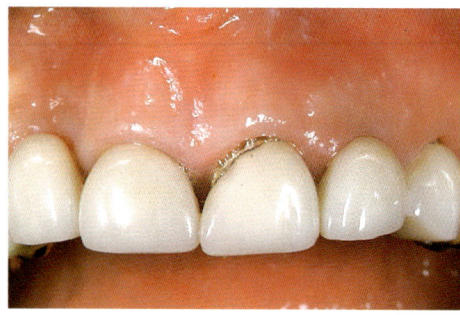

Fig 9-32 The frontal view evidences the thinness of the buccal gingiva in this area.

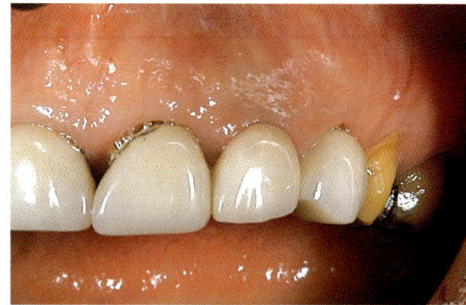

Fig 9-33 Radiographic examination has revealed a vertical root fracture on the lateral incisor that has to be extracted.

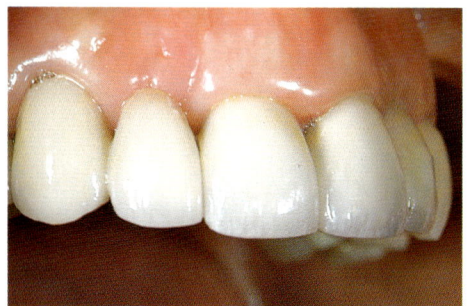

Fig 9-34 The filling of the horizontal defect required a two-stage procedure. The roll technique provided just sufficient labial tissue thickness, enabling the preparation of the coronoapical pouch.

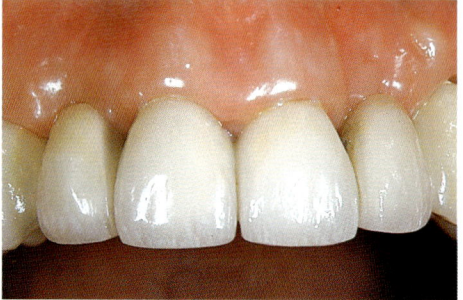

Fig 9-35 Careful examination reveals that the insertion of coralline apatite through the coronoapical pouch would have failed if an increase of tissue thickness had not been previously performed.

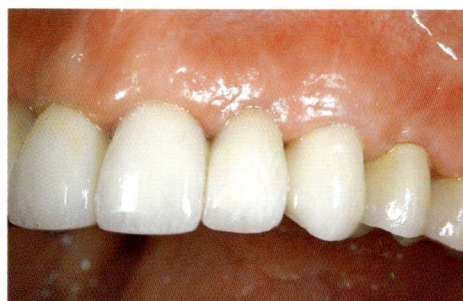

Fig 9-36 The preventive ridge augmentation by means of HA particles has maintained a satisfactory mass of bone in the area of the left lateral incisor.

giva is present, this technique is indicated to correct mild to moderate or deep horizontal defects depending upon the thickness of the connective tissue (Figs 9-31 to 9-36). The systematic creation of root prominence in an edentulous area makes this procedure, which is characterized by rapid healing, a reliable technique for the general practitioner who wishes to enhance the cosmetic results of the fixed restoration dentistry.

Onlay graft technique

The onlay procedure[13, 41] is designed to solve the most difficult problem in ridge deficiencies: moderate to severe vertical defects. It is extremely difficult to advance a flap into the air space, and the success of grafting procedures depends on the blood supply of the investing connective tissue and the biologic protection that is afforded by the walls of the pouch.

Onlay grafts are thick free gingival grafts and their use is based on established principles of wound healing. They are full-thickness grafts, which means that the total thickness of the maxillary retromolar area is used as the donor site. They gain their blood supply from a single surface during wound healing.[42]

Sequence

The site is prepared through a primary incision extending mesiodistally in the center of the crest and preserving the marginal gingiva of the adjacent teeth. Two perpendicular incisions allow for the elevation of two thin partial-thickness flaps on the buccal and lingual aspect of the defect. The graft is wedged in this recipient site and sutured (Figs 9-37 to 9-39). Seibert[41] described the use of a special scalpel blade making striations parallel to one another to the connective tissue overlying the bone. This maneuver seems to aid in ensuring a more rapid revascularization of the graft by increasing the amount of bleeding and plasma flow into the recipient site interface. Seibert noted that there is little volumetric shrinkage with this type of grafting and that it appears to be stable after 3 months. The greatest amount of shrinkage occurs within the first 6 weeks, and assessment for a second-stage procedure may be considered at that time. The procedure is indicated for moderate and severe vertical defects and to remove amalgam tattoos and pigmentation (Figs 9-40 to 9-42). The lack of sufficient blood supply and the presence of scar formation from previous surgical procedures present a contraindication.

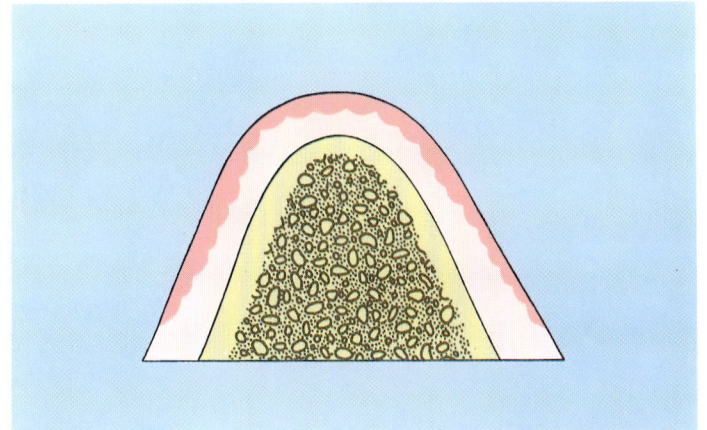

Fig 9-37 This diagrammatic representation of the recipient site indicates that an increase of the connective tissue thickness would be an asset for the success of this grafting technique.

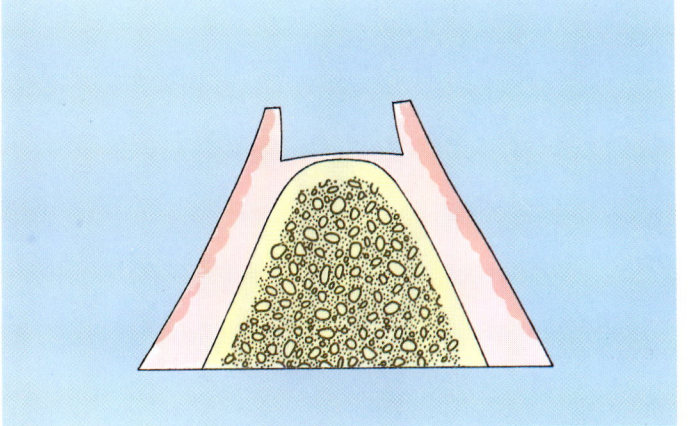

Fig 9-38 The opening of the gingival cover of the crest is realized by means of a horizontal and two perpendicular incisions permitting the elevation of their margins.

Ridge-Pontic Relationship

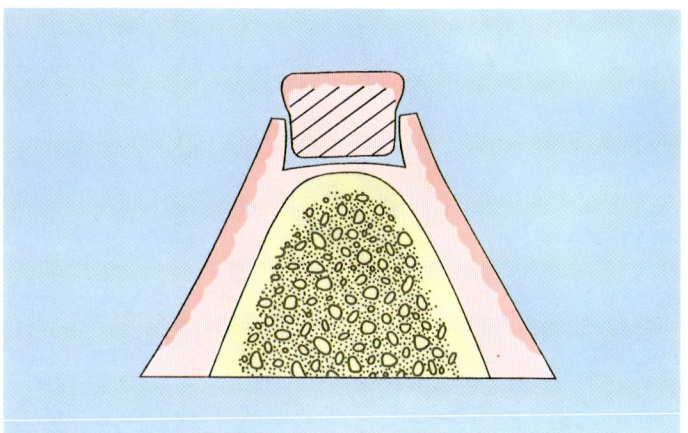

Fig 9-39 The maintenance of a free epithelial graft in the air space is made possible by its insertion in a prepared recipient site allowing vascularization. (Suggested by J. Seibert.)

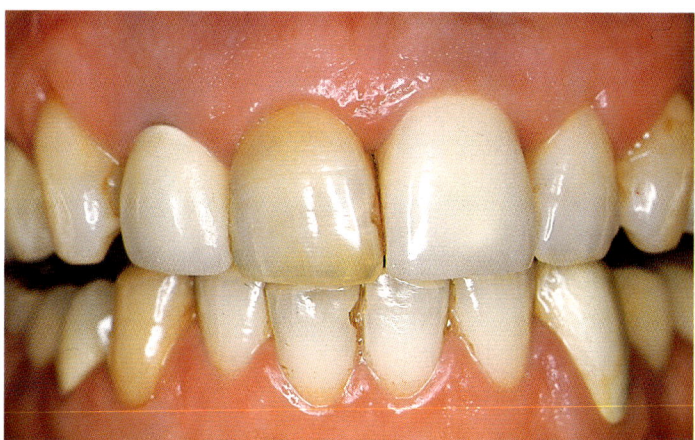

Fig 9-40 Initial clinical situation. The extraction of the lateral incisor will take away the coronal part of the buccal osseous plate.

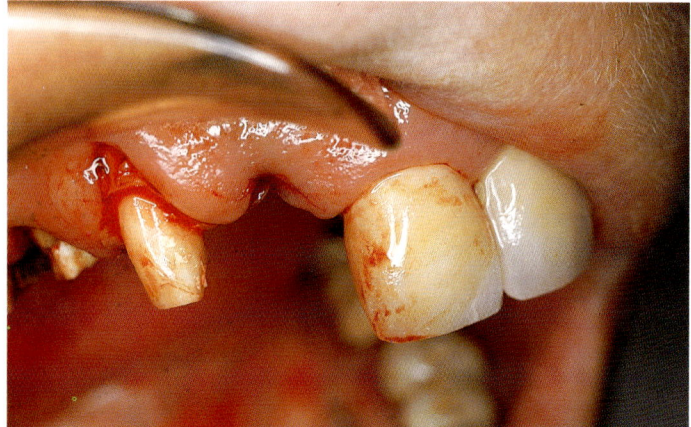

Fig 9-41 It resulted in an anesthetic vertical defect in V shape. The area was left for healing for 1 month, reopened by means of a horizontal incision, and a substantial epithelial graft was inserted into the defect.

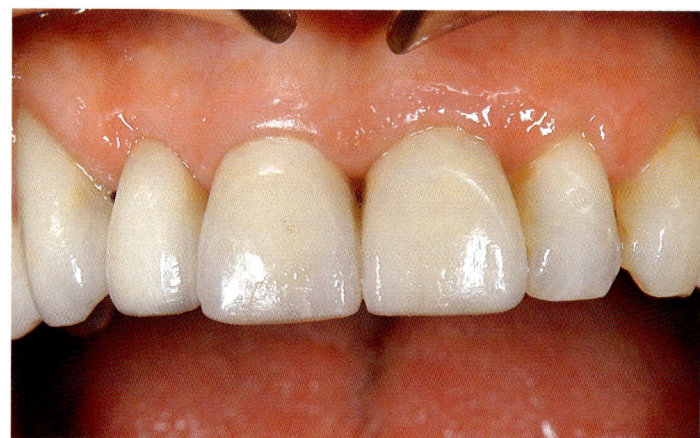

Fig 9-42 Six months later a secondary coronoapical pouch was prepared to correct the subsequent horizontal bone loss, and the case was finalized.

Metallic frame technique

To assure good control on the future reshaping of the crest in terms of volume and quality, a technique has been suggested that combines the technique of the flap with the insertion of a temporary metallic grid, which is used as a frame for HA and an osseous melted graft.[43] This technique, which requires a three-stage surgical procedure, presents a considerable advantage over the previously described techniques in the sense that the foreseen results are usually easily obtained. It also allows the prospect of restoration of severe vertical and combined vertical and horizontal defects with favorable predictability.

Sequence

Stage 1: two full-thicknesses of flap are elevated at the crest level, and an impression of the osseous topography is taken and transmitted to the laboratory. Also, periosteal stimulation is accomplished[44] and the flaps are sutured back into position. A nonprecious metallic frame will be cast, which not only adapts to the osseous topography but also restores the desired volume of the osseous ridge. The frame is rounded on the inside to allow for easy desinsertion and present openings from 5 to 9 mm^2.

Stage 2 (Figs 9-43 to 9-48): a recurrent partial-thickness flap is designed and elevated to allow for a future correct coaptation of the tissue and assure proper vascularization. The metallic frame is seated in position. Vascularization is assured by the proper design of the flap and by the endosseous vascularization that is stimulated through a small opening of the cortical plate. Dense HA *(B)* alone or mixed with autogenous bone taken from the tuberosity is introduced within the metallic frame *(A)* and the flap is sutured back in position. The remaining connective tissue is allowed to granulate.

Stage 3: 2 months later the metallic frame is removed without damaging the underlying grafted tissue, which looks fibrotic at that stage. This approach requires the collaboration of various specialists but opens a reliable approach for solving severely complex cases (Figs 9-49 to 9-52).

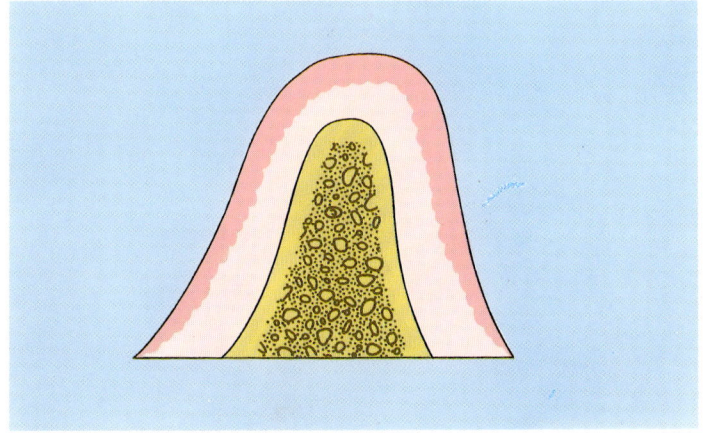

Fig 9-43 The presence of an adequate tissue thickness that has to be elevated three times is a prerequisite for the success of the metallic frame technique.

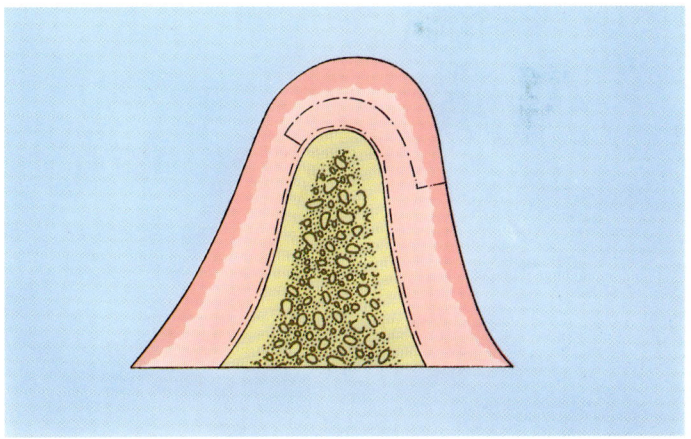

Fig 9-44 Stage 2. Diagrammatic design of the flap. This design can be used for other procedures when a lengthening of the flaps is required. It must be executed with great precision.

Ridge-Pontic Relationship

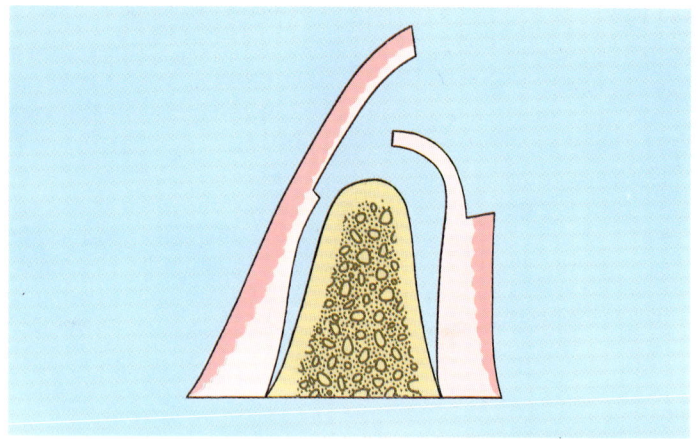

Fig 9-45 The flap is elevated and the dissection extended along both sides of the osseous crest.

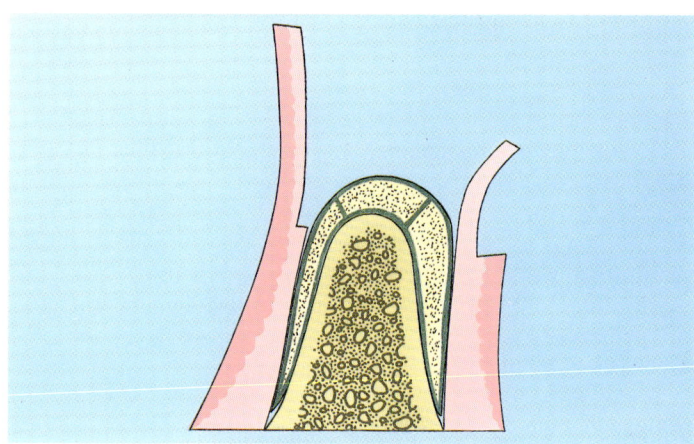

Fig 9-46 The metallic frame prepared in the laboratory according to an impression taken in the first surgical stage is inserted on a trial basis and then corrected until adaptation and stability are obtained.

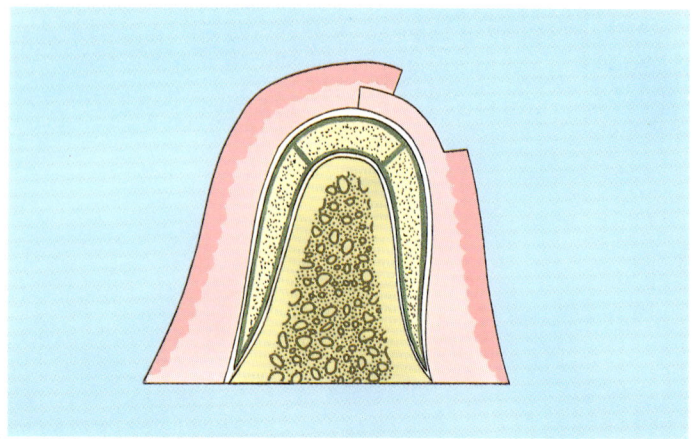

Fig 9-47 HA particle mixed with autogenous bone is incorporated into the frame and the flaps coapted. The remaining connective tissue is left for healing by granulation.

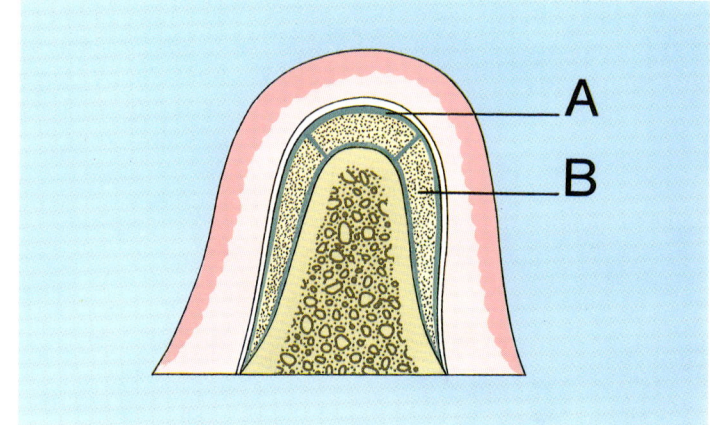

Fig 9-48 The frame is left for 3 months and then will be carefully removed in a third-stage procedure. (Suggested by P. Tardieu.)

Improved techniques for localized ridge augmentation

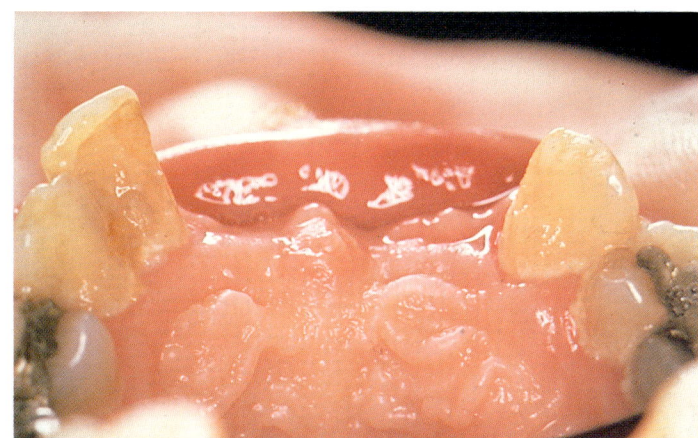

Fig 9-49 Initial clinical situation showing a significant horizontal defect. In a first-stage procedure the elevation of the flap will allow an impression of the crest anatomy for the design of the metallic frame. (Courtesy of P. Tardieu.)

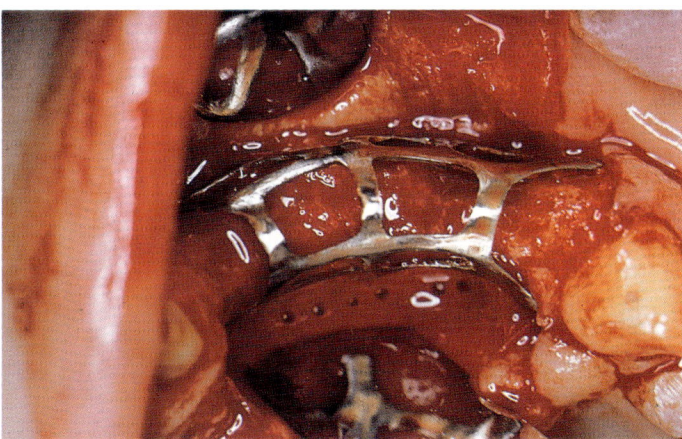

Fig 9-50 Stage 2 involves the opening of the site and the incorporation of the metallic frame. (Courtesy of P. Tardieu.)

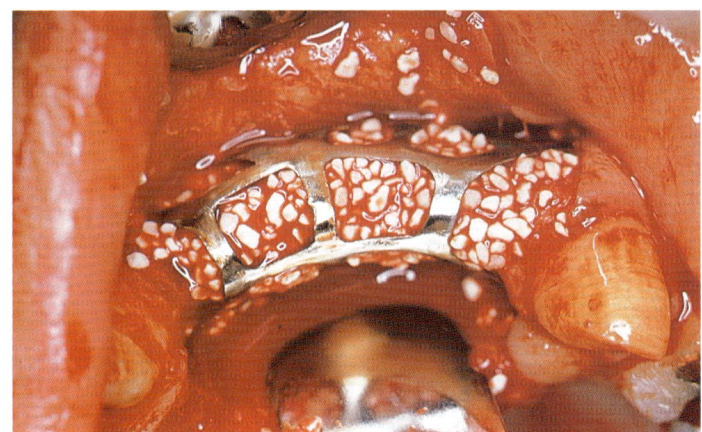

Fig 9-51 Placement of HA particles and autogenous bone. (Courtesy of P. Tardieu.)

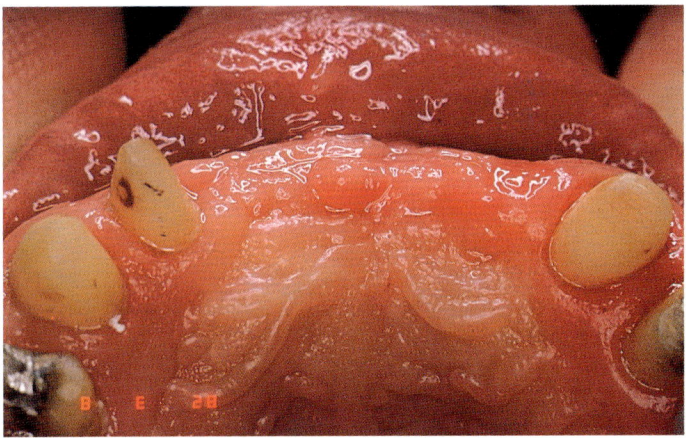

Fig 9-52 Final result after removing the metallic frame, stage 3 of the procedure, and tissue healing. (Courtesy of P. Tardieu.)

Pontic

Once the deformed partially edentulous ridge regains normal morphology by means of the aforementioned surgical procedures, prosthodontic treatment and pontic adaptation can be considered. The primary purpose of a pontic is to substitute for a missing tooth, and pontic design has to conform to the occlusal morphology and, to a great degree, to oral and labial morphology to satisfy esthetic requirements. The manner in which the pontic is adapted to the underlying soft tissue determines whether the surrounding tissues remain healthy or become diseased. The contact with the underlying tissue should be free from pressure because pressure may cause inflammation, loss of keratinized surface, ulceration, and bone resorption.

Many investigations have reported[45-48] that the inflammation of the edentulous area is probably a response to plaque accumulation on the surface of the pontic. Many advocate the specific use of highly glazed porcelain to contact the edentulous ridge,[49,50] and others have demonstrated no clinical or histologic differences in the response of the mucosa to carefully constructed pontics, whether they are gold, acrylic, or porcelain.[51,52]

The embrasure spaces adjacent to the abutment teeth should be open to allow room for interproximal tissue and access for oral hygiene.[48,53-55] Conversely, the embrasure space between two pontics should be close enough to reduce food and plaque accumulation as long as it is esthetically feasible. The gingival design of the pontic is of primary importance and, even though it has been clouded with empirical judgments, it directly depends upon the morphology of the ridge, its width, and the location of the mucogingival junction. Even if we assume that surgical corrections have improved the morphology of deformed ridges, edentulous areas do not exhibit a unique morphologic design and will require the use of a variety of pontic designs.

Pontic classification

Sanitary pontic

This type of pontic design does not come into any form of contact with the underlying tissue and leaves the proximal areas of the abutment teeth free from encumbrances, which makes oral hygiene particularly easy. This form is not recommended in areas where esthetics is concerned but may be of great help in areas where little space exists between abutments. In the posterior part of the mouth, in which the last abutment tooth is slightly mesially inclined and where a minimum band of attached gingiva exists, the sanitary pontic design may be the pontic of choice, permitting the best accessibility for oral hygiene. Because perfection does not exist, the insertion of such a type of pontic should be tested for a few days because it may become an area of food deposit and a site to which the tongue is invariably attracted.

Ridge lap pontic

This type of a pontic is considered undesirable from the point of view of tissue health and should be abandoned. Unfortunately, it is still systematically produced by technicians perplexed by tortuous crest designs that the restorative dentist did not provide by appropriate modification (Fig 9-53).

Modified ridge lap pontic

This represents the most commonly used pontic design and maintains slight contact with the underlying tissue on the buccal aspect of the ridge. This limited contact allows this area to be readily cleansed. A perfectly convex and reduced crest width is a prerequisite for this type of pontic, but depending on the underlying gingival architecture, a tendency to introduce slight concavities in the center of the gingival part of the pontic favoring plaque accumulation always exists (Fig 9-54).

Ovate pontic

The difficulty in systematically adapting the previously described pontic design to any situation, the increase in esthetic demand, and the development of efficient maintenance devices suggested to prosthodontists another type of gingival pontic design, the ovate pontic. This type of pontic requires the preparation of a concave gingival recipient site into which it could be inserted. This creates the conditions necessary to mimic the presence of the marginal and interdental papillae in assuring the requirements for maintenance purposes (Fig 9-55).

The modified ovate pontic is directly derived from the ovate and modified ridge lap pontic and is specially designed for areas of the mouth where a vertical osseous

Pontic

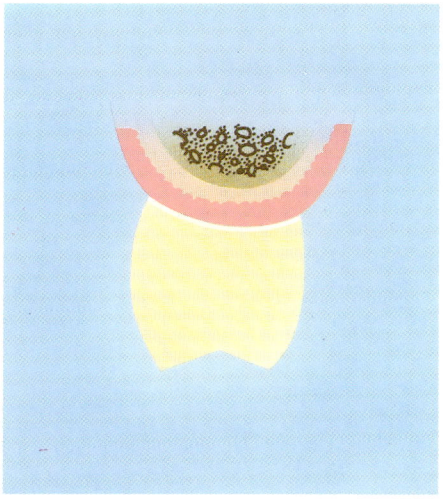

Fig 9-53 The ridge lap pontic establishes contact conforming to the anatomic design of the crest.

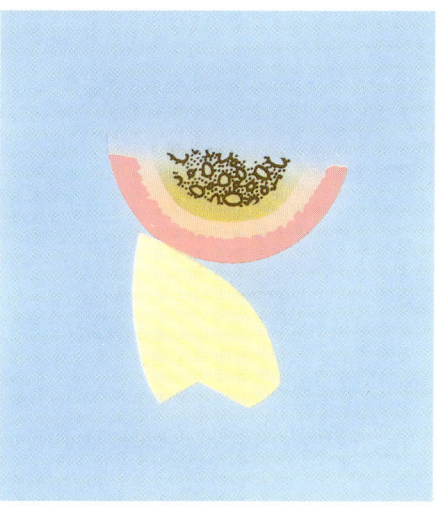

Fig 9-54 The modified ridge lap pontic establishes a selected contact on the buccal side of the crest.

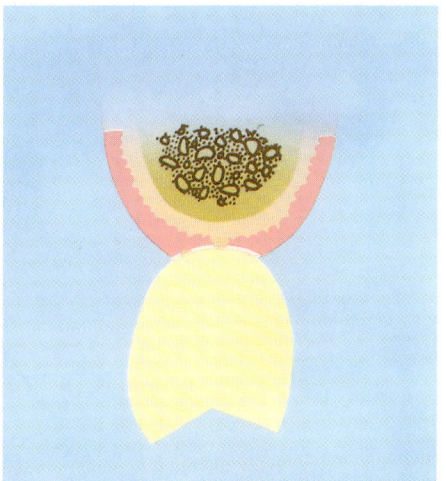

Fig 9-55 The ovate pontic restores full contact with a prepared concave recipient site permitting excellent cleaning by flossing. (Suggested by E. Rosenberg and D. Garber.)

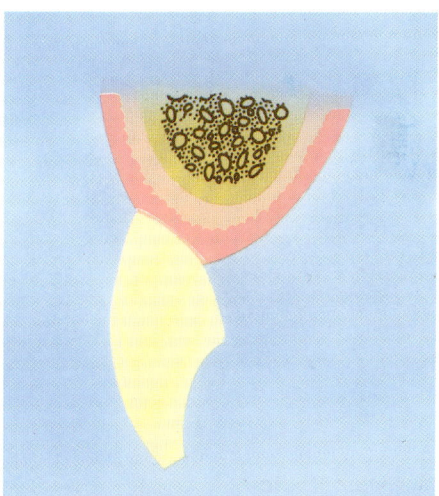

Fig 9-56 Modified ovate pontic is designed to establish identical contact with the underlying tissue when dealing with some types of vertical bone wall.

283

Ridge-Pontic Relationship

ridge exists. Like the ovate pontic design, it allows the creation of an illusive marginal and interdental gingiva (Fig 9-56). In posterior areas where we have to deal with larger, flatter, buccolingual edentulous crests, esthetics is systematically sacrificed to the imperatives of hygiene accessibility. Accessibility for oral hygiene diminishes anteroposteriorly and is directly dependent upon the patient's motivation and manual capabilities. These two factors are difficult to evaluate. They may be subject to dramatic changes depending upon life events and affect the long-term prognosis of rehabilitation.

Preparation of the recipient site

The preparation of the pontic recipient site is carried out under anesthesia after determination of the thickness of the soft tissue covering the osseous crest. A minimum thickness of 3 mm is required to perform a gingivoplasty by means of a rotary diamond instrument, sharp dissection, or electrosurgery. A concave bed is created, the diameter of which should correspond to the width of the original emerging root, and its borders mimic marginal and interdental papilla. This minor surgical preparation should precede the placement of the pontic. A dressing or provisional fixed partial denture, the gingival base of which has been relined and carefully polished, is placed over the area. The final impression can be taken at the same time and ideally the final restoration is temporarily inserted before final healing has taken place. A real esthetic improvement of the ridge–pontic relationship can be obtained by adopting the procedures described in this chapter, which can be used increasingly by the average professional (Figs 9-57 to 9-63).

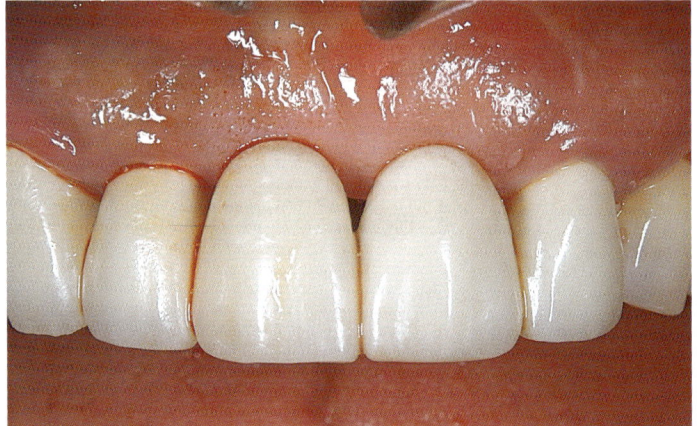

Fig 9-57 Endodontic problems on two of the abutment teeth greatly facilitated the desinsertion of this old bridge. During the sequence of endodontic treatment the pontic site was prepared by electrosurgery, the bridge relined, carefully polished, margin adaptation refined, and temporarily recemented.

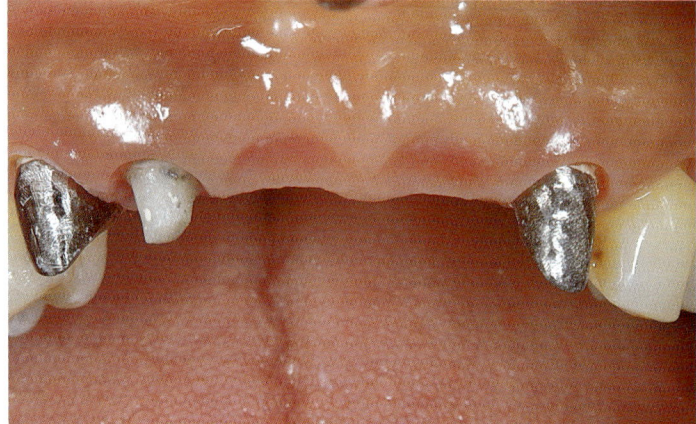

Fig 9-58 The area was left to heal for a week. Attention has been given in respecting the marginal papilla of the abutment teeth during electrosurgery.

Pontic

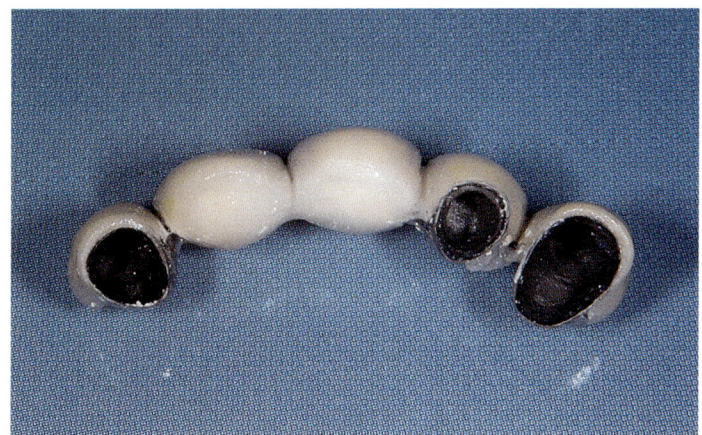

Fig 9-59 View of the gingival part of the bridge with its two well-designed ovate–modified ovate types of pontic.

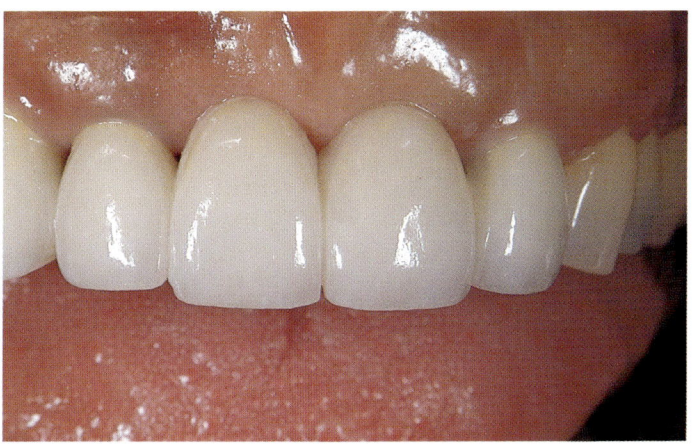

Fig 9-60 Final restoration in situ. Pontics are well seated in their prepared site. However, a better placement of the gingival zenith of the right central incisor would have improved the esthetic result.

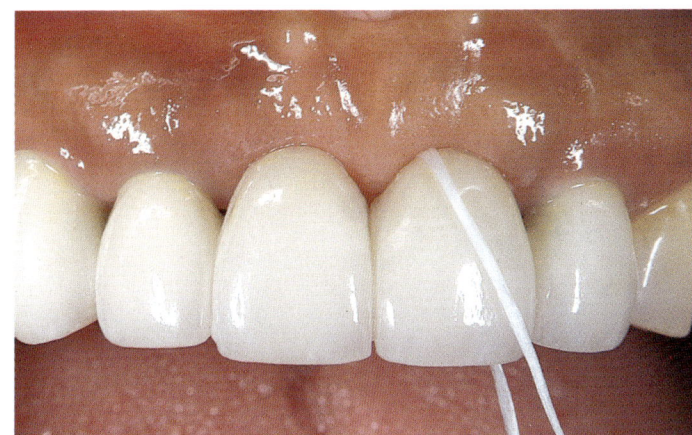

Fig 9-61 The rounded base of the pontics provides good accessibility for oral hygiene. The incisal extension of the interpontic embrasure would have permitted better visualization of the contact point.

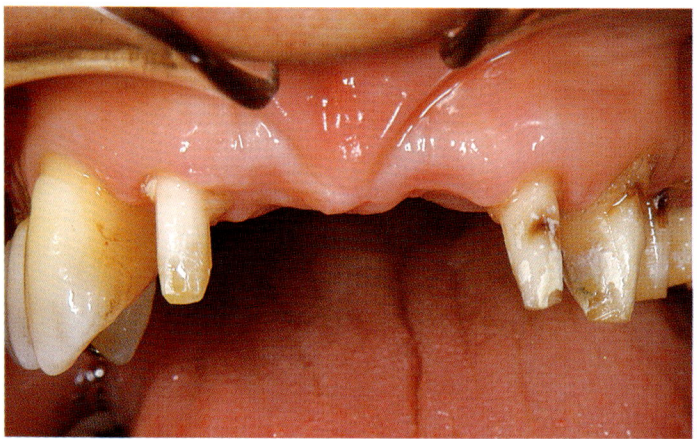

Fig 9-62 Clinical situation following preventive ridge augmentation. The incisal frenum has been left in place to maintain normal appearance between the two elements of the pontic.

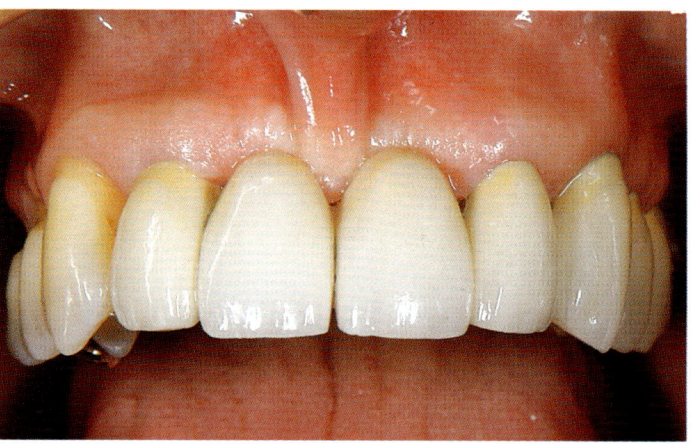

Fig 9-63 After preparation of the recipient site, a fixed partial denture is inserted and the pontics emerge nicely from the tissue. Despite periodontal surgery, tooth length remains within the limits of esthetic tolerance.

References

1. Butler. Cited by Brewer AA, Morrow RW. *Overdentures*. St. Louis, Mo: CV Mosby Co; 1975.
2. Miller PA. Complete dentures supported by natural teeth. *J Prosthet Dent*. 1958;8:924.
3. Lam RV, Poon KY. Acrylic resin root implants: A preliminary report. *J Prosthet Dent*. 1969;22:657.
4. Missika P. Les racines dentaires en carbone vitrifié. *Rev Odontostomatol*. 1977;6:15.
5. Denissen HW, de Groot K. Immediate dental root implants from dense calcium hydroxylapatite. *J Prosthet Dent*. 1979;42:551.
6. Bahat O. Preservation of ridges utilizing hydroxyapatite. *Int J Periodont Rest Dent*. 1987;6:35.
7. Quinn JH, Kent JN. Alveolar ridge maintenance with solid non porous hydroxylapatite root implants. *Oral Surg*. 1984;58:511–521.
8. Gumaer K et al. Evaluation of hydroxylapatite root implants in baboons. *J Oral Maxillofac Surg*. 1985;43:73–79.
9. Garver DG, Feuster RH, Baker RD, Johnson DL. Vital root retention in humans: A preliminary report. *J Prosthet Dent*. 1978;40:23.
10. Veldhuis AAH, Dreissen AA, Denissen HW et al. A five year evaluation of apatite tooth root as means to reduce ridge resorption. *Clin Prev Dent*. 1984;6:5.
11. Quinn JH, Kent JN. Alveolar ridge maintenance with solid non porous hydroxylapatite root implants. *Oral Surg*. 1984;58:511–521.
12. Salsbury RL, Quinn JH, Gumaer HI et al. Prevention of alveolar ridge resorption by placement of hydroxylapatite in fresh socket. *Trans Soc Biomater*. 1981;4:110.
13. Seibert JS. Reconstruction of deformed, partially edentulous ridges, using full thickness onlay grafts. I: technique and wound healing. *Compend Contin Educ Cen Dent*. 1983;4:437–453.
14. Allen EP et al. Improved techniqes for ridge augmentation: A report of 21 cases. *J Periodontol*. 1985;56:195.
15. Langer B, Calagna L. The subepithelial connective tissue graft. *J Prosthet Dent*. 1980;44:363.
16. Chaikin RW. *Elements of Surgical Treatment in the Delivery of Periodontal Therapy*. Berlin: Quintessenz, 1977.
17. Rateitschak KH, Wolf HF. *Parodontologie*. Stuttgart: Thieme; 1984.
18. Baker RD, Terry BC, Davis WH et al. Long term results of alveolar ridge augmentation. *J Oral Surg*. 1979;37:486–498.
19. Boyne PJ. Restorations of deficient edentulous ridges by bone grafting and the use of subperiosteal implants. *Int J Oral Surg*. 1974;3:278.
20. Boyne PJ, Cooksey DE. Use of cartilage and bone implants in restoration of edentulous ridges. *J Am Dent Assoc*. 1965;71:1426.
21. Mainows E, Boyne PJ, Hart G. Restoration of reaction osseous mandibles by grafting with a combination of mandible homograft and autogenous iliac narrow and hyperbaric oxygen. *Oral Surg*. 1973;35:13.
22. Frame JW. Hydroxylapatite as a biomaterial for alveolar ridge augmentation. *Int J Oral Maxillofac Surg*. 1987;16:642–655.
23. De Groot K. Bioceramics consisting of calcium phosphate salts. *Biomaterials*. 1980;1:47.
24. Jarcho M. Calcium phosphate ceramics as hard tissue prosthetics. *Clin Orthop*. 1981;157:259–278.

25. Jarcho M, Bolen CH, Thomas MB et al. Hydroxylapatite synthesis and characterization in dense polycristalline form. *J Mater Sci.* 1967;11:2027.
26. Kato K, Aoki H, Tabata T et al. Biocompatibility of apatite ceramics in mandibles. *Biomater Med Devices Artif Organs.* 1974;7:291.
27. Misiek DJ, Kent JN, Carr RF et al. Soft tissue response to different shaped hydroxylapatite particles. *J Dent Res.* 1983;62:196. Abstract.
28. Kent JN. Reconstruction of the alveolar ridge with hydroxylapatite. *Dent Clin North Am.* 1986;30:231.
29. Jarcho M, Kay JF, Gumaer KI et al. Tissue, cellular and subcellular events at a bone–ceramic hydroxylapatite interface. *J Bioeng.* 1977;1:79–92.
30. Drobeck HP, Rothstein SS, Gumaer KI, et al. Histopathologic observations for long term soft tissue responses following implantation of random shaped particles and discs of durapatite. *J Oral Maxillofac Surg.* 1984;42:143.
31. Jarcho M. Biomaterial aspects of calcium, phosphate. Properties and applications. *Dent Clin North Am.* 1986;30:25–47.
32. Metzger DS, Driskell TD, Paulsaud JR. Tricalcium phosphate ceramic: A resorbable bone implant: Review and current status. *J Am Dent Assoc.* 1982;105:1035.
33. Piecuch JF, Goldberg AJ, Shastry CV, Chrzanowski RB. Compressive strength of implanted replamineform hydroxylapatite. *J Biomed Res.* 1984;18:39–45.
34. Kenney EB, Lekovic V. Bone formation with porous hydroxylapatite in human periodontal defects. *J Periodontol.* 1976;2:76–85.
35. Abrams L. Augmentation of the deformed residual edentulous ridge for fixed prosthesis. *Compend Contin Educ Gen Dent.* 1980;1:205–214.
36. Garber DA, Rosenberg ES. The edentulous ridge in fixed prosthodontics. *Compend Contin Educ Gen Dent.* 1981;2:212–223.
37. Kaldahl WB, Tussing GJ, Wentz FR, Walker JA. Achieving an esthetic appearance with fixed prosthesis by submucosal grafts. *J Am Dent Assoc.* 1982;104:449–452.
38. Langer B, Calagna L. The subepithelial tissue graft. *J Prosthet Dent.* 1980;44:366–367.
39. Greenstein G, Jaffin RA, Hilsen KL, Berman CL. Repair of anterior gingival diformity with hydroxylapatite. *J Periodontol.* 1985;56:200–203.
40. Cohen HV. Localized ridge augmentation with hydroxylapatite: Report of case. *J Am Dent Assoc.* 1984;108:54–55.
41. Seibert JS, Cohen W. Periodontal considerations in preparation for fixed and removable prosthodontics. The Dental Clinic of North America. 1987;31:529–555.
42. Winnick AL. Periodontal and prosthetic considerations in the esthetic restoration of a cleft palate: A case report. *Int J Periodont Rest Dent.* 1987;3:75–80.
43. Tardieu PB. Reconstruction contrôlée des crêtes déformées: Technique de la grille. *J Parodontol.* 1986;5:185–194.
44. Goldman HM, Smukler H. Controlled surgical stimulation of periosteum. *J Periodontol.* 1978;49:518–522.
45. Wise M, Dykema R. The plaque retaining capacity of four dental materials. *J Prosthet Dent.* 1975;33:178.
46. Clayton J, Green E. Roughness of pontic materials and dental plaque. *J Prosthet Dent.* 1970;23:407.
47. Stein RS. Pontic–residual ridge relationship: A research report. *J Prosthet Dent.* 1966;16:283.
48. Henry P, Johnston J, Mitchell D. Tissue changes beneath fixed partial denture. *J Prosthet Dent.* 1966;16:937.
49. Glickman L. *Clinical Periodontology.* St. Louis, Mo: CV Mosby Co; 1953.
50. Cavazos E. Tissue response to fixed partial denture pontics. *J Prosthet Dent.* 1968;20:143.
51. Podshadley A. Gingival response to pontics. *J Prosthet Dent.* 1968;19:51.
52. Jones R. Pontic design in fixed prosthodontics. In Goldman H, Cohen DW, eds. *Current Therapy in Dentistry.* St. Louis, Mo: CV Mosby Co; 1970;4:259–269.
53. Tylman SD. *Theory and Practice of Crown and Bridge Prosthodontics.* 5th ed. St. Louis, Mo: CV Mosby Co; 1965.
54. Morris M. Artificial crown contours and gingival health. *J Prosthet Dent.* 1962;12:1146.
55. Johnston J, Phillips R, Dykema R. Pontic form. *Modern Practice in Crown and Bridge Prosthodontics.* 2nd ed. Philadelphia, Pa: WB Saunders Co; 1965;278–299.

Chapter 10

Mastering the Art of Tissue Management

Harold M. Shavell

Introduction

> The Little Man Who Wasn't There
>
> *As I was going up the stair*
> *I met a man who wasn't there.*
> *He wasn't there again today.*
> *I wish, I wish he'd stay away.*
>
> Hughes Mearns, 1875–1965)

To extrapolate this poem into the realm of dentistry, it might be read as follows. On the way to making final impressions, the dentist meets "a man who wasn't there" (gingival health). The absence of tissue health has given the dentist a difficult time, and the dentist fails in the attempt to make a proper impression of the boggy, prolapsed tissues. Another attempt is subsequently made, and the same failure ensues. ("He wasn't there again today.") Frustrated by the specter of the man who "wasn't there," and at this point willing to accept just about anything that even vaguely resembles a final impression, the dentist pleads for the apparition to stay away and not confront him with its reality ("I wish, I wish..."). The dentist, realizing the inability to control the tissue, proceeds nonetheless to forge ahead, consciously abjuring the "man" but secretly haunted by the ghost of what was once healthy tissue.

Atraumatic mechanical manipulation of the delicate gingival tissues during high-speed tooth preparation, retraction, and final impression making is a challenge dentistry has invented for itself. If imprudently performed, it can cause a multitude of adverse effects, not the least of which is irreversible damage to the complex dentogingival attachment region. This entire zone histologically is miniscule compared with the size of the mechanical contrivances with which we attack the area. The potential for trauma is great.

Should harm actually occur, injury to the junctional epithelium results in a series of cellular reorganizational changes at the attachment complex level that will inevitably alter gingival marginal heights. If, for example, final impressions for the maxillary anterior teeth were also "taken" (they are precisely made, not "taken") during preparation and provisionalization — adding to the chemomechanical insult to the tissues — the planned esthetics may not turn out exactly as anticipated.

Irreversible loss of interproximal tissue may have occurred; one, several, or all the papillae may have been rendered necrotic. Or perhaps just a few were only reversibly damaged, became ulcerated, and reformed at a different level and in a different shape. Because preparational trauma is not always equally distributed, not all gingival margins recede to the same degree. Add to this the possibility of hastily made "temporary" crowns with inconsistent margins and bulky, rough surfaces. Next, the entrapment of cement and possibly soft tissue tags between the edges of the ill-fitting provisional restorations and the margins of the preparation during temporary cementation seals the fate of the tissue more than it does the tooth itself. Cement spews into the sulcus, where it remains unseen and forgotten, left there to be colonized by bacteria and subsequently cause even further tissue destruction. Ironically, against this intemperate background, the final crowns are often being fabricated in the laboratory.

At the next appointment (try-in or perhaps cementation) something odd is observed. The newly fabricated crowns are no longer intracrevicular, and most margins are now readily apparent. The patient objects to the "dark lines at the gum line," and the teeth look as though they are of different lengths because of the disparate gingival levels. The dark interproximal spaces are powerful, and the eye is drawn to them. The patient does

Mastering the Art of Tissue Management

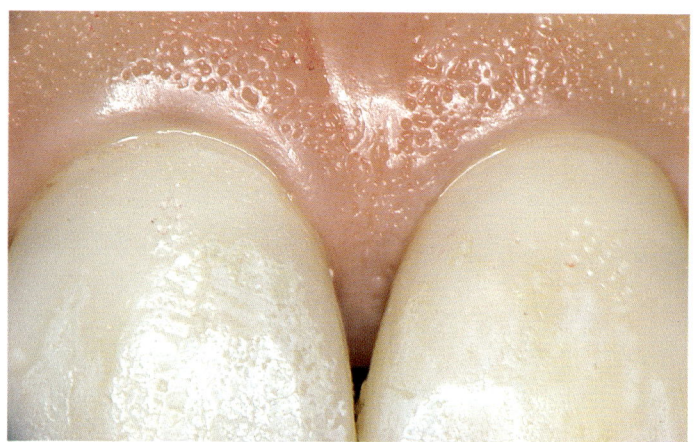

Fig 10-1a

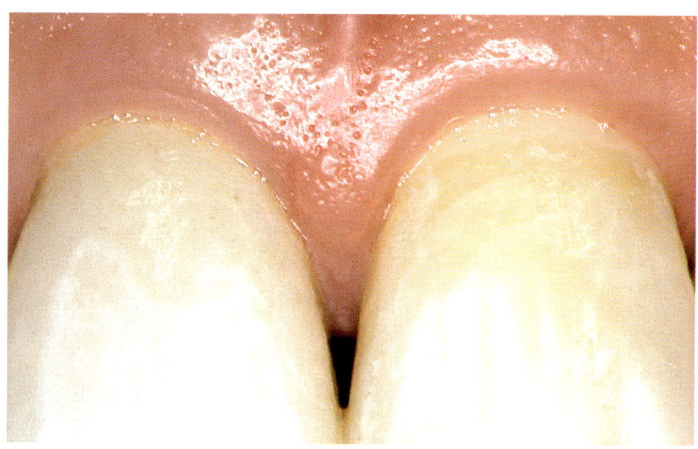

Fig 10-1b

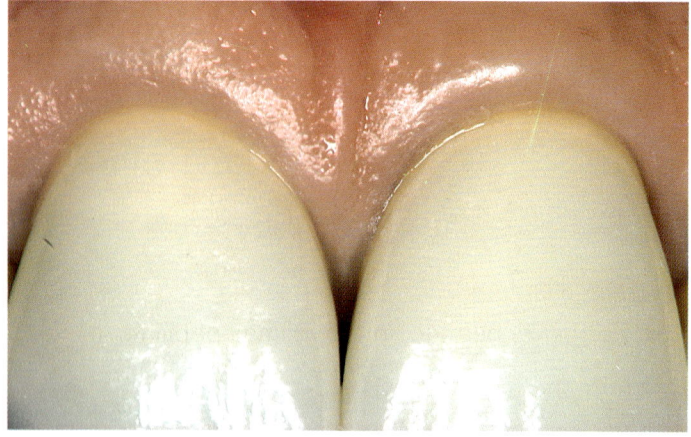

Fig 10-1c

Figs 10-1a to c The provisional restorations (10-1a and b) interface with the periodontium in a benign and respectful fashion, as do the metal ceramic restorations (10-1c). Every restoration must consider the periodontium and the occlusion.

not like the shapes or the color of the crowns. The tissues are friable and inflamed and bleed easily. The beguiled dentist searches for an explanation.

Simply stated, as dentists we are licensed to perform what in many instances we do not understand. This chapter addresses itself to these issues in the hope that some light can be shed on proper clinical tissue management to avoid unnecessary gingival trauma during mechanical maneuvers in a region where errors of a fraction of a millimeter can lead to disastrous results. Basic anatomic and morphologic guidelines will be discussed for provisional and final crown form. Instrumentation, armamentarium, retraction, and margin placement will be discussed for tooth preparation. A method of tissue protection during high-speed cutting will be presented, and the key element to predictably successful final impressions will be demonstrated. Final esthetic and functional restorative results using these techniques will be shown.

Mastering the art of seeing

It is hoped as well that some light can be shed (however small) on the processes of artistic creativity. Dentists to a great degree must objectify their thoughts as they engage in visual thinking. They then must make those thoughts visible (ie, tangible), but if they never really engage in an information-rich visual language (suffer stagnant visual infantilism), how will they ever perceive relationships, proportions, lights, shadows, form, or negative spaces? And isn't this what restorative dentistry is all about?

To understand the topographic anatomy of the healthy periodontium, to evaluate the flow of the tissues as they envelop the teeth, to perceive the entire perioprosthetic gestalt, or to deal with rehabilitational esthetics, visual thinking (not verbal) is required. It is most often an acquired talent that must be learned, but it may not be capable of being taught. It is the difference between looking and seeing. Thus, the leitmotif of this chapter will be to present its visual material descriptively, hoping to stimulate artistic, creative dentists not only to look, but to see; not only to read, but to visualize.

Visual perception is an essential precept that conveys a mystical sense of connection to nature's perfection. Nature is governed by design, and an exquisitely attentive eye can detect in out-of-the way corners traces of beauty that reflect the basic order of the universe. However, an absolute, impersonal recognition of the significance of facts is the initial prerequisite for subsequent esthetic revelation.

Periodontal esthetics

Perioprosthetic rationale

To achieve the lasting circumcoronal tissue health as well as the consistent intracrevicular margination of these labially butted metal ceramic restorations at 6 years (Fig 10-1c), the gingival tissue must be atraumatically manipulated during retraction, tooth preparation, provisionalization, and final impression making. In addition, the dentist must have a thorough knowledge of specific anatomic, occlusal, and esthetic requirements before treatment. The dentist must then be able to successfully test this knowledge in the most crucial way possible — against the tissue itself, beginning with the provisional restoration. In the examples of provisionalization shown (Figs 10-1a and b), notice the physiologic form and health of the surrounding tissues: the intracrevicular margination, the knife-like interproximal tissue, the stippling, and the lack of inflammation. Although obviously a product of atraumatic tissue management during preparation, this tissue health is also a reflection of provisional marginal seal, emergence profile, proximal concavity, labial contour, surface texture smoothness, personal oral hygiene instruction, and patient follow-through. The term *emergence profile* refers to the cervical outline of the tooth or restoration as it emerges (exits) the periodontium. It may also be thought of as *egression silhouette*. Such tissue does not just magically appear. It is earned by both doctor and patient working together for a common purpose: a healthy, peaceful coexistence between dental restoration and surrounding periodontium. An ideal restoration is the utopian reintegration of lost morphotypia.

Tissue mirrors technique

Upon provisional restoration removal (Fig 10-2), *tissue mirrors technique*. Notice the absence of inflammation, the normal-appearing interproximal papillae, the stippling, the physiologic restitution of sulcular epithelium, and the absence of retained cement, plaque, or debris in the gingival crevices. These revealing inferior-superior incisal photographs are the quintessential evaluative views of interproximal provisional tissues. Poor provisional physiologic form, open margins, and inattentive professional and/or personal oral hygiene mitigates against achieving such tissue health. To aspire to this level of tissue response, a methodology must be practiced to perfection by both dentist and patient. After initial atraumatic soft and hard tissue preparation, provisionalization, and subsequent meticulous cementation, the patient is seen weekly for tissue evaluation. Once the overt signs of labial–palatal gingival health become manifest (return to normal color, form, texture, density, crevice depth, and epithelial attachment), the provisional restorations are then removed for this direct interproximal tissue evaluation. This step generally takes place 2 to 3 weeks postprovisionalization. Final impressions are not scheduled until the interproximal tissues appear completely normal (4 to 6 weeks). A well-made, well-

Mastering the Art of Tissue Management

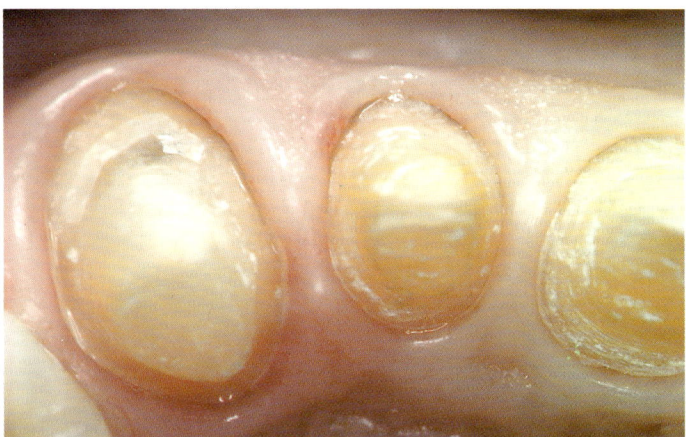

Fig 10-2a

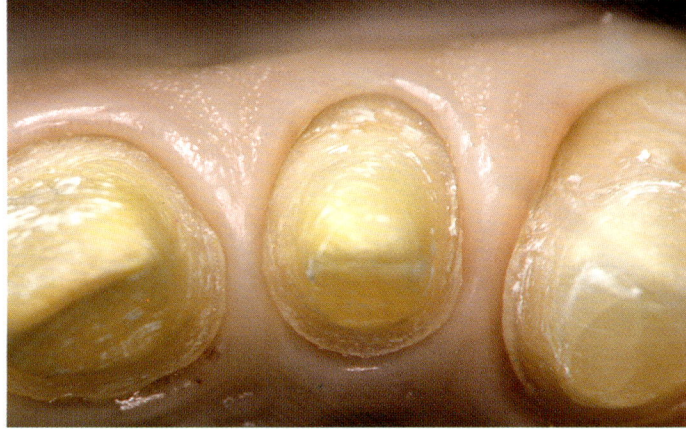

Fig 10-2b

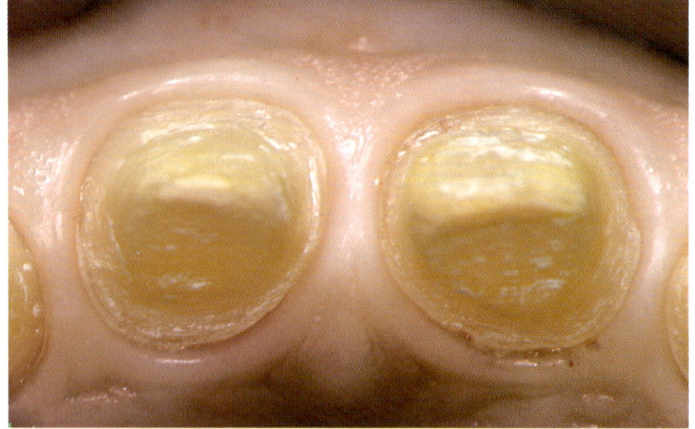

Fig 10-2c

Figs 10-2a to c The tissue talks. This periodontium indicates the peaceful coexistence that prevails between it and the provisional restorations. The principle of gingival nonviolence is illustrated. Note the interproximal papillary epithelialization and the absence of sulcular debris.

cemented provisional restoration is a storehouse of vitally important technical information and the scaffolding upon which the architecture of gingival healing takes place.

Anatomic variations

Whether the tissue management is in the maxilla or the mandible, anterior or posterior, the essential precepts of gingival nonviolence hold true. However, there are certain regional anatomic variations in provisional (and of course, final) crown form that must be considered to maintain a physiologic periodontium. For all anterior teeth (Fig 10-3c) proximal contacts occur in the incisal one third cervicoincisally and in the labial one third labiolingually. The maxillary and mandibular posterior regions (Figs 10-3a and b) are progressively broader based anteroposteriorly, and the interproximal tissues vary accordingly. Proximal contacts are always more occlusal on the mesials, and mesial contacts always more buccal than distal contacts. The cervical rise of the cementoenamel junction (CEJ) proximally is always greater on the mesial than on the distal aspect of the same tooth. It generally decreases as it proceeds posteriorly, allowing for parallel alignment of the CEJ, marginal ridges, and

Gingival displacement methods

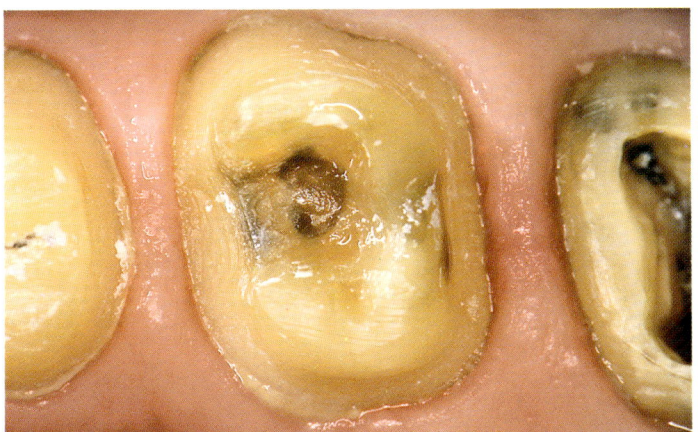

Fig 10-3a

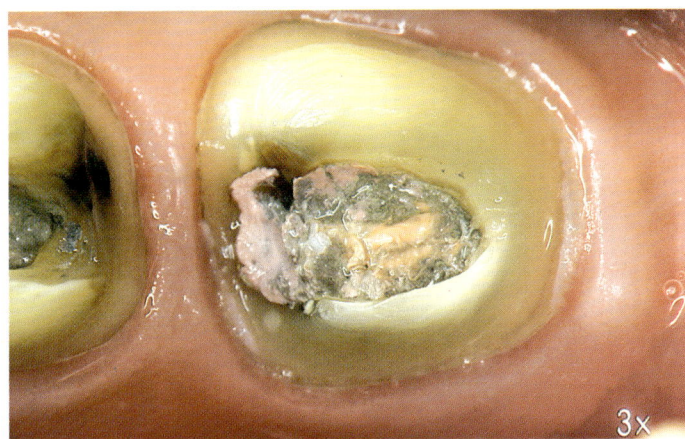

Fig 10-3b

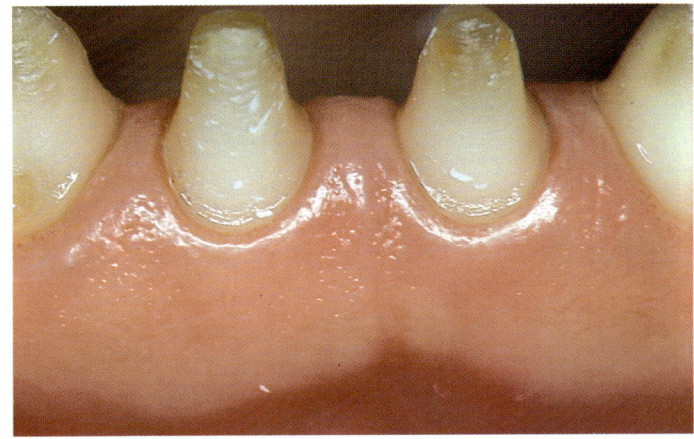

Fig 10-3c

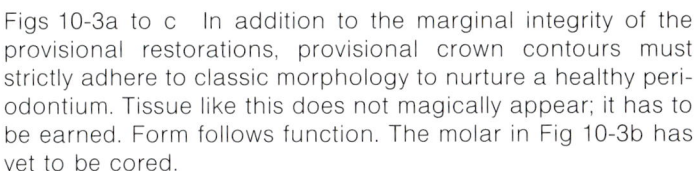

Figs 10-3a to c In addition to the marginal integrity of the provisional restorations, provisional crown contours must strictly adhere to classic morphology to nurture a healthy periodontium. Tissue like this does not magically appear; it has to be earned. Form follows function. The molar in Fig 10-3b has yet to be cored.

the underlying bony crest. Buccal contours for all teeth occur in the cervical one third or at the junction of the cervical and middle one third. Occlusal morphologic form in the mandible is trapezoidal, and in the maxilla, rhomboidal. All these criteria ultimately become manifest in the gingival architectural form shown. Structural beauty (provisional or final) must be a determining criterion if we are to achieve successful function (gingival health).

Gingival displacement methods

"Dry" retraction concept

Case 1 (Figs 10-4 to 10-12) illustrates the "dry" method of tissue retraction. In the example shown of the maxillary six anterior teeth (Fig 10-4), note the presenting cervical discoloration, which cannot be removed by prophylaxis. It will serve as a benchmark for visual comparisons of soft tissue height alteration during subsequent preparational maneuvers. The periodontium is essentially noninflammatory, there is ample attached tissue, the crevice depth is 2 to 2.5 mm, the texture is stippled, and the teeth

Mastering the Art of Tissue Management

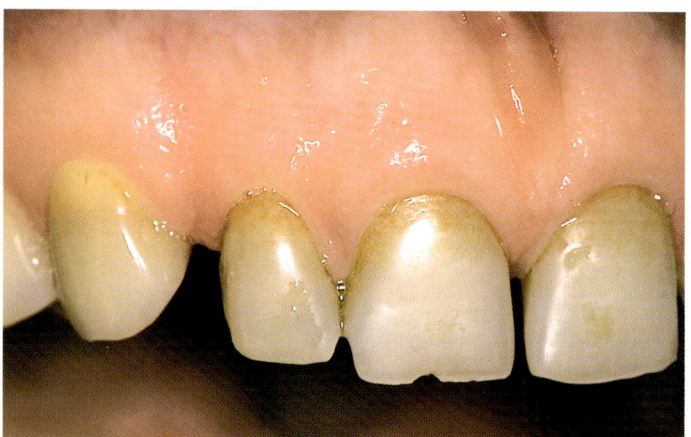

Fig 10-4a

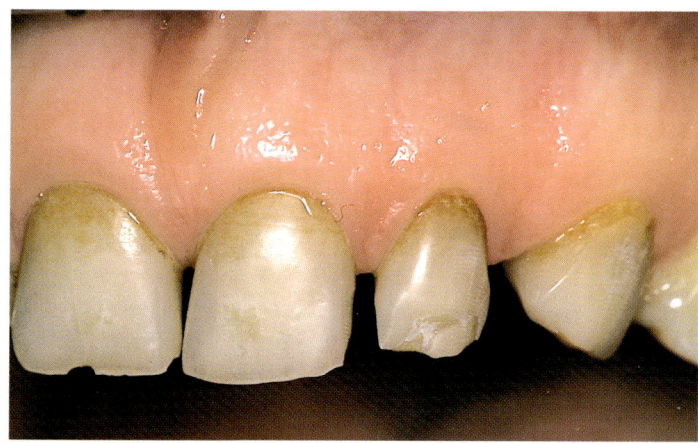

Fig 10-4b

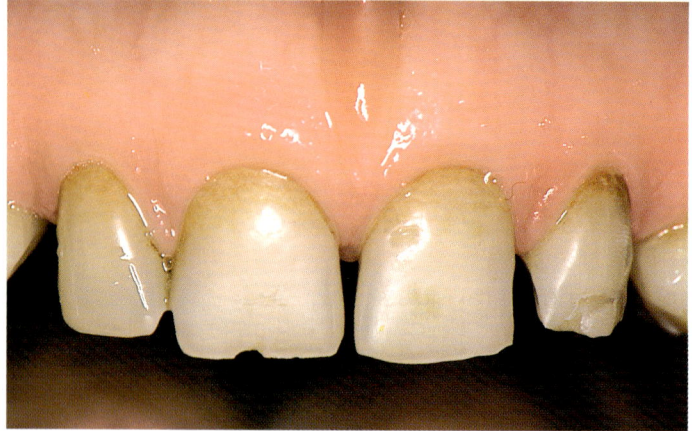

Fig 10-4c

Figs 10-4a to c Case 1 at presentation. The six anterior teeth are to be crowned. Note the cervical discoloration that will later be used to judge tissue movement. The periodontium is within normal limits and must always be addressed first.

are reasonably well aligned. All proximal contacts are initially removed to gain access to the interproximal regions; the presenting diastemata in this particular case facilitates this step. Next, *the soft tissue is always prepared before the hard tissue.* In other words, gain gingival retraction first. Then, leaving the retraction cord in place, prepare the teeth to the already retracted (and thus protected) gingival level. No attempt is made to prepare deeply within the sulcus because doing so would clearly constitute an encroachment upon (and possibly a violation of) the attachment apparatus. Instead, only the occlusal one third of the gingival crevice is entered (approximately 1 mm), and even then only

gently with the retraction cord. Having thus produced chemomechanical ischemia and retraction, and having prepared only to the retracted gingival level, all margins will become intracrevicular upon cord removal and tissue rebound. At the same time, the sulcus has been atraumatically manipulated and is laceration-free.

Retraction armamentarium

Although the retraction armamentarium is essentially the operator's choice, there are certain instruments and materials that are of great help in achieving the desired

Gingival displacement methods

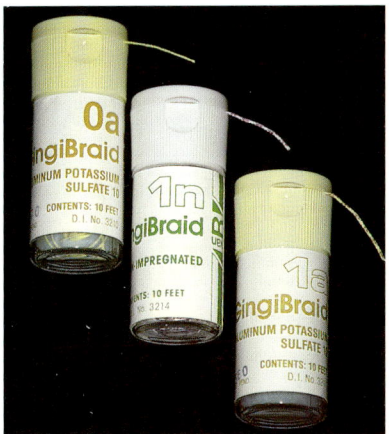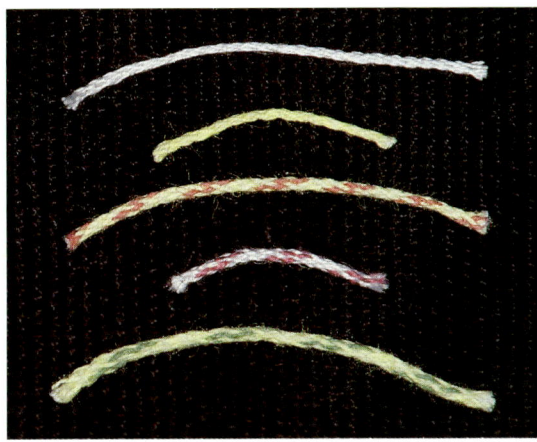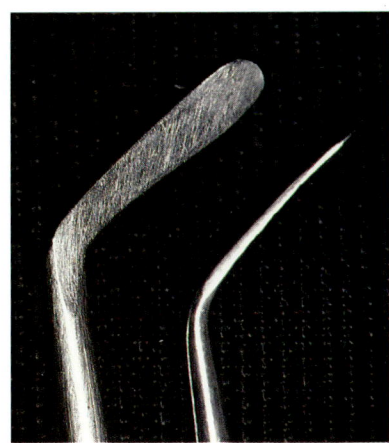

Figs 10-5a to c   The retraction armamentarium for the "dry" technique. Things are subservient to technique, which is subordinate to principle. The principle of gingival nonviolence is a sine qua non of operative and prosthodontic treatment.

results. Figure 10-5a illustrates the Gingibraid retraction cords used in the dry method, sizes 0 and 2. Although there are a variety of Gingibraid sizes and chemicals available, numbers 0 and 1 are generally employed; the cords are either nonimpregnated (n) or impregnated with potassium aluminium sulfate 10% (a). Each size has its own color code. At no time whatsoever should epinephrine be used in the retraction procedure. In Fig 10-5b, interproximal and premolar length circumferential cords are illustrated in different sizes. The white cord on the top is size 0 (n), next in succession are 0 (a), 1 (a), 1 (n), and 2 (a). The latter size is used least often and *never* as the initial retraction cord. All cords are braided, will not shred, and keep their tubular form during handling. The preferred gingival retraction instrument is the Retracta-Gard (Fig 10-5c). It is binangle, 0.5 mm thick, 3 mm wide, has smooth, rounded edges, a light, slender, polished shank for greater tactile sense, and serves a dual purpose as retractor and deflector. The key to predictable gingival esthetics is trauma-free gingival tissue, unscathed even after high-speed coarse diamond tooth preparation, and subsequent provisionalization. The additional guarding/deflecting use of the instrument will soon be apparent.

Retraction technique

In Fig 10-6, the retraction technique is demonstrated on the central incisors with a no. 1 (a) Gingibraid cord. The canines and lateral incisors have already been retracted as evidenced by the gingival ischemia and beginning apical displacement. This can conveniently be assessed via the tissue's progressive movement away from the benchmark cervical enamel discoloration seen in these and subsequent illustrations. Notice the long axis angle of the Retracta-Gard instrument as it is placed against the enamel of the left central incisor and directed gently into the sulcus in the direction from whence the cord issues (Fig 10-6a). This prevents the cord from being displaced, which has previously been tucked into position. By placing the instrument initially flat against the enamel and then engaging the innermost aspect of the cord, a rolling effect is produced, which has the effect of spinning the cord into the sulcus. To initially place the instrument peripherally against the tissue during retraction would invite slippage and laceration and would also produce a displacing effect on the cord. The retraction instrument is moved in a distal direction with a gentle tucking stroke directed mesially (Fig 10-6b). The cord is almost to place, and the retraction effect is already becoming evident. The retraction is complete for the left central incisor (Fig 10-6c). Properly sizing the

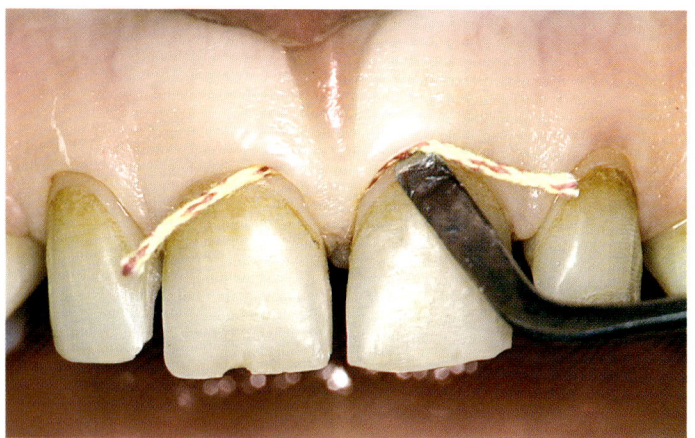

Fig 10-6a

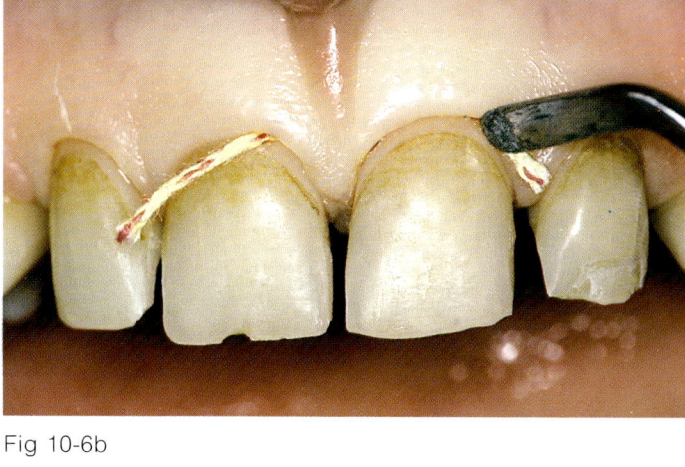

Fig 10-6b

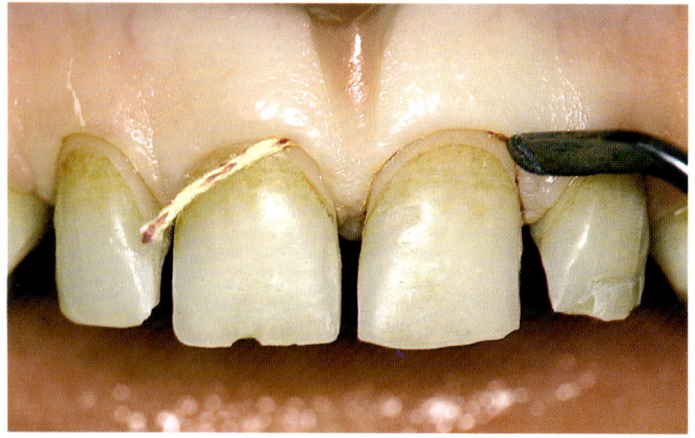

Fig 10-6c

Figs 10-6a to c The retraction technique for the maxillary left central incisor. Delicate intracrevicular tamping and tucking of healthy tissue is bloodless. Always address the soft tissue before the hard tissue.

cords is vital to avoid overlapping and consequent excessive tissue displacement; this will require intraoperative customizing of the previously cut cord. The instrument at no time is placed greater than 1 mm intracrevicularly. No encroachment must ever be made upon the junctional epithelium.

Figure 10-7 illustrates the gingival tissue of the right central incisor being retracted in the same fashion as has been described. Note the absence of clear, yellow, or red sulcular exudate. Also note the minimum depth placement of the retraction instrument intracrevicularly, the effect of the chemomechanical ischemia without resorting to problem-producing epinephrine, and the progressive retraction effect. To aid in clear field, saliva-free operation, 15 mg of propantheline bromide is taken orally 1 hour before appointment time. Major contraindications are glaucoma, prostatitis, and obstructive bowel disease. To attempt "dry" retraction in a saliva-ridden and mucous-laden environment seems pointless because it defeats the purpose and makes treatment more time-consuming and less effective. However, once the retraction cord has been placed in the sulcus free of the concerns of copious ropey saliva, partially prepared teeth, lacerated bleeding tissue, and completely obstructed vision, it may now be moistened with an adjunctive astringent. This enhances ischemia and swells

Gingival displacement methods

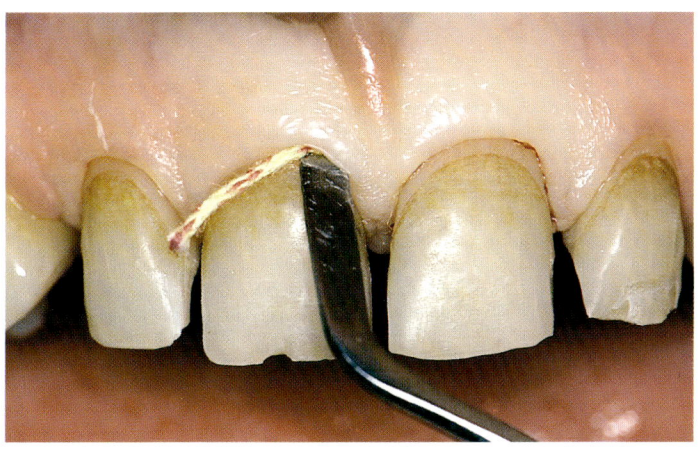

Fig 10-7a

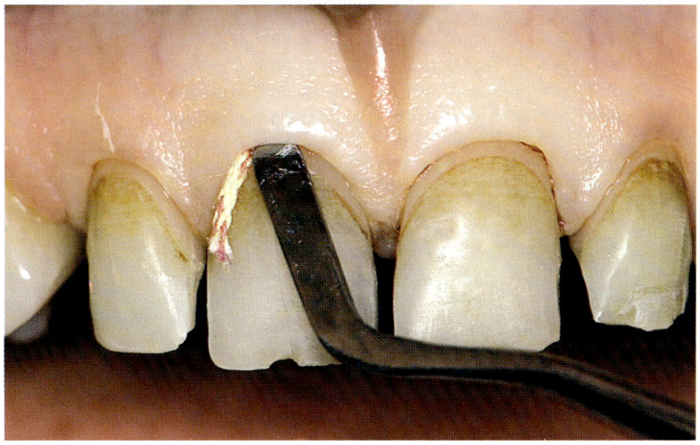

Fig 10-7b

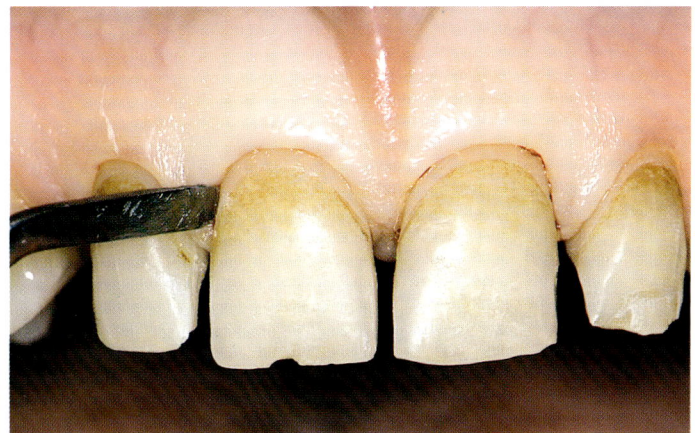

Fig 10-7c

Figs 10-7a to c The right maxillary central incisor retraction is completed. Note the amount of gingival movement compared with the (preoperative) marginal cervical discoloration.

the cord, which also serves to further enhance the mechanical retraction. As will be shown, neither during the "dry" technique nor during the "wet" technique, which follows, does the tissue ever become injured, escharotic, or necrotic. The gingival tissue may be maneuvered and manipulated, but never macerated.

Preparation armamentarium

The adjunctive astringent used to moisten retraction cords is Styptin, a 20% aluminium chloride solution in a buffered glycol concentrate (Fig 10-8b). Clinically, there is no adverse tissue reaction noted with the use of this concentration, and it has the added advantages of being colored while also possessing a gelatinous base (see Fig 10-9a). This aids in keeping the solution localized and readily visible as opposed to runny and colorless, in which case it always seems to slip unseen into the mouth where it is perceived by the patient as foul tasting. The nos. 3 and 5 Big Bite Diamonds chosen from a complete kit of six are shown in Figs 10-8a and c. Big Bite burs are slightly tapered, unusually coarse natural diamond burs that have remarkable longevity, are completely concentric at maximum speeds, and efficiently reduce tooth structure at an astonishingly rapid rate.

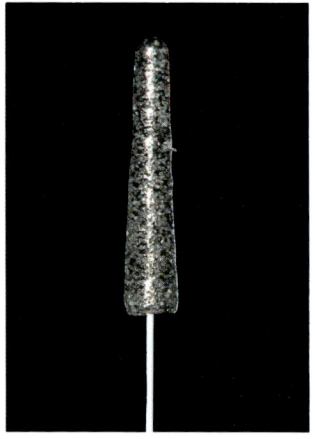 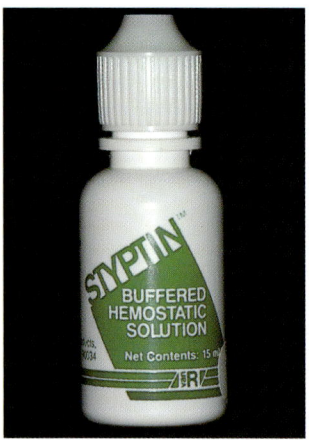 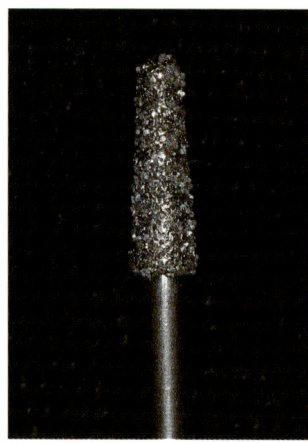

Figs 10-8a to c The adjunctive, synergistic astringent (10-8b) is 20% aluminum chloride in a buffered glycol solution. The nos. 3 and 5 Big Bite Diamond Cutting Instruments selected from a set of six (10-8a and c).

The no. 3 Big Bite Diamond (Fig 10-8a) is roughly equivalent in size to the average preparation diamond chosen by most dentists. The no. 5 Big Bite Diamond (Fig 10-8c) is two sizes larger and clearly shows the degree of coarseness needed for efficient, atraumatic tooth reduction. Indeed, this same coarseness will chew up gingival tissue as rapidly as the tooth is prepared if the tissue is inadvertently allowed to get in the way. Hence, the ironic contrast in the technique being presented: a method for gentle, protective tissue management that uses an unusually large, extremely coarse diamond running at high speed in close proximity to the tissues but yet *never* abrading them.

Preparation rationale

The ubiquitous Retracta-Gard is used to apply the gelatinous aluminum chloride over the completed retraction, thus potentiating the ischemia and swelling the Gingibraid (Fig 10-9a). A few moments later, the teeth are tamped dry and the appropriate preparation diamond is selected. In this particular case, the no. 3 Big Bite bur (Fig 10-9b) is too thin to efficiently prepare the teeth in question. The chamfer so produced would be inadequate. After slicing through the interproximal spaces, many more labiolingual axial preparational strokes will be needed to further reduce tooth structure and refine the preparations for both approximating teeth. The no. 5 Big Bite bur (Fig 10-9c) seems more appropriate for the task of tooth preparation for these particular teeth. Note how with one stroke interproximally the reduction of the right central incisor would produce an ideal preparation if the bur became more apically placed (but not touching the soft tissue). Although it is also true that perhaps similar placement of the larger no. 6 Big Bite Diamond (not shown) could be visualized as simultaneously preparing the left central incisor interproximally

Gingival displacement methods

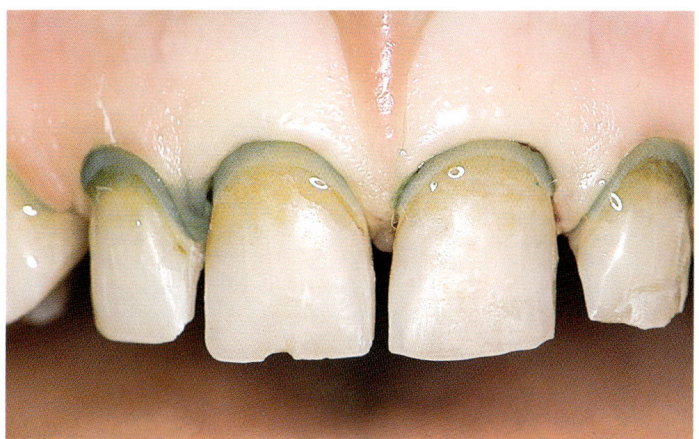

Fig 10-9a

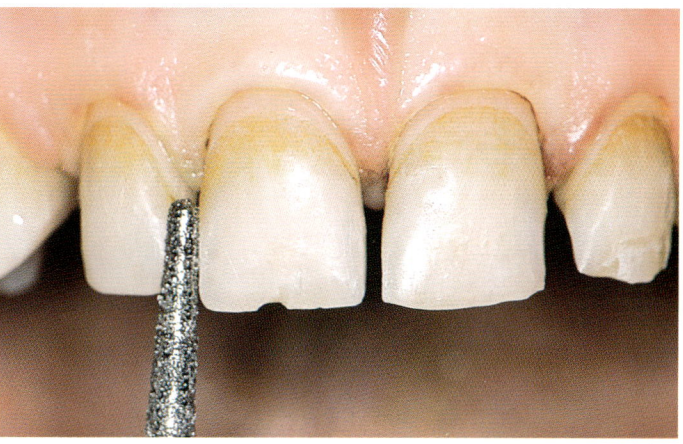

Fig 10-9b

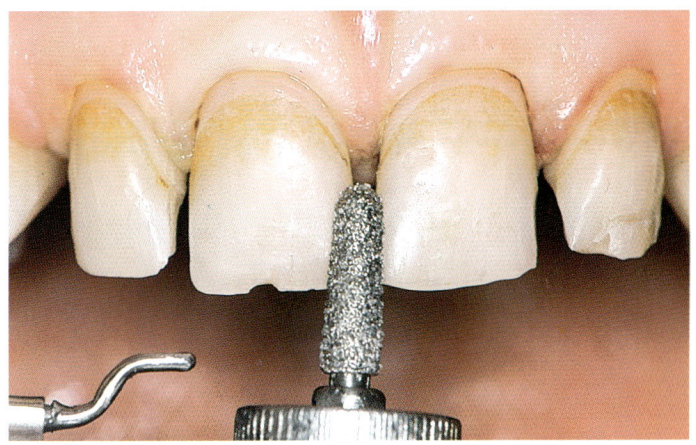

Fig 10-9c

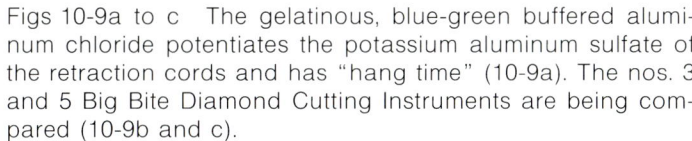

Figs 10-9a to c The gelatinous, blue-green buffered aluminum chloride potentiates the potassium aluminum sulfate of the retraction cords and has "hang time" (10-9a). The nos. 3 and 5 Big Bite Diamond Cutting Instruments are being compared (10-9b and c).

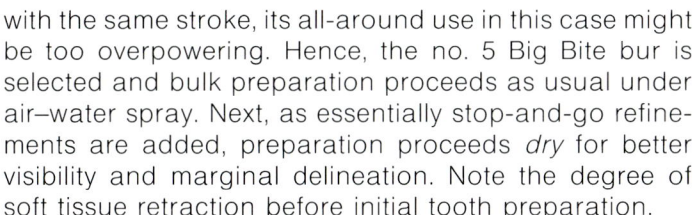

with the same stroke, its all-around use in this case might be too overpowering. Hence, the no. 5 Big Bite bur is selected and bulk preparation proceeds as usual under air–water spray. Next, as essentially stop-and-go refinements are added, preparation proceeds *dry* for better visibility and marginal delineation. Note the degree of soft tissue retraction before initial tooth preparation.

Preparation technique

With the retraction cord still in place, initial bulk preparation under air–water spray is rapidly accomplished with the appropriately selected Big Bite Diamond (Fig 10-10a). The six anterior teeth have been roughly prepared in the usual fashion to the retracted gingival level only, without any soft tissue excoriation whatsoever. Note the Retracta-Gard instrument position as it is initially placed for gingival protection. The instrument is then elevated in position for additional retraction as well (Fig 10-10b). As the no. 5 Big Bite bur is moved circumcoronally during margin placement, the Retracta-Gard is positioned in the

299

Mastering the Art of Tissue Management

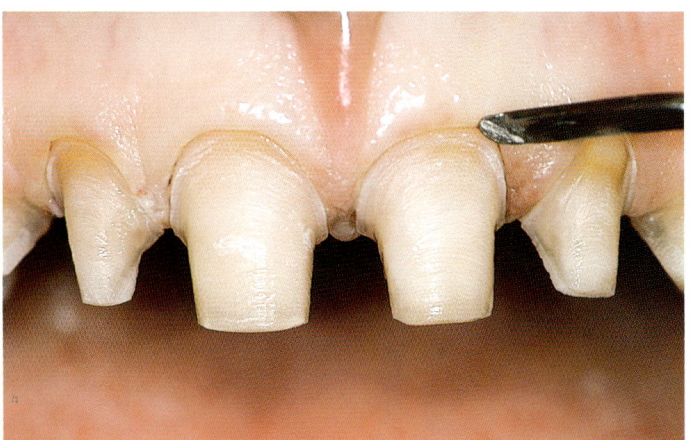

Fig 10-10a

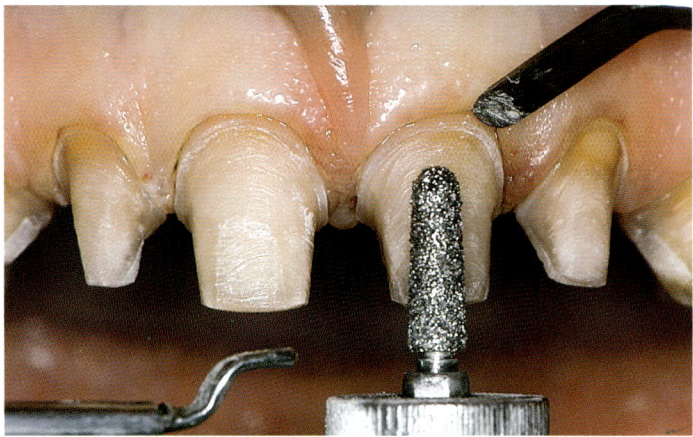

Fig 10-10b

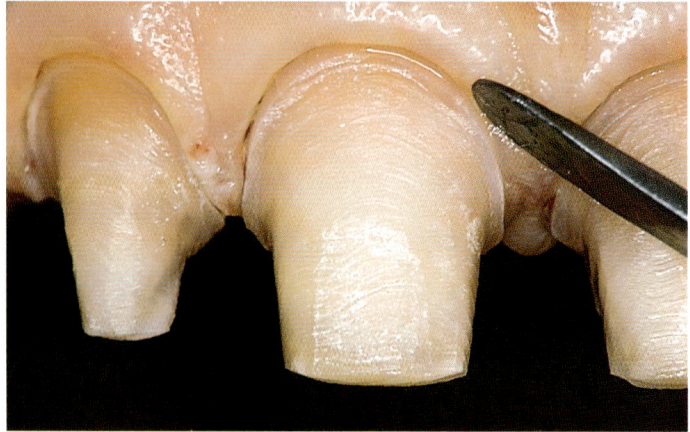

Fig 10-10c

Figs 10-10a to c   Gross preparation proceeds under air–water spray to the retracted gingival level; refinements are accomplished dry. The use of the Retracta-Gard instrument must be mastered with the nonprimary hand. Notice the unscathed tissue.

sulcus accordingly for protection. Note the scratch marks on the instrument; better here than on the tissue. A closer magnification of the Retracta-Gard instrument initially placed on the mesial aspect of the right central incisor is shown in Fig 10-10c. Note the absence of any gingival bleeding because the teeth were prepared to the retracted gingival level only while the soft tissues were concomitantly protected. Now make the comparison with Fig 10-11a where the Retracta-Gard is in the same place on the same tooth but has been rotated superiorly for additional retraction and protection. Note the ability to see all margins distinctly. The anatomic dimensional confines of the dentogingival complex within which we work are exceedingly limited and readily given to irreversible damage should the fragility of the tissues not be taken into consideration.

In Fig 10-11a, notice the clog-free nature of the Big Bite Diamonds in use, the effects of bur deflection on the Retracta-Gard, and the interproximal silhouette of the Big Bite Diamond shape, which has produced the chamfered margin. Figure 10-11b shows a close-up view of Retracta-Gard placement on the left central incisor, slightly deflecting the gingival tissue cervically. Modest cervical pressure on the instrument (Fig 10-11c) has retracted the gingival tissue a bit more in anticipation of the no. 5 Big Bite bur placement. Clearly, the margin can

Gingival displacement methods

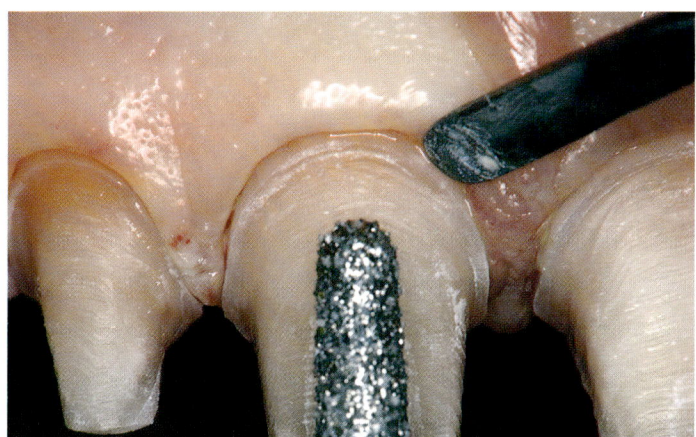

Fig 10-11a

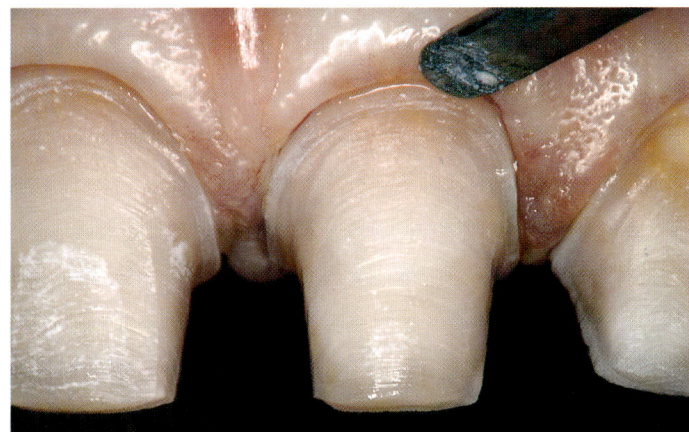

Fig 10-11b

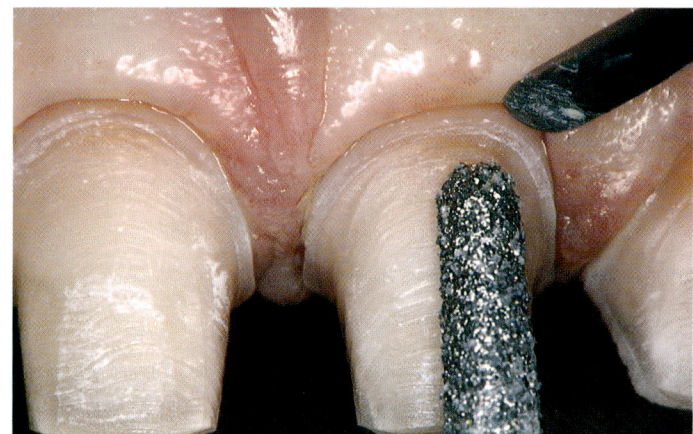

Fig 10-11c

Figs 10-11a to c   The Retracta-Gard moves simultaneously with the Big Bite bur, additionally retracting tissue and protecting the delicate dentogingival attachment complex. The handpiece is run intermittently for these refinements.

still be lowered to the Retracta-Gard surface and yet even then the coarse diamond will still not abrade gingival tissue. Not one red blood cell has been extravasated; no curettage, no crevittage, no hemorrhage. Upon cord removal and tissue rebound all margins will subsequently be approximately 1 mm intracrevicular. As discussed and illustrated in Fig 10-1, the methodology must be tested in the only place it can be proven: against the tissue itself. Hence, an observational period ensues post-provisionalization where not only are the tissues evaluated, but provisional occlusion, phonetics, and esthetics are also evaluated. However, in not following the same meticulous approach for provisional fabrication as has been suggested for tissue management, hard-won soft tissue gains will be completely reversed. The ensuing provisional restoration serves as a prequel to the final restoration.

Completed preparations

The initial tooth preparations have been completed with extremely coarse diamonds; yet, note that the soft tissue is remarkably unscathed (Fig 10-12). The no. 1 Gingibraid retraction cords are still in situ intracrevicularly and have remained as entirely free of fraying or bur impinge-

Mastering the Art of Tissue Management

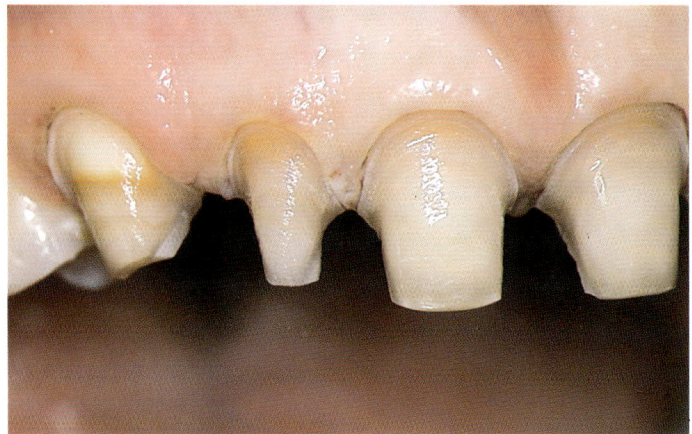

Fig 10-12a

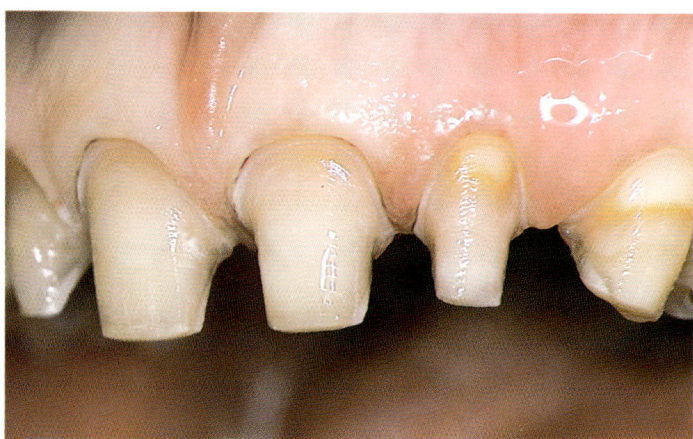

Fig 10-12b

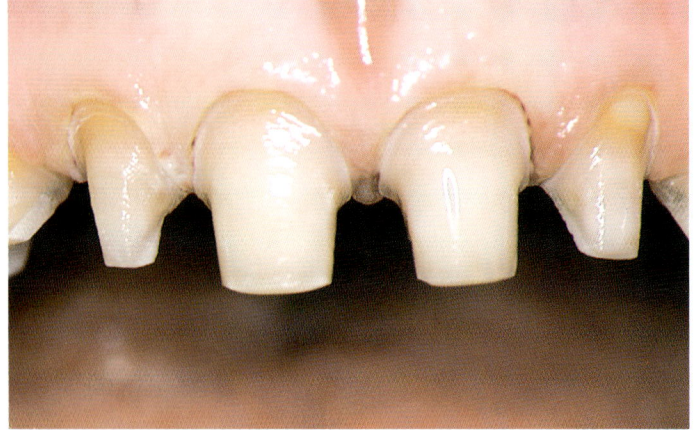

Fig 10-12c

Figs 10-12a to c Tissue mirrors technique. The teeth have undergone initial chamfer preparation to preoperatively retracted gingival tissue. Upon rebound all margins will be intracrevicular. Cords are still present.

ment as the tissue itself. The attachment apparatus has not been threatened. The teeth and tissues have been painted with a thin layer of mineral oil USP in anticipation of the direct provisionalization technique to follow. The retraction cords may remain in place until provisionalization is completed or they may be removed now (before provisionalization) to more readily proceed with marginal adaptation. In the former instance, retaining the cords within the sulcus during provisional fabrication (assuming all margins are clearly visible) and cementation assures that any overlooked cement inadvertently present in the sulcus would simultaneously be dislodged along with the retraction cords. In this fashion, complete and thorough cement debridement is effected. To be less than assiduous in this endeavor would mean that all preventive gingival maneuvers taken to this point to produce the postoperative tissue illustrated would have been performed for naught. After provisionalization completion, the patient is seen weekly for tissue checks pending final impression making. It is axiomatic that multiple tooth preparation and final impressions not be performed during the same appointment if the quality and character of the tissues seen in Figs 10-2, 10-3, and 10-22 are to be emulated.

Gingival displacement methods

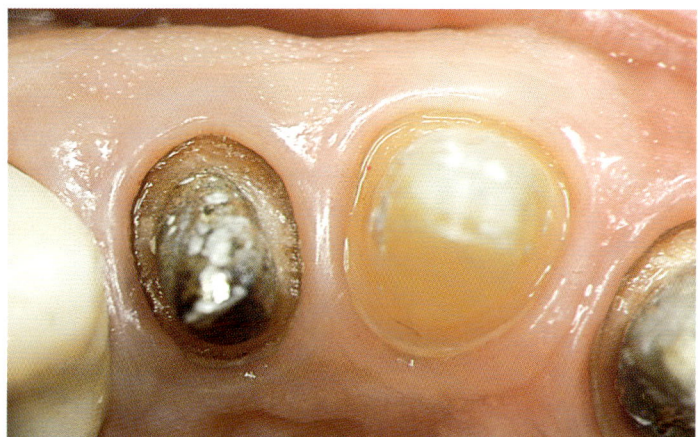

Fig 10-13a

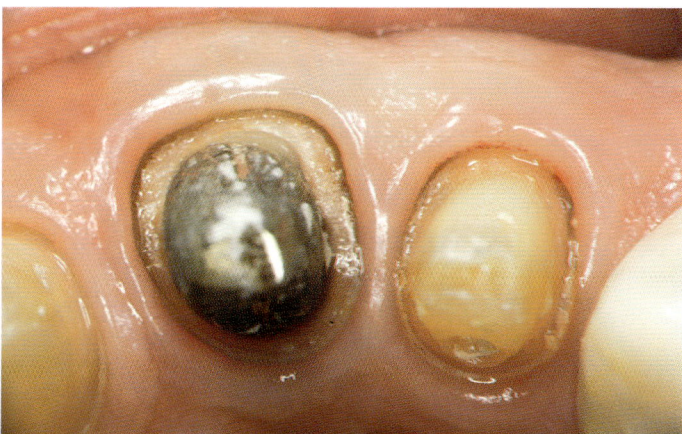

Fig 10-13b

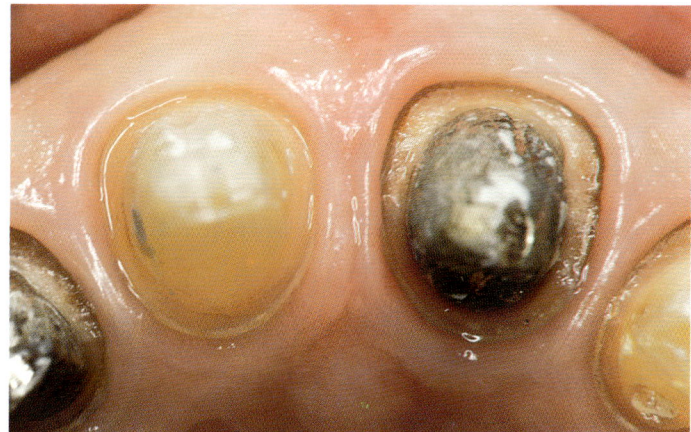

Fig 10-13c

Figs 10-13a to c Case 2 at presentation. The four anterior teeth are to be crowned. The initial preparation and provisionalization have already been previously accomplished. Note the topographic physiology of the tissue.

"Wet" retraction concept

Case 2 illustrates the "wet" method of tissue retraction (Fig 10-13). In the example, the teeth have been previously prepared, cored, and provisionalized. The patient has returned for final preparation, impression making, and provisional remargination. Note the health and beauty of the underlying periodontal tissues after provisional removal, even allowing the altered proximal contacts caused by the temporary splinting of the provisional restorations. Notice in particular the interproximal tissues as seen from the incisal view. The preparational modalities espoused herein are rational in theory and workable in fact. Good dentistry takes time to perform, but if there is not enough time to do it right to begin with, when is time ever going to be found to do it over properly? Probably never. Thrusting the imposition of an artifice upon living tissues is at best a poor compromise for missing anatomic parts. At the very least, let us be cognizant of the ensuing organic responses to our inorganic contrivances and fashion them accordingly and with care. Excellence or expedience? Restoration or ruination? The dentist who thinks in histologic, anatomic, and artistic terms (and who can make his or her thoughts tangibly visible) will always avoid doing irreversible damage to the periodontium and will garner the

Mastering the Art of Tissue Management

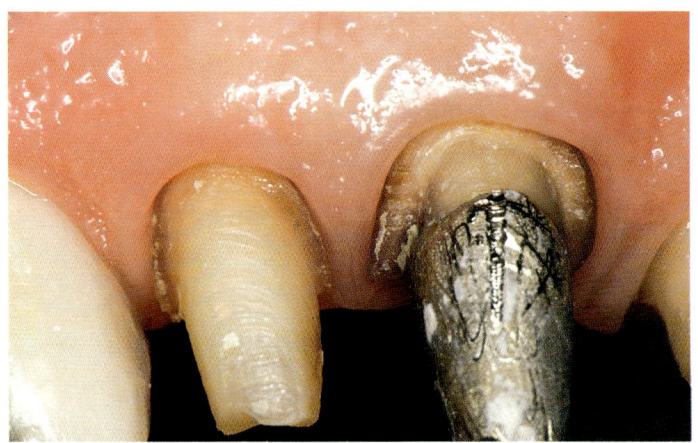

Fig 10-14a

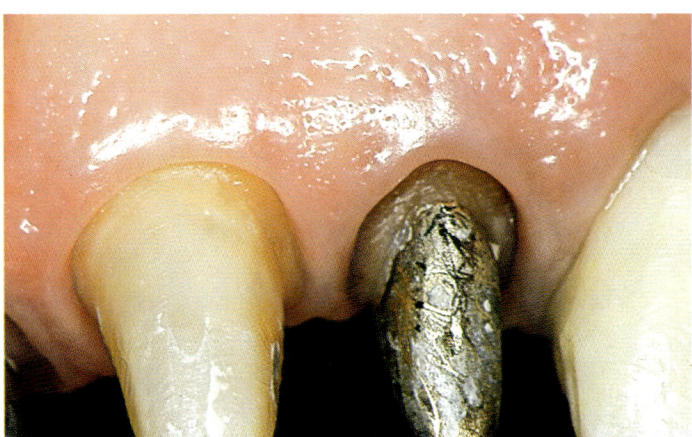

Fig 10-14b

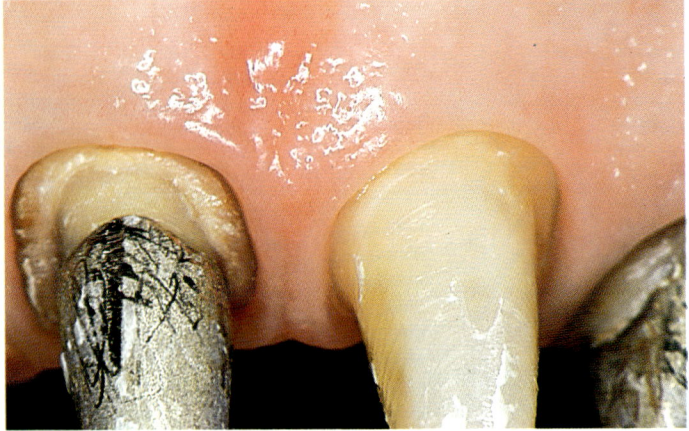

Fig 10-14c

Figs 10-14a to c The labial views of Fig 10-13. Case 2 is to be treated with the wet method of tissue retraction. Note the intracrevicular position of all margins and the absence of crevicular seepage or detritus of any kind.

respect of his or her colleagues, the patient, and ultimately the tissue itself.

In altering the incisal visual perspective of Fig 10-13 to the labial views of the same case, note in particular the crevicular response to physiologic provisionalization (Fig 10-14). The canines and both posterior quadrants have already been provisionalized. The interproximal gingival architecture is fully mature and shows no clinical evidence of inflammation, ulceration, or saucerization. Provisional crown margins are minimally intracrevicular and well adapted, as judged from the "tissue talk." However, there is a lack of chamfer depth in the preparations. In proceeding with further tooth reduction uti-

lizing the "wet" method of retraction (as in the "dry" method), *the soft tissues are addressed first* via initial retraction as has been described. The difference is that the wet retraction cords are generally dry cords that have either been soaked in astringent before placement (in which case retraction is more difficult) or dry cords that have been gelled (Fig 10-15b). In the latter case, the cord does manage to retain its integrity beacause the gel keeps the cord from becoming limp. With either technique, provisional margination, emergence profile, facial–palatal contours, and postoperative cement debridement must be meticulously executed or tissue will not respond as shown. Structural beauty must be a de-

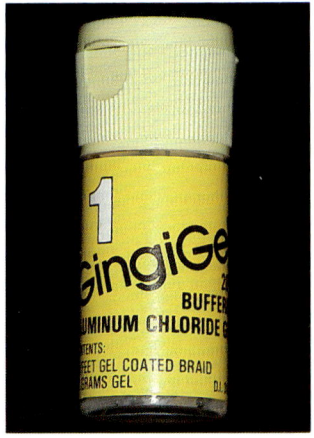 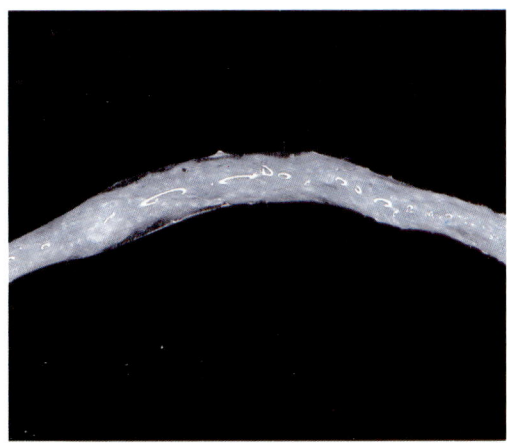 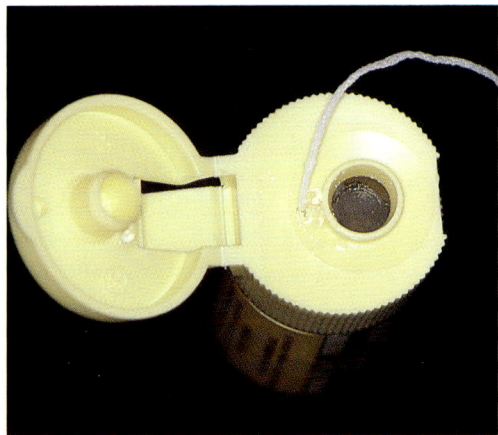

Figs 10-15a to c   Although not "wet" in the typical presoaked fashion of placing dry retraction cords in potentiating solutions, Gingigel cord emanates coated from a vial of 20% buffered aluminum chloride in a thick gel.

Retraction armamentarium

Gingigel retraction cord is a unique item that is remarkably effective. It consists of a braided cord impregnated with, and resting within, a thick gel of 20% buffered aluminium chloride. As opposed to the Gingibraid sizes previously discussed, it is not marketed in the 0 size, only sizes 1 and 2. As shown in Fig 10-15b, the no. 1 cord shown is wet but not limp or collapsed. It holds its shape while at the same time is laden with astringent gel that is carried into the crevice along with the cord. Additionally, a small quantity of the gel may be aseptically removed from the container and placed in a dappen dish for topical application during the retraction procedure. Alternatively, the gel may be introduced into the crevice before actual retraction where its viscous nature precludes rapid dissolution for lengthened astringent effect. This variation may also be used with the Gingibraid cord. Indeed, because the cord in the vial is used up in advance of the gel, a vial filled with usable 20% buffered aluminum chloride in a petroleum jelly–like gel remains. The concept of creative frugality would then have the dentist take dry Gingibraid cords cut to appropriate dimensions (interproximal, premolar circumferentials, molar circumferentials) and with a metal spatula roll them in a portion of the leftover gel that has been placed on a glass slab. This extends gel usage and at the same time creates a new kind of cord.

As opposed to Gingibraid, which can be sized, precut for efficiency, and stored in advance of treatment, Gingigel cannot be as conveniently handled. Exposure to the environment renders it tacky and difficult to handle. It must be sized and used within a few minutes for best results. However, because consummate prosthodontic tissue management is infinitely complicated in its absence, it has become the author's choice for gingival retraction.

Preparation technique

The Gingigel "wet" retraction procedure is performed exactly as has been described previously for the Gingibraid dry procedure (Fig 10-16). Note the cords in place within the crevice; there should be no overlapping. Note also the chemomechanical lateral displacement of the gingival tissues allowing for complete peripheral margin visibility. The Retracta-Gard instrument is positioned ac-

Mastering the Art of Tissue Management

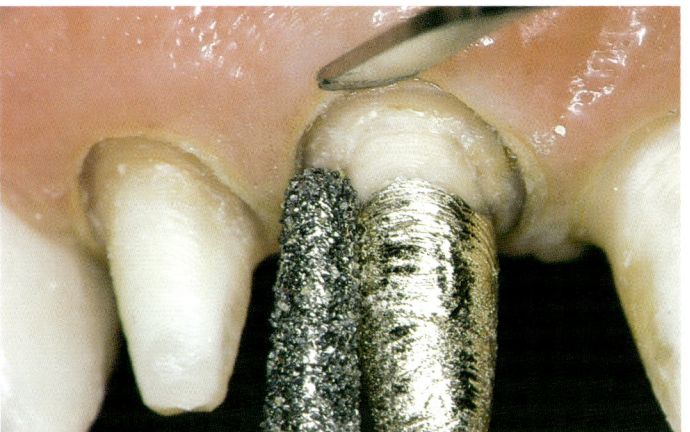

Fig 10-16a

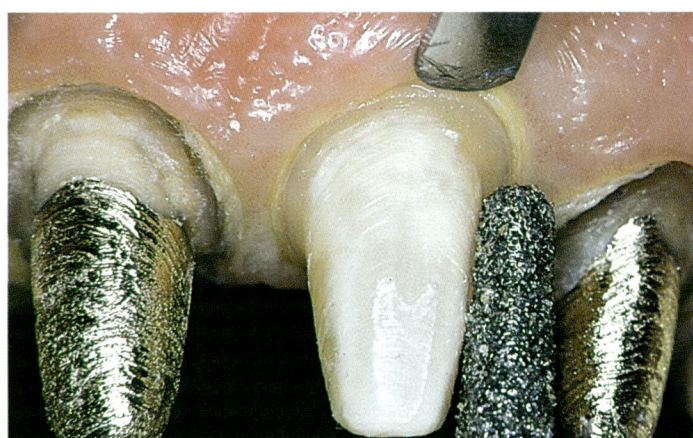

Fig 10-16b

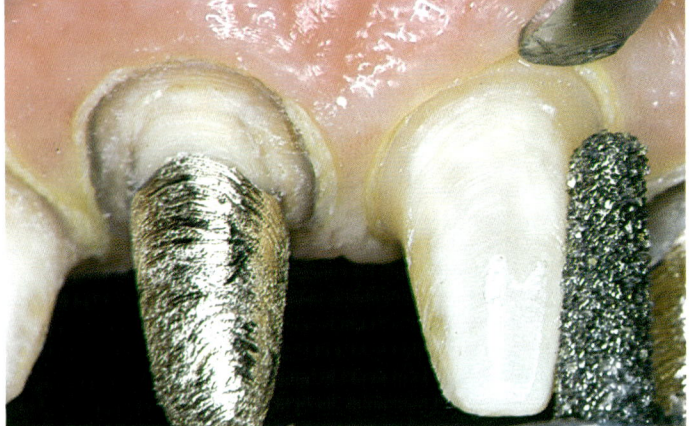

Fig 10-16c

Figs 10-16a to c The Gingigel retraction cord, Retracta-Gard, and Big Bite Diamonds can be seen performing their respective functions. Notice the trauma-free tissue despite the intracrevicular chamfer execution with extremely coarse diamonds.

cording to Big Bite bur placement for gingival deflection and protection as shown. Axial reduction and marginal chamfering are now being completed bloodlessly. The no. 4 Big Bite Diamond is perfectly placed to delineate the marginal chamfer; yet, clearly there is no soft tissue injury despite the coarseness of the diamond (Fig 10-16a). The no. 5 Big Bite Diamond is similarly placed beneath the Retracta-Gard instrument (Figs 10-16b and c), illustrating atraumatic intracrevicular margin placement while at the same time remaining supracrevicular. Therein lies the beauty of the technique. The attachment apparatus is not being violated. There is precious little room for error within the narrow confines of the gingival crevice; yet, with intelligent, painstaking preparation the seeming paradox of a large, coarse diamond and a small, delicate crevice is not as self-contradictory as it might first appear. Time taken now is never squandered; attention lavished upon gingival tissue is never wasted.

Completed preparations

The preparations for Case 2 now have been completed (Fig 10-17). All margins have been placed with care within only the occlusal one third of the sulcus. Note the gingival architectural profile: for maximum esthetics the

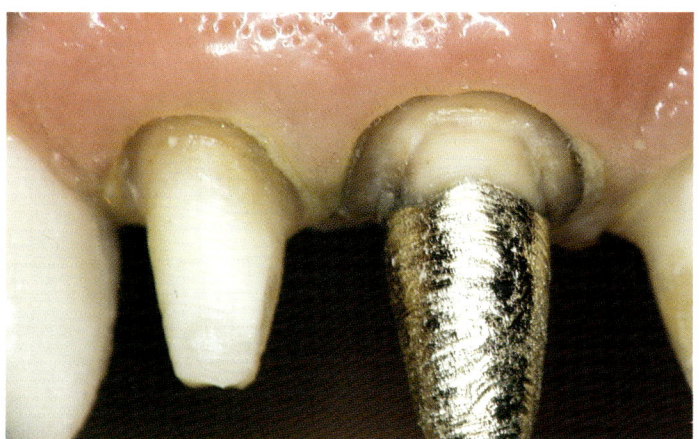

Fig 10-17a

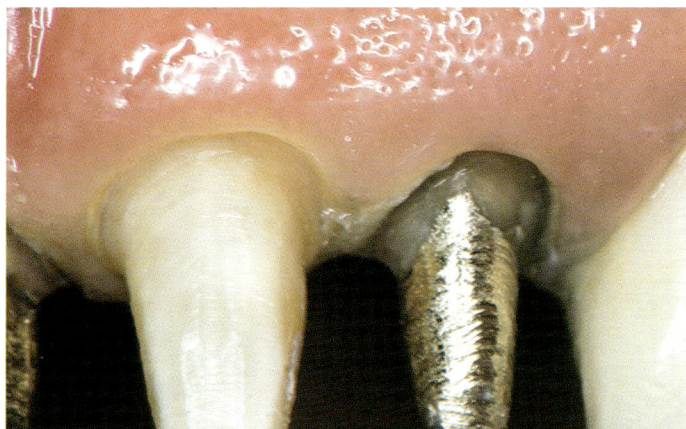

Fig 10-17b

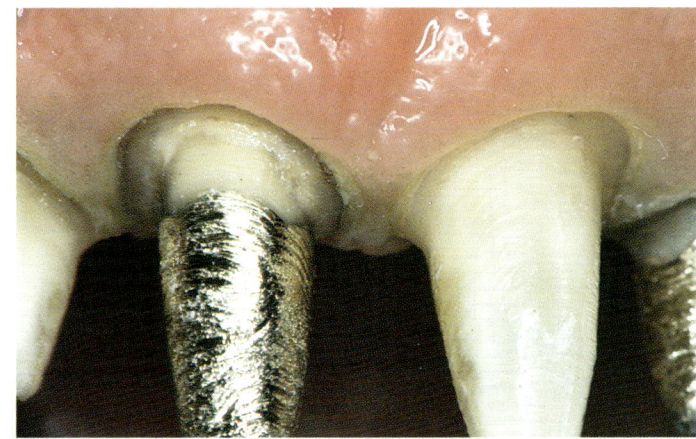

Fig 10-17c

Figs 10-17a to c The completed intracrevicular chamfered preparations. Notice the absence of even a single extravasated red blood cell, even though the preparations are within the occlusal one third of the sulcus. Retraction cords are still present.

highest point of the labial gingival tissue for each maxillary anterior tooth is always at the distolabial edge. This creates a gentle raised eyebrow effect, which aids in keeping the restoration from looking like "Chiclets" (semilunar, half moon, hemispherical, evenly rounded gingival form). Adding cervical proximal concavities to the provisional restorations and the proper emergence profile will ultimately ensure that the tissue topography thus achieved will be maintained in a healthy, functional and esthetic fashion by the ensuing restorative treatment, whether it is provisional or final. Indiscriminate margin placement, injudicious tissue management, and inattentiveness to the harmonious, bilaterally balanced flow of the gingival tissues as they specifically envelop each tooth will result in disparate gingival heights at the margins of paired restorations. This situation may be referred to as the "hi–lows," the uneven gingival crests (of matching teeth) that have been iatrogenically produced by intemperate tissue management. When this occurs, the central incisors (or lateral incisors) have different gingival heights and therefore uneven cervicoincisal lengths. This vastly complicates crown esthetics, especially when the dissimilarity occurs for each of the three pairs of anterior teeth. Nothing ever appears entirely correct in this scenario because symmetry, balance, proportion, and repeated ratio are lacking. Hence, seg-

Mastering the Art of Tissue Management

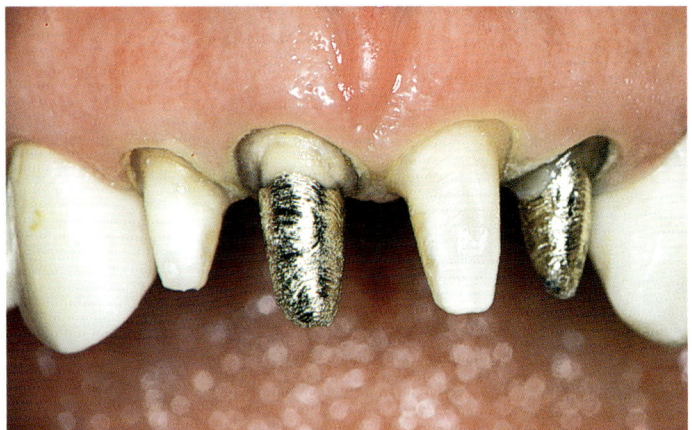

Fig 10-18a

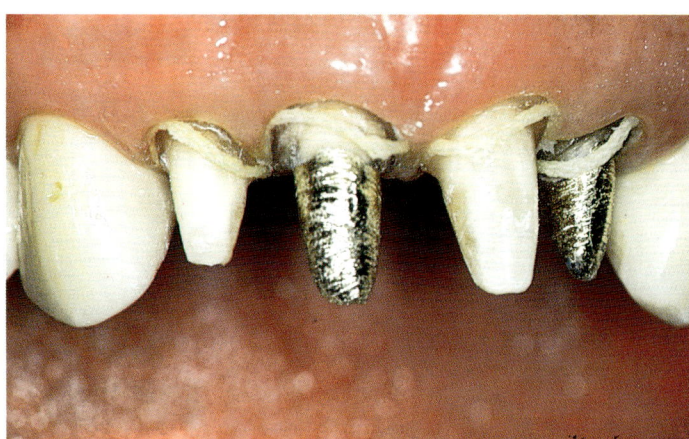

Fig 10-18b

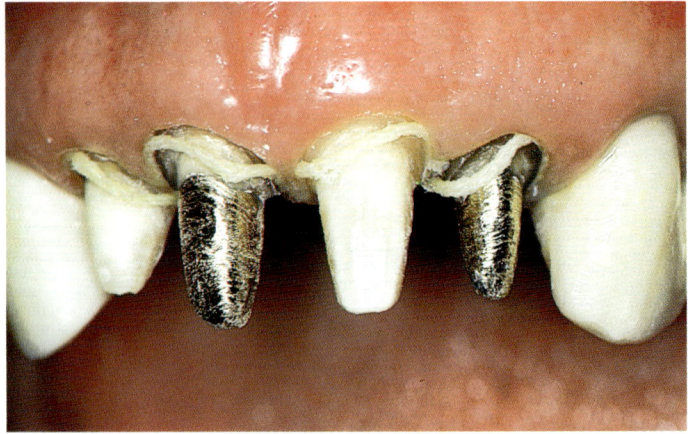

Fig 10-18c

Figs 10-18a to c   If the postpreparative tissue is in reality as healthy and atraumatic as it looks (10-18a), there should be no bleeding upon cord removal. The decisive moment (10-18b and c)—notice not only the absence of bleeding but also the untainted cords just being removed from the sulci.

regative forces overpower and dynamic unity suffers. The patient complains of color mismatch (larger objects appear brighter), unequal size of teeth (the hi–lows create cervical anarchy), and exposed margins (posttraumatic gingival recession). Clearly, proper tissue management is critically essential.

Cord removal

Sooner or later the retraction cords must be removed from within the sulci surrounding the completed preparations (Fig 10-18a), either for final impressions, prov-

isionalization or after provisional cementation. Accompanying cord removal, however, is an unfortunate phenomenon every dentist is familiar with, ie, bleeding within the sulcus, bleeding secondary to epithelial denudation from imprudent tissue management, or from the headlong rush to "prep" teeth or "take" final impressions before first achieving a state of gingival health. Bleeding need not occur—indeed should not occur—upon cord removal. Figures 10-18b and c show the decisive moment: the cords are being removed in the complete absence of any bleeding (see also Fig 10-19a). As mentioned previously, final impressions for multiple teeth are never performed on the day of preparation, thus allowing

Gingival displacement methods

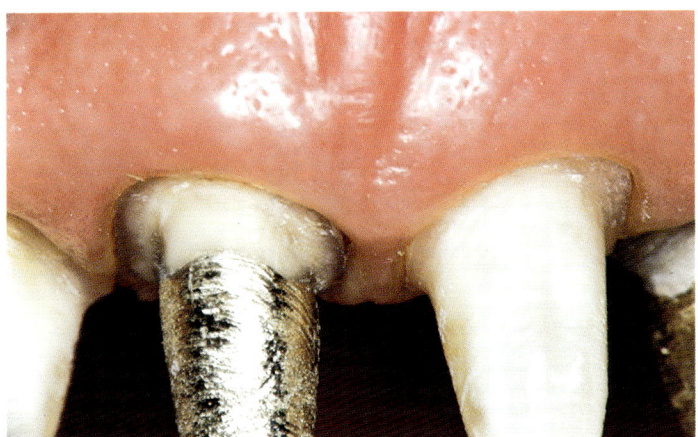

Fig 10-19a

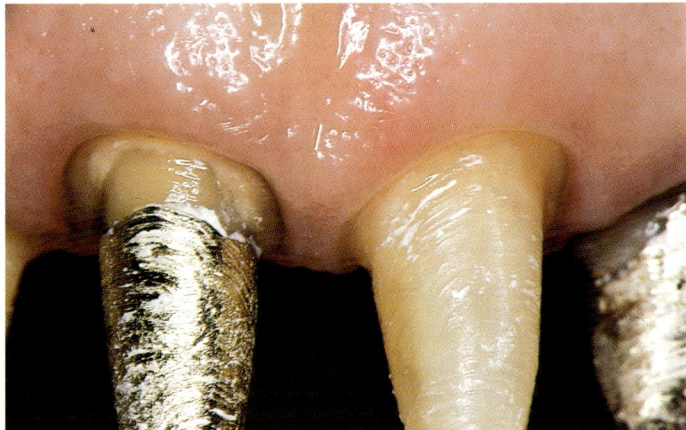

Fig 10-19b

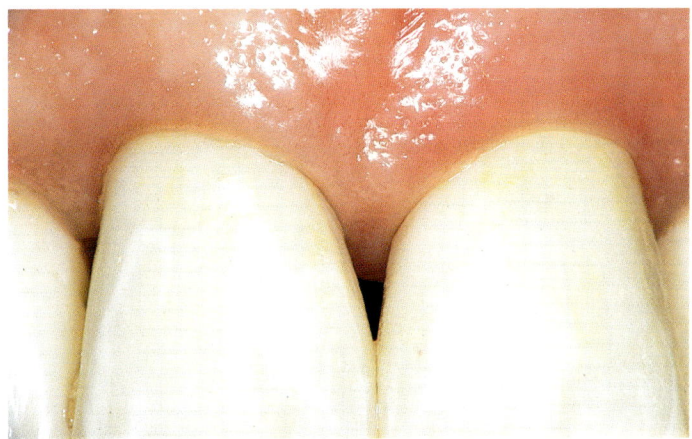

Fig 10-19c

Figs 10-19a to c   Near-normal appearing tissue immediately after cord removal (10-19a). The remargined provisional restoration at the *same* appointment (10-19c). The same area at 1 week (10-19b)—notice the absence of inflammation, the absence of retained cement anywhere within the crevice, and the intracrevicular nature of the preparations.

for critical evaluation of the gingival tissue response by the dentist. In this particular case, because the health of the provisional tissues has already been established (see Figs 10-13 and 10-14), final impressions may easily be made (Figs 10-20 and 10-21). The anatomic and physiologic considerations, retraction technique, and marginal refinements for impression making are precisely as has been described for provisionalization. There is no difference and no sudden concern for tissue that has been irritated, insulted, and violated (the abused tissue syndrome), which will in a moment reverse weeks or months of impropriety. The key to successful, atraumatic, bloodless final impressions (impressions that are really final) is the soft tissue. It is a simple truth that may not be so simply arrived at. Looked at in another fashion, bloodless, flawless final impressions are in actuality an intaglio of crevicular health. A perfect impression pays homage to perfect tissue. Perfect tissue is predictably manageable for superior esthetic achievement.

Provisionalization and follow-up

Figure 10-19a illustrates a close-up view of Fig 10-18a after the retraction cords have been entirely removed (see also Fig 10-17c). There is no seeping and no bloody

Mastering the Art of Tissue Management

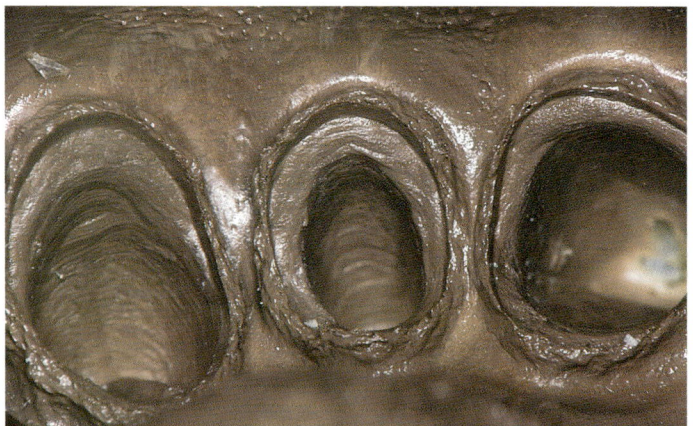

Fig 10-20a

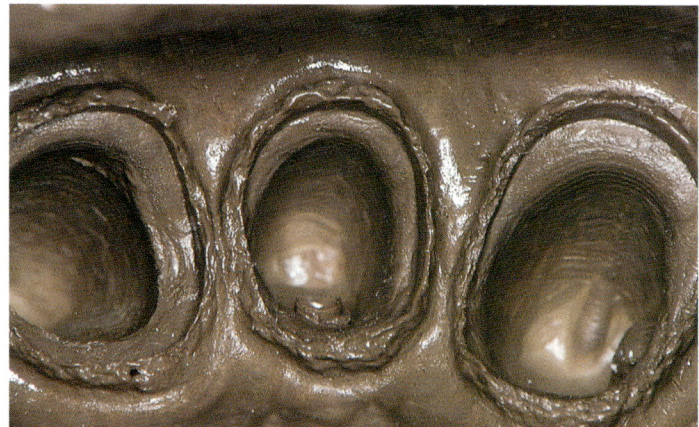

Fig 10-20b

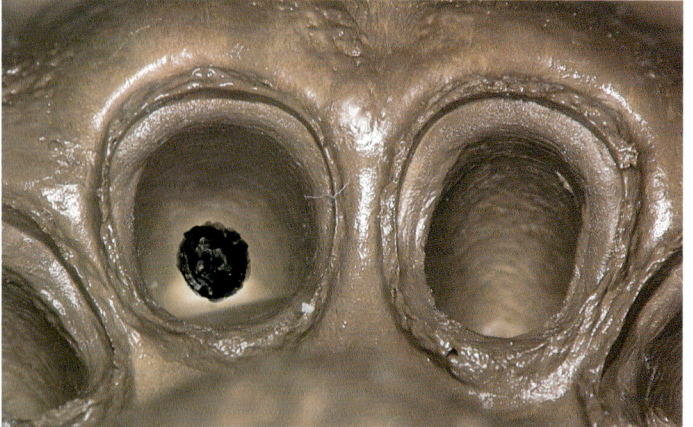

Fig 10-20c

Figs 10-20a to c   Biologic final impressions that are really final. There is no question where any margin is. Notice the intaglio of the hardly disturbed soft tissue, especially interproximally. Materials do not make impressions or mistakes ... dentists do.

moat surrounding once-proud, now besieged walls of enamel and dentin. The sulcus has been minimally distended, and it now takes little effort to syringe an impression paste into the patent crevice. There is no frantic rush to beat the bleeding caused by ulcerated, denuded, hemorrhaging, prolapsing gingival tissue. The remargined provisional restorations (Fig 10-19c) exhibit proper emergence profile, proximal concavities, marginal precision, smooth surface texture, and cervical esthetics (raised eyebrow shape, gingival heights to the distolabial). Note the tissue and intracrevicular margins *immediately* at provisional cementation. The area as it appears at 1 week is shown in Fig 10-19b. Note the interproximal tissue form and the absence of retained cement that frequently is trapped in the crevice and permitted to remain unnoticed. Subsequent acute inflammatory reaction could become chronic with time, especially if the provisional restoration must be worn for extended periods. Chronic inflammation has the potential to progress to periodontitis. Tissues become friable and impression making becomes a nightmare. Most final impressions end up being simply a brief collusion between expediency and chance. ("He wasn't there again today.") Control the tissue and you can control the case.

Biologic final impressions

Intaglio

The culmination of tooth preparation and provisionalization is biologic final impressions that are really final (Fig 10-20). The perfect impression pays homage to perfect tissue (same case as in Figs 10-13 to 10-19). There are clear, distinct, easily identified margins that are well defined. Notice the smooth flow of the impression material interproximally and the absence of papillary distortion or destruction. The impression material has entered only within 0.5 mm of the sulcus and has not endangered the integrity of the attachment apparatus, hence the term "biologic final impressions." Big Bite Diamonds produce a coarse axial surface, as can be seen in the impression; this aids in cemental retention yet at the same time can produce the smooth marginal area seen. No other rotary instruments were used (see Fig 10-22). At this juncture it must be clearly seen that the key to successful biologic impressions is in gaining and preserving the health of the gingival tissues. "Which is the best impression material?" is not the most important question to be asked. A healthy, stable, nontraumatized gingival sulcus is the real consideration. Once this is achieved (and perpetuated), the choice of impression material becomes a secondary consideration. There are many fine materials available to do the job properly; it is the operator's choice. However, even the most highly touted, the most accurate, "the best" material will do little good in a pureed crevice. Materials do not make impressions, dentists do. And dentists cannot do it with angry, noncompliant tissues that are railing at the periodontal effrontery of provisional restorations having little in common with finite provisionalization and proper wound closure (margination).

Cast

Although not of either of the cases that have been presented, this cast of a biologic final impression is yet another example of the efficacy of the methods discussed (Fig 10-21). Notice that the interproximal tissues have not been wantonly displaced and have maintained their integrity. Also note the intracrevicular nature of the marginal areas and the overall gingival topography. Examining the untrimmed cast as shown is viewing optical truth. It indicates the dentist's care and concern for gingival tissue (and generally is not a thing of beauty as any cursory inspection of the average laboratory bench would reveal). Examining the subsequently trimmed and ditched dies is viewing truth by artifice, because all tissue is removed, the emergence profile is nullified, and the dies are possibly altered in the process. They reveal nothing of the previous skirmish with the tissues or the possible quest for their preservation. The trimmed dies are as shorn of biology as many of the restorations that are made upon them. By this point in time the die (literally as well as figuratively) has assuredly been cast for technical failure. Now observe the illustrated untrimmed cast once again. For best esthetics the canines should possess the most superiorly placed gingival margins of the six maxillary anterior teeth. Next highest are the central incisors. At their level, or preferably slightly below, are the lateral incisor margins. Most importantly, gingival levels must be the same for contralateral pairs, and individual gingival heights should always be curved superiorly to the distolabial. To achieve this balance, surgical maneuvers may be required. Allow ample time for healing before impression making (approximately 4 weeks). Electrosurgical intervention is never used during final impressions because subsequent marginal tissue heights may become unpredictable. If mucogingival flaps are mandated, one should allow a minimum of 8 weeks before further restorative intervention. For optimum results, one should await complete tissue maturity before addressing (as opposed to assaulting) the sulcus.

Precementation periodontium

When all suggested surgical preparatory and restorative maneuvers have been accomplished, provisionalization completed, and the tissues brought to health, atraumatic final impressions are made and the provisional restorations are recemented. Subsequently, the patient returns for restoration try-in with the pink, firm, stippled gingival tissues as shown (Fig 10-22). Although not the same case, compare this tissue with the cast in Fig 10-21 and notice the similarity to that descriptive narrative. Also note the axial coarseness imparted by the Big Bite Diamond bur as shown in Figs 10-11a to c. This is gingival tissue as it ought to appear for either final impression making, try-in, or final cementation. The shapes of

Mastering the Art of Tissue Management

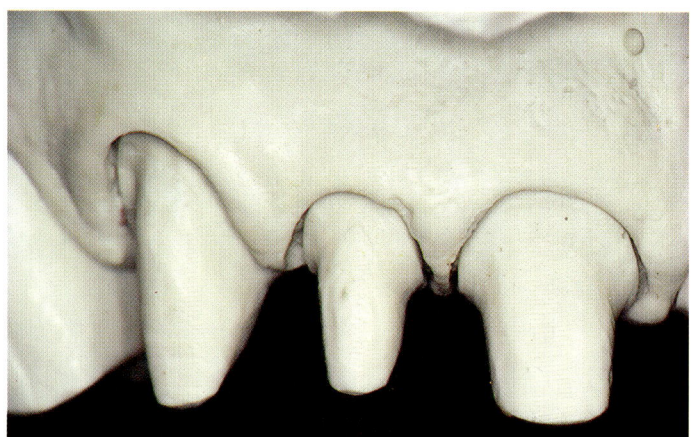

Fig 10-21a

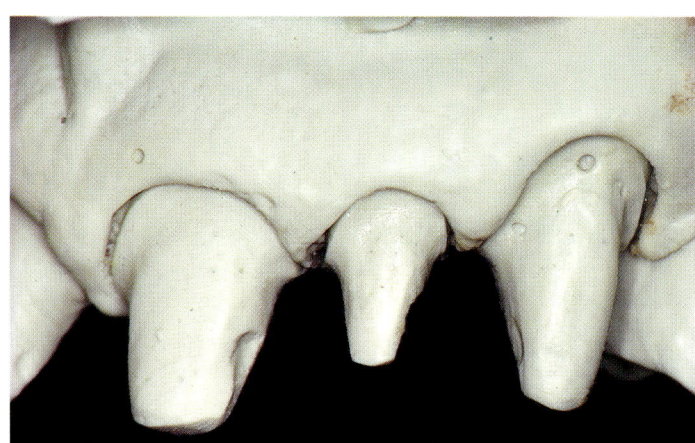

Fig 10-21b

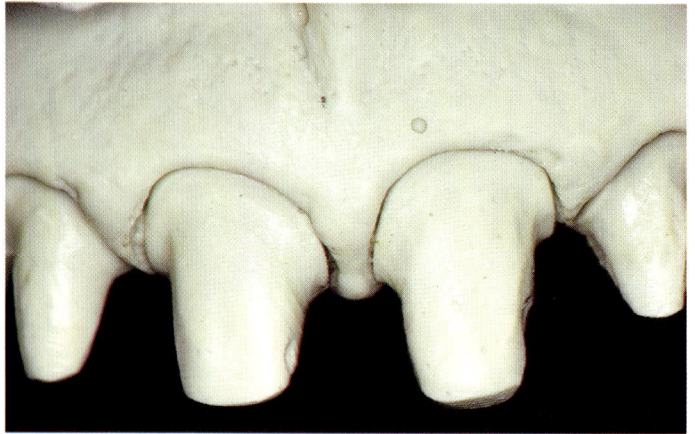

Fig 10-21c

Figs 10-21a to c   The cast of a biologic final impression. The tissues are not distorted, the preparation margins are just within the crevices—which have not been "troughed" to expose cervical areas—and the innate (or surgically corrected) gingival contour and balance of matched pairs is esthetically pleasing.

the papillae will vary according to interdental spacing and tooth morphology. No retraction is needed for final cementation when the gingivae appear as shown; the provisional restorations are "tissue friendly." Observe the mesial and distal approximal surfaces of each papilla and notice the sulcular intaglio of the emergence profile of each provisional. For all preparation appointments, before each cementation the dentinal smear layer is addressed. All dentin surfaces are scrubbed for 1 minute (per tooth) with a cotton pledget soaked in Tubulicid, then gently air-dried for 5 to 10 seconds. Next, a pledget of Tubulitec antibacterial primer is applied to all surfaces and the teeth are again air-dried for 5 to 10 seconds.

Lastly, a pledget of Tubulitec liner is applied and dried as described. Eugenol-containing cements are never used under acrylic resin provisional restorations because they destroy the acrylic resin and prevent remargination. A polycarboxylate cement should be used for provisional cementation. The Tubulitec applications (especially the liner) prevent chelation and assure easy cement removal. Painting the inside of the provisional(s) with a 50% dilution of a clear acrylic glaze also readily assures easy cement removal from the interior of the provisional. For final cementation, the same Tubulitec procedure is followed, but the liner is omitted. The interiors of the final restorations are sandblasted, and

Biologic final impressions

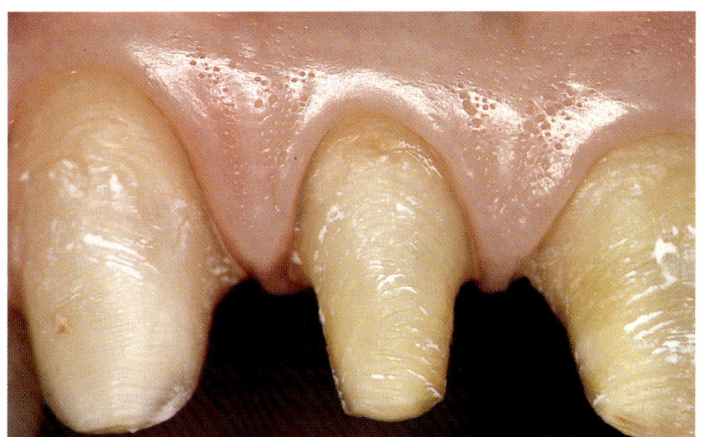

Fig 10-22a

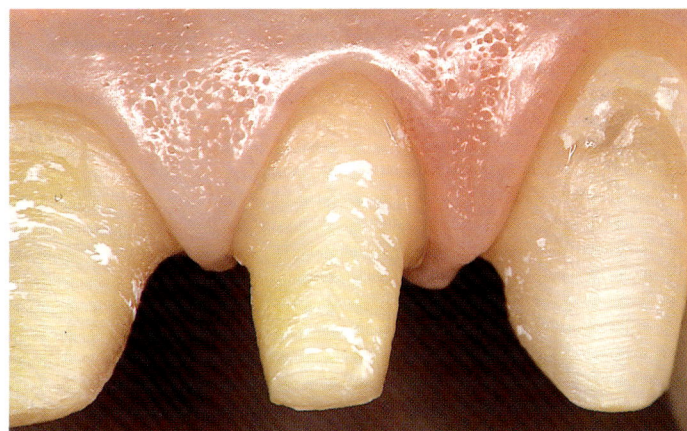

Fig 10-22b

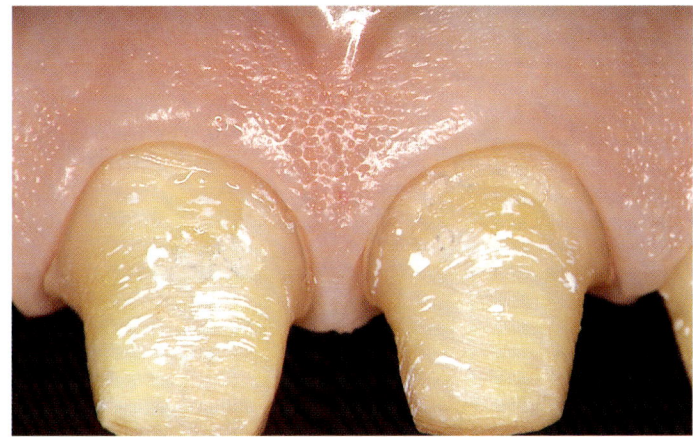

Fig 10-22c

Figs 10-22a to c The postoperative beauty of the attached periodontium. It has initially been brought to health and has remained so despite the preparation, provisionalization, cementation, removal for evaluation, recementation, final impressions, and another provisional cementation. The patient is now presenting for final crown placement.

either a zinc phosphate or a glass ionomer cement may be employed.

Structural beauty and the postcementation periodontium

Figure 10-23 illustrates final restorations in three different cases. The health of the gingival tissues is self-evident. The organic response to these metal ceramic crowns is one of peaceful coexistence; each restoration blends well with the surrounding periodontium. At 5 years (Fig 10-23a) and at 8 years (Fig 10-23c) these labially butted porcelain margins are 0.5 mm intracrevicularly. In Fig 10-23b, these labially butted porcelain margins are equicrevicular and have been in service for 4 years. Notice that in all three cases the esthetic guidelines discussed for the gingival tissues and the functional parameters for physiologic crown form have been strictly obeyed (see Fig 10-1b). Interproximal housing for the papillae has been provided courtesy of the proximal concavities of the restorations; hence, the papillae have not been forcibly evicted into bulbous malformation either facially or palatally but have been permitted to maintain their firm, gracefully pointed, V-like interproximal shape. Also note the personal hygiene of these patients as they present for preventive maintenance appointments. Each

Mastering the Art of Tissue Management

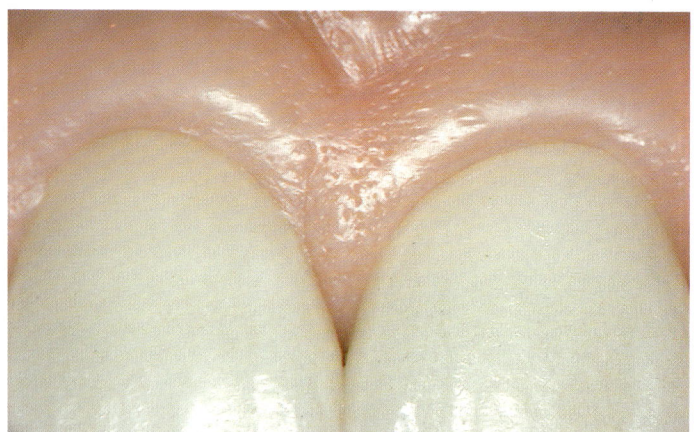

Fig 10-23a

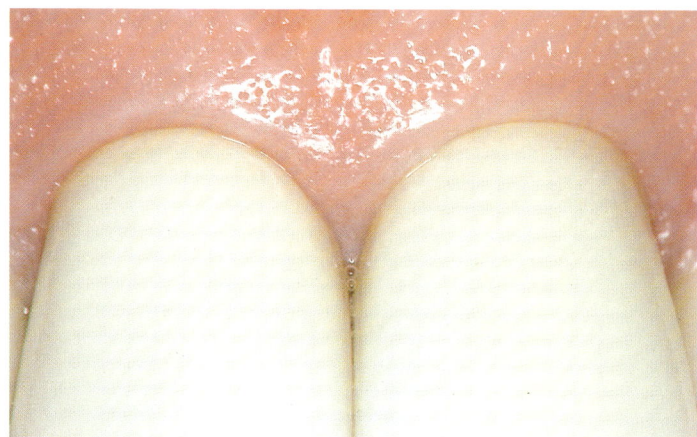

Fig 10-23b

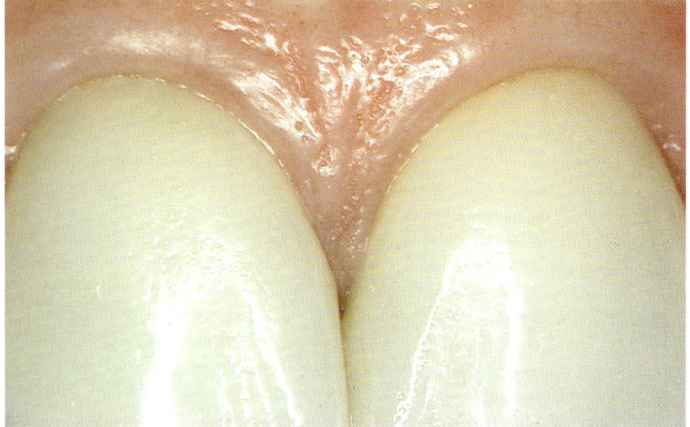

Fig 10-23c

Figs 10-23a to c Long-term tissue health surrounding ceramometal crowns. The stippled gingivae gently caress the cervical areas of meticulously fabricated, proximally concave, precisely margined restorations. The papillae are knifelike, and there is an absence of inflammation.

has been thoroughly instructed in proper 45° (angular) sulcular brushing, in flossing, and in the use of a variety of oral hygiene aids. By placing intracrevicular margins just within a healthy gingival sulcus, four things occur. The attachment complex is not violated, the patient's angular brushing reaches all marginal areas for efficient plaque removal, the gingival tissues remain stable, and the restorations are esthetic. The same may be said of equicrevicular margin placement as long as the technique of labially butted porcelain is also employed. Once again, structural beauty of the restoration and the periodontium must be a determining criterion if we are to achieve successful function.

The restorative and periodontal esthetics of a patient who had undergone periodontal (flap) surgery and complete mouth rehabilitation 11 years earlier is shown in Fig 10-24. The brand of acrylic resin used for the provisionals, the kind of impression material employed, the type of porcelain, or the articulator used all make little difference in the long run. For example (contrary to popular belief), you can do a complete mouth rehabilitation on a semiadjustable articulator just as long as you have a fully adjustable brain. What really matters is how well the techniques, materials, and instruments are used, whatever they may be. What matters is the unflinching, meticulous devotion to detail of the unstinting, caring,

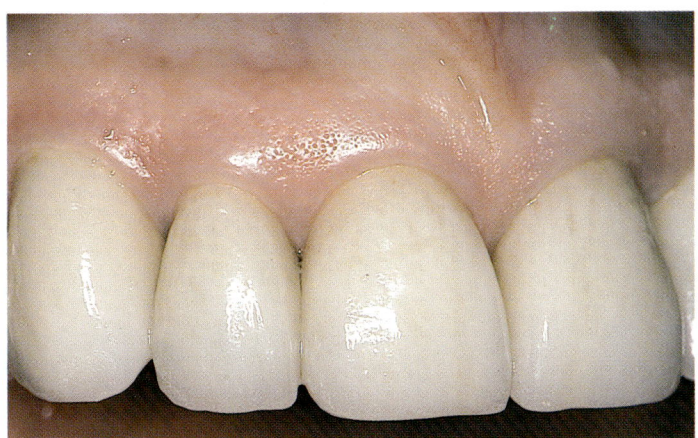
Fig 10-24a

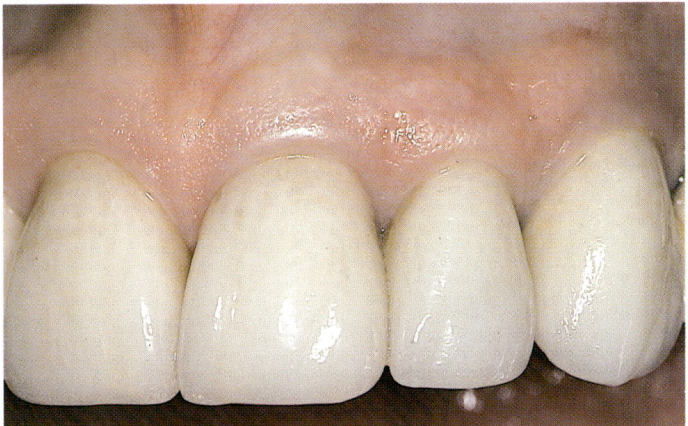
Fig 10-24b

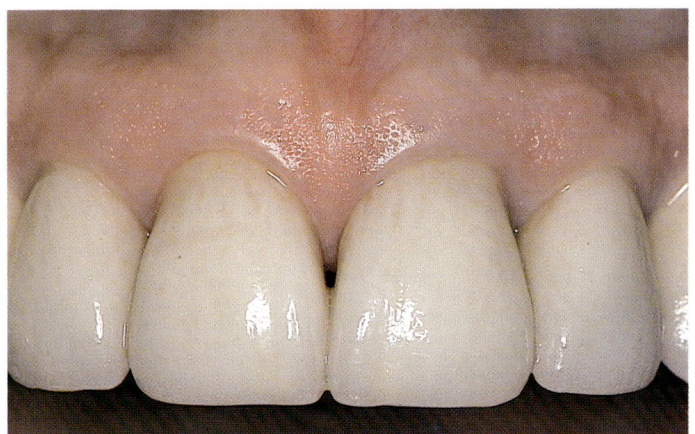
Fig 10-24c

Figs 10-24a to c Eleven-year postperiodontal and restorative esthetics. Every restoration must respect the periodontium to achieve a lasting peaceful coexistence. Note the balanced gingival heights and cervical contours of matched pairs.

creative dentist and technologist. No one is protesting the usefulness of traditional instrumentation, new methods, or advanced technology, but they must remain the servants and not become the masters of the dental profession. Structural beauty must be a determining criterion if we are ever to achieve successful function. This beauty cannot be derived solely from an instrument any more than function can, which lamentably so often is attributed to instrumentation. If Mozart were able to be queried, one doubts that he would be heard complaining about never having had a Steinway. Instruments do not create beauty, people do. Reducing the great Pavlova's cosmic dances (or the artistic nuances of gingival esthetics) to a literal discussion of vector forces and calibrated amplitudes is to nurture an ugly monster that will ultimately begin to devour its own hindquarters in an effort to destroy itself. In the final analysis, successful restorative treatment is a creative function of the intelligence, rather than an ingenuous, robotic, one-sided perception of mechanical technique only.

Mastering the Art of Tissue Management

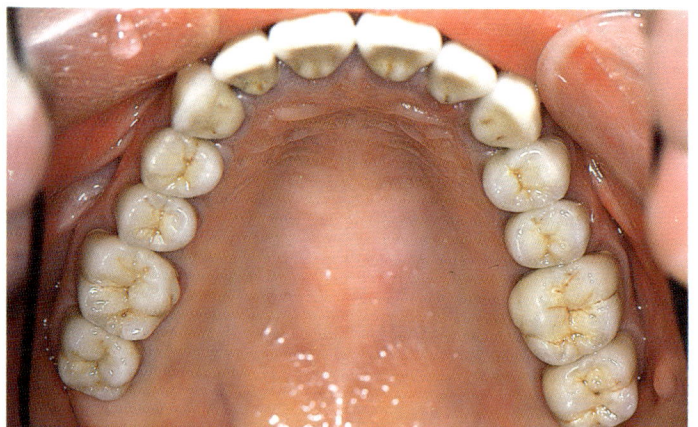

Fig 10-25a

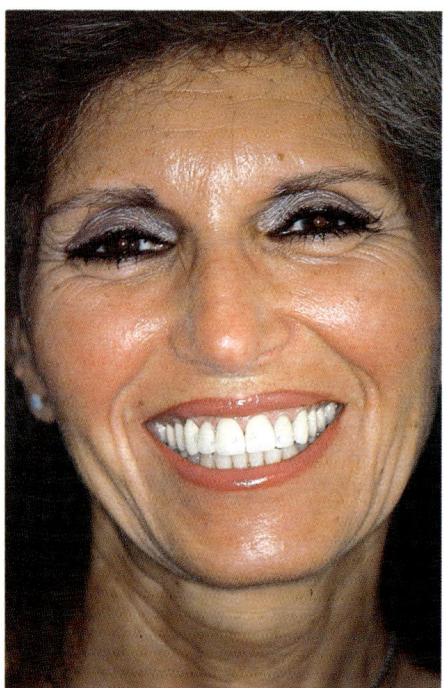

Fig 10-25b

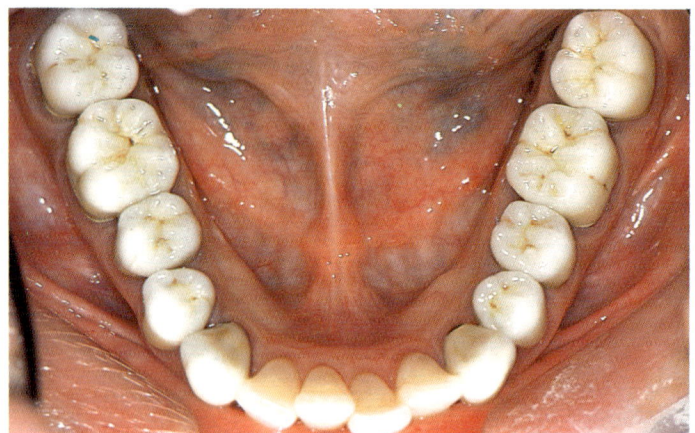

Fig 10-25c

Figs 10-25a to c   A fine example of Dr Rufenacht's global esthetic concept of harmony in art and nature (10-25b). The fundamental esthetic rules of facial, gingival, and dental composition have been satisfied. Note the cohesive and segregative forces in symmetry, balance, proportion, and dominance (ie, left and right canines and disproportionate left and right sides of the face). Also note occlusal function and its relationship to dental/facial esthetics (10-25a and c). Without properly choreographing this 28-member ballet, the visual and physical components would grievously suffer as ballerinas (cusps) collide and the ballet (occlusion) appears inimical (traumatic). Bruised and battered ballet dancers (faceted cusps) would need first aid attention (occlusal adjustment) before retraining (rehabilitation) to properly perform this beautiful *pas de deux* between form and function. However, with perseverance and an intelligent application of the global concepts in this text, it can be done. Vision will be your best asset.

Globalism and the perioprosthetic gestalt

Can creativity be taught?

Understandably, all the techniques, various methods, concern for the tissues, and effort will not produce an esthetic result if the element of artistic creativity is not present (Fig 10-25b; same patient as in Fig 10-23c). It is the unquestioning acceptance of what already exists that keeps people from being creative. A relentless, single-minded pursuit of the structural potentials inherent in classic morphology must be undertaken. The old canard "form follows function" is actually mere dogma until one realizes the higher truth that form and function are really one, inextricably interwoven, flawlessly fused, and beautifully bound (Figs 10-25a and c). To involuntarily imprison form within the mechanical contrivances born of a digital technology is to commit wholesale suffocation of artistry, visualization, and creativity. We have apparently lost the need or desire to express ourselves pictorially, graphically, and artistically as a cause-and-effect, hard-edged, unfanciful technical education has gained control of our minds. Imagery, drawing, and craftsmanship are no longer vital skills for survival in our technologically advanced culture. Hence, visualization in particular, that innate ability to recall and construct visual images within the mind, undergoes progressive disuse atrophy as we progress from child to adult and from generation to generation. Creative insight remains forever dormant in the kaleidoscopic (but malnourished) right brain hemisphere, whereas the computer-like left hemisphere is permitted to gorge on a numbers-rich (but pattern-poor) diet. How can dentistry flourish in an environment that lacks visual–spatial function, pattern perception, and fine line discrimination? What happens to the art of diagnosis and treatment planning when all the recorded information cannot be conceptualized? What is the end result of treatment when there has been no visual thinking? As dentists we must learn that how we see is just as important as what we see. The duality of the brain's function cannot be ignored.

Conclusion

Too often students and practitioners struggle to master the craft of dentistry, believing that technical skill is an end in itself, literally the sine qua non; however, craft alone may dignify but it cannot honor a dentist's effort with meaning and perhaps even grandeur. Instead of bringing one nearer to the end of the journey, technical mastery (important as it is) is only the vehicle one uses to travel the path. Just as manual skill is not a primary factor in drawing (or art in general), neither is it a primary factor in learning dental anatomy, periodontal surgery, or occlusion—contrary to popular belief. True enough, the art of dentistry, like the arts in general, cannot be taught in any formal or structured sense, but it can be learned, which is a much different thing. Conversely, we somehow believe that everything that can be learned can be taught, which is a huge fallacy and misconception. Excellence and creativity are arts won by motivation, training, and habituation. We are what we repeatedly do. Excellence and creativity are not isolated acts but rather habits of inspirational visualization prior to technical performance. Inspiration in dentistry is just as important as in poetry. Dostoevsky has said, "No man or nation can exist without a sublime ideal." The restorative dentist's sublime ideal is creative excellence in perioprosthetics. It must be the dentist's manifest imperative.

Summary

1. The integrity of the periodontium during tooth preparation and final impressions must remain inviolate. Because the margin of error for irreversible damage to the dentogingival complex during instrumentation is so extremely small, certain precautions must be taken.
2. Prepare the soft tissue before the hard tissue, ie, first gain gingival health prior to tooth preparation. Next, retract the soft tissue before preparing the teeth. Then, prepare the teeth to the retracted gingival level only (Gingibraid or preferably Gingigel).
3. Do not enter more than 0.5 mm of the crevice, which may be only one retraction cord (depending on size).
4. In addition to retracting before tooth preparation, the use of a retracting/deflecting instrument (eg, Retracta-Gard) during tooth preparation will further protect the gingivae from diamond laceration.

5. Extremely coarse diamonds will cut extremely rapidly, efficiently, and with virtually no trauma to the teeth or gingival tissues if used as described and illustrated (eg, Big Bite Diamond cutting instruments).
6. Provisional restorations must be given the same attention to detail as the ensuing final restorations or the final restorations will fail in some way.
7. Successful biologic final impressions are solely a function of the health of the soft tissue. They can be accomplished with little or no trauma to the tissues using the retracting technique discussed. They should not be made on the day multiple preparations are performed.
8. Final restorative results were illustrated that have stood the test of time both esthetically and functionally. The attendant processes of creativity were briefly mentioned.

Coda: The search for excellence

Aristotle's definition of happiness was to live "in accordance with the highest excellence." The human mind ventures out to seek the essence of this statement but brings back merely metaphor instead. Perhaps we just cannot cope with idealism. As has been explained, excellence is an art won by motivation, training, and habituation; clearly, we are what we repeatedly do. Because excellence is not an isolated mechanical act but rather a habit of inspirational visualization prior to meticulous technical performance, inspiration in dentistry is every bit as important as it is in poetry or physics.

Our profession demands that we be servants of a profound nostalgia for spatial orderliness, structural beauty, and fluidity of anatomic form. As dentists, we seek to classically protect an organ system ever on the brink of disintegration through wear, accident, or the hand of humans. We always feel a sense of sadness at the knowledge that nothing remains unviolated by time, that there is an inexorability of change. As such, we dentists must make every effort to be cognizant of the constant changes of anatomic and restorative form (no matter how slight) and hasten to implement the necessary corrections, or we can never hope to preserve structural beauty. While there is highly commendable virtue in seeking the perfect restoration, there is a unique divinity conferred in achieving its unblemished perfection.

Acknowledgment

The author would like to acknowledge the ceramic artistry of Mr Asami Tanaka.

Product list

Gingibraid, Gingigel, Styptin
   Cadco Company
   600 E. Hueneme Road
   Oxnard, CA 93033-8600

Big Bite Diamond Cutting Instruments, Retracta-Gard
   Tanaka Dental Products
   5135 Golf Road
   Skokie, IL 60077

Tubulitec System
   Global Dental Products
   PO Box 537
   2465 Jerusalem Avenue
   North Bellmore, NY 11710

Acrylic Glaze
   George Taub Dental Products
   277 New York Avenue
   Jersey City, NJ 07307

Chapter 11

Metal Ceramic Framework Design

Robert P. Berger

Introduction

This chapter is about connecting the gap between dental technology and patient health. There exists a special relationship between dental technology and good health, and among dental laboratory technicians, dentists, and patients. When a patient has a problem, the dentist must diagnose the cause of the problem and prescribe a remedy. The prescription is then given to the laboratory technician, who accepts the responsibility for fabricating the prescribed prosthesis so that it fulfills the patient's needs and solves or aids in the solution of the patient's problem. If either the dentist or the technician misses a beat, it is the patient who will suffer. It is a special relationship in which the health and well-being of the patient is a function of both the dentist and the technician and their combined abilities to diagnose, prescribe, and fabricate the correct remedy to the problem. Framework design, esthetics, and physiology are all partners in the patient's health.

Proper design of the metal ceramic framework controls the morphology of the restoration. It also promotes good oral health.

Esthetics and strength are the primary reasons why a metal ceramic restoration would be prescribed. Otherwise, technologists under the direction of the dentist would just make all-metal restorations. Fortunately, that is not what our culture is all about. Our culture has developed the desire to look natural, not reconstructed.

A metal ceramic restoration uses the best advantages of both materials, the strength of the metal, and the beauty of a veneer that defies the human eye to differentiate it from the real thing. When metal ceramic restorations are correctly constructed, the patient realizes significant benefits, not only in terms of esthetics but also in terms of oral health. Good physiology is good esthetics.

The benefits of a properly designed metal ceramic framework are as follows: *(1)* improved appearance, *(2)* absence of oral pain, *(3)* better oral hygiene, *(4)* total overall bodily health, and *(5)* a feeling of self-confidence and self-worth. When it has been decided that a metal ceramic prosthesis is the restoration of choice, it must be assured that it is made in such a way that the maximum benefits of good oral physiology and natural esthetics are achieved. Is that possible? Yes, esthetics and physiology are partners in good health.

There are three areas of framework design that promote proper construction of fixed prostheses and will ensure good oral health of the hard and soft tissues: marginal fit, contour control, and lingual metal band design. These are the factors that determine structural integrity, esthetic appearance, and the physiologic response to the fixed partial denture or individual crown.

Marginal fit

The accuracy of the marginal fit has a significant influence on maintaining the health of the hard and soft tissues. There are three types of inaccuracies pertaining to marginal fit: short margin, overexpansion, and underexpansion. A well-fitting crown placed on an abutment protects the dentinal hard tissues by sealing the prepared tooth from the bacterial environment of the oral cavity. The short margin, whether caused by a discrepancy between the preparation and the impression or an error in the fabrication of the restoration, is an open invitation to plaque attachment leading to inflammation.

Metal Ceramic Framework Design

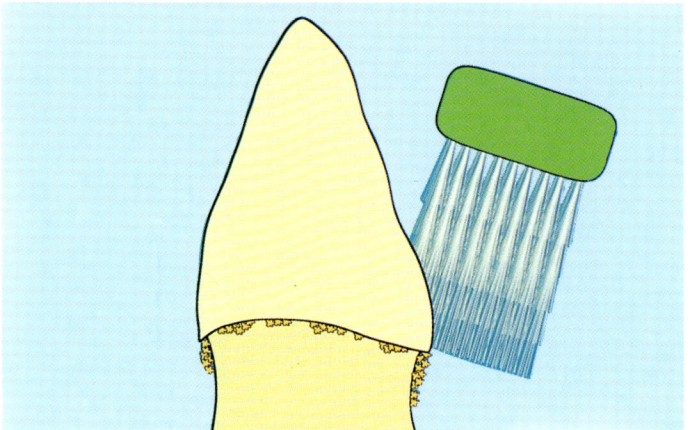

Fig 11-1 An overexpanded crown will collect plaque subgingival to the shelf created by the overhang. The plaque cannot be easily removed by the patient, a situation that can lead to inflammation of the surrounding gingival tissue.

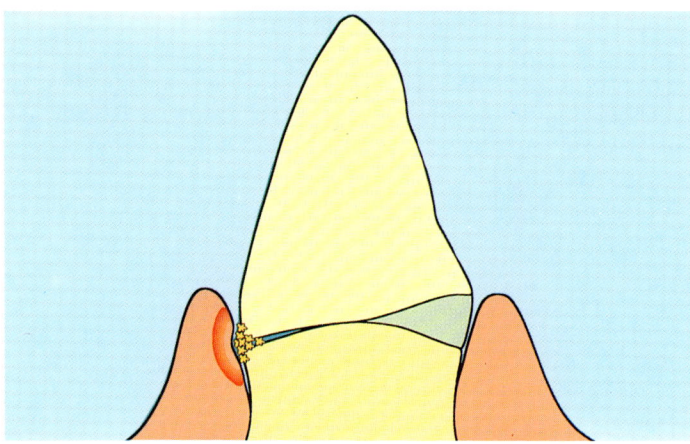

Fig 11-2 An underexpanded or overexpanded crown will always have an open margin because the periphery of the margin of this crown is different than the margin periphery of the prepared tooth.

Overexpansion

Overexpansion can cause the cast restoration to rock on the prepared tooth, opening either the facial or lingual margin, but, even more detrimental, if seated, the overexpanded restoration creates an overhang extending beyond the margin of the tooth. The overhang creates an area for plaque collection. The shelf created by the overexpansion of the casting prevents debris from being easily removed by the patient. The persistence of this condition will lead to a deterioration in the health of the surrounding tissues (Fig 11-1).

Underexpansion

Underexpansion makes fitting of the cast restoration extremely difficult because the internal dimension of the casting is smaller than the preparation. Machining the internal surface of the casting, ie, making its internal dimension larger, may allow the casting to seat fully on the prepared tooth, but it will not eliminate the physiologic negative of a short margin. The marginal periphery of an underexpanded cast crown is always smaller (less in circumference) than the marginal periphery of the prepared tooth.

Placing an underexpanded or overexpanded crown, which has been machined to fit, will always leave an exposed surface around the periphery of the prepared tooth (Fig 11-2).

Control of marginal fit

The accuracy of the fit of a crown casting can be controlled by tooth preparation, complete and accurate impressions, accurate cast pouring, use of controlled thickness cement spacers, fabrication of accurate wax patterns, and the control of investment mold expansion.

Tooth preparation

A shoulder, beveled shoulder with gingival metal band, or chamfer design is preferable. The feather-edge design should not be used except where absolutely unavoidable. Kuwata[1] illustrated that the feather-edge margin design causes an overcontour of the ceramic veneer at the gingival margin of a restoration due to insufficient tooth reduction. Shillingburg et al[2] demonstrated that the shoulder design, adequately reducing the tooth structure just above the preparation margin, allowed for the thickness of the porcelain veneer. Sufficient reduction at the gingival margin ensures that the gingival contour of the crown will be in line with the emergence profile of the tooth.

Accurate complete impressions

Full-arch impressions will allow the dental technician to construct a prosthesis that will be in balance with the patient's existing dentition by having the advantage of being able to see a full view of the patient's oral architecture. Quadrant-arch impressions will not permit the technician to make a bilateral comparison of the patient's existing morphology and leave occlusal function to guesswork.

Accurate cast pouring

Correct measurement of the gypsum water-to-powder ratio will ensure controlled expansion of the die stone, producing an exact duplication of the patient's dentition in the dental cast. The dental cast is the first step in the prosthesis fabrication process. Although the produced prosthesis may accurately fit the dental cast, an inaccurate cast will create an inaccurate fit of the prosthesis on the patient's prepared teeth. A poor physiologic result is inevitable when the prosthesis fits inaccurately.

Spacers

Cement spacer thickness must be controlled to ensure accurate fit of the cast crowns. Far too often the application thickness of the spacer is unknown. Frequently the spacer thickness is insufficient, not allowing the minimum required relief of 25 μm on the die surface.[3,4] When the relief is less than required, the crown when cemented will be prevented from fully seating on the patient's prepared tooth because of the film thickness of the cement that lines the internal surfaces of the crown. This condition will not only necessitate occlusal adjustment but will also leave the crown short of marginal seal, creating an unesthetic appearance at the junction of the crown and the tooth and leading to other physiologic problems associated with poor marginal fit.

Accurate wax patterns

A cast crown will never fit the die any better than the wax pattern that was made to generate the casting fit. Hand application of wax to the die has shown to be an extremely demanding technique. The shrinkage of inlay waxes necessitated the frustrating and sometimes inaccurate procedure of margin resealing. Antiquated inlay waxes, originally designed for making wax patterns directly in the patient's mouth, belong in the dental office. Today, progressive, highly skilled dental technicians working in modern dental laboratories use a new generation of wax known as Microcrystalline Dipping Wax (Belle de St. Claire, Chatsworth, Calif). This new formulation of wax has proven to be superior for the indirect waxing technique. Because of the low shrinkage property of the microcrystalline wax, the dipped wax coping can also be used to produce the marginal area of the pattern. When only one wax is used to construct the entire area of the pattern that contacts the surface of the die, including the marginal seal, the expansion and contraction of the wax throughout the pattern will be uniform. When expansion of the wax pattern is uniform, hygroscopic expansion of the casting investment will be uniform. Uniform pattern expansion ensures that the internal surfaces of the cast crown will equally fit all surfaces of the die. The strength and malleability of the dipping wax permit handling without distortion, and the high fusing temperature (165°F/melting point) of the new wax resists heat distortion when carving waxes, used to build contour, are added to its surface. The use of the dipped wax coping for the initial wax adaptation to the die and the sealed marginal periphery of the pattern, eliminating margin resealing, will ensure a more accurate fit of the pattern to the die and thus the casting to the die and inevitably the completed prosthesis to the patient's prepared tooth.

Metal Ceramic Framework Design

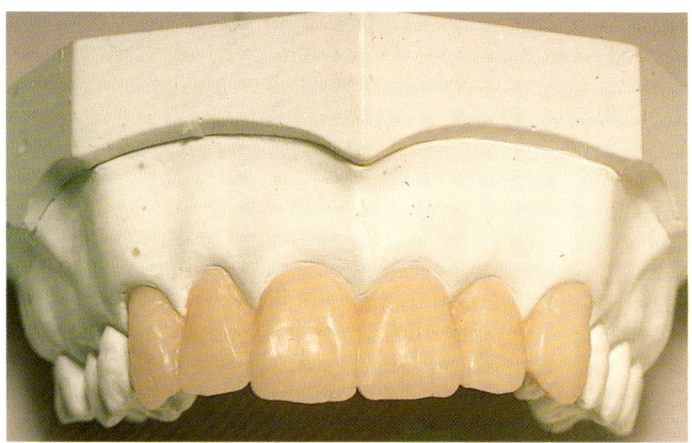

Fig 11-3 The diagnostic wax sculpture indicates the correct location of the metallic framework to ensure proper support and optimal esthetics.

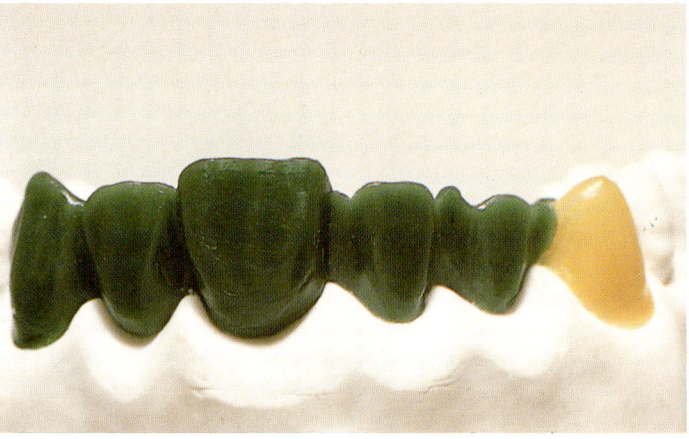

Fig 11-4 The full form wax-up, produced from an impression made of the diagnostic wax sculpture, is in the process of cutback to allow clearance for the porcelain veneer.

Investment control

Dental alloys expand when they are liquefied during melting to make a casting, and they shrink, returning to their original mass, as they solidify after filling the investment mold. The casting investment that makes up the mold for the lost wax casting technique must expand to compensate for the shrinkage of the alloy after casting. The investment can be expanded to compensate for the alloy shrinkage hygroscopically or thermally. The investment's hygroscopic expansion is determined by controlling the liquid-to-powder ratio of the investment at the time of mixing or by regulating the environmental temperature surrounding the investment during setting. The investment's thermal expansion is determined by the temperature of the burnout or preheat. Precise control of the investment's percentage of expansion is imperative if the cast crown is to fit the die, and in turn, the patient's prepared tooth, as accurately as the wax patterns fit the die.

Planning for esthetics, physiologic form, and strength

Fabricating a ceramic metal restoration is a tremendously detailed procedure that requires knowledge of structural mechanics, metallurgy, chemistry, biology, colorimetry, and esthetics. A good technician must not only possess working knowledge and experience in these areas but also must have great manual and perceptual skills. If the technician does not have this knowledge or skill, it is doubtful that the patient is going to receive a dental restoration that promotes good health and a pleasant appearance.

In fabricating the ceramic metal restoration, the technician must have a clear understanding of how the restoration will look when completed, how it is going to achieve the esthetic concerns of the patient, and how it is going to behave structurally to withstand the forces of the oral environment. The restoration must be strong yet have the natural appearance and good physiologic adaptation the patient desires. If the framework is too bulky, the porcelain will be well supported, but due to its overcontour, the prosthesis may impinge on the tissue. When the framework is overcontoured, the thickness of

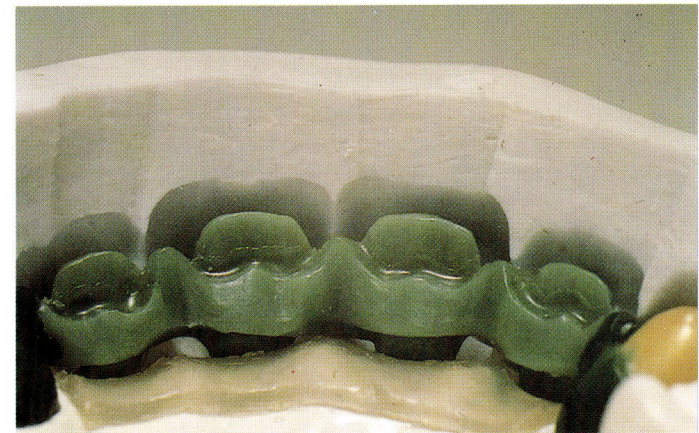

Fig 11-5 The impression of the wax sculpture can be used to align premade wax pontic patterns when developing the framework wax-up.

the ceramic veneer must be restricted, preventing it from having adequate thickness to develop the desired color.

A framework that is merely a skeleton may provide more than enough room for the porcelain veneer but will lack the needed strength to resist a flex distortion, leading to the inevitable fracture of the ceramic.

To achieve optimum esthetics, physiologic adaptation, and adequate strength, the final form must be determined before fabricating the framework. Once a diagnostic wax model has been completed (Fig 11-3), the actual wax pattern for the fixed partial denture framework may be developed by first making an impression of the diagnostic wax-up, then recreating the full form wax-up on the working model and cutting back the completed wax sculpture to create a uniform space for the porcelain veneer. Figure 11-4 shows the full form wax-up in the process of being cut back. Alternatively, the impression of the diagnostic wax sculpture can be used to create a matrix for positioning preformed wax patterns. Figure 11-5 shows the finished wax pattern with the pontics in the proper position.

Interproximal connectors: Design for strength

Fixed partial dentures rarely fail because of fracture within a pontic or abutment. The weak section is the connector area. Inadequate design of the connector can allow the framework to flex. A flex distortion of the framework will result in either a fracture in the porcelain or, in severe cases, the framework itself may fracture at the connector. The size of a connector is determined by the stresses that will be placed upon it. The greater the stress, or the longer the unsupported span between the abutments, the greater the requirement for adequate cross section of metal in the connector area.[5] In the vocabulary of structural engineering, the law of beams states that the strength of beam (its ability to support a load) is proportional to its cross-sectional area.[6]

The cross-sectional area has two factors: height and width. The law of beams also states that the height, in the direction opposing the force, is by far the more important of the two factors (Figs 11-6 and 11-7). Relating to metal framework design, this law indicates that the strength of a multiple-unit metal framework can be optimized by maximizing the height of the interproximal

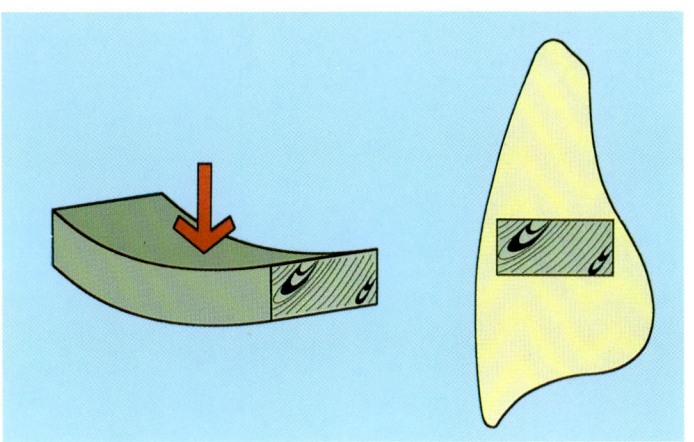 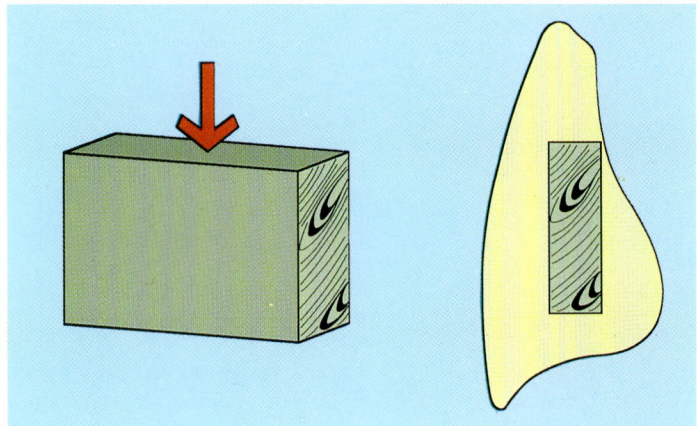

Figs 11-6 and 11-7   The law of beams states that the height in the direction opposing the force is by far more important than the width.

connector. All the multiple-unit frameworks built in laboratories use the law of beams and their strength is a function of their design rather than bulk. When we translate the structural engineer's vocabulary into the dental laboratory technician's vocabulary, the law of beams means that the occlusogingival connector cross-sectional dimension is of greater importance in providing strength through support to the prosthesis than the faciolingual dimension. This places severe demands on the design and position of the interproximal connector, for it must strongly support the pontic while still allowing adequate space for the overlying porcelain. The faciolingual placement of the connector requires careful planning because the facial aspect of the connector area must allow sufficient space for porcelain placement without sacrificing strength (Fig 11-8).

To meet the requirements of support and esthetics, the connector is developed in the lingual zone. By placing the connector on the lingual, optimal thickness of porcelain can be placed on the facial aspect in the interproximal. By placing the interproximal connector on the lingual surface, maximum strength can be achieved because the connector remains in metal, taking advantage of the greatest occlusogingival connector cross section allowable.

Interproximal design: Esthetics

How the interproximal connector is shaped, where it is placed, and how it blends to the pontic body are critical in achieving the optimum esthetics of the restoration. This is a three-dimensional consideration involving the facial form as well as the incisal and gingival aspects. To allow adequate separation of the units without exposing metal, it is essential to provide space for porcelain on both sides of the pontic body. Placing the metal framework toward the lingual allows for the creation of an adequate facial embrasure (Fig 11-9). Placing the connector toward the lingual will allow for a deep interproximal embrasure creating separation of the units, which is important to the esthetic appearance. Providing adequate space for porcelain in the interproximal zone

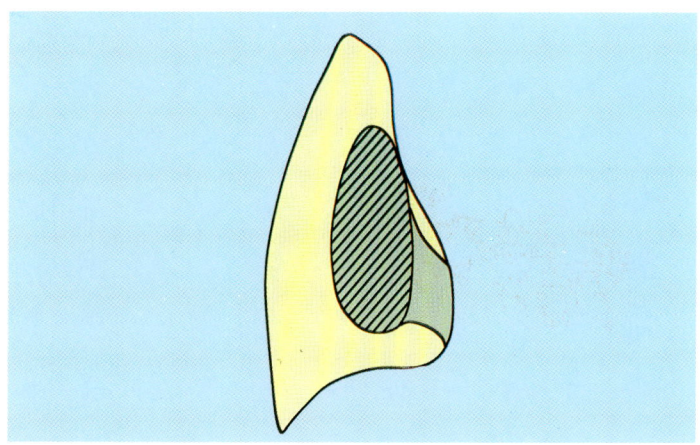

Fig 11-8 To take advantage of the law of beams, the interproximal connector is designed to resist opposing forces by having its bulk in a vertical direction.

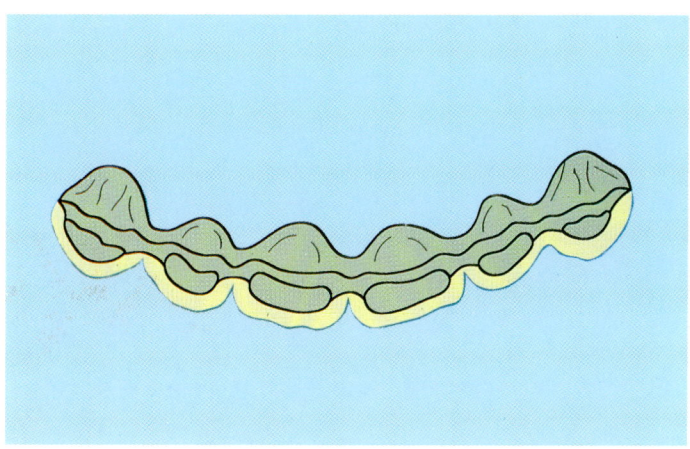

Fig 11-9 The placement of the interproximal connector must be toward the lingual to permit maximum interproximal thickness of the porcelain veneer.

will allow the correct thickness of porcelain to be veneered over the framework, ensuring vitality and color to the restoration.

Pontic–tissue relationship

Porcelain is widely recognized as being compatible with the residual ridge tissues.[7] Enough space must be provided on the tissue side of the pontic to ensure that the surface will not have concavities and that the porcelain that is in contact with the tissue can be glazed or highly polished, leaving a smooth surface to contact the ridge. Insufficient clearance for porcelain can result in opaque porcelain tissue contact. Opaque cannot be finished to a smooth surface by glazing or polishing and will leave a rough surface that will collect food and plaque, irritating and inflaming the tissue.

Designing the framework so that the junction of the metal and porcelain occurs on the bottom of the pontic should also be avoided. It is virtually impossible to provide a metal-porcelain junction that is as smooth and as resistant to plaque attachment as an all-porcelain tissue contact. Figure 11-10 shows the collection of plaque at the junction of the porcelain and metal after 11 years in the mouth. When the pontic tissue contact cannot be maintained by the patient, inflammation will occur under the restoration. When constructing the framework wax pattern, it is helpful to place a 1-mm-thick wax spacer over the residual ridge area on the working model over which the pontic can be positioned (Fig 11-11). The wax spacer will hold the wax pontic section in place while creating a uniform 1-mm space under the section. After casting, all the pontics will be a uniform 1 mm from the surface of the tissue. Providing a 1-mm space will permit adequate porcelain thickness to ensure a smooth, properly contoured, highly glazed surface.

Metal Ceramic Framework Design

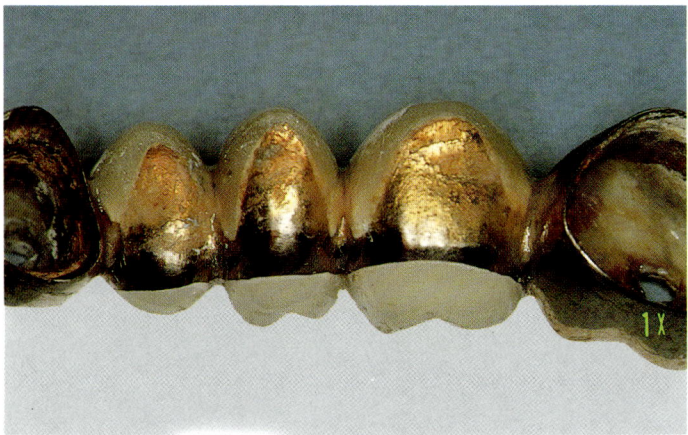

Fig 11-10 Plaque has collected at the junction of the porcelain and the metal due to the rough surface finish of the opaque where it finishes against the metallic framework (11 years postinsertion).

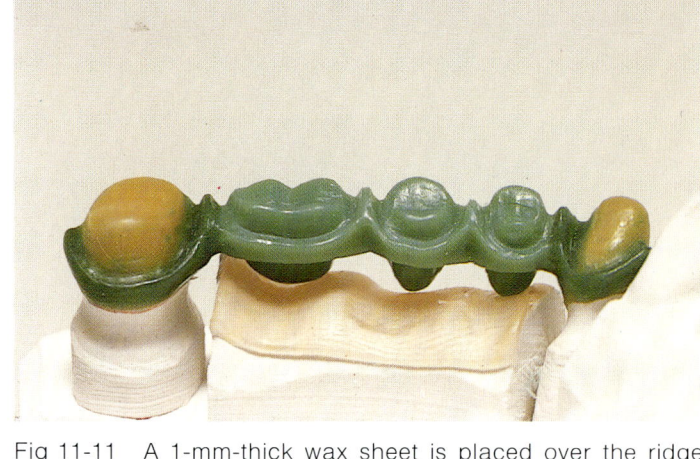

Fig 11-11 A 1-mm-thick wax sheet is placed over the ridge area of the working model before beginning the wax-up to create a uniform space for the porcelain veneer.

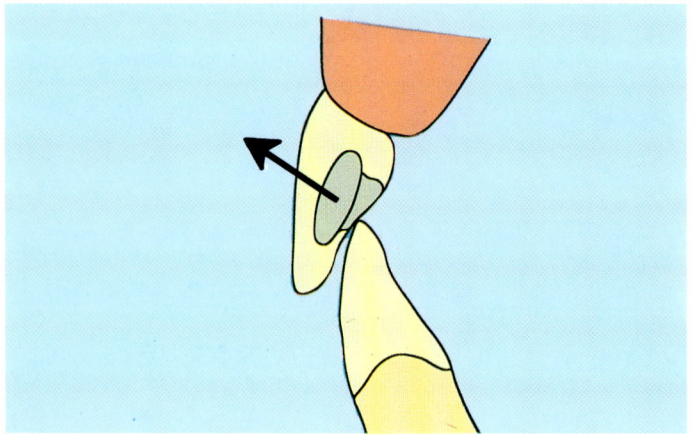

Fig 11-12 The continuous lingual metal band develops horizontal support and distributes the forces of mastication over the entire span.

Lingual metal band design

The three determinants for the implementation of the lingual metal band are strengthening, controlling the coefficient of thermal expansion, and oral hygiene.

Strengthening

Compressive strength of a metal ceramic restoration is considerable, whereas tensile strength is weak. Once cemented on the patient's prepared tooth, the metal ceramic restoration can withstand high forces to its outer surface, but during trial fitting or cementation, a metal ceramic restoration cannot tolerate outward pressure from within the coping. Placing a reinforcing band of metal on the lingual surface of individual crowns or abutments of multiple-unit frameworks strengthens the marginal periphery of the coping, preventing stress fractures from forming during fitting and cementation of the restoration. Joining the interproximal connectors of a multiple-unit framework with a continuous metal band strengthens the framework by adding bulk to the horizontal supporting beam and by distributing the forces of mastication over the entire span (Fig 11-12).

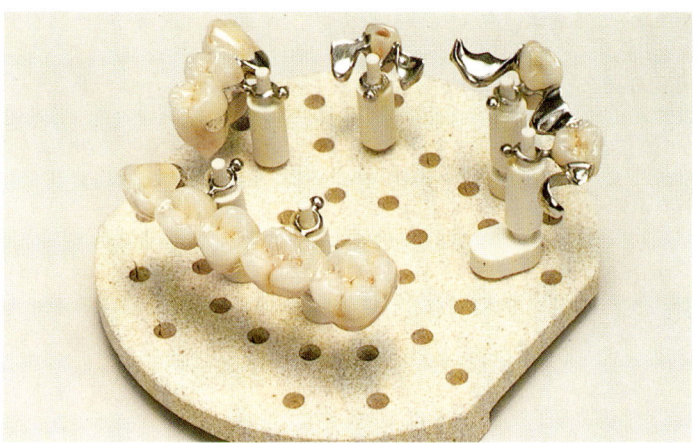

Fig 11-13 Supporting the pontic section during the firing of the porcelain prevents sag distortion. The loop wax pattern of the tray support is attached to the waxed framework and becomes part of the casting.

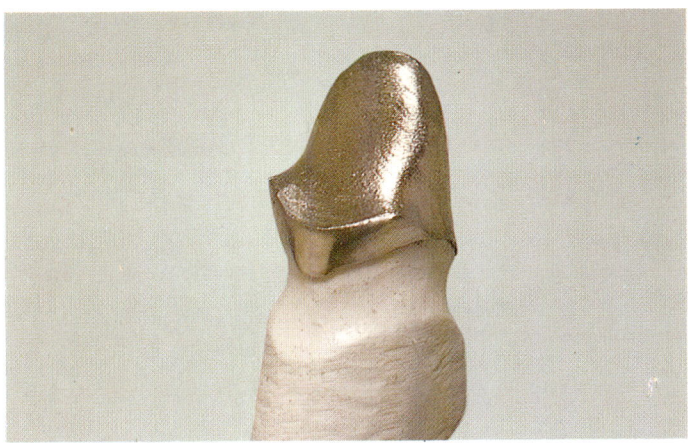

Fig 11-14 The porcelain metal finish point must be well defined in the metal framework to permit the creation of a smooth junction. There should be no doubt in the mind of the ceramist as to where the metal stops and the porcelain begins.

Coefficient of thermal expansion

When the metal ceramic framework is removed from the porcelain firing furnace, it is critical that the ceramic and the metal cool at as similar a rate as possible. There will always be a difference in the cooling rate because the ceramic always cools faster than the metal. This difference, or mismatch, in the cooling rate actually increases the physical bond of the ceramic to the metal.[8] If the metal is completely surrounded (encapsulated) by the ceramic veneer, the metal framework will be insulated by the ceramic, causing it to cool too slowly and creating too great a mismatch between the ceramic and the metal.

Too great a mismatch in the coefficient of expansion will cause the development of interface stresses between the ceramic veneer and the metallic framework. Designing the framework with exposed metal on the lingual surface of the restoration will allow the framework to cool more rapidly, avoiding the problems created by cooling mismatch. Placing a heat sink on the lingual metal band will accelerate the cooling rate of the framework. The heat sink can incorporate a firing tray support (Belle de St. Claire, Chatsworth, Calif), which in addition to drawing the heat from the metal after firing, supports the weight of the pontics during firing rather than placing firing pegs in the abutments, thus allowing the pontics to hang unsupported during the critical firing phase (Fig 11-13).

Hygiene lingual metal band

The key to maintaining good oral hygiene at the junction of the metal band and the ceramic is to produce the metal band with a sharp outer edge so that the ceramic has a definite finishing point (Fig 11-14). Plaque has a tendency to collect wherever a junction of the ceramic and metal occurs because the junction is never totally sealed. Plaque collection can be kept to a minimum by creating a well-defined metal-ceramic junction.

The band should have a definite shoulder to allow for the proper thickness of the ceramic at the junction and a well-defined outer edge to clearly indicate the exact point at which the ceramic ends and the metal begins. The shoulder should be at least 0.5 mm wide but should not exceed 1 mm in thickness. If the band is too narrow, the ceramic will be too thin where it butts into the band, creating inherent weakness and possible fracture. It will also be difficult to create a self-cleansing condition at the junction of the band and the veneer.

The external edge of the band must be well defined to provide a definite and clearly defined edge to finish the ceramic. If the edge of the junction is questionable, the ceramist will not have a clear indication of where to finish the ceramic, leaving an unsightly joint with areas of overhanging ceramic.

The porcelain-metal junction must be in a position that allows easy and thorough cleaning by the patient. The lingual band places the porcelain-metal junction in an accessible position where hygiene may be easily maintained by the patient through self-cleansing.

Conclusion

The metal framework is the essential foundation for a successful metal ceramic fixed partial denture. The framework should be rigid not by bulkiness but by design. Pontics must be supported to span the edentulous space and replace the missing dentition while still providing adequate space for a 1-mm porcelain veneer. The combined thickness of the metal and porcelain must be sufficient to achieve strength, color, and vitality without producing a prosthesis that is morphologically overcontoured. To develop a framework that meets all the requirements of physiology, esthetics, and strength, a diagnostic wax-up directs the positioning of connectors and allows planning of both form and support. A properly designed and positioned connector area should allow separation of the units by permitting the development of natural appearing labial embrasures.

At the same time, the connector must, by engineered design, provide adequate structural strength to support the porcelain. Designing and fabricating the metallic framework for a crown or a fixed partial denture require planning and an understanding of what is desired in the final form.

Fulfilling the patient's needs requires correct diagnosis, planned treatment, adequate preparation, accurate impressions, working casts, and accurate fabrication of the prosthesis. If either the dentist or the technician misses a beat, the patient suffers.

Dentists and technicians do not need to be told (but do perhaps need to be reminded) that fabrication and delivery of a fixed metal ceramic prosthesis is a team effort. The dentist and the technician must work together for the benefit of the patient.

References

1. Kuwata M. *Theory and Practice for Ceramo Metal Restoration.* Chicago, Ill: Quintessence Publ Co; 1980;4:126–127.
2. Shillingburg T, Hobo S, Whitsett LD. *Fundamentals of Fixed Prosthodontics.* Chicago, Ill: Quintessence Publ Co; 1978;3:78–80.
3. Fusayama T, Iwamoto T. Optimum cement film thickness for maximum shear resistance between teeth and restoration. *Bull Tokyo Med Dent Assoc.* 1961;8:147.
4. Campagni WV, Preston JD, Reisbeck MH. Measurement of paint-on die spacers used for casting relief. *J Prosthet Dent.* 1968;47:169.
5. Miller L. A clinician's interpretation of tooth preparation and design of metal substructures for metal-ceramic restorations. In McLean JW (ed). *Dental Ceramics: Proceedings of the First International Symposium on Ceramics.* Chicago, Ill: Quintessence Publ Co; 1983;173–176.
6. Smyd ES. The role of torque, tension and bending in prosthodontic failures. *J Prosthet Dent.* 1961;11:95–111.
7. Stein RS. Pontic-residual ridge relationship: A research report. *J Prosthet Dent.* 1966;16:251–285.
8. Mackert JR Jr. Effects of thermally induced changes on porcelain-metal compatibility. In Preston JD (ed). *Perspectives in Dental Ceramics: Proceedings of the Fourth International Symposium on Ceramics.* Chicago, Ill: Quintessence Publ Co; 1988;53–64.

Chapter 12

Porcelain Veneers: An Esthetic Therapeutic Alternative

Robert L. Nixon

Introduction

Each decade in dentistry is characterized by emerging concepts, which become generally accepted due to academic and clinical research, materials' technology, and perceived public need. In the 1980s, porcelain laminate veneers qualified for this distinction, expedited by the growing demand for esthetic dentistry. Although often hailed as "new," porcelain veneers have definite antecedents, which predate the current era.

Porcelain veneers were introduced by Dr Charles Pincus in Hollywood in the 1930s, to enhance an actor's appearance for close-ups in the movie industry. Dr Pincus attached these thin veneers temporarily with a denture adhesive powder. He then removed them after the filming for the day was completed because no adhesive system existed at that time to permanently attach them.[1]

Indirect veneering did not progress over the next several decades until Dr Frank Faunce described a prefabricated acrylic resin veneer in the 1970s, integrating the adhesion principles of Buonocore[2] and Bowen[3] with an indirect veneer alternative to porcelain.[4] These veneers were primed with ethyl acetate or methylene chloride liquid and luted to the etched tooth with a composite resin. Although the processed acrylic resin veneer initially exhibited greater stain resistance than direct composite resins of this period, debonding of the veneer occurred frequently at the veneer and luting resin interface because of inadequate chemical bond strength.[5] Additionally, wear resistance was poor, which contributed to staining.[6]

Seeking a viable alternative to indirect acrylic veneers, Simonsen and Calamia[7] as well as Horn[8] reactivated interest in porcelain veneering by reporting procedures for long-term porcelain veneer retention. Simonsen and Calamia[7] demonstrated that etching of the internal surface of the porcelain veneer allowed the veneer to be retained on etched tooth enamel as well as or better than composite resins or acrylic resin. Horn[8] advocated the use of a light-curing resin luting agent for efficacy and convenience. Further studies revealed the enhancement of the etched porcelain/luting resin bond by chemical means through pretreatment with silane.[9] Research in the recent past has shown that the bond strength of a silanated etched veneer to the luting resin is routinely greater than the bond strength of etched tooth enamel to the same luting resin.[10]

The advent of the etched porcelain laminate veneer represents the progress of several decades of research, culminating in the synthesis of the acid-etch technique and dentistry's most time-honored esthetic material, porcelain. Glazed porcelain or cast ceramics offer abrasion resistance, biocompatibility with gingival tissues, long-term color stability, and esthetic attractiveness. The creative initiative of the dentist is coordinated with the ceramic skill of the laboratory technician to achieve attractive predictable results. The inherent advantages of laboratory-fabricated veneers are numerous, such as relative thinness (0.4 to 0.6 mm), precise fit, anatomic accuracy, gradient shading, and appropriate surface texture. Overall, the esthetics and longevity of porcelain veneers surpass any indirect or direct resin alternative at this time.

From this background, the clinical and laboratory techniques have undergone continuing refinements.[11–13] Because porcelain veneers are relatively technique-sensitive,[14] detailed educational materials have recently been published to help clarify the nuances of the clinical approach.[15,16]

This chapter provides a comprehensive description of the clinical technique for porcelain laminate veneers. In a broader sense, it is designed to present porcelain laminate veneers as a viable esthetic alternative to traditional metal ceramic and all-ceramic crowns in certain clinical situations.

Case evaluation

The cornerstone of every good treatment plan is an accurate diagnosis. An esthetic treatment plan requires an esthetic diagnosis. The truly esthetic dentist devises an attractive dental composition not only from stereotypical guidelines of form and function but also as an organic expression of personality, status, life-style, gender, occupation, and other characteristics that distinguish one individual from another. The smile is perceived as an integral part of the face and, in a larger sense, of the whole person. It is an expression of beauty, youth, age, or persona. In addition, the esthetic dentist must have an awareness of contemporary fashions, a perception of patient expectations and self-image, and the creativity and technical skill to orchestrate this information into a successful therapeutic result.

An initial step in determining patient desires is to provide a written questionnaire to be answered. Properly structured, this questionnaire provides a focus from which a personalized treatment plan is eventually derived. Having patients elaborate on their questionnaire responses is a good starting point for the clinical evaluation. Perceived smile deficiencies are noted, and the desired image that is sought is discussed in great detail. In short, each patient is encouraged to articulate both smile likes and dislikes. The key concern is the patient's desires. Sometimes the desires are blatantly obvious; other times they are deceptively subtle.

Moving from the verbal to the visual, patients are invited to scan a photo album of assorted faces and smiles from completed cases to further clarify subjective preferences. If a photo album of completed cases has not been assembled, then close-up clippings of fashion models or celebrity smiles can be substituted. Smile books for dentistry currently on the market can also be used, as can brochures, videotapes, color slides, or articles that vividly illustrate the dynamics of esthetic dentistry.

The esthetic and morphopsychologic factors that must be thoroughly evaluated to formulate treatment recommendations appropriate to the needs of any patient are systematically discussed in Chapters 1 to 4. This primarily objective information, once discovered, must now be harmoniously integrated with the patient's subjective desires to finalize the treatment plan. In other words, the treatment plan must represent a symbiotic balance between a patient's needs and a patient's desires.

Tooth color must be discussed in a general way and then selected specifically for each patient. The patient's perception of tooth color during the selection process can be greatly enhanced by multiple tooth "smile guides." These are six porcelain denture teeth, luted together, and made up of four maxillary incisors in one shade (eg, Vita A2) and two canines in a slightly darker shade (eg, Vita A3). They provide the patient with a realistic "collective" color, rather than merely one or two shade guide buttons that are customarily used. Smile previewing through computer-assisted dental imaging represents a new high-tech system capable of clarifying further a patient's preferences for contour and color in a dramatic way.

Staff enthusiasm, knowledge, and finesse in guiding patients through this important introductory phase can be a significant asset toward establishing the necessary rapport. Generally, some constructive guidelines concerning specific smile parameters emerge from exposure to these visual stimuli.

The final phase of the case evaluation is to unify the objective analysis of clinical data with the patient's subjective desires. Throughout this delicate interaction, it is important to remain sensitive to the patient's responses as they are guided to the optimal treatment plan. Reciprocally, the patients must orient *us* through this refinement process by means of self-observations. In this manner, patient expectations can be effectively coordinated with the ultimate treatment plan.

Indications for porcelain veneers

1. Multiple discolored teeth.
2. Multiple teeth with enamel defects and unsatisfactory tooth color (Figs 12-1 and 12-2).
3. Multiple teeth with spacing and unsatisfactory tooth color (Figs 12-3 and 12-4).
4. Multiple worn or foreshortened teeth.

Indications for porcelain veneers

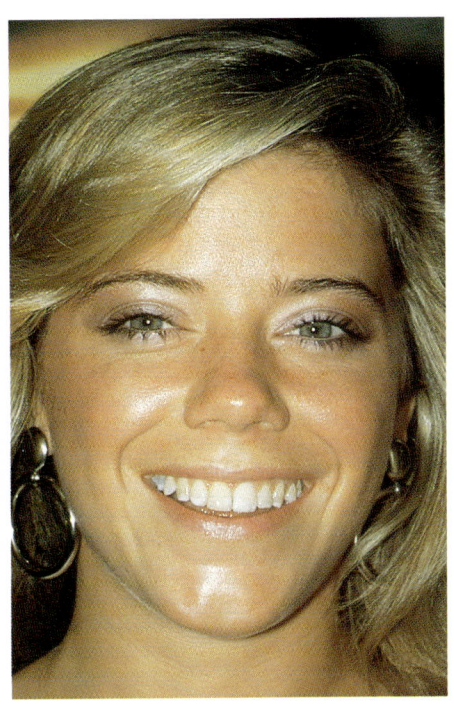

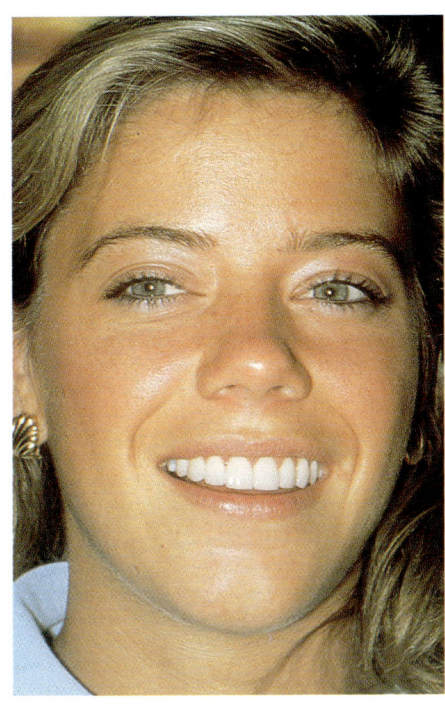

Fig 12-1 Before placement of eight maxillary porcelain veneers, this pretty young woman displayed yellowish, mottled teeth.

Fig 12-2 After placement of the porcelain veneers she displays a radiant smile. This esthetically pleasing result can be achieved routinely with the clinical technique to be described.

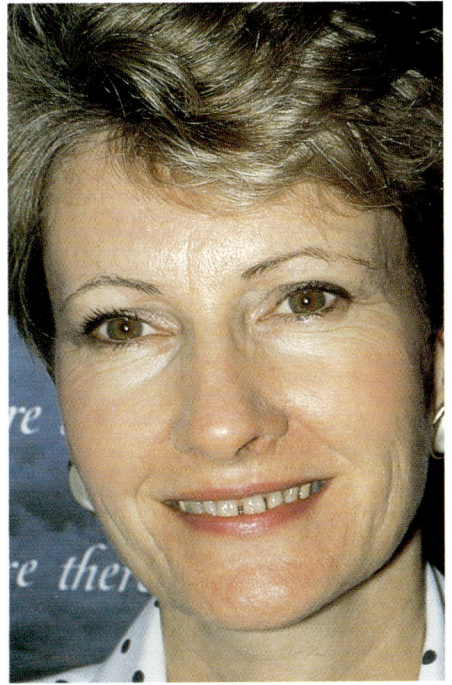

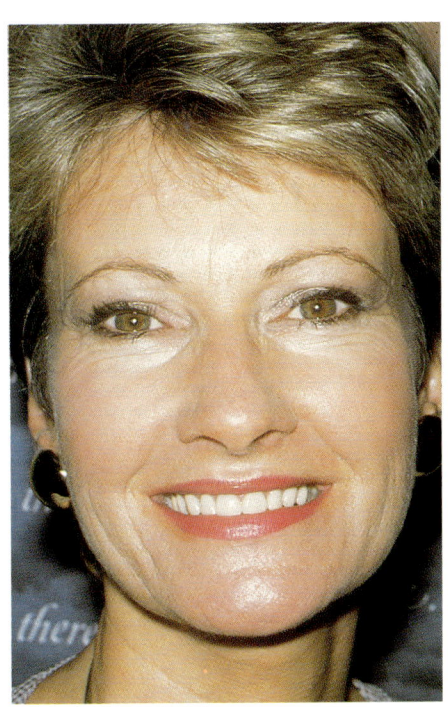

Fig 12-3 An attractive woman presents a pretreatment condition of both discolored and spaced maxillary teeth.

Fig 12-4 After receiving eight maxillary porcelain veneers, her entire face "lights up" from her attractive new smile.

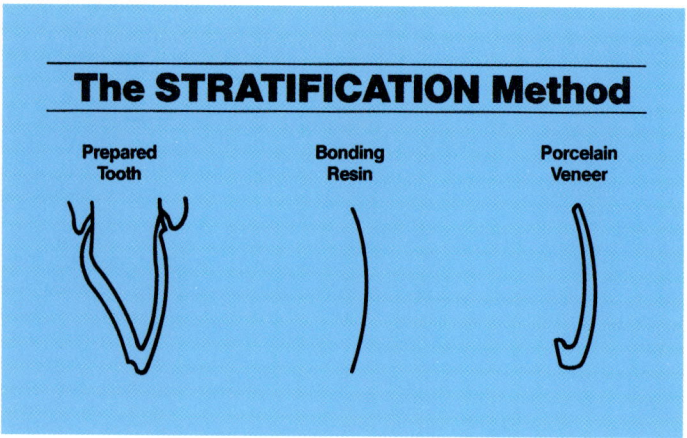

Fig 12-5 Stratification method is based on the concept that the tooth, the resin cement, and the porcelain veneer must be manipulated precisely for optimal clinical results.

5. Multiple misaligned teeth and unsatisfactory tooth color.
6. Teeth with generalized facial discoloration from amalgam shine-through.

Contraindications for porcelain veneers

1. Teeth with defective enamel over the entire crown.
2. Teeth with insufficient coronal tooth structure (less than one half of coronal tooth structure remains).
3. Teeth that are still actively erupting.
4. Teeth exhibiting severe crowding.
5. Teeth in which an intracoronal resin restoration would suffice.
6. Teeth exhibiting extreme occlusal trauma or wear.

Porcelain veneer indications are generally based on color change and, to a certain degree, on contour and alignment modifications. Porcelain veneer contraindications usually stem from insufficient enamel to ensure a durable, long-term cement bond or extreme tooth crowding. Dentitions with extensive wear from bruxism are also poor candidates for porcelain veneering.

Stratification method

Stratification is the process of forming in layers (Fig 12-5). A porcelain veneer that is bonded to a tooth with a resin cement is an example of stratification. The layers are as follows: inner layer, the tooth; middle layer, the resin cement; and outer layer, the porcelain veneer.

Various principles, which enhance control of porcelain veneer color by correlating tooth preparation, resin interface space, and porcelain veneer formulation, have been discovered through clinical research. The dynamic application of these principles to the complex area of porcelain veneer coloration is called the stratification method. The collective impact of the stratification meth-

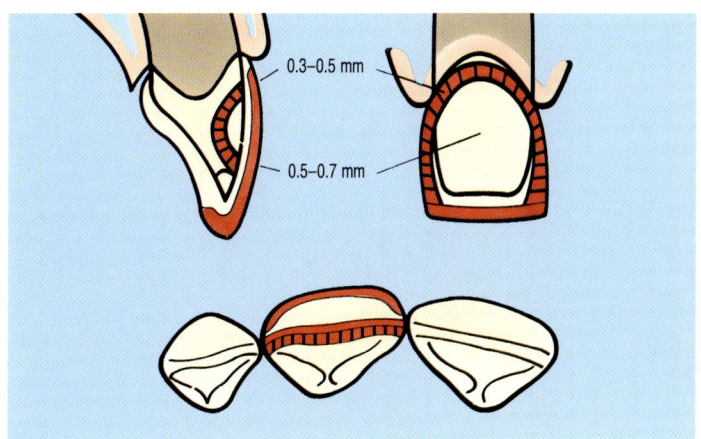

Fig 12-6 Stratification method—facial tooth preparation for most cases is 0.3 mm deep in the cervical one third and 0.5 mm deep in the remaining two thirds. For profound color change, up to 0.5 mm depth in the cervical area and 0.7 mm in the remaining facial surface is advisable.

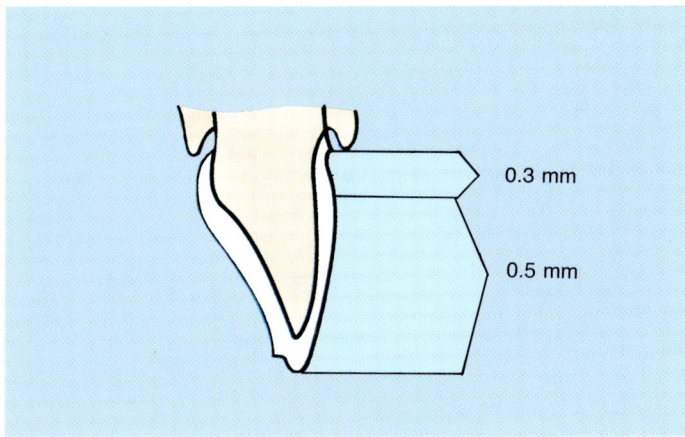

Fig 12-7 Stratification method—for a two-shade color shift in all teeth, a 0.3-mm tooth reduction in the cervical one third and a 0.5-mm tooth reduction in the remainder of the facial surface are sufficient.

od is best understood by examining the manipulation of each of the three layers.

Tooth preparation

Without graded tooth preparation, color control is inconsistent, and overbulked veneers are the rule. Graded tooth preparation rests on the principle that the greater the color change, the greater the misalignment toward the facial, or the greater the occlusal function, the greater the amount of tooth reduction. Two levels of graded tooth preparation are necessary to create space: one level for a moderate color change (the universal preparation) and another level for profound color change (Fig 12-6).

For moderate color change, defined as two shades or less, a two-plane facial reduction of 0.3 mm in the cervical one third and 0.5 mm in the incisal two thirds is indicated. This is considered the universal preparation because more than 90% of the cases necessitate this preparation (Fig 12-7). For profound color change, defined as three shades or more, including tetracycline and endodontically discolored teeth, a deeper biplane facial reduction is desirable. For all teeth except mandibular incisors, at least 0.4-mm enamel reduction in the cervical area and at least 0.6-mm enamel reduction along the remaining facial surface are indicated (Figs 12-8 and 12-9).

Mandibular incisors cannot be reduced more than 0.3 mm cervically and 0.5 mm on the remaining facial surface without substantial dentin exposure (Fig 12-10). Color control for mandibular incisors will be developed through greater emphasis on resin interface space and intrinsic veneer opacity.

In summary, the rationale for graded tooth preparation is to create sufficient space to totally convert the existing tooth color to the desired veneer color without undesirable overcontouring or color compromise.

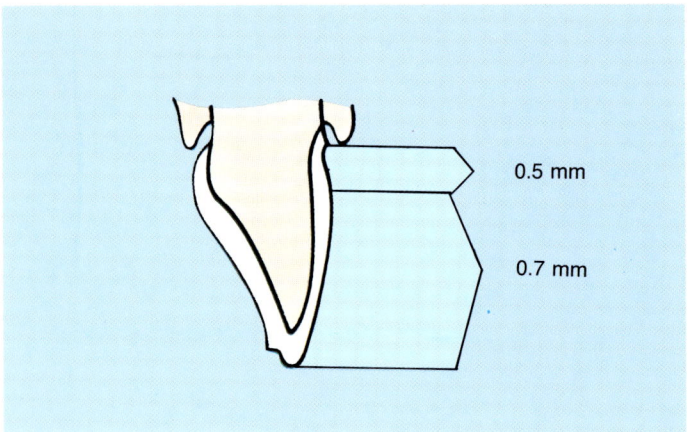

Fig 12-8 Stratification method—for the larger enamel-plated teeth, tooth reduction levels of 0.5 mm in the cervical one third and 0.7 mm in the remaining facial surface are possible when the color change is profound.

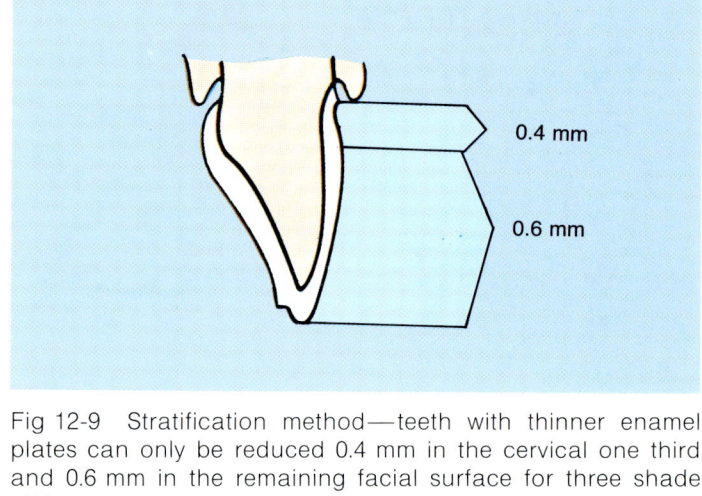

Fig 12-9 Stratification method—teeth with thinner enamel plates can only be reduced 0.4 mm in the cervical one third and 0.6 mm in the remaining facial surface for three shade shifts or more.

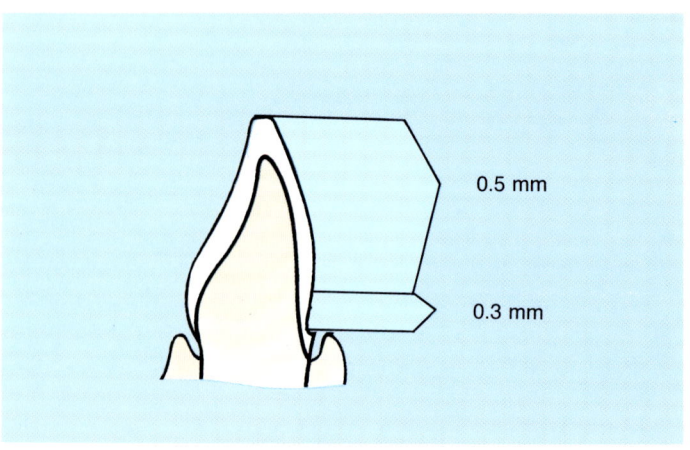

Fig 12-10 Stratification method—mandibular incisors, with the thinnest enamel plates, are confined to 0.3-mm cervical depths and 0.5-mm remaining facial depths, even with three shade shifts or more. Color correction will depend more on resin spacer and porcelain formulation.

Resin interface space

Just as graded tooth preparation was based on the degree of color shift between the prepared tooth color and the intended veneer color, in a similar manner, graded resin interface space is also related to this change. In the stratification method, this is perhaps the most significant factor in controlling veneer color, with tooth preparation and porcelain veneer formulation ranking a close second and third.

Before coordinating resin interface space with tooth preparation and with porcelain veneer formulation, it is advantageous to discuss light reflection and veneer vitality: the greater the surface reflection (specular reflection) of light off the surface of a porcelain veneer (as with a mirror), the lower the vitality of the veneer. The greater the internal reflection (diffuse reflection) of light (as with a natural tooth), the more vital the veneer becomes. In effect, this means that a veneer formed with a highly opaque porcelain will mask undesirable tooth color but display limited vitality due to the predominance of surface light reflection. By contrast, a more translu-

Stratification method

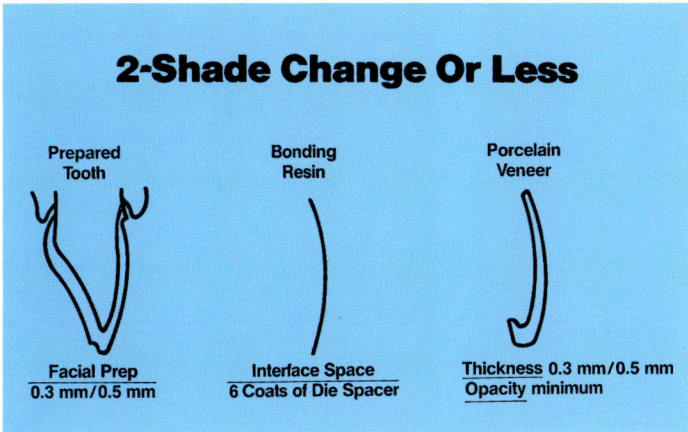

Fig 12-11 Stratification method—correlated with the tooth preparation for a two-shade shift or less is resin spacing of 0.1 mm and a relatively translucent porcelain veneer.

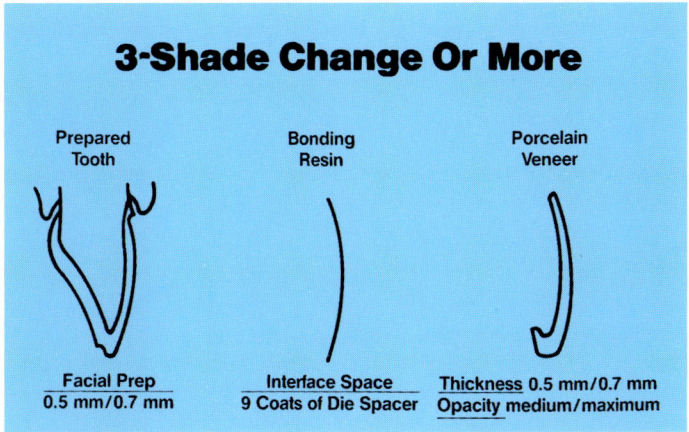

Fig 12-12 Stratification method—in a three-shade shift or more, along with the appropriate tooth preparation, a 0.1 to 0.2 mm die spacer is advocated. The porcelain veneer must increase in opacity as well.

cent porcelain allows considerably more light transmission and reflection internally, which significantly enhances vitality. However, at an average veneer thickness of 0.6 mm, the translucent porcelain allows some of the undesirable color of teeth with profound discoloration to bleed through. If neither opaque nor translucent porcelain produces both the desired color and vitality by itself, how can porcelain veneers simulate natural teeth against the backdrop of profoundly discolored teeth? The stratification method offers a solution to this seeming dilemma by:

1. Using graded resin interface space to allow the resin to dilute the tooth discoloration, ie, the principle utilized for graded tooth preparation is also applicable to graded resin interface space: the greater the color change, the greater the resin interface space.
2. Fabricating porcelain veneers with graded opacities.

For moderate color changes of two shades or less, graded resin interface space is accomplished by applying six coats of die spacer (one coat is assumed to be approximately 10 to 15 µm) as uniformly as possible over the entire preparation surface of veneer dies or a solid model, except for a 1-mm zone at the finish line and the incisal edge (Fig 12-11). This 1-mm unrelieved zone is established to retain accurate veneer seating and to minimize excessive resin cement film thickness at the margins.

For profound color changes of three shades or more, twelve die spacer coats are recommended (Fig 12-12). Again, the 1-mm zone at the margin remains free of die spacer. More than twelve die spacer coats up to 18 coats (0.2 mm) are reserved for the most severely discolored teeth, such as tetracycline and endodontically stained teeth. The rationale of using graded die spacer to occupy a portion of the space, created by graded tooth preparation, is to permit the resin cement color to dilute the tooth discoloration to a sufficient degree that the overlying porcelain veneer can establish the desired color and retain a high degree of vitality. In short, the resin cement value (lightness or darkness), hue (color), and chroma (intensity of color) will exert a decisive influence on the establishment of the desired color without sacrificing vitality because of the graded resin interface space.

Porcelain Veneers: An Esthetic Therapeutic Alternative

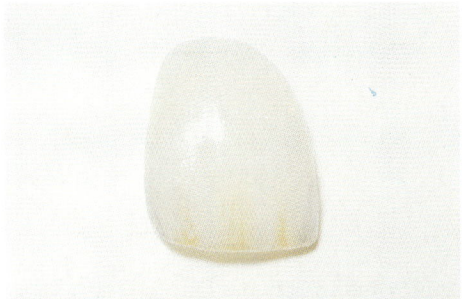

Fig 12-13 Stratification method—a typical porcelain veneer for a three-shade color shift or more is formulated with medium to high opacity. It is also more highly characterized, especially in the incisal zone and cervical zone.

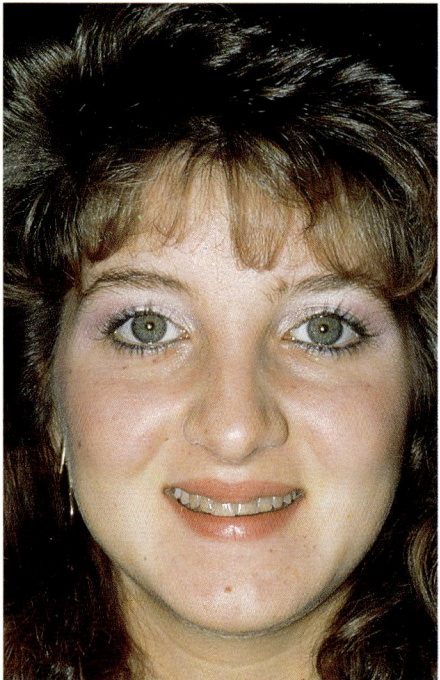

Fig 12-14 Stratification method—a young woman with dark tetracycline-stained teeth before placement of eight maxillary porcelain veneers.

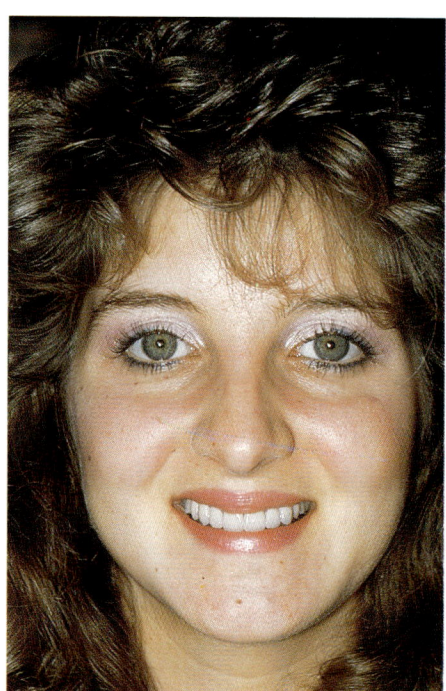

Fig 12-15 Stratification method—the striking improvement in her smile is obvious. The stratification method greatly simplifies difficult cases such as this one.

Porcelain veneer formulation

For a given case, the ceramist must formulate a porcelain veneer that will contain graded opacity appropriate to the desired color change. This could range from virtually no color change to a profound color correction of tetracycline or endodontically discolored teeth. The brand of porcelain used, the degree of opacity or pigmentation of the porcelain, the method of establishing the graded opacity, and the layered characterization of the porcelain veneer varies with the ceramist. In general, for a two-shade color change or less, the porcelain of choice tends to be relatively translucent (see Fig 12-11). For a three-shade shift or more, it is preferable to use a more opaque porcelain. To produce a polychromatic, natural tooth color gradation in the more opaque veneers, the veneers are more highly characterized than a porcelain crown (Fig 12-13).

Verification of the stratification method is apparent in the results of case after case, which demonstrate lively, natural color (Figs 12-14 and 12-15).

Tooth preparation and impression taking

Advantages of tooth preparation

The main advantage of tooth preparation is control over

a number of factors, which, if left haphazard, can seriously jeopardize the biologic and esthetic final result. Correct tooth preparation initiates control of the following:

1. Contour.
    a. Emergence angle.
    b. Margin.
    c. Facial profile.
2. Color without overbulking.
3. Margin placement for concealment.
4. Veneer seating for placement and bonding.
5. Definitiveness of margin for the technician.
6. Porcelain bulk for occlusal loading.
7. Glaze preservation in finishing procedures.
8. Tooth recontouring for misalignment correction.
9. Enamel etch by removing fluoride-rich layer.

Tooth preparation will vary somewhat from tooth to tooth, depending on tooth size, tooth alignment, and existing enamel. For example, a maxillary central incisor would require more tooth preparation than a mandibular incisor. A protruding tooth would necessitate more tooth preparation than a correctly aligned tooth. A younger tooth, with minimal enamel wear, would permit more tooth preparation than an older tooth with considerable enamel wear.

It is assumed that before porcelain veneering is undertaken, restoration of all carious lesions, replacement of all failing restoratives, and eradication of all periodontal disease has been completed on all teeth to be veneered. Pumice all teeth to be veneered to remove any extrinsic stain. Make a shade determination for the veneers based on as much patient input as possible if this important decision was not made during case evaluation. Any occlusal abnormalities should also be corrected before starting.

The stratification method is now employed to determine the correct amount of tooth preparation. Note the shade(s) of the existing teeth to be veneered, and lower it one shade because of tooth preparation, eg, if the unprepared teeth are A3, then assume they will be A3.5 after preparation. Based on the guidelines of the stratification method, if the veneer shade is A1, then a 0.5-mm emergence/0.7-mm facial plane preparation should be made in the thickest teeth and 0.4-mm/0.6-mm and 0.3-mm/0.5-mm in the thinner and thinnest teeth. If the veneer shade is A2, however, this would necessitate only a two-shade shift (from A3.5 to A2), and a 0.3-mm emergence/0.5-mm facial plane preparation would be used. As an additional example of stratification method logic, if the shade of the unprepared teeth is A2 and the prepared teeth become A3, then no matter how light an A shade the patient selects, the preparation would still be 0.3-mm/0.5-mm. Estimating the shade of the prepared tooth to be one shade darker than the unprepared tooth to determine the amount of tooth preparation is correct for the majority of teeth. Occasionally, the prepped tooth violates this estimate, being more than one shade darker or remains the same shade or gets lighter. In these situations, the final preparation is always determined by the actual shade of the prepared tooth. Sometimes this necessitates changing a 0.3-mm/0.5-mm preparation into a 0.5-mm/0.7-mm preparation to properly control color.

Tooth preparation for maxillary anterior teeth

It is much easier to visualize tooth preparation in enamel if the teeth are prepared dry: periodically (every 15 seconds) a water–air syringe spray is activated to wash away powdered tooth cuttings and cool the tooth. The lack of a continual water-mist introduces much greater control and obviates inadvertent overpreparation. If dentin is exposed, water spray must be activated for pulpal health. Anesthesia, which may or may not have been necessary up to this point (based on patient subjectivity), should be administered at this time, as a general rule.

Before initiating tooth preparation, it is necessary to determine where to place the gingival margin. The advantages of a slightly supragingival margin (0.5 mm) are numerous, such as minimal tissue trauma in preparation, lessened likelihood of exposing dentin, reduced probability of tissue retraction for impression taking, greater control of surface contamination during bonding, easier access for marginal finishing procedures after placement, reduced probability of contour alterations in the bonded restoration (potentiating gingival inflammation), and improved patient accessibility for soft tissue maintenance procedures. Therefore, with the exception of pronounced tooth discoloration or a patient who is obsessive about disguising the margin, it is highly desirable to place the margin slightly supragingival in enamel. In cases in which a 0.5-mm supragingival margin has been prepared, as previously stated, placement of retraction cord is usually unnecessary.

Porcelain Veneers: An Esthetic Therapeutic Alternative

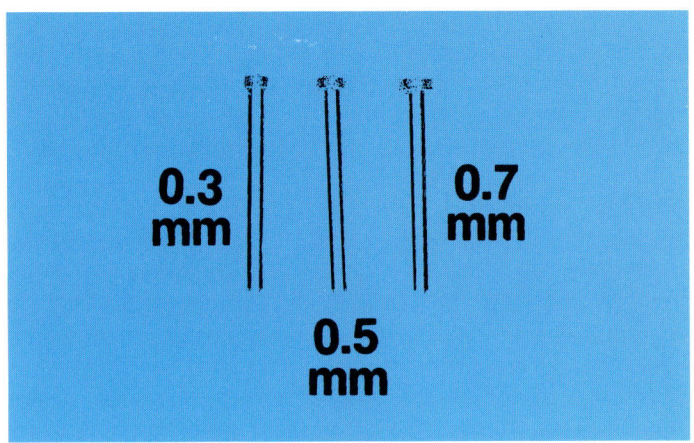

Fig 12-16 Tooth preparation sequence—the 0.3-mm, 0.5-mm, and 0.7-mm self-limiting depth-cutting disks provide controlled facial reduction. They are part of the Nixon Porcelain Veneer Kit 2 (Brasseler).

Tooth preparation sequence: Maxillary teeth

To control the depth of the facial tooth preparation and remain primarily in enamel for bond strength and reliability of marginal seal, self-limiting, depth-cutting disks are used. These depth-cutting disks permit 0.3-mm, 0.5-mm, and 0.7-mm cuts to be placed anywhere on the facial surface (Fig 12-16). In more than 90% of the cases, the 0.3-mm and 0.5-mm depth-cutting disks are used because the color change is two shades or less.

To illustrate the correct sequence of tooth preparation in stages, a maxillary right central incisor tooth has been colored white. The distal one half of the facial surface will be prepared to graphically demonstrate the tooth preparation sequence. In everyday clinical practice, both mesial and distal surfaces would be prepared according to this sequence (Figs 12-17 to 12-22).

Placement of depth cuts

Whether a single tooth or multiple teeth are to be prepared, the 0.3-mm depth-cutting disk (or infrequently the 0.5-mm depth-cutting disk for profound color change) is used first to place a uniform horizontal depth cut from the mesioproximal line angle to the distoproximal line angle. This horizontal cut should be placed in the cervical one third of the tooth and preferably at least 3 mm from the cementoenamal junction. If multiple teeth are to be veneered, then the 0.3-mm depth cuts are placed as described on each of these teeth. The 0.3-mm depth-cutting disk is now replaced by the 0.5-mm depth-cutting disk (or infrequently the 0.7-mm depth-cutting disk for profound color change). The 0.5-mm depth-cutting disk is now used on all teeth to be veneered to place two additional depth cuts. One horizontal depth cut is placed midfacially from the mesioproximal line angle to the distoproximal line angle. The other horizontal depth cut is placed in the incisal one third of the facial surface, approximately 3 mm from the incisal edge. This horizontal depth cut also extends from the mesioproximal line angle to the distoproximal line angle (see Fig 12-17).

Gingivoproximal preparation

To establish the veneer margin, using a long, tapered medium or fine grit snub-nosed diamond bur, prepare a definitive chamfer (0.3 to 0.4 mm in depth) uniformly 0.5 mm supragingival from the gingival margin. Begin at the height of the free gingival margin and prepare the chamfer margin to the distal papilla tip. Then prepare the chamfer margin to the mesial papilla tip (see Figs 12-18 and 12-21).

Continue the definitive chamfer finish line from the

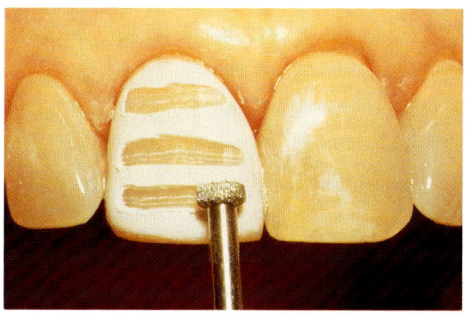

Fig 12-17 Tooth preparation sequence—depth cut placements, appropriate to the maxillary central incisor in this case, are illustrated. The cervical horizontal depth cut is 0.3 mm. The midfacial and incisal depths cuts are 0.5 mm.

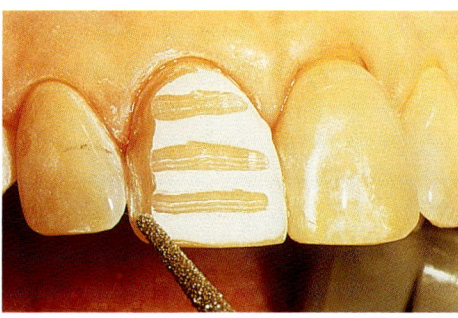

Fig 12-18 Tooth preparation sequence—the gingivoproximal chamfer finish line is illustrated on the distal one half of the tooth. Note that the finish line is slightly supragingival, has an indentation or elbow below the papilla tip, and does *not* penetrate into the contact zone.

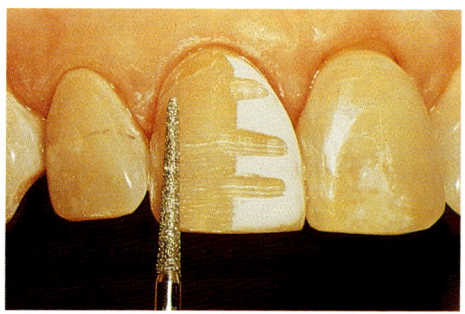

Fig 12-19 Tooth preparation sequence—facial reduction is accomplished by removing the depth cuts and "rolling" the proximal corners into the preestablished chamfer finish lines, eliminating any sharp line angles.

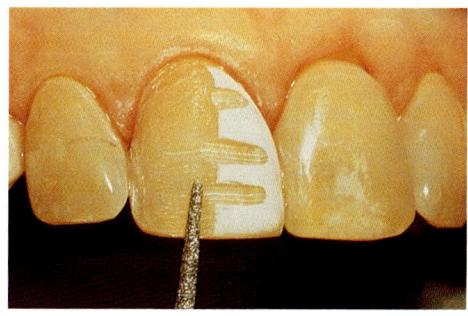

Fig 12-20 Tooth preparation sequence—facial reduction in the incisal one fourth is sometimes incomplete due to placing the incisal depth cut too high. If this situation occurs, correct it with further reduction.

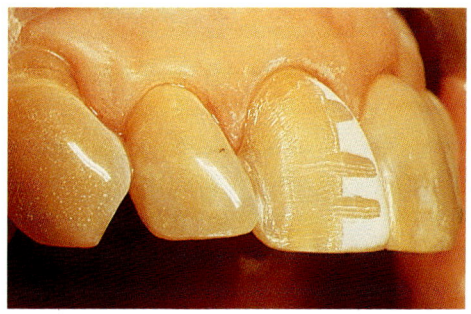

Fig 12-21 Tooth preparation sequence—side view of the completed gingivoproximal and facial reduction of the distal one half of the tooth. Note that the finish line resembles a dog leg, to hide the margin and facilitate veneer finishing.

distal papilla tip to the beginning of the contact zone, far enough lingually, to hide the veneer margin when viewed from the side of the tooth. This produces an elbow-like cut, which translates into the "wings" of the forthcoming veneer, which will conceal the margin from an unesthetic display (see Fig 12-21). Without breaking into the tooth contact from the labial, carry the definitive chamfer from the elbow cut incisalward to the incisal embrasure, cutting just labial (0.2 mm) to the entire contact zone. The tooth contact is left intact with a narrow island (0.2 mm) of proximal tooth structure, just labial to the contact zone, remaining unprepared (see Figs 12-18 and 12-21). This sliver of unprepared tooth structure just labial to the contact is significant because it permits a small separation between the veneer margin and the adjacent tooth or veneer. This slight separation, which is not perceptible to a casual observer, permits access for finishing the cemented veneer to remove resin cement flash or an irregular porcelain ledge (see Fig 12-22). Naturally, the same type of definitive chamfer is

Porcelain Veneers: An Esthetic Therapeutic Alternative

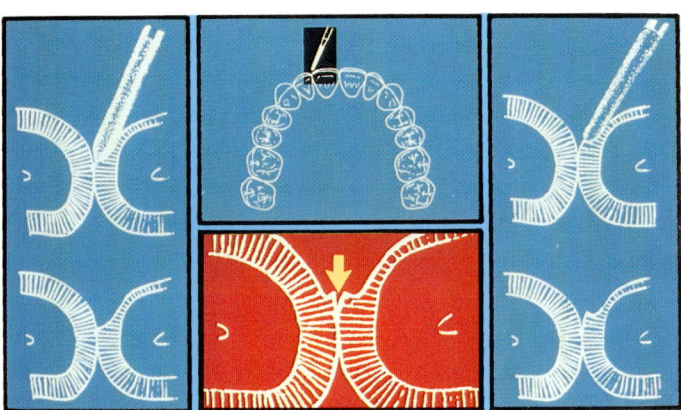

Fig 12-22 Tooth preparation sequencea—a diagrammatic representation of tooth preparation at the contact zone *(arrow)* emphasizes the correct placement of the proximal finish line. It also demonstrates the advantage of a snub-nosed diamond bur tip (Nixon Porcelain Veneer Kit 2) over a bullet-nosed diamond bur tip. The snub-nosed diamond bur tip produces a cavosurface angle of 110° to 120° or more. The bullet-nosed diamond bur tip cuts a 135° angle and tends to thrust into the contact zone.

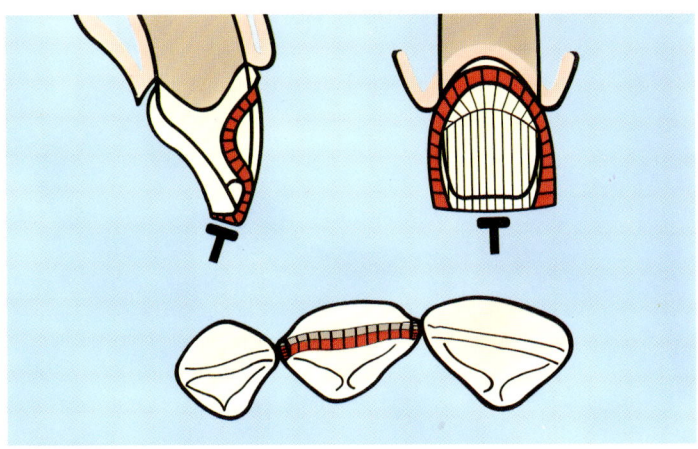

Fig 12-23 Tooth preparation sequence—a diagrammatic representation of the incisal reduction for a tooth that will not be lengthened and will have a porcelain incisal edge. Note the angle toward the lingual edge of the edge-reducing disk. It is 30° to 40° off perpendicular to the long axis of the tooth toward the lingual.

placed from the mesial papilla tip to the end of the incisal embrasure in clinical practice before beginning facial reduction. The purpose of establishing the entire gingivoproximal definitive chamfer margin before beginning facial depth cut removal is to avoid overpreparation, which often occurs when facial reduction is begun first. The no. 850-014 diamond bur from the Nixon Porcelain Veneer Kit II (Brasseler) is recommended for the gingivoproximal preparation for most teeth. The no. 850-016 diamond bur in the Nixon Porcelain Veneer Kit II is used occasionally for larger teeth in the proximal preparation.

Facial preparation

Based on the stratification method, remove 0.3 mm of enamel (0.5 mm for profound color change) in the cervical one third, blending this enamel reduction into the gingival chamfer. Avoid overreduction or underreduction by preparing until the depth cuts just disappear. Paralleling the remaining facial surface, remove from 0.5 mm of the facial enamel (0.7 mm for profound color change),

depending on the stratification method guidelines. Again, use appropriate depth cuts as a precise measurement to gauge tooth reduction. Use a no. 850-014 Brasseler diamond bur (medium grit). Be sure to round off any sharp angles that develop during facial preparation, such as the facioproximal line angles or the facioincisal line angle. These sharp angles create potential stress zones, which render porcelain more prone to fracture (see Fig 12-19). Check facial reduction in the incisal one third. Sometimes it is not fully prepared, resulting in a labialization of the incisal edge. If a mirror check from the incisal reveals this underreduction, remove more tooth structure (see Fig 12-20). Adequate facial preparation allows room for matching, modifying, or masking of various tooth colors, and it makes it unnecessary to perceptibly overcontour the veneer.

Tooth preparation sequence: Maxillary teeth

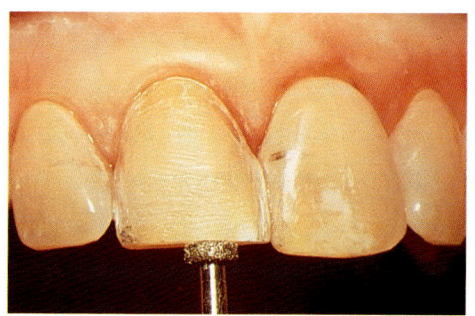

Fig 12-24 Tooth preparation sequence —the incisal reduction of 1 mm is correct, but the angle of the disk is incorrect. By not tilting the cutting surface lingually, no resistance form is created to withstand functional edge fracture.

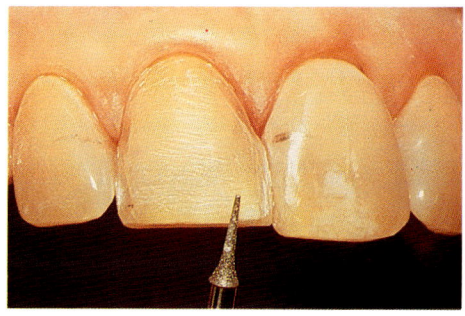

Fig 12-25 Tooth preparation sequence —to avoid stress concentration, which could result in eventual porcelain fracture, the facioincisal angle, which becomes sharp after facial preparation, is rounded off.

Incisal preparation

Before completing the final stage of basic tooth preparation, the incisal preparation, it is necessary to evaluate each tooth in regard to the esthetic treatment plan. If porcelain is to cover the incisal table, it is essential to allow for sufficient porcelain bulk in the preparation design to resist functional failure due to crack propagation in the porcelain. This ranges from 0.75 to 1.5 mm, depending on the severity of occlusal loading, with 1.0 mm being a generally accepted average incisal thickness of porcelain. Additionally, it is necessary to terminate the incisal margin in such a manner as to protect against marginal "peel" (progressive fatiguing of the bonding resin over time until cohesive failure occurs, resulting in incisal fracture of the bonded veneer). This requires developing resistance form in the incisal preparation by either ending it at the linguoincisal line angle after reducing the incisal table more toward the lingual to provide added support to the restoration, or by ending it at the beveled facioincisal line angle to provide support from the incisal table of the tooth.

Bearing these factors in mind, for maxillary incisors, if the teeth are not to be lengthened and the facial reduction has resulted in an incisal table of less than 1 mm width, then the incisal edge should be reduced approximately 1 mm or more for central incisors and 0.75 mm or more for lateral incisors. The reduction of the incisal table should not be done perpendicular to the long axis of the tooth but about 30° to 40° off perpendicular toward the lingual (Figs 12-23 and 12-24). This slight angulation toward the lingual provides resistance form against porcelain edge fracture and a sharp finish line for the ceramist to form a porcelain butt margin against. The facioincisal angle, which becomes sharp from the facial reduction, must now be rounded off or it will create an area of stress under the veneer (Fig 12-25).

If the maxillary incisors are not to be lengthened and facial reduction leaves an incisal table greater than 1 mm in width, then the sharpened facioincisal line angle can be given a 30° bevel, and the termination of that bevel on the incisal table serves as the incisal finish line. In other words, when a thicker incisal table exists after facial reduction, the porcelain veneer does not need to fully replace the incisal edge. Rather, it can merge with the incisal boundary of a 30° bevel of the resultant facioincisal line angle. This alternative incisal preparation is a reliable way of preserving existing incisal length.

If the maxillary incisors are to be lengthened up to 2 mm and the incisal table is less than 1 mm in width, then the incisal table is reduced in a 30° to 40° plane toward the lingual until the incisal table width reaches

Porcelain Veneers: An Esthetic Therapeutic Alternative

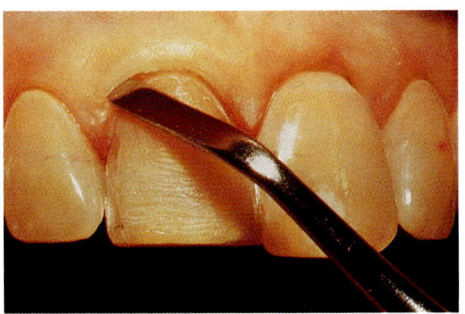

Fig 12-26 Tooth preparation sequence—if a subgingival margin is necessary to hide extremely dark teeth, prepare the chamfer to the edge of the unretracted gingival margin. Then, delicately retract the gingiva with one or two strands of thin, braided cord.

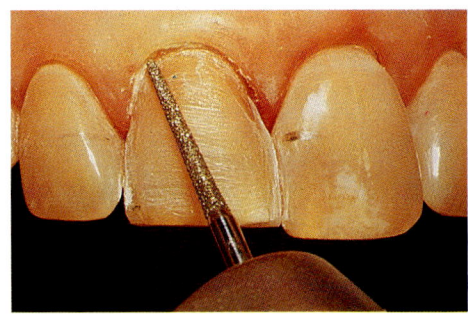

Fig 12-27 Tooth preparation sequence—following atraumatic retraction of gingiva, carefully extend the chamfer finish line, prepared to the unretracted gingiva, approximately 0.75 to 1.0 mm apically. Avoid going more than 1 mm subgingival due to problems of finishing access, contamination, and soft tissue irritation.

1 mm or more. The added tooth length desired will be accomplished by additional incisal porcelain in the veneer. If the incisal table after facial reduction is 1 mm or more in width and the tooth is to be lengthened, then the existing incisal table is lightly beveled 30° to 40° toward the lingual. The added length will be built into the incisal of the porcelain veneer.

Because of its role in anterior guidance, the canine is best handled one of two ways. If the existing incisal length and shape are satisfactory, then a "window" preparation is advisable because it does not alter anterior guidance in any way. A window preparation of the canine incisal table, which is usually twice the width of the incisal table of incisors following facial reduction, is accomplished by undermining the incisal table and removing about one third of the incisal table toward the facial. This is done by pointing the snub-nosed diamond bur downward (from cervical to incisal) and running the tip from the mesioproximal chamfer terminus to the distoproximal chamfer terminus, with the tip following at all times the line of the incisal table. By creating a continuous 360° finish line, essentially on the facial surface, the preparation roughly resembles a window, hence the name window preparation.

If the canine is worn at the incisal edge and the treatment plan is to restore the tooth to a more rounded incisal shape and lengthen it, then a different incisal preparation is advisable. Perform at least enough tooth reduction by angling 30° to 40° toward the lingual to permit 1.0 to 1.5 mm incisal thickness in the porcelain veneer in the area of incisal guidance, as well as at least 1 mm thickness in the remaining areas of the incisal table. The sharp linguoincisal angle from this incisal preparation will be the finish line for the ceramist to form a butt porcelain margin. As with the maxillary incisors, the facioincisal line angle is rounded off. [Note of caution: there is no advantage to carrying the incisal chamfer several millimeters onto the lingual surface.] Naturally long teeth, eg, canines with blunted papillae or periodontally involved teeth treated with flap therapy, require maximal interproximal penetration without undercuts to hide margins. Veneer seating is best accomplished by a direct facial line of insertion or an incisofacial rotation. In the incisofacial rotation, the incisal porcelain of the veneer is seated first and acts as a pivot, and the cervical portion of the veneer is gradually seated by rotating the veneer into place with gentle finger pressure. Neither of these preferred seating methods is served by having a lingual chamfer, which is several millimeters cervical to the linguoincisal line angle. This creates a considerably more incisal line of insertion and increases the probability of fracture of the thin proximal wings on seating, incomplete seating of the veneer, an open lingual margin in fabrication to permit seating, and fracture of the thin lingual extension during placement or subsequent function.

Occlusal preparation for premolars involves two variations from the maxillary anterior tooth preparations. Carry the chamfer finish line about 1.0 to 1.5 mm onto the occlusal surface to a depth of about 0.75 mm. This will "hood" the cusp and diminish greatly the possibility of shear fracture. Carry the distal chamfer only to the distal line angle not within 0.2 mm of the contact. This surface is not seen from a frontal or side view. This little adjustment simplifies finishing and polishing of this surface, which becomes increasingly difficult the more posteriorly the veneers are placed.

If a subgingival finish line is to be prepared because of severely discolored teeth, as mentioned, at the outset of tooth preparation an atraumatic retraction cord should be placed (Fig 12-26). The gingival chamfer is then carried slightly subgingival (maximum of 1 mm) from its original location at the gingival crest (Fig 12-27). Anesthesia for cord placement may or may not be necessary depending on subjective pain tolerance of the patient.

Even if subgingival margins are not placed, unless there is a 0.5 mm or more supragingival margin, thin braided retraction cord should be placed beneath the gingival crest on all prepared teeth. After placement of the cord, the gingival chamfers on all teeth are examined. It is possible that one or more teeth require additional chamfer definition at the gingival margin. Chamfer redefinition is carried out at this time, before impression taking, to ensure definitive margins that can be readily visualized and fabricated by the ceramist.

With the retraction cord in place around all prepared teeth and chamfer margins definitive around the entire periphery, the teeth are carefully inspected to ensure that no undercuts exist for the facial or incisofacial path of insertion. If any are present they are removed at this time. Additionally, any obtrusive bulge areas must be flattened to avoid "headlight" show-through of the underlying tooth color or opaque-bonding resin. All resin restorations in the prepared teeth should be carefully reassessed and replaced if they are substandard. Careful scrutiny of tooth structure sometimes reveals surface caries, fractures, or hypocalcified areas. These potential problem sites must be evaluated and resolved, particularly if they are at the margin of the veneer. Marginal integrity is of paramount importance to the longevity of a porcelain veneer. Finally, 1-μm metal strips are passed between each contact to ensure that the contacts are not bound. Bound contacts hinder veneer cementation. If any contacts are bound, lighten them with ultrafine diamond-coated strips.

Dentin considerations

If during the course of tooth preparation an "island" of dentin is exposed but the chamfer margin remains in enamel, the freshly exposed surface dentin should be sealed with two thin coats of a dentin-bonding adhesive cured independently. This will seal the dentinal tubules from bacterial invasion in the interim from the preparation appointment to the placement appointment. This procedure should be performed before impression taking so that the layers of adhesive are accounted for in the impression. It is advisable to caution the patient to refrain from extremely cold or hot beverages or food, until the veneers are placed, to minimize postpreparation discomfort.

If cervical caries, erosion, or abrasion exists, necessitating placement of the veneer margin outside the enamel, a glass ionomer restorative or a hybrid composite restorative with shallow mechanical retention is desirable as a subsurface to the veneer. This "sandwich" technique is more likely to preserve the marginal seal of the veneer over a period of time.

Gloss temporization

Many cases requiring color change but little alteration in alignment can endure porcelain veneer preparation and not be terribly unesthetic. The teeth often appear shorter, flatter, but acceptable for the short interval of 1 or 2 weeks before placement. To enhance the appearance of the prepared teeth by illusion, it is convenient to merely polish the facial surface lightly with medium and fine aluminum oxide disks. This yields a shiny surface, rather than the matte finish produced by diamond burs, but does not remove the diamond surface striations. Because of the surface luster this technique produces, it is called gloss temporization. For the maxillary anterior teeth, in the tooth preparation sequence, before and after preparation are shown in Figs 12-28 and 12-29. Note that they have been gloss-temporized and the mandibular anterior teeth have been equilibrated at the

Porcelain Veneers: An Esthetic Therapeutic Alternative

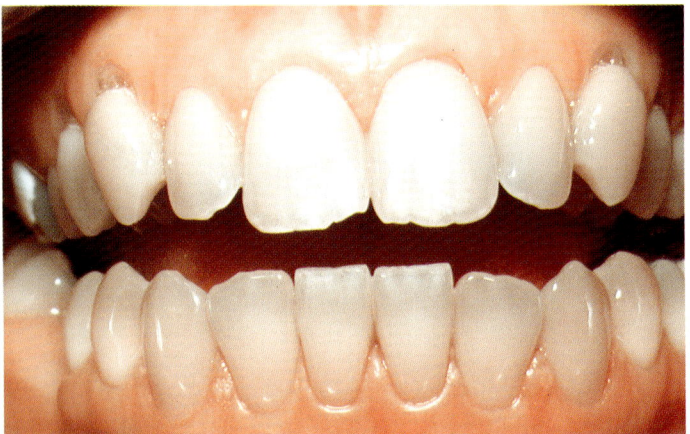

Fig 12-28 Tooth preparation sequence—appearance of the six maxillary anterior teeth before any tooth preparation.

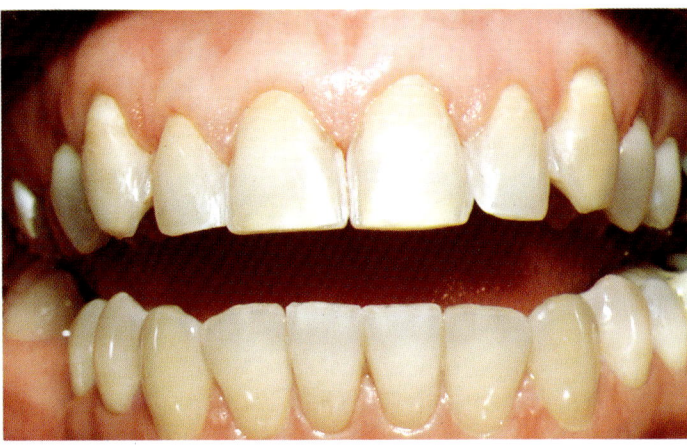

Fig 12-29 Tooth preparation sequence—appearance of the same six maxillary anterior teeth after tooth preparation. Observe the shiny reflective appearance of the facial surfaces, produced by light polishing with aluminum oxide disks. Note also the restoration of the cervical erosions in the canines with glass ionomer.

incisal edge. For a more complex method of temporization with composite resins or acrylic, see "Resin temporization" following "Impression taking."

Tooth preparation sequence: Mandibular teeth

Mandibular anterior teeth differ from maxillary anterior teeth in that they have thinner enamel plates, flatter gingival emergence profiles, require less esthetic emphasis in the cervical one third, and, most importantly, require disruption of centric occlusion and anterior guidance. Consequently, certain modifications are instituted for preparation of mandibular teeth to make provision for occlusal loading as well as contour and color correction.

Before initiating any tooth preparation, it is advisable to eliminate any premature, edge irregularities and compressions by careful occlusal equilibration.

Incisal clearance

To initiate tooth preparation for depth control, place two depth cuts (rather than three depth cuts as in maxillary teeth) in all mandibular anterior teeth. One depth cut of 0.3 mm is placed approximately at the junction of the middle and the cervical one third of the teeth from mesioproximal line angle to distoproximal line angle. The other depth cut of 0.5 mm is placed approximately 4 mm from the existing incisal table.

If the tooth makes contact in centric occlusion, take the tooth out of occlusion by 0.5 mm for mandibular incisors and 0.7 mm for canines, paralleling the plane of the existing incisal table insofar as possible. The 0.5-mm and 0.7-mm depth cutting disks can be used for controlling the depth of this reduction by placing two vertical cuts into the incisal table, one third the distance from the mesial and distal edges. The incisal table reduction will take the incisors out of occlusion by 0.5 mm and the canines by 0.7 mm. A second preparation cut is then made, paralleling the facial surface, to the depth of the 0.5-mm depth cut. The intersection of these two preparation cuts will generally create an incisal clearance at the facioincisal line angle of at least 0.75 mm

Tooth preparation sequence: Mandibular teeth

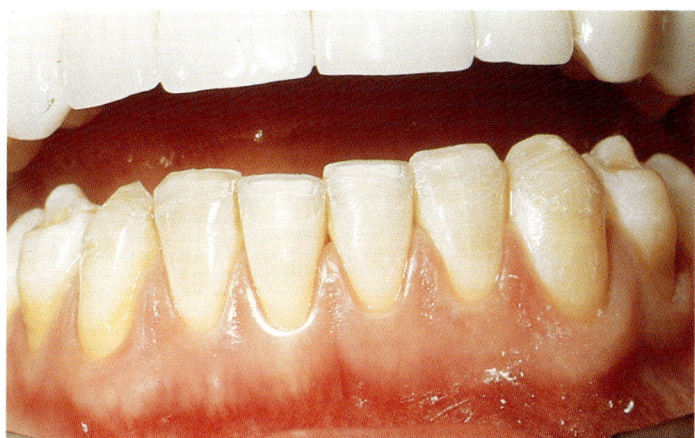

Fig 12-30 Tooth preparation sequence—to create incisal clearance for mandibular teeth, incisors and canines are prepared first on the incisal table, then parallel to the facial surface, as described in the text. Here is how the teeth appear after this reduction. Note the 0.3-mm cervical one third depth cut has not yet been placed.

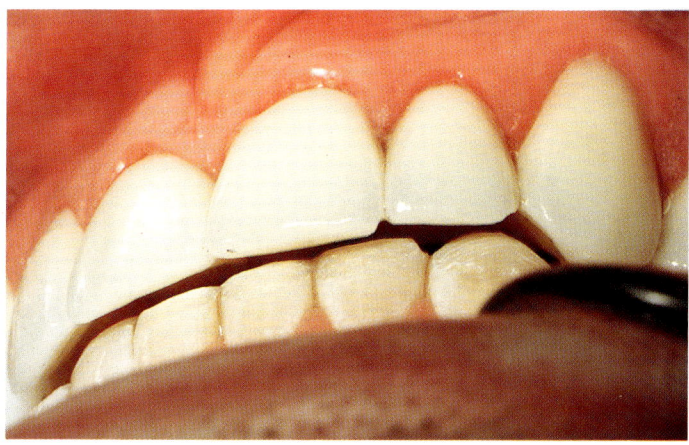

Fig 12-31 Tooth preparation sequence—the adequacy of the initial incisal clearance is assessed by having the patient close tightly in centric occlusion. The 1-mm rubber tongue of a Flexible Clearance Guide (Belle de St. Claire) is an excellent means of verifying clearance.

for the incisors and at least 1.0 mm for the canines (Fig 12-30). To verify the incisal clearance, the patient should close in centric occlusion, and the estimated clearance distance should be carefully checked for adequacy (Fig 12-31). For heavier occlusions, increasing the incisal clearance to 1.0 mm for incisors and 1.5 mm for canines may be advisable. The preparation cuts for incisal clearance have completed the tooth preparation of the incisal one third of the mandibular teeth.

Gingivoproximal and facial preparation

The gingival chamfer is now begun in enamel, even if it is supragingival. The mandibular tooth gingival margin is not nearly as esthetically relevant as the maxillary tooth gingival margin. Therefore, for ease of impression taking and moisture control, as well as access for finishing, when bonding the veneers the gingival chamfer is routinely placed entirely in enamel, even if it creates a slightly supragingival margin. The chamfer in mandibular incisors is not as pronounced as with maxillary incisors, being a maximum of 0.3 mm, because of the thinner enamel plate. The Brasseler no. 850-014 is well designed for this fine cut. The proximal chamfer preparation is similar to that for maxillary incisors with the exception of the depth. It should be 0.4 mm as it extends from the papilla tip incisally to the embrasure. From the papilla tip to the tooth contact, the chamfer moves slightly lingually to hide the margin (dog leg effect) but remains just facial to the tooth contact to retain the contact in its entirety. Cervical facial reduction for mandibular incisors is less severe than maxillary incisors, being in the 0.3 mm range. If a severe discoloration must be corrected by the veneer, approximately 0.1 to 0.2 mm must be added to the veneer to compensate for the insufficient tooth reduction depth, as suggested by the stratification method. The facial reduction has already been accomplished in the incisal one third from the two-plane preparation required for occlusal clearance. Therefore, the facial reduction involves merely blending the middle one third of the facial surface with the cervical reduction and the incisal clearance reduction. This generally averages between 0.4 and 0.6 mm in depth. Therefore, the facioincisal line angle is slightly rounded for stress reduction, but the linguoincisal line angle is left sharp to allow a butt joint marginal termination by the ceramist (Fig 12-32).

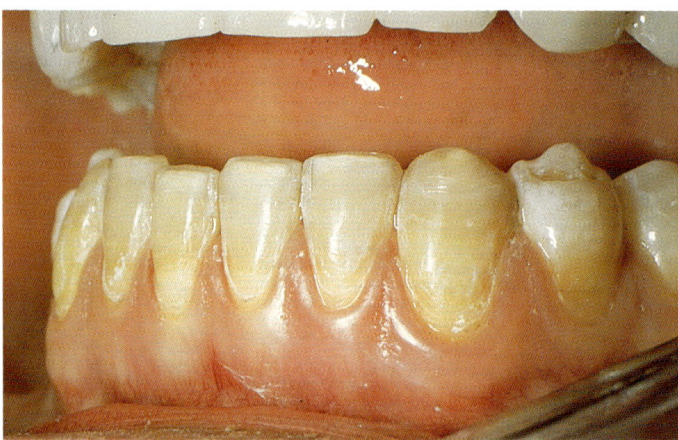

Fig 12-32 Tooth preparation sequence—appearance of six mandibular anterior teeth, as photographed from the left side, after completion of tooth preparation. Observe the slightly (0.5 to 1 mm) supragingival finish lines, as well as the "dog leg" gingivoproximal finish line, on the mesial surface of the right central incisor.

The same general guidelines exist for the canines as for the incisors, except that the cuts are deeper due to a thicker enamel plate and increased functional stress upon the porcelain from canine-protected dentitions. Gingival preparation is supragingival about 0.5 mm and preferably in enamel. Chamfer depths are 0.3 mm along the gingival and 0.4 mm interproximally. Facial preparation depth averages 0.5 mm until the incisalmost one third is reached, and then it is increased to provide for occlusal loading, as previously described. The facioincisal line angle is rounded. Because the occlusion is totally disrupted by mandibular veneer tooth preparation, careful precautions should be taken to reestablish, in porcelain, precise occlusal function. In many cases the color of the teeth is the main reason for veneers, and the preexisting occlusion is normal. To sustain a physiologically acceptable occlusion with the newly placed veneers, it is advisable to do the following:

1. Send pretreatment maxillary and mandibular stone casts to serve as contour guides for the ceramist fabricating the veneers. Send along checkbites for articulator mounting of the casts to further aid in reestablishing correct occlusion. Face-bow transfers and registrations to allow the case to be mounted on a fully adjustable articulator can also be performed.
2. Give sufficient tooth reduction in the critical occlusal zone to prevent inadequate porcelain bulk, which could cause veneer fracture. With insufficient tooth reduction veneers with adequate porcelain bulk could create occlusal prematurities.
3. Keep the time between the preparation appointment and the placement appointment short (1 week) to avoid supereruption of the teeth. A temporary bite guard, to be worn except when eating, can be created for longer interappointment periods.

The result of precise tooth preparation and accurate veneer formulation and placement is an esthetically attractive dentition, which in no way violates function or soft tissue health. Such a dentition is shown in Figs 12-33 and 12-34.

Tooth preparation for spaced teeth

Because no contact exists with spaced teeth, the proximal preparation is changed from a chamfer to a long

Tooth preparation sequence: Mandibular teeth

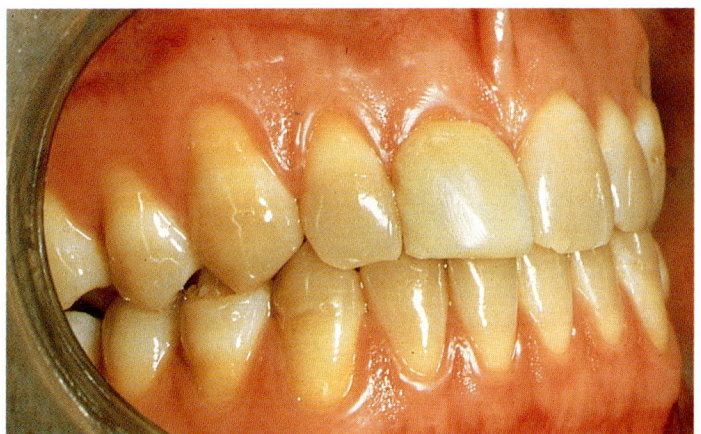

Fig 12-33 Tooth preparation sequence—pretreatment profile appearance of the maxillary and mandibular dentition.

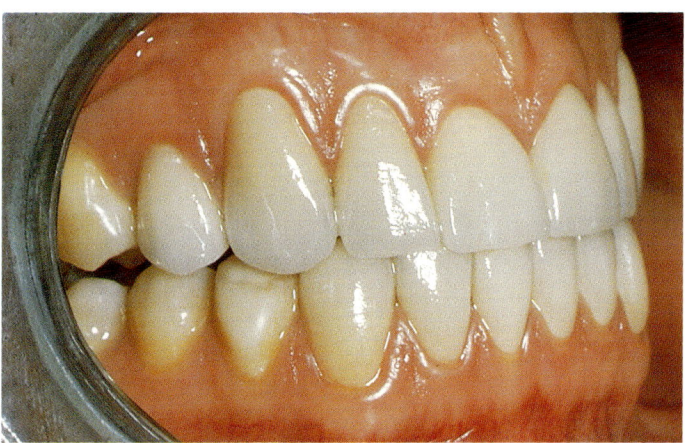

Fig 12-34 Tooth preparation sequence—posttreatment appearance of Fig 12-33. The patient has received eight maxillary and six mandibular porcelain veneers. Note the lack of overcontouring, the unseen margins (except along the gingival margin of the mandibular teeth), and the striking color change.

bevel. This bevel will terminate at the linguoproximal line angle and eliminate any proximal convexity that would create an undercut for a facial line of insertion. This involves carrying the gingival chamfer along the papilla tip until the linguoproximal line angle is nearly reached and then using the side of the diamond bur to flatten (bevel) the remaining proximal surface incisalward. The proximal surface is flattened by repeated passages of the diamond bur, until the long bevel reaches the linguoproximal line angle along the entire proximal surface.

Another modification in tooth preparation for spaced teeth involves removing more enamel (0.2 mm) at the facioproximal line angles to narrow the illusory width of the facial surface and prevent the "block" tooth look.

Partial veneer tooth preparation

Teeth with unesthetic spaces, whether single or multiple, where the existing tooth color is acceptable, need not be corrected by a complete facial veneer. Instead, a more conservative method of treatment is possible with partial veneers. These add-on porcelain restorations require little or no tooth preparation. The proximal tooth surface, transisting into the facial and lingual surfaces, produces a natural tooth finish line for a partial porcelain veneer. If a developmental groove is slightly accentuated on the facial surface near the proximal line angle, an imperceptible margin is created, and the partial veneer blends nicely into the recipient tooth. Color is relatively easy to derive because the partial veneer projects extending tooth color in a chameleon effect, rather than masking a disharmonious color. The "taco shell" wraparound effect of the partial veneer, along with the high bond strength of etched porcelain and the minimal occlusal stress brought to bear on this restoration, make the partial porcelain veneer a useful option in the esthetic repertoire.

Impression taking

Before taking final impressions of the prepared teeth, carefully evaluate all aspects of the tooth preparations, especially concealment of the margins between the papilla tip and beginning of the contact zone, and the adequacy of the gingival chamfer. Check the occlusion

Porcelain Veneers: An Esthetic Therapeutic Alternative

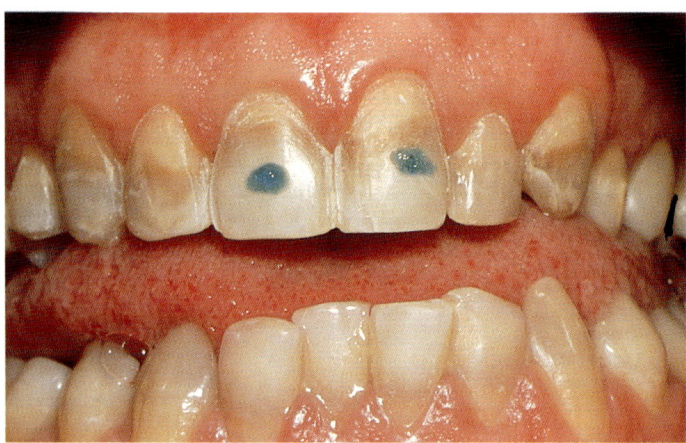

Fig 12-35 Resin temporization—because preparation of eight maxillary teeth dramatized the discoloration, it was decided that temporary resin veneers would be placed. Note the limited area of etching (away from the finish lines), to permit "spot bonding" of the veneers.

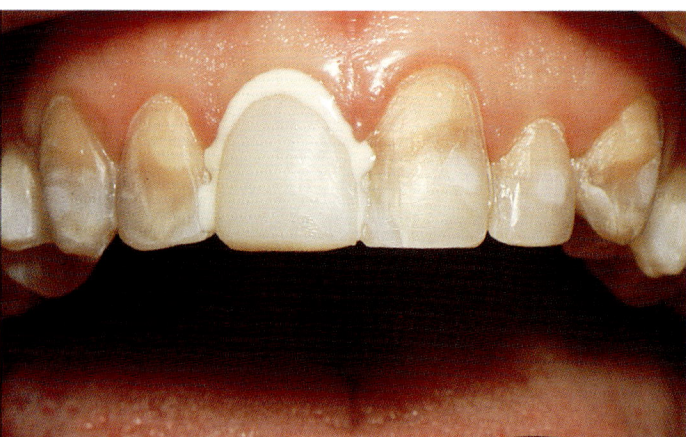

Fig 12-36 Resin temporization—to improve the temporary resin veneer color against the background of the discolored prepared teeth, a white, lightly filled color modifier is recommended. The peripheral excess of the modifier cleans up quickly with a small sponge or cotton pellet before light curing.

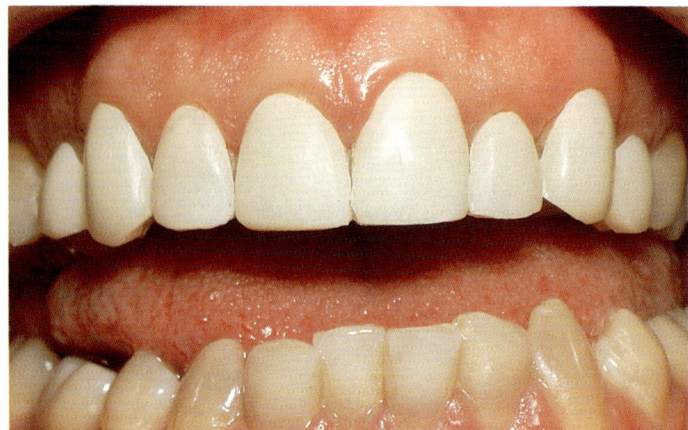

Fig 12-37 Resin temporization—appearance of the eight maxillary temporary resin veneers after "spot bonding." The patient is cautioned against any vigorous chewing on the veneers to avoid accidental dislodging.

scrupulously in centric contact, as well as excursive movements, to verify that there is adequate clearance for the porcelain material. Be sure to seal any freshly exposed dentin with two thin coats of a light-curable halophosphorus ester dentin bonding agent.

As previously stated, if the gingival chamfer is less than 0.5 mm supragingival and retraction cord has not already been placed for deeply stained teeth, gently place a thin, braided retraction cord to expose a dry, unprepared zone (0.5 mm) cervical to the gingival chamfer finish line. If the chamfer finish line is indistinct in any area, define it further before taking the impression. If cord is already in place due to a subgingival chamfer finish line, delicately deepen its seat to the degree necessary to fully expose the finish line for an accurate impression.

For impression taking use a reliable polyvinylsiloxane impression material with good dimensional stability and high tear resistance. If hydrocolloid is used, two impressions should be taken. Use light viscosity material to syringe along the entire gingival and proximal finish lines. Load a full-arch tray with medium or heavy viscosity material, and seat the tray carefully. After complete setting of the material has occurred, remove the tray. Examine the impression for good gingival, interproximal, and facial detail. If voids are discovered, retake the impression because the porcelain veneer will display the tooth veneer margin and be unesthetic. Be careful not to place the tray too far lingually to avoid tray penetration. For tooth veneering of more than one or two anterior teeth, a full-arch impression is recommended. Take an accurate counterimpression (alginate is acceptable here) and checkbites.

The impression may be sent to a laboratory for margin delineation or a stone model can be made in the office, the margins defined by the dentist, and the trimmed model sent to the laboratory. All models made in the office should incorporate a model and die hardener (eg, Stalite-Buffalo Dental Co) to improve its handling at the laboratory. Occasionally, a pencil delineation of the interproximal and incisal margins of the trimmed stone cast provides the ceramist with a sure guideline in vague areas. A second pour stone model may be useful to provide the ceramist with gingival contours (this model is not ditched) in certain cases.

Resin temporization

If the prepared teeth are unsightly to the patient because of contact openings, incisal irregularities, and/or generalized darkening of discolored teeth, a temporary facioproximal "splint" of a polishable resin can be fabricated. A thin, vacuum-formed acetate shell of the pretreatment stone model is made, trimmed to remove the lingual surface and 1 mm along the gingival margin of the facial surface, and loaded with a light-curable polishable resin in the spaces of the teeth to be temporized. The shell is placed against the prepared teeth, fully seated with finger pressure, and freed of all excess resin at the gingival and the incisal. The temporary splint is then light-cured, the vacuum-formed shell removed, and the resin finished carefully at the gingival margin to prevent tissue irritation. The incisal resin is also adjusted to an acceptable esthetic and phonetic alignment and checked for correct occlusion in excursive moments. Finally, the temporary splint is polished carefully to enhance the overall appearance and soft tissue response. The splint can then be carefully sectioned into individual veneer units, with a thin disk, to allow dental floss passage between preparation and placement visits.

The prepared teeth are now "spot-etched" in a 2- to 3-mm zone in the center of the facial surface, away from the margins (Fig 12-35). The etchant is rinsed away, the tooth is dried, and a bonding agent is placed over both the etched and unetched enamel of the preparation. The etched zone will provide an area to "spot bond" the veneers to place for the 1- or 2-week period until the veneers are ready to be placed. The bonding agent on the unetched enamel creates a temporary seal to minimize fluid contamination during this period.

The veneers are best bonded with a white color modifier, from a resin tint kit, because a more pleasing color is usually achieved by the white modifier against darkly discolored teeth. Also, this lightly filled, fluid-like material is rapidly removed around the resin veneer with a brush or sponge before light-curing it to establish a bond. Additionally, because it is lightly filled, the white color modifier is easily dislocated from the unetched and etched enamel at the placement visit (Fig 12-36).

The resin provisional veneers provide a sense of security to the patient because they are reasonably esthetic and conceal the dark underlying color or preparation defects of the teeth (Fig 12-37). The patient must be cautioned to avoid any hard biting on the veneers to avoid having them accidentally pop off.

The provisional veneers will be removed from the spot-etched enamel at the placement visit by dislocating the nonbonded peripheral resin and carefully gross reducing the bonded resin or film of white modifier with fine diamond burs, followed by disks to avoid removing any underlying enamel. This leaves the original preparation unaltered, expecially at the margins.

Resin provisional veneers are time-consuming and, at times, difficult to formulate to the patient's satisfaction. Because of these factors, an additional fee for provisional resin veneers, above the fee for the porcelain veneers per se, should be rendered.

Patients should be instructed and encouraged to perform exquisite oral hygiene between the preparation visit and the placement visit. This home care intensity should produce a favorable soft tissue condition for veneer placement.

Laboratory communication

With any indirect technique the end result is directly proportional to the quality of technical performance by the dentist and the technician and the thoroughness of communication between these individuals concerning the specifics of a given case. Logically, if both the dentist and the technician perform with technical excellence but insufficient communication exists to define the subtleties of the case, the end result will almost always show a degree of compromise. Porcelain veneers are no exception to this general rule. Close coordination between the dentist and the ceramist is vital for consistent success with porcelain veneers. The sine qua non of this informational exchange is a definitive laboratory prescription, supplemented by 35 mm slides, pretreatment models, direct color detailing by the ceramist if possible, color conveyance diagrams, and shade guide tabs, sent with accurate final impressions.

Laboratory prescription

A complete laboratory prescription consists of the following:

1. Shade(s) of prepared teeth: incisors, canines, premolars.
2. Shade gradation of veneers: cervical, body, incisal.
3. Appropriate interface space in die spacer coats.
4. Translucency/opacity level of veneers.
5. Veneer surface anatomy, texture, gloss.
6. Veneer length, contacts, incisal shape.

Shade of prepared teeth

Probably the most frequently missing element in the average laboratory prescription for multiple porcelain veneers is the shade(s) of the prepared teeth. Most of the color control of a case hinges on knowing this variable. Veneer die spacing, translucency/opacity, and thickness are closely related to the differential between prepared tooth color and the designated veneer color. The stratification method is based on using the resin cement layer and the porcelain veneer to attain a predictable veneer color. Without specifying the background color of the prepared teeth to be veneered, this system becomes highly unpredictable.

The color of the prepared teeth is best communicated by selecting a shade guide tab, which most closely approximates each tooth grouping (incisors, canines, and premolars). If in doubt, select the darker of the two shade guide tabs that the prepared tooth color falls between. If the prepared teeth fall outside the shade tab ranges or have unusual color variations (tetracycline-stained teeth), it is best to take a 35 mm slide or a high-quality Polaroid picture of the teeth, with the closest matching shade guide adjacent to these teeth. Sending these data to the technician is immensely helpful in conveying atypical colorations precisely, and permits him to more readily counteract them in processing the case.

Shade of veneers

The designated veneer color for multiple units is often given as a mere shade tab designation, such as A2 or 65. Most shade tabs do not match natural teeth in the cervical or incisal. It is much more realistic to "color map" on schematic tooth diagrams three zones, ie, body, cervical, and incisal. The body shade can be a shade tab designation, but, because of the dilution effect of veneer characterization when it is tried in with resin cement, it is often helpful to slightly overemphasize the cervical and incisal to create lifelike gradation or polychromatism. For example, if a natural-appearing A2 veneer is sought for a young to middle age patient, it is constructive to designate an A3 cervical shade and a medium to heavy outlined translucency in the incisal one fourth and proximal corners of the veneer. For single veneers color mapping is essential in conjunction with multiple photographs or slides.

It is also helpful to slightly overcompensate in shade value to account for patient variability in approving the color selection chairside, as well as dentist-technician variability in communication. In the example of the A2 case, the veneer body shade is adjusted to A1.5 in the laboratory prescription. This allows the dentist to easily lower the value chairside with darker resin cements. However, if the patient opts for a lighter color, it is readily attained without resorting to a strong opaque resin that deadens the vitality of the veneers.

It is important to build as much color gradation as possible (more than 80%) into the porcelain veneer to avoid relying on the unpredictable coloration of resin cements. Resin cements should be used primarily to alter the value or to raise the chroma of the veneers.

Die spacer

To permit flexible chairside adjustment of value, chroma, and, to some extent, opacity, color shift-related die spacing has evolved in stages. Ceramist Dan Materdomini of DaVinci Dental Studios, Canoga Park, California, and I have experimented with a number of die spacer thicknesses over the last several years. In an attempt to simplify and standardize the vast majority of multiple unit cases, we have suggested that, routinely, a 0.1-mm die spacer (eight or nine coats for most commercial die spacers) be used for all cases requiring a two-shade shift or less, eg, A3 to A1, B4 to B2, D3 to D2. For color shifts of greater than two shades and profoundly stained teeth (tetracycline), die spacing up to 0.2 mm is recommended. Many commercial laboratories have found numerous die spacing coats to be tedious and time-consuming. With the introduction of a new light-cured die spacer system, time for die spacer placement is greatly reduced. To allow for accurate veneer seating during cementation, it is advantageous to terminate die spacing approximately 0.5 to 1.0 mm short of the finish line.

Translucency/opacity level

Closely correlated with controlled die spacing is the degree of translucency or opacity of the veneers. The trend is toward translucent, more highly characterized porcelains, combined with increased die spacing. This minimizes the loss of vitality accompanying the use of more highly opaque porcelains. Porcelains vary from manufacturer to manufacturer and veneer formulations from ceramist to ceramist. Therefore, it is impossible to standardize formulations for all porcelains and ceramists. In this area, art must interact with science and experience with inherent skill. In general, the desire to preserve lifelike vitality in veneers has led to a pattern of graded dilution of opaque porcelains by 25% to 80% with translucent porcelains, accompanied by increased die spacing.

With a standardized tooth preparation of 0.3 mm ± 0.2 mm in the cervical one third of normally aligned teeth, and 0.5 ± 0.2 mm in the remaining area of the facial surface, die spacing and slightly increased veneer thickness (relative to surface tooth reduction) can further enhance predictable color and vitality without gross overbulking.

Other important variables that are often excluded are surface anatomy, texture, and gloss. Surface anatomy prior to tooth preparation for veneering or surface anatomy of the remaining unprepared teeth should be evaluated. Designations, such as light, medium, and heavy surface anatomy, can be of use, particularly if the dentist sends a few samples that display what these terms mean to the specific technician. As important as veneer color is, if surface anatomy and texture are inadequate or inappropriate, the entire case can appear flat. Surface texture can be described as smooth, normal, or rough. High gloss, particularly if nonveneered teeth have a duller matte finish, can create an artificial appearance. Specify high gloss or matte finish.

Length, contacts, and incisal shape

Finally, although not directly related to color communication, several additional variables should be clarified. The veneer length relative to the prepared teeth, the contact zone (long or short) especially for space closures, the tooth shape (tapered, square), and the incisal shape (round, square, variable) are specifics that translate into individualized tooth borders, which effectively frame the new veneer color.

Occlusion and stone models

Especially when mandibular veneers are placed, but also for certain maxillary teeth, such as canines and premolars, the occlusion must be precise. Pretreatment stone models with accurate bite registrations allow the ceramist to follow contours closely when refashioning the mandibular teeth with veneers. The same precise occlusal concepts that characterize full coverage systems are operative with porcelain veneers. If occlusal variations are necessary, they should be noted clearly in the laboratory prescription and marked on the pretreatment stone model.

Pretreatment stone models give the ceramist, among other things, a clear representation of gingival emergence profiles and gingival architecture (thick or thin). This one benefit alone is of immense importance in re-establishing periodontally sound contours in the veneers. Therefore, whether they are used for planning a case, as a guide to tooth preparation or occlusion, or for cervical contours of the tooth and the soft tissue, pretreatment stone casts are eminently useful, as an accompaniment to a thorough, esthetically sound laboratory prescription.

Veneer try-in for individual and collective fit

Initial veneer inspection

Upon receiving the etched porcelain veneers from the laboratory, the dentist should thoroughly inspect each veneer to determine if any imperfections are present. The porcelain veneers are fragile before bonding and should be handled with care. Check each veneer for crack or craze lines. Then seat each veneer individually and check for marginal fit. After each veneer has been individually checked, seat the veneers sequentially on the master cast until all veneers are in place. Frequently, the veneers will readily seat without interference. Occasionally, an interproximal interference or an overextended margin will necessitate delicately modifying the veneers, with microfine diamond burs, silent stones, or rubber wheels. Do not force the veneers into position because they can fracture or crack. If the veneer evaluation reveals any flaws that are not correctable, return the veneers and master cast to the laboratory for refabrication.

Veneer color, if assessed against the master cast, will vary considerably depending on the color of the stone or die material. To determine the veneer color effectively, place the veneers on a white towel and compare them with a shade button. Note whether the veneers are similar in value or higher or lower. Note how contralateral teeth compare with each other, eg, central and lateral incisors, canines, etc. If the color is relatively close, carefully used tinted, translucent, or opaque resin cements can adjust the color in the appropriate direction. As discussed previously, it is preferable to have a veneer slightly lighter than the desired shade. Subtle darkening (lowering the value) of the veneer one shade level is readily achieved with current porcelain resin cements.

If examination of the veneers reveals an unetched area (glossy appearance) on the underside of the veneer, especially at the margin, return the veneer to the laboratory for reetching or chairside etch with a porcelain etchant after protecting the glazed surface by beading with sticky wax.

The fit of porcelain veneer margins should be accurate, particularly if a definitive preparation was performed. Small marginal deficiencies can be bridged by the porcelain resin cement. However, this could lead to resin discoloration and possible plaque accumulation if the resin is not polished in finishing procedures. So if marginal deficiencies are frequent and large, return the case to the laboratory and have it done again. A discussion concerning why the deficiencies are present, to such an extent, is in order between the dentist and the ceramist. Possibly a change in technique on the part of either or both parties would bring about a greatly improved result.

Chairside try-in sequence for individual and collective fit

If a careful evaluation of all of the check points has been made and the veneers are acceptable, the veneers are then ready to be placed on the patient. We can now try-in the veneers on the patient for fit and select the resin cement to be used to achieve our intended veneer color. Basically, the try-in phase consists of three separate

Chairside try-in sequence for individual and collective fit

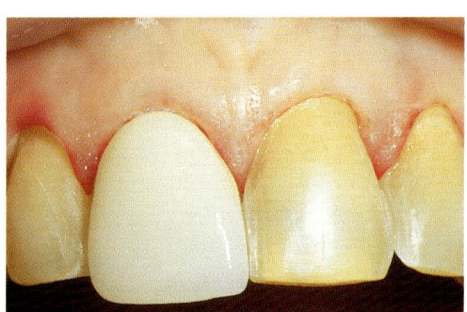

Fig 12-38 Chairside try-in sequence for individual fit—returning to the case prepared in Fig 12-29, after the prepared teeth are clean and isolated, each veneer is placed dry on the prepared tooth to check the marginal fit. The right central incisor veneer is being evaluated for marginal fit here.

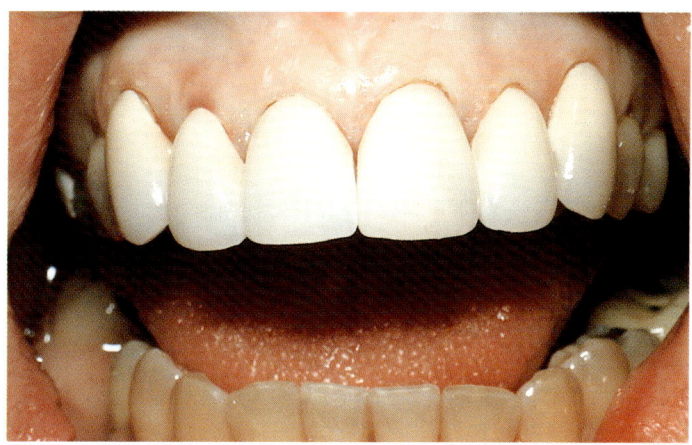

Fig 12-39 Chairside try-in sequence for collective fit—all six maxillary porcelain veneers are seated with glycerin to test the proximal fit. If any of the veneers move when slight pressure is applied to an adjacent veneer, proximal binding exists. The proximal porcelain of these veneers must be delicately reduced until no movement occurs.

steps: *(1)* dry try-in of each individual veneer for marginal fit; *(2)* wet try-in of all veneers collectively with a clear liquid medium, such as water-soluble glycerin, for proximal fit; and *(3)* resin cement try-in of one or several veneers for color match to the appropriate color standard for the case. The following sequence is recommended:

1. Isolate the teeth with cotton rolls and/or lip retractors. Remove any resin provisional veneer by dislocating the resin near the unetched margins with a sharp instrument. Then spot grind carefully the bonded remnant of the temporary resin to thin it. Remove the remaining resin with disks, thus exposing the enamel without reducing it to any degree.
2. Clean the teeth with fine flour of pumice and remove interproximal surface contamination with floss or yarn passage.
3. Except where the margin is 0.5 mm supragingival or more, place braided retraction cord subgingivally to prevent sulcular moisture or bleeding from contaminating the surface.
4. Try each veneer in dry to determine marginal accuracy. Adjust the veneer margin where indicated (Fig 12-38).
5. Fill the internal etched surface of the porcelain veneers with water-soluble glycerin to minimize dislodgement if a vertical position is assumed. Try-in the porcelain veneers on the appropriate teeth in sequential fashion (Fig 12-39). If any porcelain veneer resists seating due to binding interproximally, remove the veneer. Do not force it into place because the veneer may fracture. Working over a foam pad and under magnification, use a microfine diamond bur, rubber wheels, or silent stones, and carefully reduce the proximal surface. Reduction is delicately continued until the veneer seats properly. Do not use 8 or 12 fluted carbide burs for the reduction because they will "catch" and fracture the veneer. Be sure to restore the glaze in the adjusted areas by using the smallest grit microfine diamonds (10 to 20 μm), 30 fluted polishing burs, ultrafine disks, and porcelain polishing pastes.
6. Remove all veneers except for one central incisor veneer when the fit, insertion sequence, and seating of the veneers have been verified.

Veneer try-in for color/color modification

The indications for porcelain veneers are primarily multiple teeth with discolorations, enamel defects, spaces, or moderate malpositioning. In acknowledgment of the ongoing advances in porcelain technology, such as closer color matching of shade guides, polychromatic shade variance at an average 0.5-mm thickness, graded opacity built into the veneer in direct proportion to the degree of tooth discoloration, and finer marginal adaption for improved fit, most multiple porcelain veneer cases require only a single porcelain resin cement shade, whether it be a single opaque shade or a single translucent shade. The coloring of the porcelain veneer itself, particularly if the tooth preparation and laboratory communication previously recommended are used, essentially does the work. In other words, the porcelain veneer plays the major role in establishing the ultimate polychromatic veneer color, whereas the porcelain resin cement is used to fine tune the color of the veneer by slightly lightening, darkening, tinting, or opaqueing it.

Porcelain resin cements

Porcelain resin cements should have basic properties and esthetically related characteristics in the ranges given in Table 12-1.

Table 12-1 Optimal properties of porcelain resin cements

Good physical properties	
Filler % by weight	65–75
Water sorption (mf/cm²)	0.6–0.8
Polymerization shrinkage (% by volume)	0.5–1.6
Film thickness (μm)	10–25
Bond strength (psi)	2200–3000
Medium viscosity	
Honey consistency or thixotropic	
Too low viscosity	
Veneer slump and marginal voids (watery)	
Too high viscosity	
Veneer fracture (putty)	
High film thickness-resin line	
Suitable spectrum of translucent shades, opaque shades, and tints	
Light-curable with optional chemical curing capability	
Color-stable	
Polishable: hybrid finish	

Porcelain resin cements should possess physical properties in the ranges listed in Table 12-1. Although a medium viscosity resin cement is preferred in general, because it most represents the optimal blend of physical properties and handling characteristics, it is fitting to identify the three categories of resin cements by viscosity: firm viscosity resin cement, medium (thixotropic) viscosity resin cement, and fluid viscosity resin cement. All of these viscosities can be useful under certain clinical conditions. A resin cement is classified by the simple but useful test of quickly extruding about 3 mm of the material from its syringe or squeeze bottle dispenser, placed horizontal above a cement pad. Note the immediate response of the material. If it does not slump but retains its extruded shape for 5 seconds or more, it is a firm viscosity resin cement. If it slumps to the surface of the pad but does not spread out appreciably over the surface, it is a medium viscosity resin cement. If it slumps rapidly to the surface of the pad immediately after extrusion and starts to visibly spread out over the surface, it is a fluid viscosity resin cement.

Porcelain resin cements should have several translucent shades, several opaque shades, and appropriate color-modifying tints to achieve optimal veneer coloring. In many cases this can be accomplished through the use of a single resin cement, as stated previously. In other cases it may involve mixing resin cements to achieve the desired effect. Concerning color stability with the passage of time, a note of caution must be sounded concerning composite resins in general. Most, if not all, composite resins undergo two fundamental color shifts beneath a porcelain veneer. The first color shift, which occurs concomitantly with light-activated polymerization, is primarily (if not entirely) related to the amine initiator, which interacts with camphoroquinone, to generate free radicals in the first stage of polymerization. Depending on the chemical composition of the amine (aromatic or aliphatic) and the concentration level, the color shift can be perceptible. In practical terms, a resin cement could lighten one shade or darken one shade after visible light-curing. Depending on the relative translucency of the porcelain veneer and the underlying tooth color, this could produce a significant variance from the appearance of the porcelain veneer, as evaluated with uncured resin cement at try-in.

The second color shift that occurs over a longer period of time (24 hours to several months) has been described as "lucency" by Dr Harry Albers. Dr Albers observed that the camphoroquinone, which is initially a urine yellow color, gradually turns clear like water with the passage of time. The chemistry of a given resin cement and the concentration level of the camphoroquinone determine the ultimate extent of this color shift. On a clinical level, this color change results in a more lucent or transparent resin cement color as the camphoroquinone becomes clear. If the teeth being veneered are not profoundly discolored, the color shift is relatively innocuous to the esthetics of a given case. However, if the teeth are badly discolored, then a perceptible darkening of the veneer color can occur to such a degree that a patient may respond adversely to this esthetic regression and request a remake.

To evaluate any given resin cement for the degree of these color shifts, it is advisable to compare, side by side, all resin cement shades both uncured and light-cured.

The immediate color shift can be identified by observing the color comparison, after a 60- to 120-second curing period. For the delayed color shift, the cured resin cement samples can be put aside for 3 or 4 weeks, and then again compared with the uncured resin cement shades and the 60- to 120-second cured resin cement shades. If significant (more than one half shade) color shifts occur in these trials, serious consideration should be given regarding the advisability of using such a resin cement clinically.

Try-in for color

To verify the collective fit of the porcelain veneers, glycerin was recommended as a wetting agent to prevent the veneers from falling off. It is also used as a starting point for color modification and determination of the degree of opacity of the veneers. Recently developed water-soluble try-in gels, which match the resin cement colors but are not light-activated, are even more appropriate for color trials. Place one central incisor veneer on the prepared tooth with either glycerin or a light, clear try-in gel. This veneer is used as a starting point for selection of the appropriate porcelain resin cement. If the stratification method of laboratory communication was used and a 0.3-mm/0.5-mm preparation was made for a two-shade shift or less, the try-in veneer color will frequently match the intended shade closely. If this occurs, then select the lightest translucent porcelain resin cement from the resin cement kit. Ideally, this resin cement would be virtually clear or colorless to closely match glycerin or the gel. If the try-in is lighter than the intended shade, select a porcelain resin cement that is darker to approximately the same degree. If the try-in veneer color is darker than the intended shade, mix one part of a light opaque porcelain resin cement with about ten parts of the light translucent resin cement; or take a small amount of an intense white color modifier for opacity and mix it into the light translucent resin cement. (A ratio of ten parts porcelain resin cement to one part intense white color modifier is often a usable mix.) If a resin cement kit with the water-soluble nonlight-activating gels or pastes is used, this same mix could be formulated without messy resin cement cleanup, or shielding the veneers from the dental headlight. If the try-in color is lacking in saturation (too low a chroma), then add a small amount of the appropriate tint to the light translucent resin cement or water-soluble gel or paste. For example, if the Vita Lumin B range was being sought, add a small amount of yellow tint because it is a predominantly yellow shade grouping. Whatever the porcelain resin cement mix used, note the proportions of each component and place a small amount aside for duplication to formulate a larger batch for bonding on the veneers.

Once a porcelain resin cement or porcelain resin cement mix has been selected, load the other central incisor porcelain veneer with this resin cement and carefully place it on the tooth. Be sure to lower the dental headlight to chin level to avoid premature polymerization of the resin cement. If the new water-soluble try-in gels, which color copy the resin cement, are used, light protection is not necessary. Also, avoid exposing the resin cement to any intense ambient room light for the same reason. Using a sponge or cotton pellet, wipe away the gross resin cement excess around the margins of the veneer. A comparison can now be made between the trial resin veneer and the shade guide of the intended veneer color. In most cases there will be a close match. If additional color adjustment is necessary, the adjacent try-in veneer can be removed from the tooth, washed thoroughly with water, and loaded with a second porcelain resin cement or resin cement mix, which compensates for the color deficiency of the first trial resin cement veneer. If the water-soluble gels or pastes are used, all veneers can be placed and the color evaluated. The veneers and prepared teeth are cleaned by washing them with a copious water spray from the dental syringe.

Match Color	Resin Cement	Veneer
	light "colorless"	minimum opacity in desired shade or ½ shade lighter
	translucent in color range of desired shade	

Fig 12-40 Try-in for color/color modification—general guidelines for veneer body shade, translucency/opacity level, and initial trial resin cement selection are given for matching tooth color or making it one shade lighter.

Color modification guidelines

Depending on the degree of color shift, ie, one-shade shift or match color, two-shade shift, three-shade shift or more, certain general guidelines can be defined to expedite resin cement selection for any given case. As mentioned, it all hinges on knowing the body shade of the prepared teeth (and any extreme variations) and the desired body shade of the veneers. This color difference will define whether the case should be placed in the category of matching color or lightening just one shade, modifying color or lightening approximately two shades, or masking color or lightening three shades or more. Before each category is discussed, review the laboratory prescription recommendations. This is of particular importance regarding overcompensation in value, ie, a lighter veneer shade than the shade selected by the patient.

Matching color

To match existing tooth color or lighten the tooth one shade, a minimum opacity veneer is chosen to allow a significant portion of the background tooth color to show through. Generally, it is prudent to ask for a veneer that is one half shade lighter than the actual shade requested for the case. If these variables (translucency/opacity and value of the actual veneer shade) are programmed in this manner, the resin cement selection narrows to either a light, clear translucent cement, or a light, translucent resin cement with greater chroma in the dominant color for that shade range. For example, Vita A range veneers might require more reddish brown, Vita B more yellow, etc (Figs 12-40 to 12-44).

Modifying color

To modify the prepared tooth color by two shades, a minimum opacity veneer that is one half shade lighter is again chosen if the prepared tooth color is no darker than the Vita 3 range, ie, A3, A3.5, B3, C3, D3. However, if the prepared tooth is darker than the Vita 3 range but a two shade shift is still planned, the veneer should be formulated with medium opacity and one shade lighter than the designated shade for the case. Because of the compensation in the veneer formulation for the color

Modify Color	Resin Cement	Veneer
2 shades or less	lighter than desired shade and with correct tint in color range of desired shade plus a small amount of opaque resin or opaque color modifer	minimum to medium opacity— ½ to 1 shade lighter than desired shade

Fig 12-41 Try-in for color/color modification—general guidelines for veneer body shade, translucency/opacity level, and initial trial resin cement selection are given when making the prepared teeth two shades lighter.

Mask Color	Resin Cement	Veneer
	opaque with tint to block discoloration and emphasize dominant color of desired shade	medium to maximum opacity 1 to 1½ shades lighter than desired shade

Fig 12-42 Try-in for color/color modification—general guidelines for veneer body shade, translucency/opacity level, and initial trial resin cement selection for a three-shade shift or more are given.

shift, the resin cement selection generally becomes a translucent cement, but lighter than the designated shade in the dominant color for that shade range. For example, if C4 prepared teeth were being converted to C2 porcelain veneers, then the laboratory prescription would be for medium opacity C1 veneers. The resin cement selected would be a translucent grayish cement that is slightly lighter than C2 value.

If the initial trial resin cement yields too dark a color, a small amount (10%) of a light opaque resin or white color modifier resin is added to impart a degree of opacity. If the trial resin cement color is too light, then a darker translucent cement in the dominant color range is substituted for the initial trial cement. If the trial cement color is too low in chroma, a trace (5%) of a color modifier resin in the dominant color range is added. In the case of the C4 to C2 conversion previously mentioned, the color modifier would be gray (Figs 12-43 to 12-46).

Masking color

For a three-shade shift or more, to correct the color of profoundly stained teeth, a medium to maximum opacity veneer is requested that is at least one shade lighter than the selected shade for the case. Again, increased die spacer up to 0.2 mm is an asset to neutralizing the dark, undesirable tooth background (Fig 12-42).

The initial trial resin cement is relatively light and opaque, with a slight tint that emphasizes the dominant color for the shade range selected. Athough no exact formula exists for adjusting color in these difficult cases, in general, if the color is too dark, a white resin modifier must be added in degrees, at the expense of vitality. To counteract this, the illusion of veneer color gradation is created by overemphasizing the cervical and incisal areas with layered porcelain veneer formulations and/or more intense surface staining (Figs 12-47 and 12-48). Figure 12-48 shows the natural color gradation in the mandibular anterior veneers.

Once the resin cement selection has been finalized, the porcelain resin cement or resin cement mix used on one or both of the central incisor veneers must be completely removed from the etched surface(s) of the veneers(s). This can be accomplished with alcohol, acetone, or methyl chloride. Alcohol is preferred because of its lower cost and less toxicity. The veneers are initially cleared of gross resin cement on the etched surface by

Porcelain Veneers: An Esthetic Therapeutic Alternative

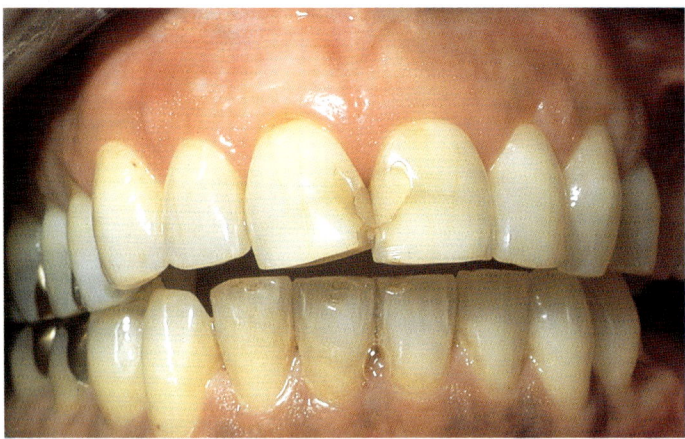

Fig 12-43 Try-in for color/color modification—this case illustrates matching color. The two central incisors, which exhibit worn and chipped incisal edges, discolored restorations, and slight overlap due to crowding, will receive two porcelain veneers that closely match the two lateral incisors in color.

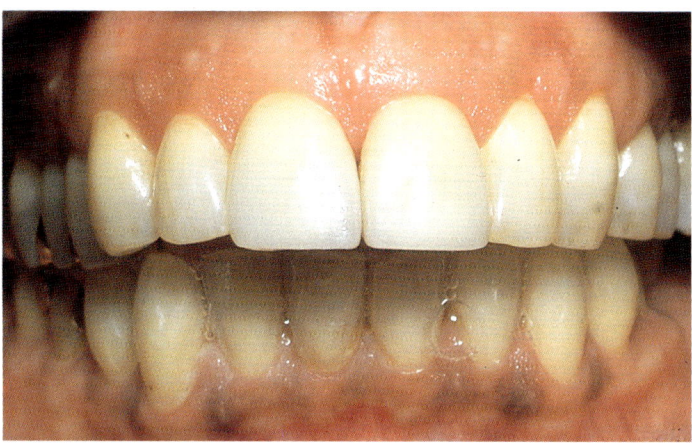

Fig 12-44 Try-in for color/color modification—the case shown in Fig 12-41 after placement of two central incisor porcelain veneers. The color is harmonious.

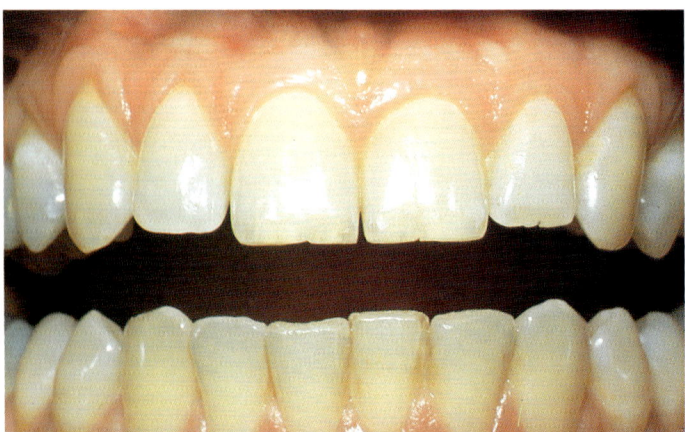

Fig 12-45 Try-in for color/color modification—pretreatment appearance of teeth with an unesthetic brown color. The treatment plan was to lighten the teeth two shades by placing eight maxillary porcelain veneers. The only other esthetic modification was to lenghthen the incisors slightly.

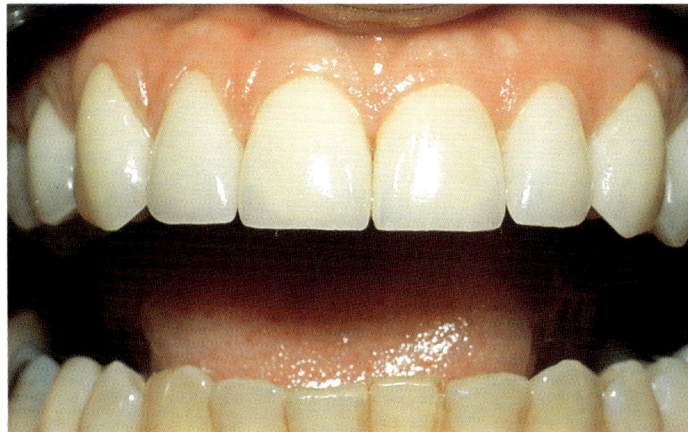

Fig 12-46 Try-in for color/color modification—after esthetic modification of the maxillary dentition, shown in Fig 12-44, with eight porcelain veneers, the color is considerably lighter and brighter. Note the healthy gingival response to correctly contoured, polished porcelain.

Veneer try-in for color/color modification

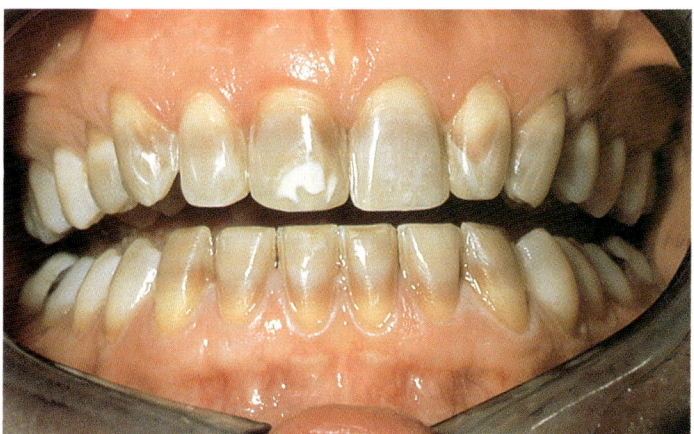

Fig 12-47 Try-in for color/color modification—appearance of a severe tetracycline-stained case before placement of eight maxillary and six mandibular porcelain veneers.

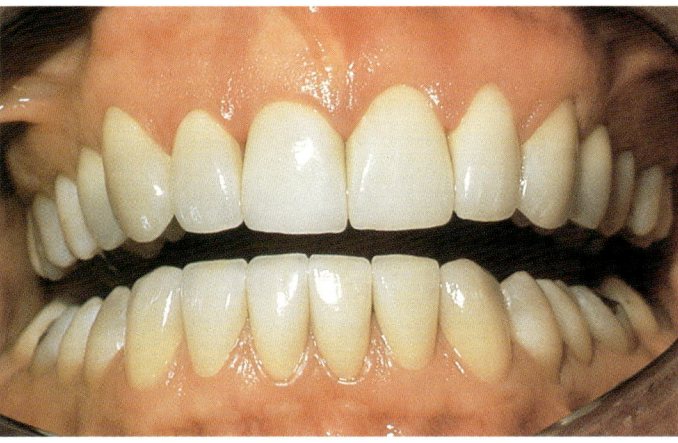

Fig 12-48 Try-in for color/color modification—posttreatment appearance of Fig 12-47. Note the dramatic color shift, the favorable soft tissue response, and the polychromatic color in the mandibular anterior porcelain veneers.

placing them, one at a time, in a dappen dish of alcohol and "scrubbing" the etched surface with a small brush (such as an acid-etch brush used for liquid enamel etchants or a small, soft toothbrush). A small foam sponge can also be used. Then the veneers are transferred into another dappen dish of alcohol to remove any additional traces of resin cement remnants (no turbidity in the alcohol solution). Any residual resin cement that is tenacious can be removed by ultrasonic cleaning with alcohol, acetone, or methyl chloride for 2 to 3 minutes or by placing phosphoric acid etchant inside the veneer for 30 seconds and rinsing the veneer thoroughly with water. The glycerin soaked veneers from the try-in for fit can be cleaned by a vigorous water–air spray on the etched surface, over the sink or a plastic cup, or they can be placed in a beaker of water in the ultrasonic cleaner for 2 to 3 minutes. Water-soluble gels or pastes can be readily removed from tooth surfaces and etched veneer surfaces with a thorough water-air spray. All veneers must be completely clean and dry on the etched surfaces before proceeding to final cementation. Regarding resin cement or glycerin removal from the etched surfaces, one should not use cotton pellets or Q-tips, becase unnoticed cotton fibers can cling to the etched surfaces and create a potential for marginal leakage. Instead of resin cement try-ins, if water-soluble color matching gels are used, the clean up of the veneers with alcohol is avoided. The inside surfaces of the veneers need merely to be thoroughly washed with water from a syringe and dried.

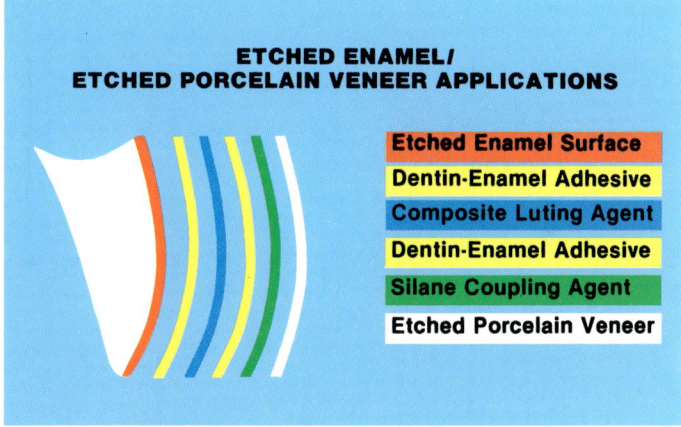

Fig 12-49 Cementation and finishing—diagrammatic representation of the correct order of surface applications of materials from the tooth to the veneer. Dentin-enamel adhesive refers to the most currently desirable materials for conditioning the enamel and dentin.

Cementation and finishing

Remove all porcelain resin cement that may have remained on any tooth from the try-in with an alcohol soaked cotton pellet or sponge cube and an interproximal polishing strip. If a water-soluble color gel was used, wash off the teeth with water for 20 seconds. If necessary, pumice again, but be careful not to traumatize the gingiva and induce bleeding. Check the position of the retraction traction cord to ensure that all finish lines are exposed; if not, retract the tissue again in those areas. Check the interproximal contacts of all teeth to be veneered by passage of thin metal strips. If any contact resists metal strip placement, lighten but do not open the contact by two or three passages of an ultrathin, diamond-coated metal strip. This will allow metal strip passage between the interproximal surfaces. If any existing resin restorations are to be bonded to, lightly roughen that portion of the restoration on which the veneer will be placed with a fine diamond bur to expose "fresh" bond sites. If the restorations are hybrids, with soluble glass filler, etch them for 30 seconds with a buffered, 9.5% hydrofluoric acid etchant, or use an intraoral air polisher. Finally, place metal strips along the mesial and distal proximal surfaces of the first tooth or two teeth (generally the central incisors) to be bonded to protect the adjacent teeth from inadvertent etching during the next step. The metal strips should be placed just under the papilla tip of the adjacent teeth to protect the entire proximal surface of these teeth.

A diagrammatic representation of the surface treatment and material applications for the tooth and veneer is given in Fig 12-49. This sequence will now be elaborated on, first for the tooth and then for the veneer, to explain thoroughly the cementation and finishing of porcelain veneers.

Before etching the enamel it is beneficial to determine if any dentin will be covered by the veneer. There are two reasons for this: *(1)* to confine the phosphoric acid etchant to the enamel if this is desirable, and *(2)* to treat the dentin with the appropriate bonding materials to improve bond strength and lessen or eliminate marginal leakage.

To identify the dentin, colored dyes have been developed that color the collagen of the dentin preferentially. These dyes, when placed on a tooth for a brief time (10 to 15 seconds), stain the dentin surface (Fig 12-50). However, when the tooth is vigorously washed with a water–air syringe flash, no discoloration occurs on the enamel surface due to the lack of available collagen (Fig 12-51). Once the lightly stained dentin areas are revealed, the enamel etching gel can be placed carefully so as to avoid etching the exposed dentin. Depending on the method of conditioning the dentin for the resin cement, this may be desirable. The following sequence for conditioning the tooth and the veneer for cementation is suggested. Etch all enamel that the veneer will cover for 15 to 30 seconds with a phosphoric acid gel etchant (or other acid-etching material), keeping the etchant off the dentin if indicated (Fig 12-52). Wash the tooth vigorously with water for 20 seconds to remove all traces of the etching solution (Fig 12-53).

The surface stain of the dentin is now removed with a mild solution of sodium hypochlorite to prepare for dentin conditioning (Fig 12-54). The remains of the sodium hypochlorite solution is washed away with water, and the tooth is thoroughly dried (Fig 12-55).

Currently, dentin conditioning agents that improve bond strengths of resin materials to dentin and the marginal seal of the resin are in the state of continued refinement. Smear layer removal or alteration, followed by tubular penetration with hyprophilic resins (both chemical-curing and light-curing), represents the optimal system at this time. In the context of porcelain veneer cementation, it is advisable to utilize one of the later generation dentin conditioning systems to enhance bond strength and marginal insolubility of the veneers to the dentin (Fig 12-56).

Returning to the chairside sequence, once the enamel has been etched and the dentin conditioned, the tooth is now ready to have the veneer cemented.

To properly prepare the porcelain veneers for cementation, place them in the proper bonding sequence with the etched surfaces up. Be sure the etched surfaces are clean and dry. Identify the veneers by numbers, if necessary, to avoid misplacement of similarly shaped veneers.

Silanate the veneers if they have not been already silanated by the laboratory to slightly augment chemically the considerable (2000 to 2500 psi) micromechanical bond strength derived from the etching of the porcelain veneers. Follow the manufacturer's directions for placing these silananting agents (see Fig 12-49). Apply a thin film of a light-cured dentin-enamel adhesive liner to the etched surface of the veneer. Do not light-cure.

Cementation and finishing

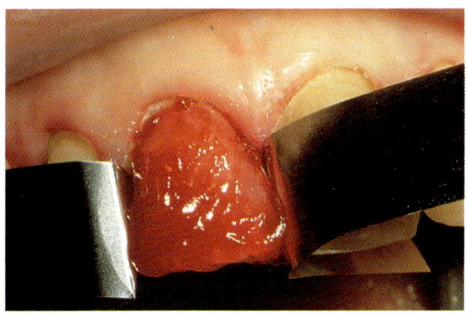

Fig 12-50 Cementation and finishing—dentin-detecting dye has been placed over the entire prepared surface of the right central incisor. It preferentially stains the dentin surface and thereby reveals the location of dentin for appropriate material conditioning during cementation. Note the placement of metal strips interproximally to isolate this tooth.

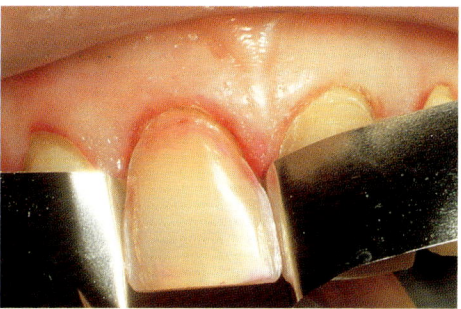

Fig 12-51 Cementation and finishing—after the tooth in Fig 12-50 has been washed thoroughly for 30 seconds, the enamel retains none of the dye because the dye is dentin-specific. The dentin is identified by light surface staining that does not wash off with water.

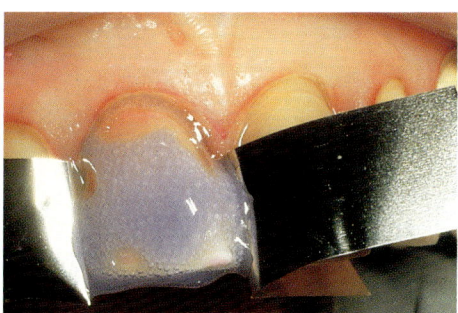

Fig 12-52 Cementation and finishing—enamel etchant gel is carefully placed with a fine-tipped syringe, avoiding the dentin areas identified by the reddish stain.

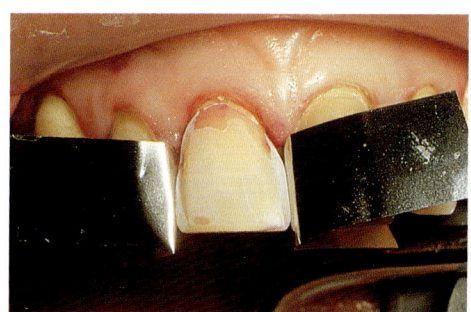

Fig 12-53 Cementation and finishing—once the etched enamel has been thoroughly washed with water, the frosted etch pattern, free of stain, is demonstrated. The reddish stain on the dentin is still present, however.

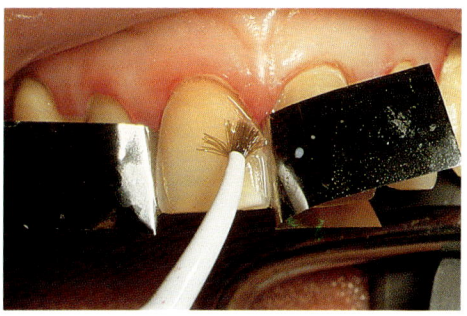

Fig 12-54 Cementation and finishing—reddish stain of the dentin disclosing dye is removed, with a soft microtipped brush syringe containing a mild sodium hypochlorite solution.

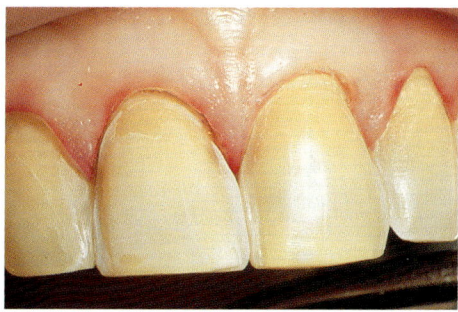

Fig 12-55 Cementation and finishing—after removal of the stain with sodium hypochlorite, the tooth is washed thoroughly for 20 seconds and dried. It is now ready to receive the appropriate dentin and enamel surface applications in preparation for cementation.

Porcelain Veneers: An Esthetic Therapeutic Alternative

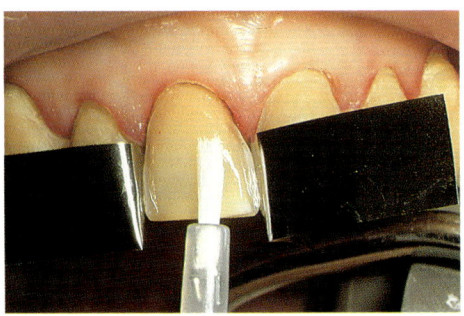

Fig 12-56 Cementation and finishing—dentin–enamel conditioners and adhesives, which etch enamel, disrupt the dentin smear layer, and penetrate into the altered surfaces, are in the state of constant refinement. Higher bond strengths and reduced marginal leakage are the benefits of these later generation materials. The final stage of the dentin–enamel adhesive sequence is shown.

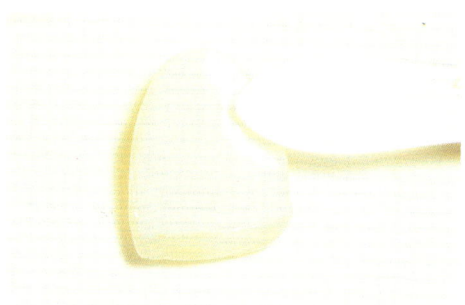

Fig 12-57 Cementation and finishing—loading the veneer with an adequate amount of resin cement is important. Once the veneer is initially loaded with resin cement, it should be "leveled" to the margin with a thin metal instrument and checked for air pockets in the mesioincisal and distoincisal corners.

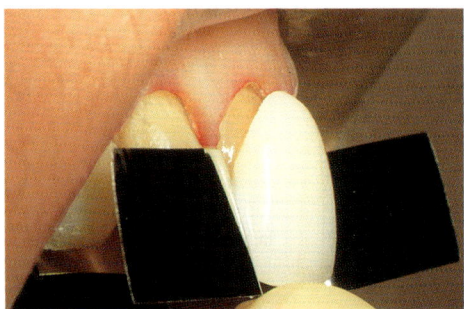

Fig 12-58 Cementation and finishing—seating a veneer with incisal edge in porcelain is accomplished by means of an incisofacial pivot. First, the incisal porcelain contacts the incisal edge of the prepared tooth and acts as a vertical stop. Then, the veneer is seated proximally and cervically with gentle finger pressure.

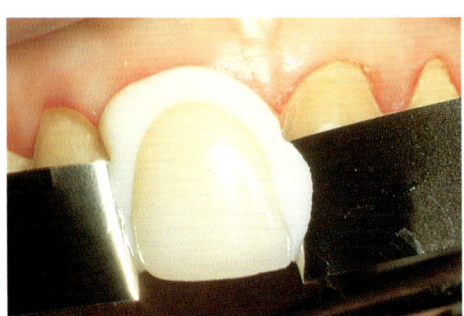

Fig 12-59 Cementation and finishing—appearance of a veneer that has been completed seated. Observe the generous amount of excess resin cement at the margins.

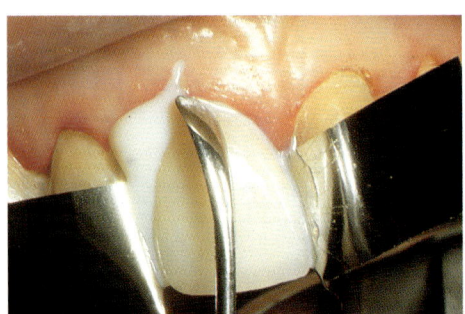

Fig 12-60 Cementation and finishing—systematic removal of the gross, uncured resin cement excess, before light curing, simplifies postcementation finishing. For medium viscosity resins, a thin-bladed instrument is effective.

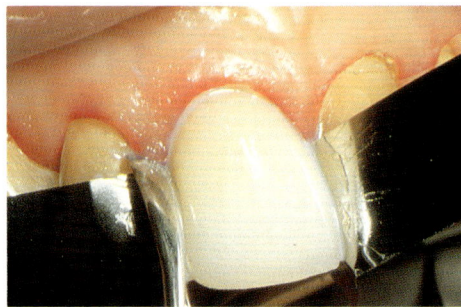

Fig 12-61 Cementation and finishing—gross resin cement excess is reduced considerably along the gingival margin by a second passage of the thin-bladed instrument.

Cementation and finishing

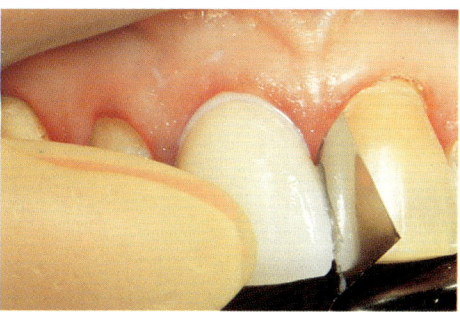

Fig 12-62 Cementation and finishing—while the veneer is held in place on the distal one half of the facial surface, the thin metal strip is drawn lingually to remove resin cement excess interproximally.

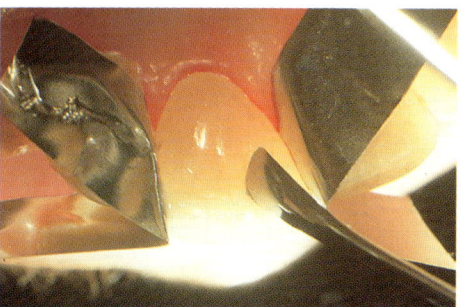

Fig 12-63 Cementation and finishing—excess resin cement is removed from the lingual margin with the same instrument shown in Figs 12-60 and 12-61. Care must be taken to avoid removing all excess resin cement in this area particularly, because marginal voids will readily result.

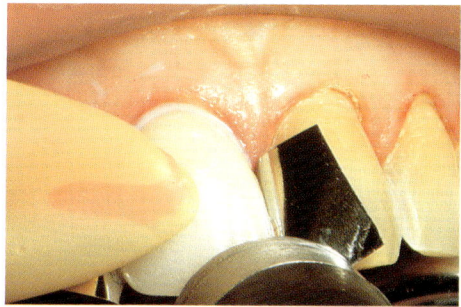

Fig 12-64 Cementation and finishing—while the veneer is held firmly in the distal area of the facial surface, the veneer is "tacked" by light curing a small segment of the facial surface at the mesioincisal edge. This stabilizes the veneer during additional uncured resin cement removal.

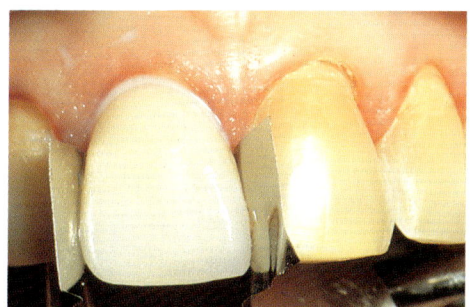

Fig 12-65 Cementation and finishing—with the veneer now partially bonded for stability, the thin metal strip is drawn lingually with a college pliers to remove resin excess along the distal proximal surface.

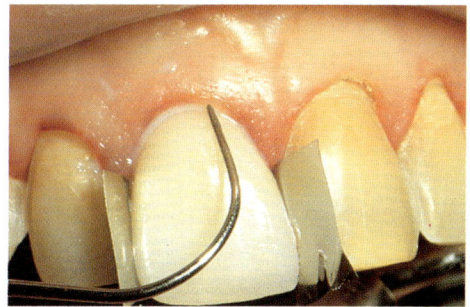

Fig 12-66 Cementation and finishing—additional removal of excess resin cement is accomplished along the gingival finish line with an explorer tip. A small bead of excess resin should always remain before curing to prevent voids.

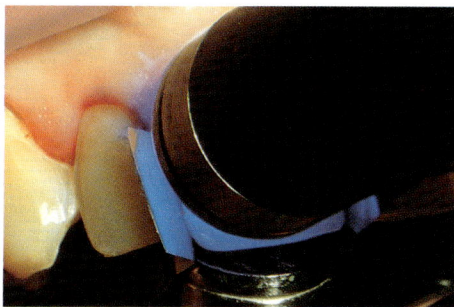

Fig 12-67 Cementation and finishing—facial and incisal surfaces of the veneer are light-cured with two wide angle tips for 60 seconds to ensure complete polymerization.

Place the veneers in a light-shielded holder or a light-protected area.

Because the central incisor veneers are the key to the correct placement of subsequent veneers in multiple veneer cases, they should be bonded first. To accomplish this, load both central incisor veneers with the porcelain resin cement selected during the color try-in. Be sure to put enough resin onto the etched surface of the veneer to fill the veneer completely, ie, level to the veneer edge. Distribute the resin if necessary with a brush or a thin-bladed instrument (Fig 12-57), and check for air pockets at the mesioincisal and distoincisal corners. If any air bubbles are visible, pop them with a sharp explorer.

Seat the veneers from the incisofacial or facial, using the porcelain incisal edge (if present) as a guide to seating (Fig 12-58). With gentle finger pressure, complete the preliminary seating of the veneers. Excess resin cement will be expressed along the entire margin (Fig 12-59). Remove the resin cement excess initially with a thin-bladed instrument (Fig 12-60). After partial removal of the resin cement excess has been achieved with one passage, remove additional gingival resin cement gross excess with a second passage (Fig 12-61). With a faciolingual passage of an ultrathin metal strip, most of the gross resin cement excess on the mesioproximal is removed (Fig 12-62). In preparation for curing, place the thin metal strips interproximally on the distal of both central incisor veneers. With a finger covering the distal one half of the facial surface of the veneer, exert light pressure upward and inward toward the midline. If any additional resin cement excess extrudes at the midline, pass a thin metal strip lingually to remove most of the excess. Do not remove the metal strip, but leave it in place at the midline.

Normally, this midline, mesioproximal metal strip would be pulled lingually until it was removed. Then, the left central incisor veneer, loaded with resin cement, would be placed on the left central incisor, as has just been described. This would allow the veneers to be placed and cemented by light-curing in pairs. This ensures accurate placement at the midline and expedites the cementation process. However, for the sake of precise illustration, the right central incisor veneer will be used to demonstrate all of the cementation and finishing sequence, rather than both central incisors together, as would be done normally.

Remove gross resin cement from the linguoincisal margin with a thin-bladed instrument (Fig 12-63). Be sure to leave a thin bead of excess resin cement in this area to prevent possible voids along this area of the margin.

Tack the veneer in place by light-curing it at the mesioincisal edge for 20 seconds (Fig 12-64). This step will ensure that a veneer will not move or dislodge while the remaining resin cement excess at the margin is thinned out. Pull the metal strip on the distoproximal suface lingually to remove gross cement excess there (Fig 12-65). Before completely light-curing the remaining part of the veneer, feather out the remaining gross cement excess cervically and interproximally with a pigtail explorer (Fig 12-66). The gingival and interproximal portions of the facial surface of the veneer are now cured for 40 to 60 seconds. To prevent possible incomplete cure, the incisal edge is also cured for 30 seconds from the lingual (Fig 12-67). This should cure all material, but if the veneer is thick and opaque and the resin cement is dark, a longer cure time may be necessary. Porcelain resin cements cannot be overcured.

After complete curing of the resin cement through the porcelain veneer, the interproximal metal strips are removed. The placement of these strips interproximally during light-curing ensures the passage of finishing disks and strips to remove excess resin cement. Using scalers or interproximal carvers, remove excess resin cement from the gingival margin and the interproximal margins. The porcelain-glazed surface will permit easy "flicking off" of the excess porcelain resin cement in most areas (Fig 12-68).

Interproximal finishing is initiated with medium finishing disks, followed by medium gapped finishing strips, and graduated to fine or superfine disks and strips. If binding occurs initially, preventing the passage of even the fine or superfine strips, lightly separate the contact by torquing the adjacent tooth with a metal instrument while a dental auxiliary slides an ultrafine metal strip through a couple of times (Fig 12-69). Infrequently, it may be necessary to resort to controlled separation. An anterior separator is superb for this purpose. Cautiously activate the separator to avoid porcelain veneer fracture. A sound precaution in preventing interproximal "splinting" with resin cement is to always cover the interproximal surfaces of adjacent teeth with metal strips when etching. If the resin cement is lodged against unetched enamel, it will not bond to it.

It is imperative that the interproximal margins be void of excess porcelain resin cement and smooth to allow

Cementation and finishing

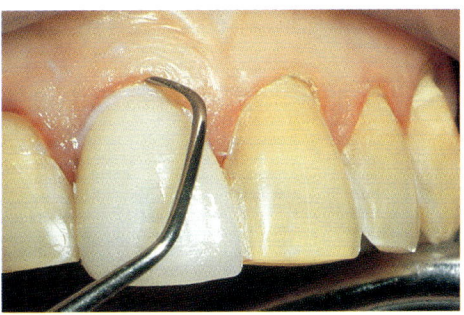

Fig 12-68 Cementation and finishing—light-cured resin cement excess can be removed, to a large extent, at the gingival margin with a scaler or curette.

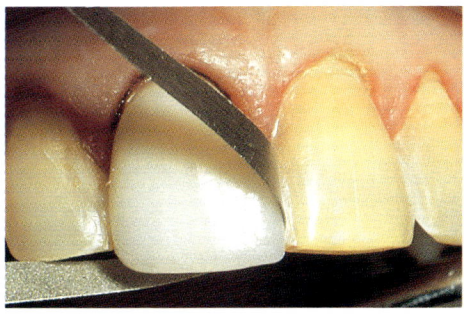

Fig 12-69 Cementation and finishing—if the interproximal resin cement flash inhibits finishing with disks and strips, a thin, diamond-coated abrasive strip can be used initially to remove the flash.

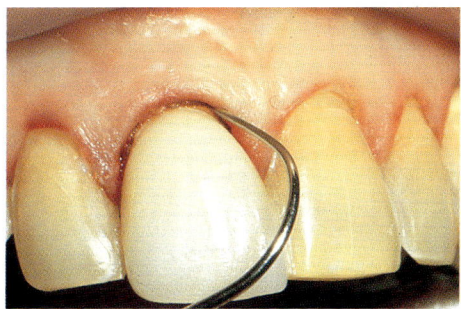

Fig 12-70 Cementation and finishing—cervical resin cement excess should be completely removed, as carefully determined with an extremely sharp, fine-tipped explorer. If not removed, the undetected excess can cause gingival inflammation.

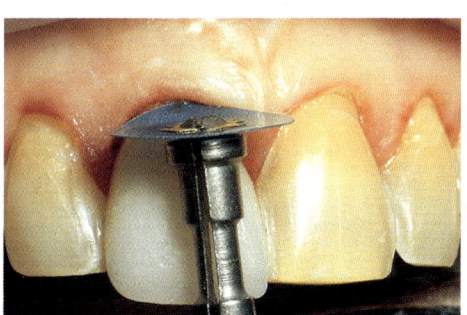

Fig 12-71 Cementation and finishing—if thin resin cement flash is present, a flexible aluminum oxide disk with a back action motion should be used to feather it away. The abrasive material is on the underside of the disk in this illustration.

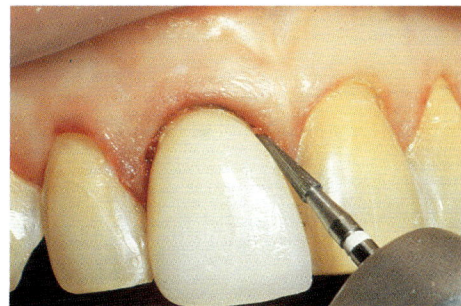

Fig 12-72 Cementation and finishing—academic research substantiates the need for microfine diamond burs and 30 fluted carbide burs to remove small porcelain overhangs at the margin and to polish the porcelain. This 30 fluted carbide bur should be utilized at high speed with no water mist to avoid overheating the resin or porcelain. It should be used with a feather touch and should be used only for light polishing, never finishing.

complete seating of the adjacent veneers and to avoid undesirable plaque accumulation. Finalize interproximal polishing with fine or superfine finishing disks and strips, flexible rubber polishing cups, and porcelain-polishing pastes. Determine that all margins are undetectable with a sharp, fine-tipped explorer (Fig 12-70). If resin cement flash is still present, remove it entirely as previously described (Fig 12-71).

If porcelain "ledging" requires adjustment, use microfine diamonds with a copious water spray at slow speed, sharp-edged rubber and silicone wheels, 30 fluted carbide burs without water spray at high speed, and porcelain-polishing paste to renew the glaze (Fig 12-72). Normally, if this case were not planned for sequence photography to illustrate the fine points of the technique, both central incisor veneers would have been cemented simultaneously. The remaining veneers of a multiple unit case are cemented in contralateral pairs, ie, lateral incisors, canines, and premolars.

Once all the veneers are cemented and finished completely at the margins, evaluate the veneers collectively. Check centric occlusion and all excursive contacts with fine articulating paper. If the occlusion requires adjustment, make corrections with an appropriate fine diamond bur followed by microfine diamond burs and 30 fluted carbide burs under copious water spray to prevent crazing of the porcelain. Avoid removing the porcelain glaze on facial surface if possible, except where a deflective contact occurs at the facioincisal line angle.

Eight maxillary porcelain veneers have been placed to improve the color of the brownish teeth used for technical discussion (Fig 12-73). The positive emotional reaction, improved self-image, enhanced feeling of well-being that the patient experiences subsequent to these esthetic makeovers are difficult to put into words. It is wisely stated that "if a picture is worth a thousand words, then a radiant smile must be worth at least twice as many."

Figures 12-74 and 12-75 portray one of many patients who have had a new dimension of beauty added to their appearance through the exciting, new medium of porcelain laminate veneers.

Maintenance of porcelain veneers

Maintenance of porcelain veneers consists of periodic reexamination of the veneers as well as the contiguous hard and soft tissue. Patient receptivity to oral hygiene instruction and posttreatment monitoring is optimal. It is a golden opportunity for the dentist and staff to translate this heightened oral consciousness into a progressive program for the future, including prevention, nutritional counseling, definitive restorative dentistry, and maintenance of the veneers. It is beneficial to contact a patient within 30 days of initial veneer placement. The soft tissue around the veneers is frequently irritated from finishing procedures. This inflammatory reaction is usually transient, assuming the periodontal tissues were healthy before porcelain veneering. However, if the veneer margin has a porcelain "ledge," the veneer is overcontoured, the porcelain surface has been roughened, or extraneous resin cement flash is still present, a localized gingivitis may persist. The causative factor(s) for any such residual gingivitis should be diagnosed and eliminated at this follow-up appointment by recontouring and polishing of the porcelain or removal of the excess resin cement. The patient should continue to be followed up at 2-week intervals until the gingival tissue is healthy. A naturally glazed porcelain surface, with the correct emergence profile and an undetectable butt margin, is arguably the most biocompatible surface in the oral cavity. Consequently, if repeated attempts to resolve a localized gingivitis around a veneer fail despite performing the aforementioned corrective measures and verifying correct soft tissue management on the part of the patient, then the veneer should be removed and replaced.

At the initial follow-up appointment, all veneer margins should be carfully checked with a sharp explorer, not only along the gingival margin but also proximally and incisally. If a perceptible catch occurs, a microfine diamond bur and a 30 fluted carbide bur, followed by porcelain-polishing paste, should be used to eradicate it. If a marginal void is detected, a small diamond bur should be used to make a shallow penetration into the void. The enamel surrounding the void is then etched for 30 seconds, and a polishable resin, which color matches the veneer, is placed to repair the void. The resin "patch" should be polished to a high luster. If a small amount of resin cement flash is discovered, it can be delicately milled away with a microfine diamond bur or a multi-

Maintenance of porcelain veneers

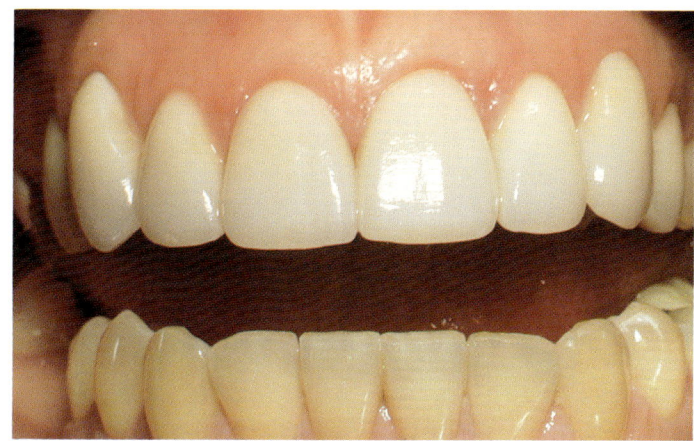

Fig 12-73 Cementation and finishing—posttreatment appearance of the maxillary anterior teeth used for the technical sequences is shown. Six maxillary porcelain veneers have been placed to brighten the teeth considerably.

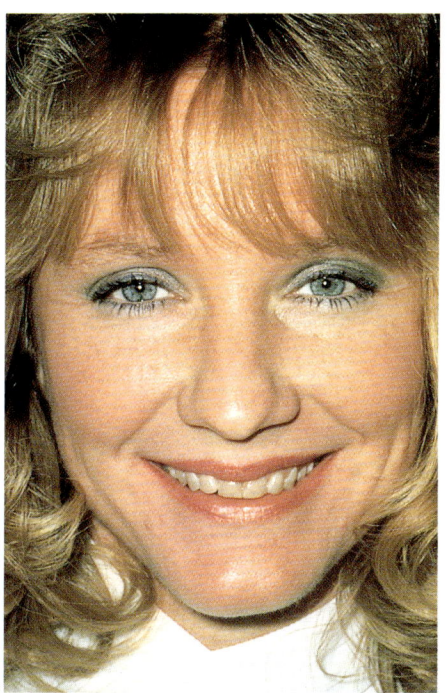

Fig 12-74 A portrait of an attractive young woman whose smile is an injustice to her overall beauty.

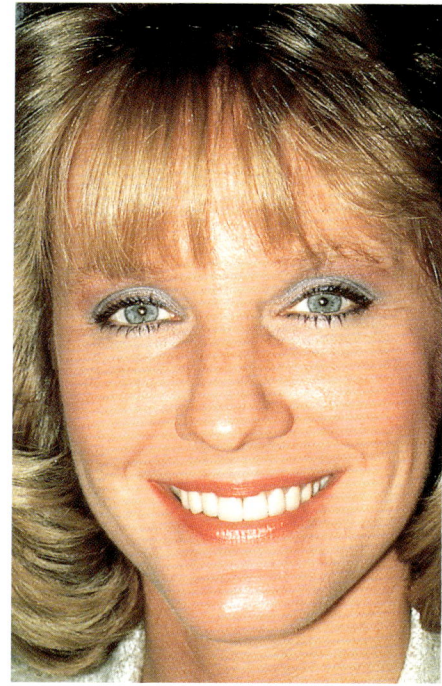

Fig 12-75 A vibrant transformation in her appearance has resulted from the "magic" of a porcelain veneer makeover. Dramatic results like this can become routine with mastery of the porcelain veneer technique.

fluted carbide bur and polished to a high luster with appropriate disks, strips, and resin-polishing pastes.

Any occlusal prematurities should be adjusted to prevent porcelain checking of natural tooth wear. Centric occlusion, straight protrusive, lateral protrusive, and lateral excursion should be checked with fine articulating paper. As a general rule, unless a canine is missing or an abnormal occlusion is present, anterior guidance should be canine-protected without veneer interferences. If any interferences are present, they should be removed, and the porcelain glaze restored with polishing procedures.

In recall appointments subsequent to veneer placement, the dental hygienist should not routinely polish the porcelain surface with any form of pumice (even fine pumice) to avoid altering the surface glaze and roughening the porcelain. If polishing of porcelain is necessary, due to surface abrasion, a silicone polishing wheel followed by a porcelain-polishing paste should be used at conventional speed with the surface kept moist. If any porcelain is discovered around any veneer, it should be brought to the dentist's attention, and a correction of the problem should be instituted. Scaling around the veneer margin should be performed as with a natural tooth. However, indiscriminate scaling of the facial surface of a veneer, due to carelessness, is to be condemned. The porcelain facial surface is inherently smooth and will remain stain-free if the porcelain was properly fabricated and finished. Therefore, there is no justification for arbitrarily manipulating it like natural teeth because the surface should be optimal after placement and finishing.

In addition to avoidance of mechanical abrading of the porcelain surface during prophylaxis procedures, the dental hygienist should not use acidulated fluoride solutions on any porcelain surface. Several reliable research studies have shown that the glaze is marred and the surface progressively roughened. Nonacidulated fluoride solutions are acceptable for porcelain. Finally, the Prophy-Jet is contraindicated for porcelain veneers because of the possibility of surface disturbance of the glaze or porcelain stains. Porcelain veneers that are correctly fabricated, placed, and finished are essentially self-maintaining for the foreseeable future.

References

1. Pincus CR. Building mouth personality. *J South Calif Dent Assoc.* 1938;14:125–129.
2. Buonocore MG. A simple method of increasing the adhesion of acrylic filling materials to enamel surfaces. *J Dent Res.* 1955; 34:849–853.
3. Bowen RL. Properties of a silica-reinforced polymer for dental restorations. *J Am Dent Assoc.* 1963;66:57–64.
4. Faunce FR, Myers DR. Laminate veneer restoration of permanent incisors. *J Am Dent Assoc.* 1976;93:790–792.
5. Fleming JE, Bayne SD, Spence P, Taes CG. Forty-five month clinical evaluation of extracoronal laminate veneer performance. *J Dent Res.* 1984;63:1082. Abstract.
6. Cannon M. Surface resistance to abrasion of performed laminate resin veneers. *J Prosthet Dent.* 1984;52:323–330.
7. Simonsen RJ, Calamia JR. Tensile bond strength of etched porcelain. *J Dent Res.* 1983;62:297. Abstract.
8. Horn HR. Porcelain laminate veneers bonded to etched enamel. *Dent Clin North Am.* 1983;17:671–684.
9. Calamia JR, Simonsen RJ. Effect of coupling agents on bond strength of etched porcelain. *J Dent Res.* 1984;63:162–362.
10. Hsu C, Stangel I, Nathanson D. Shear bond strength of etched porcelain. *J Dent Res.* 1985;64:296. Abstract.
11. Haywood VB, Heymann HO, Andreaus SB. Polishing porcelain veneers: An SEM analysis. *J Dent Res.* 1987;66:289. Abstract.
12. Haywood VB, Heymann HO, Scurria MS. Experimental instrumentation for polishing porcelain intraorally. *J Dent Res.* 1988;67:377. Abstract.
13. Haywood VB, Heymann HO, Scurria MS. Efficacy of stones for polishing porcelain intraorally. *J Dent Res.* 1989;68:395. Abstract.
14. Christensen GC. Veneering of teeth: State of the art. *Dent Clin North Am.* 1985;29:373–391.
15. Garber DA, Goldstein RE, Feinman RA. *Porcelain Laminate Veneers.* Chicago, Ill: Quintessence Publ Co; 1988.
16. Nixon RL. *The Chairside Manual for Porcelain Bonding.* Wilmington, Del: BA Videographics; 1987.

Index

A

Aging,	
accidental	67, 69
biologic	67
chronologic	75
programmed	67, 69
Analog	170, 177
Anatomy, perioral	213
Arch form	98
Articulator	177, 314
"Axi path" recorder	170, 176

B

Balance	24, 85, 87, 94, 96
Beauty,	
essential	13, 14
natural	12, 13
structural	64, 313, 315
Bennett movement	174–176
Bennett shift	172
Biologic width	225
"Bridging" phenomenon	253

C

Cast	311, 321
Cementation	313, 360
Cementoenamel junction (CEJ)	138–142, 226, 228, 292
Centric relation	145, 146
Characterization	117, 177, 189
Collagen	242, 264
Composition,	
dental	15
dento-facial	15
facial	15
Concept,	
dry retraction	293
SAP	116
wet retraction	303
Contact,	
anatomy of	115
occlusal	146–148
proximal	117, 119, 140, 292

D

Dehiscence	238
Dental,	
composition	15
midline	84, 85
morphology	107
Dentin consideration	312, 343
Disclusion	153
Dominance,	28
individual	30, 31, 83, 111
psychologic	30, 31

segmental	30, 31, 83, 111
strong	29, 30
weak	29

E

"Egression silhouette." *See* emergence profile.	
Embrasure	120, 121, 127, 145, 330
Emergence profile	225, 291, 306, 312, 321, 337, 352
Eruption,	
delayed	227
forced orthodontic	229
passive	226
Esthetics,	
origins of	12
perception of	13
periodontal	291
principles of	15
schematic framework of	14
Esthetics and function	59
Esthetics and morphopsychology	37
Expansion,	
hygroscopic	322
over	320
under	320

F

Facial,	
composition	15
midline	84, 85
morphopsychology	39
sagging	21, 70–73
sculpture	211
Fenestration	238
Flap,	
coronally positioned	250
double papilla	248
full thickness	242, 253, 279
laterally positioned	241
split thickness	244
Forces,	
cohesive	16, 17, 29
segregative	16, 18, 29
vital	39
Function,	
bioesthetic	183
incising	167
lateral chewing	172

G

Gingival,	
contour	124
displacement	293
flange	267
flap	273
groove	123
health	124
height	126, 127
margin	122
morphology	121
mucosa	124
pigmentation	123
recession	226, 237
trauma	290
zenith	125
Gradation	104, 140
Graft,	
free gingival	253
onlay	277
subepithelial or connective tissue	254, 269
Groove,	
facial	67
gingival	123
labial	67, 70, 71
mento-labial	67
naso-labial	67, 70, 71
Guidance,	
anterior tooth	153
canine	153
condylar	160
incisal	153
posterior tooth	155

H

Head posture	69, 70
Hinge axis	162
Hydroxyapatite	270

I

Illusion	127
Implant,	
endosseous	267
material	269
Impression	311, 321, 347
Intaglio	311
Interproximal,	
connectors	323
design	324
space. *See* embrasure.	

L

Line,	
axial	94, 95
commissural	81–83, 86
CPC	97
gingival	84, 85
lip	76, 77
occlusal frontal	82
tooth contact	118, 119, 140
Lips	57, 70, 71, 103, 150

M

Mandibular incisor,	
contour	112
dimension	114, 142, 143
function	138
Margin placement	225, 314, 337
Marginal fit	319, 352, 353
Mastication	167
Maxillary canine,	
contour	112
function	141
mesio-distal width	113
morphopsychological significance	117
Maxillary incisor,	
contour	112
function	138
incisogingival length	114, 116, 145
mesio-distal width	113, 114
morphopsychological significance	117
Modiolus	101
Molars	143
Morphology,	
contact point	118
dental	107
gingival	121
Morphopsychologic,	
appraisal	34
equilibrium	41
interpretation	45
types	34–36, 38
Morphopsychology	33
Mouth	55, 57, 58
Movement,	
Bennett	174–177
mandibular	162, 163
muscle	214
Muscle,	
buccinator	214
caninus	214
characteristics	211
facial	214
mentalis	214
orbicularis	214
platysma	214
quadratus labii inferioris	214
quadratus labii superioris	214
retraining exercise	73, 74, 77, 84, 214
risorius	214
tone	211
triangularis	214
zygomaticus	214
Muscular activity	211, 212

O

Occlusal,	
loading	181
plane	82, 165
Occlusion,	
development of	152
overloaded	181
physiology of	145
traumatic	153
vertical dimension of	151
Opacity	336, 351
Overbite,	
horizontal	148, 149
vertical	148, 149

P

Pantograph	163
Papilla,	
interdental	122
incisive	96–98, 101
marginal	122
Pontic,	
classification	282
ridge relationship	263
tissue relationship	282, 325
Porcelain,	
resin cement	354
veneer	329
veneer formulation	336
veneer try-in	354
Position,	
intercusp	145, 146
rest	152
speaking	150
Procedure,	
flap	273
pouch	275
Proportion, golden	20, 21, 23, 87
Provisionalization	309

R

Rapid extrusion	229
Receptors	42
Recession. *See* gingival recession.	
Restoration,	
anterior	189
posterior	190
Retraction. *See* retraction technique.	
Rhytidectomy	72
Ridge,	
augmentation	270
collapse	264
morphology	264
nasio-labial	60, 70

S

Segments	33
Self image	59, 366
Sexual type	42, 116, 117
Smear layer	312
Smile,	
components of	77
exercise	214
line	77
perfect	85
symmetry	80, 82
Space,	
anterior negative	80
free way	151
lateral negative	80, 100
Spacer	321, 351
Spee, Curve of	165
Stratification	332
Sublimation	64, 85
Sulcus	225, 228, 311

T

Technique,	
envelope	254
metallic frame	279
retraction	294, 303
roll	270
tissue mirrors	291
Tegumental relief	44
Temporization	289, 349
Texture,	
skin	44, 108
tooth	108, 351
Tissue,	
management	289
pontic relationship	325
Tooth,	
arrangements	96
contour	113, 225, 337
genetics	145
lengthening	229
preparation	121, 297–302, 320, 333, 336–347
structure	108
visibility	73
Translucency	336, 351

U

Unit, dentogingival	225
Unity	16
Upper lip curvature	78

V

Visual perception. *See* visualization.

Visualization	13, 317

Vertical dimension of occlusion. *See* occlusion.

W

Wilson, Curve of	165

Y

Youth,	
extension	47
factor	63

Z

Zone,	
affective	47
cerebral	48
facial	39
instinctive	52